HANDBOOK OF
Clinical Obstetrics
The Fetus & Mother

Dedication

To Sharon, Kelie, Brynne, and Sharon-Andrea with greatest love and gratitude.
                                                                                                    ~E. Albert Reece MD, PhD, MBA

To the memory of my father, who was the best role model anyone could have had, and my mother, who always gave me love and support (despite her never quite understanding what I did for a living).
                                                                                                    ~John C. Hobbins MD

HANDBOOK OF
Clinical
Obstetrics
The Fetus & Mother

E. Albert Reece MD, PhD, MBA
Vice President for Medical Affairs, University of Maryland, and
John Z. & Akiko K. Bowers Distinguished Professor and
Dean, School of Medicine,
Baltimore, Maryland

John C. Hobbins MD
Professor of Obstetrics and Gynecology
University of Colorado School of Medicine
University of Colorado Health Sciences Center
Denver, Colorado

FOREWORD BY
Norman F. Gant Jr. MD
Professor and Chairman Emeritus
University of Texas Southwestern Medical School
Executive Director, The American Board of Obstetrics and Gynecology
Dallas, Texas

THIRD EDITION

Blackwell
Publishing

© 2007 by Blackwell Publishing Ltd
Blackwell Publishing, Inc., 350 Main Street, Malden, Massachusetts 02148-5020, USA
Blackwell Publishing Ltd, 9600 Garsington Road, Oxford OX4 2DQ, UK
Blackwell Publishing Asia Pty Ltd, 550 Swanston Street, Carlton, Victoria 3053, Australia

The right of the Author to be identified as the Author of this Work has been asserted in
accordance with the Copyright, Designs and Patents Act 1988.

All rights reserved. No part of this publication may be reproduced, stored in a retrieval system, or
transmitted, in any form or by any means, electronic, mechanical, photocopying, recording or
otherwise, except as permitted by the UK Copyright, Designs and Patents Act 1988, without the
prior permission of the publisher.

First published 1995 © J.B. Lippincott Company
Second edition 2007

1 2007

Library of Congress Cataloging-in-Publication Data

Clinical obstetrics : the fetus & mother handbook / [edited by] E.
    Albert Reece, John C. Hobbins. – 2nd ed.
      p. ; cm.
    Rev. ed. of: Handbook of medicine of the fetus & mother. c1995.
    Includes bibliographical references and index.
    ISBN-13: 978-1-4051-5609-7
    ISBN-10: 1-4051-5609-0
      1. Pregnancy–Handbooks, manuals, etc.   2. Obstetrics–Handbooks, manuals, etc.   I. Reece,
    E. Albert.   II. Hobbins, John C., 1936– .   III. Handbook of medicine of the fetus & mother.
      [DNLM: 1. Pregnancy Complications.   2. Embryonic Development.   3. Fetal
    Development.   4. Fetal Diseases.   5. Pregnancy.
    WQ 240 C63975 2006]
    RG551.H36 2006
    618.2–dc22

2006021155

A catalogue record for this title is available from the British Library

Set in Sabon 9/12 pt by SNP Best-set Typesetter Ltd., Hong Kong

Commissioning Editor: Stuart Taylor
Development Editor: Rebecca Huxley
Production Controller: Kate Charman
Production Editor: Karin Skeet

For further information on Blackwell Publishing, visit our website:
http://www.blackwellpublishing.com

The publisher's policy is to use permanent paper from mills that operate a sustainable forestry
policy, and which has been manufactured from pulp processed using acid-free and elementary
chlorine-free practices. Furthermore, the publisher ensures that the text paper and cover board
used have met acceptable environmental accreditation standards.

Blackwell Publishing makes no representation, express or implied, that the drug dosages in this
book are correct. Readers must therefore always check that any product mentioned in this
publication is used in accordance with the prescribing information prepared by the manufacturers.
The author and the publishers do not accept responsibility or legal liability for any errors in the
text or for the misuse or misapplication of material in this book.

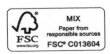

Contents

Part VII: Methods of Evaluation of Fetal Development and Well-being

Part VIII: Fetal Therapy

Part IX: Maternal Biological Adaptations to Pregnancy

Part X: Maternal Diseases Complicating Pregnancy

Contributors

Kjersti Aagaard-Tillery MD, PhD
MFM Fellow, Division of Maternal–Fetal Medicine, University of Utah, Salt Lake City, UT, USA

Eli Y. Adashi MD
Dean of Medicine and Biological Sciences, Brown Medical School, Providence, RI, USA

Erol Amon
Professor and Director, Department of Obstetrics, Gynecology, and Women's Health, Division of Maternal–Fetal Medicine, St Louis University, St Louis, MI, USA

Janet I. Andrews MD
Associate Maternal–Fetal Medicine, Department of Obstetrics and Gynecology, University of Iowa, Iowa City, IA, USA

Teresita L. Angtuaco MD, FACR, FAIUM, FSRU
Professor of Radiology, Obstetrics, and Gynecology, Director, Division of Imaging and Chief of Ultrasound, Department of Radiology, University of Arkansas for Medical Sciences College of Medicine, Little Rock, AR, USA

R. Lee Archer MD, FAAN
Associate Professor, Department of Neurology, University of Arkansas for Medical Sciences College of Medicine, Little Rock, AR, USA

Masoud Azodi MD
Assistant Professor, Department of Obstetrics and Gynecology, Yale University School of Medicine, New Haven, CT, USA

Ray Bahado-Singh MD
Professor, Department of Obstetrics and Gynecology, Division of Maternal–Fetal Medicine, Wayne State University/Hutzel Women's Hospital, Detroit, MI, USA

Robert H. Ball MD
Associate Professor, Department of Obstetrics, Gynecology, and Reproductive Sciences and Radiology, UCSF Fetal Treatment Center, San Francisco, CA, USA

Frederick C. Battaglia MD
Professor Emeritus, Departments of Pediatrics and Obstetrics–Gynecology, University of Colorado School of Medicine, University of Colorado at Denver and Health Sciences Center, Perinatal Research Center, Aurora, CO, USA

Pamela D. Berens MD
Associate Professor, Department of Obstetrics, Gynecology, and Reproductive Sciences, University of Texas Medical School – Houston, Houston, TX, USA

Matthew J. Bizzarro MD
Assistant Professor, Department of Pediatrics, Yale University School of Medicine, New Haven, CT, USA

D. Ware Branch MD
Professor and H.A. & Edna Benning Presidential Endowed Chair, Department of Obstetrics and Gynecology, University of Utah Health Sciences Center, Salt Lake City, UT, USA

Robert L. Brent MD, PhD, DSc
Distinguished Professor, Departments of Pediatrics, Radiology, and Pathology, Thomas Jefferson University and Alfred I. duPont Hospital for Children, Wilmington, DE, USA

Stephen R. Carr MD
Associate Professor, Department of Obstetrics–Gynecology, Division of Maternal–Fetal Medicine, Brown University, Women and Infants' Hospital, Providence, RI, USA

Tim Chard MD, FRCOG
Professor of Obstetrics and Gynaecology, St Bartholomew's Hospital and the Royal London School of Medicine and Dentistry, West Smithfield, London, UK

Frank A. Chervenak MD
Professor and Chairman, Department of Obstetrics and Gynecology, Weill Medical College of Cornell University, New York, NY, USA

Judith L. Chervenak MD, JD
Of Counsel, Heidell, Pittoni, Murphy & Bach, LLP, New York, NY, USA

Edward K.S. Chien MD, FACOG
Assistant Professor, Department of Obstetrics and Gynecology, Women and Infants' Hospital of Rhode Island, Brown University, Providence, RI, USA

Erin A.S. Clark MD
Chief Resident, Department of Obstetrics and Gynecology, University of Utah Hospital, Salt Lake City, UT, USA

Steven L. Clark MD
Director of Perinatal Medicine, Hospital Corporation of America, St. Marks Hospital, Salt Lake City, UT, USA

Richard B. Clark BSM, MD
Professor Emeritus, Departments of Anesthesiology and Obstetrics and Gynecology, University of Arkansas for Medical Sciences College of Medicine, Little Rock, AR, USA

Wayne R. Cohen MD
Chairman, Department of Obstetrics and Gynecology, Jamaica Hospital Medical Center, Professor of Clinical Obstetrics and Gynecology, Weill–Cornell Medical College, Jamaica, NY, USA

Donald R. Coustan MD
Chace/Joukowsky Professor and Chair, Department of Obstetrics and Gynecology, Brown Medical School
Chief Obstetrician and Gynecologist, Women and Infants' Hospital of Rhode Island, Providence, RI, USA

Luis E. De Las Casas MD
Staff Pathologist, Pathology Professional Services, El Paso, TX, USA

Alan H. DeCherney MD
Chief, Reproductive Biology and Medicine Branch, National Institute of Child Health and Human Development, National Institutes of Health, Bethesda, MD, USA

Patricia L. Devers MS, CGC
Perinatology Research Branch, National Institute of Child Health and Human Development, National Institutes of Health, Department of Health and Human Services, Wayne State University School of Medicine, Detroit, MI, USA

Gary A. Dildy MD
Associate Professor, Division of Maternal–Fetal Medicine, Department of Obstetrics and Gynecology, University of Utah School of Medicine, UT, USA

Offer Erez MD
Research Associate, Perinatology Research Branch, National Institute of Child Health and Human Development, National Institutes of Health, Department of Health and Human Services, Wayne State University School of Medicine, Detroit, MI, USA

Frederick U. Eruo MD, MPH
Instructor, Department of Obstetrics and Gynecology, University of Cincinnati, Cincinnati, OH, USA

Jimmy Espinoza MSc MD
Assistant Professor, Department of Obstetrics and Gynecology, Wayne State University/Hutzel Women's Hospital, and Perinatology Research Branch, National Institute of Child Health and Human Development, National Institutes of Health, Department of Health and Human Services, Detroit, MI, USA

Mark I. Evans MD
President, Fetal Medicine Foundation of America
Director, Comprehensive Genetics
Professor of Obstetrics and Gynecology, Mt. Sinai School of Medicine New York, NY, USA

Fred H. Faas MD
Staff Physician, VA Hospital, Professor of Medicine, University of Arkansas for Medical Sciences, Little Rock, AR, USA

Lynda B. Fawcett PhD
Assistant Professor, Department of Pediatrics, Alfred I. duPont Hospital for Children, Wilmington, DE, USA

Helen Feltovich MD, MS
Minnesota Perinatal Physicians, Abbott Northwestern Hospital, Minneapolis, MN, USA

Alan W. Flake MD
Professor, Departments of Surgery and Obstetrics and Gynecology, University of Pennsylvania School of Medicine, Ruth and Tristram C. Colket Jr. Chair of Pediatric Surgery and Director, Children's Institute of Surgical Science, Children's Hospital of Philadelphia, Philadelphia, PA, USA

Alfred D. Fleming MD, FACOG
Professor and Chairman, Department of Obstetrics and Gynecology, Creighton University School of Medicine, Omaha, NE, USA

Jean-Claude Fouron MD, FRCP
Professor, Department of Pediatrics, Université de Montréal, Director of the Fetal Cardiology Unit, Division of Pediatric Cardiology, Hôpital Sainte-Justine, Montréal, QC, Canada

Lara A. Friel MD, PhD
Fellow, Division of Maternal–Fetal Medicine, Department of Obstetrics and Gynecology, Wayne State University/Hutzel Women's Hospital, Detroit, MI, USA

Sandro Gabrielli MD
Attending Physician, Prenatal Medicine, S. Orsola-Malpighi University Hospital, Bologna, Italy

Henry L. Galan MD
Associate Professor, Department of Obstetrics–Gynecology, Department of Maternal–Fetal Medicine, University of Colorado Health Sciences Center, Denver, CO, USA

Norman F. Gant Jr. MD
Professor and Chairman Emeritus, University of Texas Southwestern Medical School, Executive Director, American Board of Obstetrics and Gynecology, Dallas, TX, USA

Ronald S. Gibbs MD
Professor and Chairman, E. Stewart Taylor Chair in Obstetrics and Gynecology, Department of Obstetrics–Gynecology, University of Colorado School of Medicine, Denver, CO, USA

Luís F. Gonçalves MD
Director of Prenatal Diagnosis, Perinatology Research Branch, National Institute of Child Health and Human Development, National Institutes of Health, Department of Health and Human Services, Bethesda, MD, and Detroit, MI,
Assistant Professor, Department of Obstetrics and Gynecology, Wayne State University/Hutzel Women's Hospital, Detroit, MI, USA

Ian Gross MD
Professor of Pediatrics, Department of Pediatrics, Yale University School of Medicine, New Haven, CT, USA

Andrée Gruslin MD, FRCS
Associate Professor, Division of Maternal–Fetal Medicine, Department of Obstetrics and Gynecology, University of Ottawa, Ottawa, ON, Canada

James E. Haddow MD
Vice President and Medical Director, Foundation for Blood Research, Scarborough, ME, USA

Zion J. Hagay MD
Professor and Chairman, Department of Obstetrics and Gynecology, Kaplan Medical Center, Rehovot, Israel

Michael R. Harrison MD
Professor of Surgery and Pediatrics, Director, Fetal Treatment Center, Department of Surgery, University of California, San Francisco School of Medicine, San Francisco, CA, USA

Jean C. Hay BSc(Hons), MSc
Associate Professor of Anatomy (retired), Department of Human Anatomy and Cell Science, University of Manitoba, Winnipeg, MB, Canada

Alan Hill MD, PhD
Professor, Department of Pediatrics, University of British Columbia,
Consultant Pediatric Neurologist, British Columbia's Children's Hospital, Vancouver, BC, Canada

Washington Clark Hill MD, FACOG
Chairman, Department of Obstetrics and Gynecology,
Director, Maternal–Fetal Medicine, Sarasota Memorial Hospital, Sarasota,
Clinical Professor, Department of Obstetrics and Gynecology, University of South Florida, College of Medicine, Tampa, Clinical Professor, Department of Clinical Sciences, OB-GYN Clerkship Director-Sarasota, Florida State University College of Medicine, Tallahassee FL, USA

John C. Hobbins MD
Professor, Department of Obstetrics and Gynecology, University of Colorado School of Medicine, Health Sciences Center, Denver, CO, USA

Calla Holmgren MD
Fellow, Maternal–Fetal Medicine, Department of Obstetrics and Gynecology, University of Utah, Salt Lake City, UT, USA

Carol J. Homko PhD, RN
Assistant Professor, Department of Obstetrics, Gynecology, and Reproductive Sciences, Temple University Hospital, Philadelphia, PA, USA

Judy M. Hopkinson PhD, IBCLC
Associate Professor, Department of Pediatrics, Baylor College of Medicine, Houston, TX, USA

Thomas D. Horn MD, MBA
Chairman, Department of Dermatology, Professor, Departments of Dermatology and Pathology, University of Arkansas for Medical Sciences College of Medicine, Little Rock, AR, USA

Jerri L. Hoskyn MD
Assistant Professor, Department of Dermatology, University of Arkansas for Medical Sciences College of Medicine, Staff Physician, Central Arkansas Veterans' Hospital Administration, Little Rock, AR, USA

Karen A. Hutchinson MD
Director of Medical Education, Bridgeport Hospital, Bridgeport, CT, USA

Philippe Jeanty MD, PhD
Tennessee Women's Care, PC, Nashville, TN, USA

Helen H. Kay MD
Professor and Chair, Department of Obstetrics and Gynecology, University of Arkansas for Medical Sciences College of Medicine, Little Rock, AR, USA

Maureen Keller-Wood PhD
Professor and Chair, Department of Pharmacodynamics, College of Pharmacy, University of Florida, Gainesville, FL, USA

Charles S. Kleinman MD
Professor of Clinical Pediatrics in Obstetrics and Gynecology, Columbia University College of Physicians and Surgeons/Weill Medical College of Cornell University, Chief, Pediatric Cardiac Imaging, New York – Presbyterian Hospital, Division of Pediatric Cardiology, Babies Hospital, New York, NY, USA

Soheila Korourian MD
Associate Professor, Department of Pathology, University of Arkansas for Medical Sciences College of Medicine, Little Rock, AR, USA

Michelle W. Krause MD, MPH
Assistant Professor of Medicine, Division of Nephrology, Department of Internal Medicine, University of Arkansas for Medical Sciences College of Medicine, Little Rock, AR, USA

Juan Pedro Kusanovic MD
Research Associate, Perinatology Research Branch, National Institute of Child Health and Human Development, National Institutes of Health, Department of Health and Human Services, Wayne State University School of Medicine, Detroit, MI, USA

Matthew Laughon MD, MPH
Assistant Professor, Department of Pediatrics, Division of Neonatal/Perinatal Medicine, The University of North Carolina at Chapel Hill, Chapel Hill, NC, USA

Gustavo F. Leguizamón MD
Assistant Professor, Chief, High Risk Pregnancy Unit, Department of Obstetrics and Gynecology, CEMIC University, Buenos Aires, Argentina

Juliana M.B. Leite MD
Nashville, TN, USA

Charles J. Lockwood MD
The Anita O'Keefe Young Professor and Chair, Department of Obstetrics, Gynecology, and Reproductive Sciences, Yale University School of Medicine, New Haven, CT, USA

Curtis L. Lowery MD
Professor and Director, Maternal–Fetal Medicine, Department of Obstetrics and Gynecology, University of Arkansas for Medical Sciences College of Medicine, Little Rock, AR, USA

Barbara Luke ScD, MPH, RN, RD
Professor of Nursing, Obstetrics, and Pediatrics, School of Nursing and Health Studies, University of Miami, Coral Gables, FL, USA

Laurence B. McCullough PhD
Professor of Medicine and Medical Ethics, Center for Medical Ethics and Health Policy, Baylor College of Medicine, Houston, TX, USA

Maurice J. Mahoney MD, JD
Professor, Departments of Genetics, Pediatrics, and Obstetrics, Gynecology and Reproductive Sciences, Department of Genetics, Yale University School of Medicine, New Haven, CT, USA

Anita C. Manogura MD
Fellow, Maternal–Fetal Medicine, Department of Obstetrics and Gynecology, University of Maryland, Baltimore, MD, USA

Jennifer L. Melville MD, MPH
Assistant Professor, Department of Obstetrics and Gynecology, University of Washington
School of Medicine, Seattle, WA, USA

Howard Minkoff MD
Chairman, Obstetrics and Gynecology, Maimonides Medical Center,
Distinguished Professor, Obstetrics and Gynecology, SUNY Downstate, Brooklyn,
NY, USA

Fernando R. Moya MD
Director of Neonatology, Coastal AHEC, Wilmington,
Professor, Department of Pediatrics, University of North Carolina, Chapel Hill, NC, USA

Thomas D. Myles MD
St. Louis University, Richmond Heights, MO, USA

Jennifer R. Niebyl MD
Professor and Head, Department of Obstetrics and Gynecology, University of Iowa Roy
J. and Lucille A. Carver College of Medicine, Iowa City, IA, USA

Jyh Kae Nien MD
Fellow, Perinatology Research Branch, National Institute of Child Health and Human
Development, National Institutes of Health, Department of Health and Human Services,
Bethesda, MD, and Detroit, MI, USA

The late Carl A. Nimrod MB, BS, FRCS(C)
Formerly Professor and Chair, Department of Obstetrics and Gynecology, University of
Ottawa, Ottawa, ON, Canada

Chien Oh MD
Fellow of Maternal–Fetal Medicine, Department of Obstetrics, Gynecology, and
Reproductive Sciences, University of Maryland, Baltimore, MD, USA

Lawrence W. Oppenheimer MB, FRCOG, FRCS(UK), FRCS(C)
Associate Professor, Division of Maternal–Fetal Medicine, Department of Obstetrics and
Gynecology, University of Ottawa, Ottawa, ON, Canada

Michael J. Paidas MD
Associate Professor, Department of Obstetrics, Gynecology, and Reproductive Sciences,
Co-Director, Yale Blood Center for Women and Children, Yale University School of
Medicine, New Haven, CT, USA

Glenn E. Palomaki
Director of Biometry, Foundation for Blood Research, Scarborough, MA, USA

Santosh Pandipati MD
Instructor-Fellow, Maternal–Fetal Medicine, University of Colorado Health Sciences Center,
Denver, CO, USA

Trivedi Vidhya N. Persaud MD, PhD, DSc, FRCPath(Lond)
Professor Emeritus, Department of Human Anatomy and Cell Science, University of Manitoba, Winnipeg, MB, Canada

Christian M. Pettker MD
Instructor and Clinical Fellow, Division of Maternal–Fetal Medicine, Department of Obstetrics, Gynecology, and Reproductive Sciences, Yale University School of Medicine, New Haven, CT, USA

Gianluigi Pilu MD
Associate Professor, Department of Obstetrics and Gynecology, Prenatal Medicine, S. Orsola-Malpighi University Hospital, Bologna, Italy

Mladen Predanic MSC, MD
Fellow, Division of Maternal–Fetal Medicine, Department of Obstetrics and Gynecology, Weill Medical College of Cornell University, New York, NY, USA

Vivek Raj MB, BS, MD, MRCP(UK)
Associate Professor,
Interim Director, Division of Gastroenterology, University of Arkansas for Medical Sciences College of Medicine, Little Rock, AR, USA

E. Albert Reece MD, PhD, MBA
Vice President for Medical Affairs, University of Maryland, and John Z. & Akiko K. Bowers Distinguished Professor and Dean, School of Medicine, and Professor, Departments of OB/GYN and Reproductive Sciences; Medicine; and Biochemistry and Molecular Biology; Baltimore, MD, USA

Nicola Rizzo MD
Professor of Obstetrics and Gynecology, Prenatal Medicine, S. Orsola-Malpighi University Hospital, Bologna, Italy

Paula K. Roberson PhD
Professor and Chair, Biostatistics, Colleges of Medicine and Public Health, University of Arkansas for Medical Sciences College of Medicine, Little Rock, AR, USA

Roberto Romero MD
Chief, Perinatology Research Branch, Intramural Division, National Institute of Child Health and Human Development, National Institutes of Health, Department of Health and Human Services, Bethesda, MD, and Detroit, MI, USA

Michael G. Ross MD, MPH
Professor and Chairman, Department of Obstetrics and Gynecology, Harbor–UCLA Medical Center, Torrance, CA, USA

Stacy A. Rudnicki MD
Associate Professor of Neurology, University of Arkansas for Medical Sciences College of Medicine, Little Rock, AR, USA

Benjamin P. Sachs MB, BS, DPH, FACOG
Obstetrician-Gynecologist-in-Chief,
Harold H. Rosenfield Professor of Obstetrics, Gynecology, and Reproductive
Biology, Harvard Medical School, Department of Obstetrics/Gynecology, Beth Israel
Deaconess Medical Center, Boston, MA, USA

Joaquin Santolaya-Forgas MD, PhD
Professor, Wayne State University/Hutzel Women's Hospital, Department of Obstetrics and
Gynecology, Perinatology Research Branch, National Institute of Child Health and Human
Development, National Institutes of Health, Department of Health and Human Services,
Detroit, MI, USA

Peter E. Schwartz MD
John Slade Ely Professor of Gynecology, Yale University School of Medicine, New
Haven, CT, USA

Sudhir V. Shah MD, FACP
Professor of Medicine, Division Director of Nephrology, University of Arkansas for Medical
Sciences College of Medicine, Little Rock, AR, USA

Eyal Sheiner MD
Attending Physician, Department of Obstetrics–Gynecology, Soroka University Medical
Center, Faculty of Health Sciences, Ben-Gurion University, Beer-Sheva, Israel

Bashir S. Shihabuddin MD
Assistant Professor, Department of Neurology, University of Arkansas for Medical Sciences
College of Medicine, Little Rock, AR, USA

Baha M. Sibai MD
Professor, Department of Obstetrics and Gynecology, University of Cincinnati College of
Medicine, Cincinnati, OH, USA

Robert M. Silver MD
Professor, Department of Obstetrics–Gynecology,
Division Chief, Maternal–Fetal Medicine, University of Utah, Salt Lake City, UT, USA

Joe Leigh Simpson MD
Ernst W. Bertner Chairman and Professor, Department of Obstetrics and Gynecology,
Professor, Department of Molecular and Human Genetics, Baylor College of Medicine,
Houston, TX, USA

Antonio V. Sison MD
Chairman, Department of Obstetrics and Gynecology, Robert Wood Johnson
University Hospital at Hamilton, Medical Director, Robert Wood Johnson
OB/GYN Group, Hamilton, NJ, USA

Amanda Skoll MD, FRCSC
Associate Professor, Division of Maternal–Fetal Medicine, Department of Obstetrics and
Gynecology, University of British Columbia, Vancouver, BC, Canada

Daniel W. Skupski MD
Associate Professor, Obstetrics and Gynecology, Weill Medical College of Cornell University, New York, NY, USA

Michelle Smith-Levitin MD
Director, High Risk Pregnancy Center, North Shore University Hospital, Manhasset, NY, USA

Jessica Spencer MD
Fellow in Reproductive Endocrinology and Infertility, Department of Gynecology and Obstetrics, Emory University, Atlanta, GA, USA

Richard L. Sweet MD
*Professor and Vice Chair,
Director, Women's Center for Health, University of California, Davis Medical Center, Sacramento, CA, USA*

Kirsten von Sydow PhD
Clinical Psychologist, University of Hamburg, Psychological Institute, Private Psychotherapy Practice, Hamburg, Germany

Brian J. Trudinger MB, BS, MD, FRANZCOG, FRCOG, FRCS(Ed)
Professor of Obstetrics and Gynecology, University of Sydney at Westmead Hospital, Sydney, NSW, Australia

Anthony M. Vintzileos
Professor and Chair, Department of Obstetrics, Gynecology, and Reproductive Sciences, University of Medicine and Dentistry of New Jersey–Robert Wood Johnson Medical School, New Brunswick, NJ, USA

Ronald J. Wapner MD
Professor, Department of Obstetrics and Gynecology, Drexel University College of Medicine, Philadelphia, PA, USA

Carl P. Weiner MD, MBA, FACOG
K.E. Krantz Professor and Chair, Department of Obstetrics and Gynecology, University of Kansas School of Medicine, Kansas City, KS, USA

Paul J. Wendel MD
*Associate Professor,
Medical Director of Labor and Delivery, Division of Maternal–Fetal Medicine, Department of Obstetrics and Gynecology, University of Arkansas for Medical Sciences College of Medicine, Little Rock, AR, USA*

Danny Wilkerson MD
Assistant Professor, Departments of Anesthesiology and Obstetrics and Gynecology, University of Arkansas for Medical Sciences College of Medicine, Little Rock, AR, USA

Arnon Wiznitzer MD

Professor and Chairman, Department of Obstetrics and Gynecology, Soroka University Medical Center, Faculty of Health Sciences, Ben-Gurion University, Beer-Sheva, Israel

Kenneth H.H. Wong MD, MBA

Physician, Division of Reproductive Endocrinology and Infertility, Kaiser Permanente, Fontana, CA, USA

Charles E. Wood PhD

Professor and Chair, Department of Physiology and Functional Genomics, University of Florida, Gainesville, FL, USA

Linda L.M. Worley MD

Associate Professor, Departments of Psychiatry and Obstetrics and Gynecology, University of Arkansas for Medical Sciences College of Medicine, Little Rock, AR, USA

Yuval Yaron MD

Director, Prenatal Genetic Diagnosis Unit, Genetic Institute, Tel Aviv Sourasky Medical Center, affiliated to Sackler Faculty of Medicine, Tel Aviv University, Tel Aviv, Israel

Lami Yeo MD

Associate Professor of Obstetrics and Gynecology,
Director of Perinatal Ultrasound,
Director of Fetal Cardiovascular Unit,
Department of Obstetrics, Gynecology, and Reproductive Sciences,
Division of Maternal–Fetal Medicine, University of Medicine and Dentistry of New Jersey–Robert Wood Johnson Medical School, New Brunswick, NJ, USA

Edward R. Yeomans MD

Associate Professor, Department of Obstetrics, Gynecology, and Reproductive Sciences, University of Texas-Houston Health Science Center, Lyndon B. Johnson General Hospital, Houston, TX, USA

Foreword

When asked to write the foreword to the third edition of *Clinical Obstetrics—The Fetus & Mother*, I had two immediate thoughts, the first being that I liked the new title better than the former title, *Medicine of the Fetus & Mother*. The second was that those already acquainted with the former title might not recognize the new one. As I had no control over either, I was pleased that I at least could remind readers of the importance of this current work.

When considering a new or forward-thinking idea, concept, or treatise, it is often a good idea to consider where we have been and where we are going. This is especially true when considering clinical obstetrics, which today means both fetus and mother.

Although the fetus could be evaluated prior to the early 1960s, the methods were crude when considered retrospectively. Auscultation and radiography were the primary tools and little could be accomplished to alter fetal outcome other than by delivery. This changed in 1961 with Lily's pioneering work with the use of amniocentesis to manage Rh-isoimmunization.

In less than one professional lifetime, the fetus has become our patient, not just the mother. This rapid evolution has been helped by pioneers in electronic fetal heart rate monitoring, such as Edward Hon, and of course by the use of ultrasound and Doppler evaluations of the fetus. In this last field it is important to acknowledge individuals such as Ian Donald in the United Kingdom. He struggled in the 1960s to develop ultrasound as a useful clinical tool when many of our colleagues in radiology considered such machines to be toys. Certainly, as is obvious in the current textbook, the authors' efforts over the past two decades have proven Dr. Donald right. Many of their own studies have formed the basis for maternal and actual fetal therapy.

It is critically important to recognize in the current textbook that maternal–fetal medicine now encompasses the areas of conception and fetal growth, extending into the neonatal time period. It is now apparent that the basic fundamental biology of conception likely will lead to a better understanding of stem cell biology and basic immunology. Finally, an entire new field of study is developing in understanding how fetal/neonatal illness may result in adult disease(s) many years after birth.

Both the student of obstetrics and the practitioner should read this third edition of what is becoming an essential update of maternal–fetal knowledge. Today's practice is founded upon the principles and practices so clearly presented in this book. This third edition provides the proof that learning can be fun!

Norman F. Gant Jr. MD
2006

Preface

The field of clinical obstetrics and maternal–fetal medicine is undergoing major advances, with rapid strides being made.

The first edition was introduced as the fulfillment of a concept: to combine into one source maternal medicine—an established field focusing primarily on medical complications of pregnancy—and the rapidly evolving field of fetal medicine. The acceptance of this single source book has been overwhelming. The text has been embraced not only by clinical obstetricians but also by maternal–fetal medicine specialists, resident physicians in training, medical students, and others who use the book primarily for its comprehensive obstetrical coverage.

However, this edition is not only entirely revised, but now has a strong clinical emphasis, while maintaining a scholarly orientation that is expected to be appealing to both clinicians and academicians. The new book title, *Clinical Obstetrics— The Fetus & Mother*, reflects the new orientation of this edition.

This text is a treatise in obstetrics and maternal–fetal medicine. It discusses subjects from the time of conception to delivery, including the normal processes and disease states of the fetus, as well as diagnostic and therapeutic measures that can be used to effect fetal well-being. The fetal medicine section includes prenatal diagnosis and places a strong emphasis on the biology of early pregnancy and the fetal–placental unit, fetal development, and variations in normal embryonic and fetal growth. The influence of teratogens, infections, and fetal diseases on outcome is also discussed. Extensive coverage is given to the prenatal diagnosis of congenital malformations using a variety of modalities, both noninvasive and invasive. The various biophysical and biochemical means of evaluation of fetal well-being are also discussed in great detail. The application of fetal therapy, both surgical and medical, is presented, with limited coverage on the evolving field of gene and cell therapy. In addition, maternal medical complications of pregnancy are thoroughly covered.

This book is designed to provide readily accessible information. The overall balance, scope, content, and design fully serve the needs of academic subspecialists, obstetricians, and house staff physicians, as well as other keen students of medicine.

E. Albert Reece MD, PhD, MBA
John C. Hobbins MD
2006

Preface to the first edition

The field of maternal–fetal medicine has been recognized as the academic arm of obstetrics since the 1970s. In recent years, the specialty has flourished and now encompasses many other allied fields, including genetics, teratology, diagnostic imaging, endocrinology, fetal physiology, and pathology. Various technological advances now permit *in utero* diagnosis, as well as both medical and surgical treatment of the fetus.

This handbook has been designed to complement the textbook *Medicine of the Fetus & Mother*. It is our hope that clinicians will turn to this handbook for assistance and guidance as they encounter the complex and often perplexing issues involving care of the fetus and mother. This handbook is intended to provide the practicing obstetrician with succinct, clinically focused and easily retrievable information regarding both the maternal and fetal complications of pregnancy. Each chapter focuses on a specific aspect of maternal–fetal medicine and highlights current modalities for diagnosis, evaluation, and treatment.

E. Albert Reece MD
John C. Hobbins MD
Maurice J. Mahoney MD
Roy H. Petrie MD, ScD

Acknowledgments

The editors are deeply indebted to all of the contributors, who have invested an enormous amount of time and energy in this project. We count ourselves extremely fortunate to have colleagues and friends who are willing to make this type of investment. The collective efforts have resulted in an entirely revised and most up-to-date book series.

We truly appreciate the invaluable efforts of Ms. Veronika Guttenberger, project specialist in the College of Medicine at the University of Arkansas for Medical Sciences, who assisted in coordinating this entire project. We remain grateful and indebted to her. Carol Homko, PhD, from Temple University School of Medicine made invaluable editorial contributions to this project and we are most appreciative of her assistance.

Finally, we are greatly appreciative of the editors at Blackwell Publishing Ltd., especially Ms. Rebecca Huxley and Dr. Stuart Taylor, for their wise counsel and enduring patience.

The collective efforts of all who contributed to this project are a true testimony of scholarship, commitment, and selflessness. Our lives have been touched by the willingness of everyone to be so generous in sharing their time and talents. Thank you very kindly.

We want to especially acknowledge and thank our good friend and colleague the late Dr. Carl Nimrod, MB, BS, FRCS(C), who contributed so generously to this book series and prior editions. His untimely death saddens us all, but his life and scholarly contributions will brighten our memories.

E. Albert Reece MD, PhD, MBA
John C. Hobbins MD
2006

Part I

Conception and Conceptus Development

1 Early conceptus growth and immunobiologic adaptations of pregnancy

Kenneth H.H. Wong and Eli Y. Adashi

Reproduction will only be successful if a multitude of intricate sequences and interactions occur. This reproductive process begins with the formation of individual male and female gametes. Following gamete formation, a mechanism must be provided to ensure that these gametes attain close proximity to each other so that fertilization may take place. After successful fertilization, the newly formed embryo must develop correctly and, finally, implant in a nourishing environment.

Fertilization

Embryonic development begins with the process of fertilization, the union of individual male and female gametes (Fig. 1.1). The fusion of two haploid cells, each bearing 22 autosomes and one sex chromosome, creates an offspring whose genetic makeup is different that of from both parents. Fertilization consists of a regulated sequence of interactions that will ultimately result in embryo development (Fig. 1.2).

Preimplantation embryo

The initial phases of embryonic growth following fertilization are concerned with rapid cell division (Fig. 1.3). This initial increase in cell numbers is critical in establishing a sufficient number of cells in the embryo, which can then initiate differentiation. These cells are known as blastomeres. Beginning with the first division approximately 24–30 hours after fertilization, the blastomeres become smaller with successive divisions. Approximately 3 days after fertilization, the berry-like mass of cells, termed the morula, enters the uterus.

The next event in embryo development is the formation of a fluid-filled cavity, the blastocele. With blastocyst formation, there is a partitioning of cells between an inner cell mass, the embryoblast, and an outer mass of cells, the trophectoderm. After entering the uterus, the developing blastocyst floats inside the endometrial cavity for about 2–3 days. The embryo begins implantation approximately 6 days

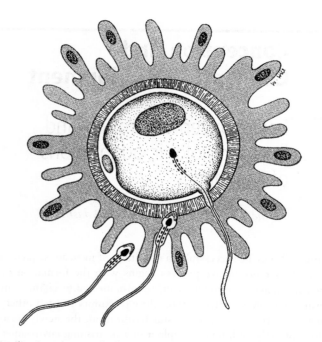

Figure 1.1 Fertilization. A sperm is shown penetrating an oocyte. The spermatozoon must first undergo capacitation. Next, the sperm must penetrate the cumulus (the investment of cells and matrix surrounding the oocyte). After cumulus penetration, the sperm binds to the zona pellucida via specific receptors. The plasma membranes of the sperm and oocyte fuse. The sperm and tail of the sperm enter the oocyte, leaving the sperm's plasma membrane.

after fertilization, while the primitive germ layers develop between days 6 and 8. Following initial implantation, the embryo is completely imbedded within the endometrium by approximately 8–9 days after ovulation. Immediately following adhesion, the blastocyst begins penetration into the endometrial epithelium and stroma (Fig. 1.4).

Immunobiologic adaptations of pregnancy

The primary role of the immune system is to protect the body from invasion by foreign organisms and their toxic products. This requires an ability to discriminate between self and nonself antigens, so that immune destruction can be targeted against the invading organism and not against the animal's own tissues. In pregnancy, the antigenically foreign fetus grows in its mother for 9 months, unharmed

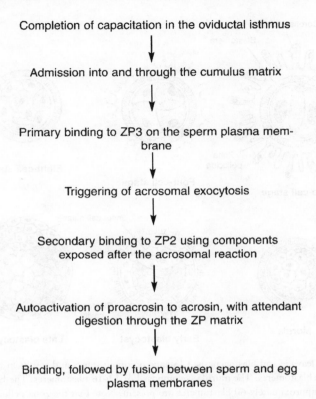

Completion of capacitation in the oviductal isthmus

↓

Admission into and through the cumulus matrix

↓

Primary binding to ZP3 on the sperm plasma membrane

↓

Triggering of acrosomal exocytosis

↓

Secondary binding to ZP2 using components exposed after the acrosomal reaction

↓

Autoactivation of proacrosin to acrosin, with attendant digestion through the ZP matrix

↓

Binding, followed by fusion between sperm and egg plasma membranes

Figure 1.2 Proposed sequence for mammalian gamete interaction. ZP, zona pellucida. (Adapted from ref. 35, with permission.)

by her immune system. Clearly, immune adaptations must occur in pregnancy that are central to the survival of the fetus while maintaining the mother's ability to fight infection.

Immune circuit

It is clear from the foregoing discussion that, in normal pregnancy, fetal growth progresses side by side with the development of a number of immune mechanisms that function at several levels. These can be summarized by constructing an immune circuit (Fig. 1.5A). The first stage in this circuit is the exposure of the maternal

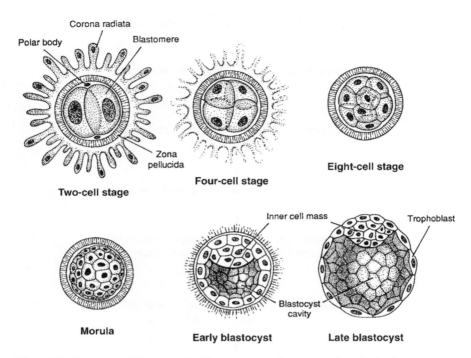

Figure 1.3 Cleavage and blastogenesis. Cleavage occurs in stages and results in the formation of blastomeres. The morula is composed of 12–16 blastomeres. The blastocyst forms when approximately 60 blastomeres are present. Note that the zona pellucida has disappeared by the late blastocyst stage. Until the zona pellucida is shed, the developing embryo essentially does not increase in size.

immune system to both fetal trophoblast and leukocytes. This could potentially lead to immune recognition and the development of cell-mediated and antibody responses to fetal antigens, which in turn would lead to rejection of the fetus (placenta). However, this circuit is broken at several stages (Fig. 1.5B). First, on the basis of current evidence, the maternal immune system does not recognize the trophoblast because it either fails to express HLA or expresses HLA-G. Second, although fetal leukocytes can be recognized by maternal immune cells, only antibody responses occur because the placenta's production of Th2 cytokines downregulates cell-mediated immunity. Finally, the production of antipaternal antibodies is not harmful because the placenta filters out these antibodies before they reach the fetal circulation. Thus, it is the combination of these many immune adaptations of pregnancy that ensures the success of the fetus.

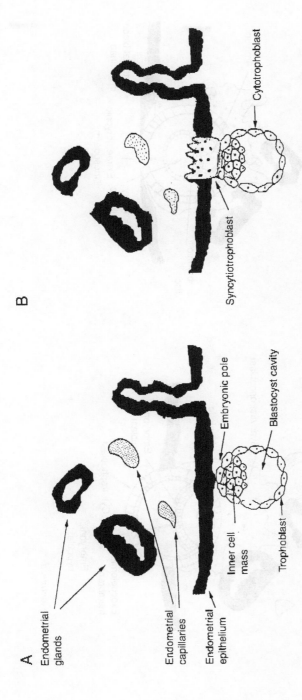

Figure 1.4 Implantation. (A) After floating free for 2 days, the polar trophectoderm of the embryo apposes the endometrial epithelium. (B) Penetration begins with rapid proliferation and differentiation into two cell types, the cytotrophoblast and the syncytiotrophoblast. The syncytiotrophoblast, a multinucleated mass of cells with no cell boundaries, extends through the endometrial epithelium to penetrate the stroma. (C) The inner cell mass differentiates into the epiblast, which gives rise to the mesoderm and ectoderm, and the hypoblast, which gives rise to the endoderm. (D) The embryo becomes completely embedded 7–13 days after ovulation.

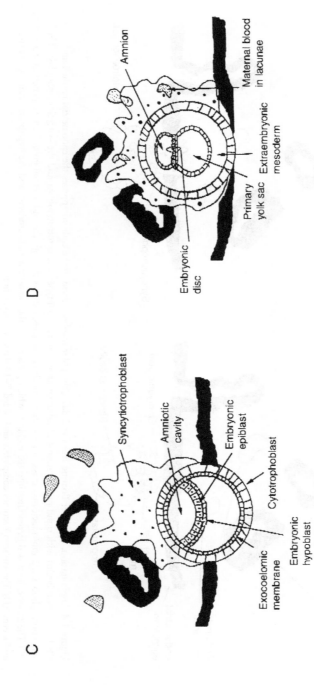

Figure 1.4 *Continued*

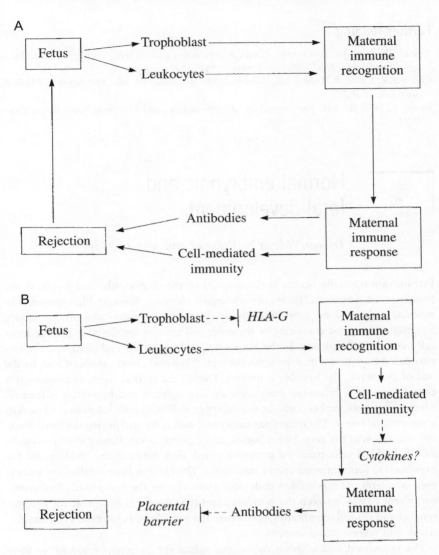

Figure 1.5 (A) Immune responses in pregnancy that could lead to rejection of the fetus. (B) Immunoregulatory mechanisms in pregnancy that prevent the rejection of the fetus.

Further reading

Adashi EY, Rock JA, Rosenwaks Z, eds. *Reproductive endocrinology, surgery and technology.* Philadelphia, PA: Lippincott-Raven, 1996.

Creasy RK, Resnik R, Iams J, eds. *Maternal–fetal medicine,* 5th edn. Philadelphia, PA: W.B. Saunders, 2004.

Knobil E, Neill JD, eds. *The physiology of reproduction,* 2nd edn. New York: Raven Press, 1994.

2 Normal embryonic and fetal development

Trivedi Vidhya N. Persaud and Jean C. Hay

Fertilization normally occurs in the ampulla of the uterine tube and results in the formation of a zygote. The zygote undergoes cleavage, forming blastomeres. The morula, composed of approximately 16 blastomeres, enters the uterine cavity, forming a blastocyst consisting of the outer cell mass or trophoblast and the inner cell mass or embryoblast. As the blastocyst implants in the endometrium, the trophoblast differentiates into the syncytiotrophoblast and cytotrophoblast and, by the end of this week, the hypoblast appears. During the second week, implantation is completed, and a bilaminar embryonic disk of epiblast and hypoblast is formed. The primary yolk sac becomes the secondary or definitive yolk sac as hypoblast cells grow out and line it. The trilaminar embryonic disk is formed during the third week, differentiation of the germ layers begins, and a primitive circulatory system is established. Epiblast cells from the primitive streak pass between the epiblast and the hypoblast to form intraembryonic mesoderm. The epiblast is now called the embryonic ectoderm. The primitive node also gives rise to the notochord. Embryonic mesoderm passes between the ectoderm and the endoderm except at the oropharyngeal and cloacal membranes, and where the notochord is located. The primitive streak will regress and disappear.

The notochord and adjacent mesoderm induce the overlying ectoderm to form the neural plate, which gives rise to neural folds. The neural folds fuse to form the neural tube with a central neural canal, the anterior neuropore (closes between days 25 and 26 of gestation), and the posterior neuropore (closes by day 28). Intraembryonic mesoderm forms the somites. A somite is composed of a dermatome, which contributes to the dermis, a myotome, which gives rises to skeletal muscle, and a sclerotome, the precursors of the vertebrae and the ribs. Finally, it forms the lateral mesoderm in which spaces develop and coalesce, forming a horseshoe-shaped intraembryonic coelom, which gives rise to the pericardial, pleural, and peritoneal cavities. This coelom splits the lateral mesoderm into a somatic and a splanchnic layer. The embryonic somatic mesoderm and ectoderm form the body walls, and the embryonic splanchnic mesoderm and endoderm will form the primitive gut and the structures derived from it.

Chorionic villi, a core of extraembryonic mesoderm covered with cytotrophoblast and syncytiotrophoblast, develops around the chorionic sac. Blood vessels first appear in the extraembryonic mesoderm as clusters of mesenchymal cells (blood islands) acquire lumina. As the vessels develop and sprout, the intra- and extraembryonic vessels are linked. Paired endothelial heart tubes develop and fuse to form a single contractile heart tube and, by the end of the third week, a primordial or primitive circulation is established between the embryo and the chorion.

The embryonic period extends from the beginning of the fourth week to the end of the eighth week. By the end of this period, the embryo has acquired characteristic human features. In the fourth week, the embryonic disk undergoes folding, which converts the flat embryonic disk into a cylindrical embryo. The dorsal part of the yolk sac is incorporated into the embryo to form the primitive gut. Folding in the transverse axis results in the somatopleure forming the lateral and ventral body walls. The pericardioperitoneal canals become the future pleural cavities. The fetal period extends from the beginning of the ninth week until birth. The main features of this period are the growth and differentiation of those tissues and organs that began their development in the embryonic period.

By the fourth week, the facial primordia appear: six pairs of pharyngeal arches (the fifth pharyngeal arch is absent); the pharyngeal grooves or clefts between the arches; and the pharyngeal pouches. The first (mandibular) arch gives rise to the maxillary and mandibular prominences. The second (hyoid arch) enlarges and grows caudally, ultimately fusing with the upper thoracic wall to give the neck a smooth contour. The first pharyngeal groove becomes the external auditory meatus. The mandible is derived from intramembranous ossification. The first pair of pouches forms the tympanic cavity and pharyngotympanic tube. The first pharyngeal membrane forms the tympanic membrane. The second pair of pouches is associated with development of the palatine tonsils. The dorsal portions of the third pouch form the inferior parathyroid glands; the ventral portions form the thymus. The dorsal portions of the fourth pouch form the superior parathyroid glands; the small ventral portions of the fourth pouches and the rudimentary fifth pouches form the ultimobranchial bodies, which are incorporated into the thyroid gland to form the parafollicular cells. The thyroid diverticulum, which forms in the floor of the pharynx, grows caudally and becomes functional by the 12th week of gestation. The parafollicular cells are derived from the ultimobranchial bodies.

The primordia of the face (the frontonasal prominence, the maxillary prominences, and the mandibular prominences) merge mainly during the fifth to eighth weeks to form the facial structures. The adult derivatives are as follows: the frontonasal prominence – the forehead, dorsum, and apex of the nose; the lateral nasal prominences – the alae of the nose; the merged medial nasal prominences (intermaxillary segment) – the columella, philtrum of the upper lip, the maxilla that bears the incisors (the premaxilla), and the primary palate; the maxillary prominences –

the lateral portions of the upper lip, the upper cheeks and face, the rest of the maxilla, and the secondary palate; and the mandibular prominences – the lower lip, lower cheeks and face, and the mandible. The palate develops from two primordia: the primary palate, a wedge-shaped mesodermal mass from the innermost aspect of the intermaxillary segment (fifth week); and the secondary palate from the medial aspects of the maxillary prominences (sixth week). Fusion of the primordia of the palate begins in the ninth week and is completed by the 11th week in males and the 12th week in females. The larynx and trachea develop from the laryngotracheal tube. A lung bud develops at the caudal end of the tube, and this soon bifurcates to give two bronchopulmonary or lung buds. The right lung bud develops two secondary buds, and the left lung bud gives rise to one secondary lung bud; these buds demarcate the future lobes of the lung. Dichotomous branching forms the air-conducting passages, the bronchi and bronchioles.

The primordial (primitive) gut is divided into the foregut, midgut, and hindgut. The foregut derivatives are the pharynx and its derivatives, the lower respiratory tract, the esophagus, the stomach, the duodenum, proximal to the common bile duct, and the liver, biliary tract, gallbladder, and pancreas. The liver arises as an endodermal bud from the most caudal part of the foregut; this hepatic diverticulum extends into the septum transversum, divides into a larger cranial part, the primordium of the liver, and a smaller caudal part, which will form the gallbladder and cystic duct. The pancreas develops from dorsal and ventral pancreatic buds. The ventral pancreatic bud forms as an evagination of the hepatic diverticulum, and the dorsal pancreatic bud is derived from the proximal part of the duodenum. The two pancreatic ducts usually anastomose to form a single pancreatic duct. The spleen is derived from mesenchymal nodules located in the dorsal mesogastrium.

The intermediate mesoderm forms the nephrogenic cords. From the nephrogenic cords, three successive sets of excretory organs develop: the pronephros, the mesonephros, and the metanephros. The pronephros, a transitory nonfunctional structure, regresses leaving the pronephric ducts that will become the mesonephric ducts. The mesonephros serves as a temporary, excretory organ, which degenerates by the end of the embryonic period. In the male, the mesonephric ducts form some components of the reproductive system. In the female, the mesonephric ducts degenerate, except for vestigial remnants. The permanent adult kidney, the metanephros, develops in the fifth week and is functional 2–3 weeks later. The ureteric bud develops from the mesonephric duct. The ureteric bud forms the ureter, renal pelvis, calyces, and collecting tubules. The nephrons are derived from the metanephric blastema. At birth, the nephrons, approximately one million in each kidney, are formed. No new nephrons are formed after birth. The urinary bladder is derived from the cranial part of the urogenital sinus.

The genetic sex of the embryo is determined at fertilization. The Y chromosome has a testis-determining effect on the indifferent gonad. Under its influence, the primary sex cords differentiate into seminiferous tubules. Absence of a Y chromosome results in the formation of an ovary. The type of gonad determines the sexual differentiation of the genital ducts and external genitalia. Two pairs of genital ducts develop in both sexes: mesonephric (wolffian) ducts and paramesonephric (müllerian) ducts. Some mesonephric tubules near the testis persist and are transformed into efferent ductules or ductuli efferentes, which connect the rete testis to the epididymis. The mesonephric duct becomes the ductus epididymis and the vas deferens. The part of the mesonephric duct between the duct of this gland and the urethra becomes the ejaculatory duct. In the male, the paramesonephric ducts largely degenerate, except for a few vestigial remnants. In female embryos, the mesonephric ducts regress, and the paramesonephric ducts give rise to the female genital tract. The cranial unfused ends of the paramesonephric ducts form the uterine tubes. The caudal portions of the ducts converge and fuse in the midline to form the uterovaginal primordium, which gives rise to the uterus, cervix, and possibly part of the vagina. The uterovaginal primordium induces the formation of paired, endodermally derived outgrowths from the urogenital sinus. These fuse to form a solid vaginal plate, which eventually canalizes to become the vagina. Another view is that the uterus and upper third of the vagina are formed from the uterovaginal primordium and surrounding mesenchyme, while the lower two-thirds of the vagina is presumed to be derived from the vaginal plate and the surrounding mesenchyme. Early in the fourth week, a genital tubercle develops ventrally to the cloacal membrane. This elongates to form the phallus. By the sixth week, labioscrotal swellings and urogenital folds develop on each side of the future urogenital membrane. The phallus will form the penis. The urogenital folds fuse with each other along the ventral (under) surface of the penis and form the penile urethra. The paired labioscrotal swellings grow toward each other and fuse to form the scrotum. In the female, because of the absence of androgens, feminization of the indifferent external genitalia occurs. The phallus elongates rapidly at first but, as its growth gradually slows, it becomes the relatively small clitoris. The unfused urogenital folds form the paired labia minora, whereas the labioscrotal swellings give rise to the labia majora. The caudal portion of the urogenital sinus gives rise to the vestibule of the vagina.

The development of the heart begins as the paired endocardial heart tubes fuse to form a single median endocardial heart tube. The heart tube differentiates from cranial to caudal into: the bulbus cordis, ventricle, atrium, and sinus venosus. The bulbus cordis represents the arterial end of the heart. The sinus venosus represents the venous end of the heart. The heart tube bends to form a U-shaped bulboventricular loop. The atrium and the sinus venosus come to lie dorsal to the bulbus cordis, truncus arteriosus, and ventricle. Partitioning of the atrioventricular canal, the atrium, and the ventricle begins about the middle of the fourth week and is essentially complete by the end of the seventh week.

The neural tube gives rise to the central nervous system. The cranial part of the neural tube forms the three primary brain vesicles: the forebrain vesicle (prosencephalon), the midbrain vesicle (mesencephalon), and the hindbrain vesicle (rhombencephalon). These will form the adult derivatives of the brain. The lumen of the neural tube forms the ventricles of the brain. The spinal cord develops from the caudal part of the neural tube. The hypophysis develops from the neurohypophysis (a downgrowth from the floor of the diencephalon) and the adenohypophysis (an ectodermal outgrowth from the roof of the stomodeum).

By the end of the fourth week, the limb buds appear. The overlying ectoderm at the apex of each limb bud forms the apical ectodermal ridge, which induces mesenchymal proliferation. The flattened hand and foot plates develop five mesenchymal condensations (digital rays), which will give rise to the metacarpals, metatarsals, and phalanges. Programmed cell death or apoptosis is responsible for the degeneration of the loose mesenchyme between the digital rays which separates the fingers and toes. By the seventh week, endochondral ossification begins. The skull consists of the neurocranium (surrounds the brain) and the viscerocranium or facial skeleton. The flat bones surrounding the brain form the membranous part of the neurocranium, and the cartilaginous part gives rise to the bones of the base of the skull.

Further reading

Carlson BM. *Human embryology and developmental biology*, 3rd edn. Philadelphia, PA: Mosby, 2004.

Cochard LR. *Netter's atlas of human embryology*. Teterboro, NJ: Icon, 2002.

Drews V. *Color atlas of embryology*. New York: Thieme Medical Publishers, 1995.

England MA. *Color atlas of life before birth*. Chicago, IL: Year Book Medical, 1983.

Hinrichsen KV, ed. *Human embryologie*. Berlin: Springer Verlag, 1995.

Larsen WJ. *Human embryology*, 3rd edn. New York: Churchill Livingstone, 2001.

Moore KL, Persaud TVN. *The developing human. Clinically oriented embryology*, 7th edn. Philadelphia, PA: W.B. Saunders, 2003.

Moore KL, Persaud TVN, Shiota K. *Color atlas of clinical embryology*, 2nd edn. Philadelphia, PA: W.B. Saunders, 2000.

O'Rahilly R, Müller F. *Human embryology and teratology*, 3rd edn. New York: Wiley-Liss, 2001.

Sadler TW. *Langman's medical embryology*, 9th edn. Baltimore, MD: Lippincott Williams & Wilkins, 2004.

Part II   Pregnancy and the Fetoplacental Unit

3   Normal and abnormal placentation

Soheila Korourian and Luis De Las Casas

The placenta is crucial for fetal growth and survival. It performs the most important functions of many somatic organs before birth.

Table 3.1 Percentiles, means, and standard deviations (SD) for placental weights from 36 to 42 weeks' gestation (term placentas).

Gestational age (weeks)	Percentile								
	Mean	SD	3	5	10	25	50	75	95
36	447	110	270	291	320	369	440	508	628
37	467	107	303	324	349	390	452	531	660
38	493	103	320	335	365	420	484	560	675
39	500	103	330	350	379	426	490	564	683
40	510	100	340	360	390	440	501	572	685
41	524	100	358	379	403	452	515	583	705
42	532	99	370	388	412	460	525	592	700

Modified and adopted from Kraus FT, Redline RW, Gersell DJ, et al. AFIP Atlas of non tumor pathology: Placental pathology. Washington DC: American Registry of Pathology, 2004. The original data are derived from Boyd T, Gang D, Lis G, et al. Normative values for placental weights (N = 15463) (Abstract). Mod Pathol 1999;12:1.

Gross appearance of the normal term placenta

A normal placenta is a disk-shaped organ which, at term, measures approximately $19 \times 18 \times 4 \pm 1$ cm in greatest dimension and weighs 480 ± 120 g (Table 3.1). The fetal surface is steel gray and is covered by a glistening membrane. The maternal surface should be intact. A three-vessel umbilical cord, measuring 55 ± 15 cm in length and 3.7 ± 1 cm in diameter, inserts in the center or slightly off center. The membrane is translucent and glistening. Serial sections of the placenta show blood-rich, homogenous, beefy-red parenchyma. Small infarcts measuring less than 10% of the volume can be identified at the edge of the placenta. Minute amounts of blood clot might be present at the maternal surface.

Infarct

A term placenta consists of 40–60 functional units. These units receive oxygenated blood from the branches of the maternal spiral arteries. Each lobular unit depends on its own spiral artery. Thrombosis of the spiral arteries results in infarction of the dependent unit. Central or large (≥25% of placenta) infarcts and those occurring in the first and second trimester are more significant and can cause fetal demise.

Retroplacental hematomas and placental abruption

Retroplacental hematomas are clots located in the decidua between the placental floor and the muscular wall of the uterus. Retroplacental hematoma is related to, but not synonymous with, placental abruption. Placental abruption is an acute clinical syndrome characterized by pain, uterine tetany, fetal distress, and sometimes consumption coagulopathy. It occurs in 1.1% of pregnancies. It is associated with 20–40% fetal mortality rates and accounts for 10% of all stillbirths and 5% of maternal deaths.

Placental inflammation and intrauterine infections

Placental inflammation is common. Different patterns of inflammation are associated with different routes of infection. Ascending infection, commonly caused by bacteria, induces acute inflammation of the membrane (chorioamnionitis) and umbilical cord (funisitis). Hematogenous infections, usually caused by viruses, induce inflammation of the villous parenchyma.

Hydrops fetalis and placental hydrops

Hydrops fetalis is a state of profound generalized fetal edema with marked accumulation of fluid in the subcutaneous tissue and in all body cavities.

Immune hydrops
This condition used to be the most common cause of hydrops, and is caused by severe hemolytic anemia that results from the transplacental passage of maternal Rh antibodies to the Rh antigen-negative fetus.

Nonimmune hydrops
A heterogeneous group of conditions is responsible for nonimmune hydrops. Most causes can be categorized as cardiac failure, anemia, or hypoproteinemia.

Disorders of uterine implantation

Placenta previa
In placenta previa, implantation is in the lower uterine segment with some tissue near or overlying the uterine cervical os. Complete previa occurs when the placenta completely covers the cervical os. Partial previa occurs if the edge of the placenta is within 2 cm of the os.

Placenta accreta, increta, and percreta
In these conditions, anchoring villi implant on the uterine smooth muscle without intervening decidua. In placenta accreta, the villi are limited to the superficial myometrium; in increta, the villi extend into the myometrium; and in percreta, the villi extend to or through the uterine serosa.

Peripheral cord insertion

Membranous insertion (velamentous insertion)
In membranous (velamentous) insertion, the umbilical cord terminates in the membrane rather than in the chorionic disk. It occurs in 1.3–1.6% of pregnancies.

Maternal diseases affecting the fetus

Diabetes mellitus

The gross and microscopic features of the placenta vary considerably. Approximately 50% of placentas of diabetic mothers are of normal weight and size, and have normal gross and microscopic features. However, those placentas that are abnormal are larger, thicker, more friable, and heavier than normal placentas of the same gestational age, and the umbilical cord is often notably thicker.

Acquired thrombophilia

Acquired thrombophilia, especially the presence of antiphospholipid antibodies, promotes intraplacental clotting.

Toxic damage to the placenta

The placentas of women who smoke more frequently show necrotic damage. Women who smoke have a higher incidence of placenta previa, abnormalities of the placenta, and fetal malformations.

Multiple pregnancies

Multiple pregnancies are common and their rate is increasing because of assisted reproductive technology (ART). Twins are classified as dizygous (fraternal) or monozygous (identical).

All dizygous twins have dichorionic placentas (diamniotic dichorionic: DiDi). A monozygous twin can show any type of placentation depending on the time of splitting in the blastocyst. If the split occurs between days 3 and 8, there will be a diamniotic monochorionic placenta (DiMo). If a split occurs after formation of the amnion (days 8–13), this results in monoamniotic monochorionic (MoMo) twins.

Meconium staining

True meconium staining results from exposure of the placenta to meconium for several hours. Damage to the fetus increases with length of exposure to meconium.

Abnormal amniotic fluid volume

The presence of an excess of amniotic fluid is called hydramnios or polyhydramnios. A diminished amount of fluid is called oligohydramnios. Amniotic fluid provides the medium for free fetal movements and a cushioning effect to prevent possible fetal injury.

The most common significant anomalies associated with hydramnios are anencephaly, spina bifida, esophageal atresia, nonimmune hydrops, and various abnormal karyotypes.

The most common cause of oligohydramnios is leakage of the amniotic fluid caused by the premature rupture of the membranes. Oligohydramnios can cause amniotic band syndrome.

Gestational trophoblastic disease

There is a heterogeneous group of gestational and neoplastic conditions of trophoblastic origin. The incidence of gestational trophoblastic disease varies widely among different populations. It is reported to occur in 8.3 in 1000 pregnancies in some areas of Asia and South America compared with 0.1–0.6 in 1000 in the USA. The incidence of this disease is higher in women older than 40 and is also increased in those younger than 20.

Further reading

American College of Obstetricians and Gynecologists Committee on Obstetric Practice. Placenta accreta. Committee Opinion No. 266. *Obstet Gynecol* 2002;99:169–170.

Barash A, Dekel N, Fieldust S, et al. Local injury to the endometrium doubles the incidence of successful pregnancies in patients undergoing in vitro fertilization. *Fertil Steril* 2003;79:1317–1322.

Benirschke K, Kaufmann P. Pathology of the human placenta, 3th edn. New York, NY: Springer; 1995:151–181.

Benirschke K, Kaufmann P. Pathology of the human placenta, 4th edn. New York, NY: Springer, 2000.

Charnock-Jones DS, Burton GJ. Placental vascular morphogenesis. *Best Pract Res Clin Obstet Gynecol* 2000;14:953–968.

Cross JC, Werb Z, Fisher SJ. Implantation and the placenta: key pieces of the development puzzle. *Science* 1994;266:1508–1518.

Doss BJ, Greene MF, Hill J, et al. Massive chronic intervillitis associated with recurrent abortions. *Hum Pathol* 1995;26:1245–1251.

Duley L. Pre-eclampsia and hypertension (Update). *Clin Evid* 2003;9:1584–1600.

Favre R, Dreux S, Dommergues M, et al. Nonimmune fetal ascites. *Am J Obstet Gynecol* 2004;190:407–412.

Fox H. Pathology of the placenta, 2nd edn. *Major problems in pathology*. Philadelphia, PA: WB Saunders; 1997:54–60.

Goldenberg RL, Hauth JC, Andrews WW. Intrauterine infection and preterm delivery. *N Engl J Med* 2000;342:1500–1507.

Greer IA. Thrombosis in pregnancy: maternal and fetal issues. *Lancet* 1999;353:1258–1265.

Jauniaux E, Nessmann C, Imbert C, et al. Morphological aspects of placenta in HIV pregnancies. *Placenta* 1988;9:633–642.

Knisely AS. The pathologist and the hydropic placenta, fetus, or infant. *Semin Perinatol* 1995;19:525–531.

Kraus FT, Acheen VI. Fetal thrombotic vasculopathy in the placenta: cerebral thrombi and infarcts, coagulopathies, and cerebral palsy. *Hum Pathol* 1999;30:759–769.

Rand JH, Wu XX, Andree HA, et al. Pregnancy loss in the antiphospholipid-antibody syndrome – a possible thrombogenic mechanism. *N Engl J Med* 1997;337:154–160.

Redline RW, O'Riordan MA. Placental lesions associated with cerebral palsy and neurological impairment following term birth. *Arch Pathol Lab Med* 2000;124:1785–1791.

Rodriguez MM, Chaves F, Romaguera RL, et al. Value of autopsy in nonimmune hydrops fetalis. *Pediatr Dev Pathol* 2002;5:365–374.

Shih IM, Mazur MT, Kurman R. Gestational trophoblastic disease and related lesions. In: *Blaustein's pathology of female genital tract*, 5th edn. New York, NY: Springer-Verlag, 2002.

Williams MA, Hickok DE, Zingheim RW, et al. Low birth weight and preterm delivery in relation to early-gestation vaginal bleeding and elevated maternal serum alpha-fetoprotein. *Obstet Gynecol* 1992;80;745–749.

4 Fetoplacental perfusion and transfer of nutrients

Henry L. Galan and Frederick C. Battaglia

This chapter discusses the aspects of perinatal physiology that are reasonably well established and of most importance.

The relationship between fetal and maternal oxygenation is complex in that a number of factors determine the "normal" umbilical venous PO_2 in any species. These factors include: (1) placental oxygen consumption; (2) uterine and umbilical blood flows; (3) placental permeability; (4) the pattern of placental perfusion (i.e., concurrent, crosscurrent, countercurrent); (5) maternal arterial PO_2 and hemoglobin concentration; and (6) the shape of maternal and fetal oxygen dissociation curves.

One important factor affecting uterine blood flow is the absence of autoregulation in the uterine vascular bed leading to an almost fully dilated bed. Thus, from a clinical perspective, maternal hypotension must be regarded as a direct causal factor in producing a reduction in uterine and placental blood flow and should be avoided. Uterine vasculature is also unresponsive to changes in PO_2 or PCO_2. Maternal PO_2 administration has no effect on uterine or umbilical blood flows, and umbilical venous PO_2, representing the most oxygenated blood of the fetus, increases significantly.

Recent studies have shown that in pregnancies complicated by intrauterine growth retardation (IUGR) maternal oxygen administration benefits the fetus, as demonstrated by an increased fetal blood PO_2 and oxygen saturation. Doppler velocity waveform measurements of the fetal descending aorta suggest a reduced placental impedance during maternal oxygen therapy.

The decrease in fetal PO_2 in late gestation does not imply increasing fetal hypoxia because, associated with this, there is an increasing hemoglobin concentration as gestation progresses. For this reason, measurements of fetal oxygen content are particularly useful because they are independent of gestational age.

The placenta is very active metabolically. It has an oxygen consumption and glucose utilization rate similar to brain tissue. Data demonstrate that the maternal–

fetal glucose concentration difference increases as gestation advances. The increased transplacental glucose gradient is one means of accommodating the increased glucose requirements of the rapidly growing fetus.

In all mammalian species, placental growth is much more rapid than fetal growth in early gestation; placental growth then either stops or continues at a very low rate during the latter part of gestation. Although the growth rate of the human placenta decreases, its maturation continues. Fetal growth, on the other hand, is largely exponential throughout gestation. Key aspects of fetal growth include not only the rate of change in fetal body weight but also the changing body composition as gestation advances. This is particularly striking for the human fetus, which grows by approximately 1.5% each day. Because water has no caloric density and fat has the highest caloric density of tissues, the human fetus has a relatively high caloric accretion rate. Also, because fat is nitrogen free and 78% carbon, the human fetus has a relatively low nitrogen accretion rate in late pregnancy but builds up large carbon stores in fat and glycogen.

The net umbilical uptake represents the dietary supply of nutrients to the fetus. The major nutrients that the fetus receives include glucose, lactate, and amino acids. Glucose and the essential amino acids are derived from the maternal circulation.

The nonessential amino acids are a far more complicated issue, with tracer studies showing that some amino acids are produced within the placenta in large amounts with a relatively small component coming from direct transplacental transport.

Both glucose and lactate have been shown to have fairly high oxidation rates during fetal life. If their transport is increased, their contribution to oxidation will also increase, sparing the utilization of amino acids as metabolic fuels. Conversely, during maternal fasting, placental glucose transport is decreased and amino acid oxidation increased. Fatty acids and ketone bodies cross the placenta in man and in several other species, maintaining relatively small transplacental concentration gradients. Fatty acids are used largely for carbon accretion in white fat depots and are not oxidized extensively during fetal life.

Doppler velocimetry is useful for managing the fetus with IUGR. It can also be used to calculate umbilical vein volume blood flow, which determines oxygenation and nutrient delivery. Absolute umbilical vein volume flow is reduced by mid-gestation in fetuses with IUGR. The ability to calculate volume blood flow will provide the opportunity to better understand nutrient flux across the human placenta.

Further reading

Ferrazzi E, Bozzo M, Rigano S, et al. Temporal sequence of abnormal Doppler changes in the peripheral and central circulatory systems of severely growth restricted fetuses. *Ultrasound Obstet Gynecol* 2002;19:140–146.

Gill RW, Kossoff G, Warren PS, et al. Umbilical venous flow in normal and complicated pregnancy. *Ultrasound Med Biol* 1984;10:349–363.

Lyall F, Greer IA, Young A, et al. Nitric oxide concentrations are increased in the fetoplacental circulation in intrauterine growth restriction. *Placenta* 1996;17:165–168.

Marconi AM, Paolini C, Cetin I, et al. The impact of gestational age and of intrauterine growth upon the maternal–fetal glucose concentrations difference. *Obstet Gynecol* 1996;87:937–942.

Myatt L, Eis ALW, Brockman DE, et al. Endothelial nitric oxide synthase in placental villous tissue from normal, pre-eclamptic and intrauterine growth restricted pregnancies. *Hum Reprod* 1997;12:167–172.

Pardi G, Cetin I, Marconi AM, et al. The venous drainage of the human uterus: respiratory gas studies in normal and fetal growth retarded pregnancies. *Am J Obstet Gynecol* 1992; 166:699–706.

Regnault TRH, de Vrijer B, Battaglia FC. Transport and metabolism of amino acids in placenta. *Endocrine* 2002;19:23–41.

Rigano S, Bozzo M, Ferrazzi E, et al. Early and persistent reduction in umbilical vein blood flow in the growth-restricted fetus: a longitudinal study. *Am J Obstet Gynecol* 2001; 185:834–838.

Sparks JW, Girard J, Battaglia FC. An estimate of the caloric requirements of the human fetus. *Biol Neonate* 1980;38:113–119.

Wilkening RB, Meschia G. Fetal oxygen uptake, oxygenation, and acid–base balance as a function of uterine blood flow. *Am J Physiol* 1983;244:H749–H755.

5 Endocrinology of pregnancy and the placenta

Alan DeCherney, Jessica Spencer, Tim Chard, and Karen A. Hutchinson

The corpus luteum

This forms from the ovulated follicle, lasts for 14 days, and then undergoes luteolysis if no pregnancy occurs. The trophoblast produces human chorionic gonadotropin (hCG), which sustains the corpus luteum, and this, in turn, stabilizes the pregnancy.

Estrone, estradiol, and estriol

Estrone (E_1), estradiol (E_2), and estriol (E_3) all share an 18-carbon estrone nucleus.
1 E_1 predominates during the menopause.
2 E_2 predominates during the ovulatory years.
3 E_3 is produced almost exclusively by the placenta during pregnancy.

Progesterone

Progesterone functions include relaxation of uterotubal musculature, inhibition of T-cell tissue rejection, and maintenance of uterine blood flow.

Maternal immune system changes

These include:
1 type 1 T helper to type 2 T helper (Th1 to Th2) cytokine deviation;
2 changes in maternal CD4+ and CD8+ cells;
3 deletion of alloreactive B cells;
4 uterine natural killer (NK) cell activity.

Fetal immune system changes

These include:
1 replacement of major histocompatibility complex (MHC)-I with human leuko-cyte antigen (HLA)-G and -E;
2 expression of high levels of Fas ligand.

Key maternal cardiovascular adaptations

These include:
1 physiological anemia caused by an increase in blood volume by 40% but only a 33% rise in red blood cell count;
2 angiotensin II resistance in normal pregnancy, causing a mild hyponatremia with a lower plasma osmolality;
3 lowering of blood pressure by approximately 20 mmHg but an increase in peripheral vascular resistance and heart rate.

Nutrition and the fetus

The fetal glucose level is usually 10–20 mg/mL lower than that of the mother. High levels of human placental lactogen (hPL) (see Human chorionic somatomam-motropin, below) favor an insulin-resistant environment. Obesity will increase a woman's chances of infertility, miscarriage, diabetes, hypertension, preeclampsia, and risk for Cesarean delivery.

Hypothalamic and pituitary development in the fetus

The hypothalamic nuclei are differentiated by 14 weeks and the portal system is completed by 19–21 weeks. The pituitary gland develops from oral ectoderm anteriorly and neuroectoderm posteriorly. The anterior portion of the pituitary will differentiate into five cellular subtypes: thyrotrophs, corticotrophs, somatotrophs, gonadotrophs, and lactotrophs. The posterior pituitary will produce oxytocin and vasopressin. Interestingly, analogous pituitary-like hormones have been histochemically localized to the syncytiotrophoblast and analogous hypothalamic-like hormones have been localized to the cytotrophoblast (see below).

GnRH, FSH and LH, and the gonads

Secretion of gonadotropin-releasing hormone (GnRH), follicle-stimulating hormone (FSH), and luteinizing hormone (LH) begins at between 9 and 10 weeks' gestation and peaks at around 20–22 weeks.

The male fetus

Testes, which consist of Leydig cells that produce testosterone (critical for *internal* secondary sexual development), form at approximately 6 weeks. Dihydroxytestosterone (DHT) is converted from testosterone by 5α-reductase in target tissues and is critical for *external* secondary sexual development. Müllerian-inhibiting substance (MIS) is produced by the Sertoli cells in the testes and inhibits müllerian system development.

The female fetus

The fetal ovary can be histologically recognized by gestational week 10. Unlike the male gonad, its hormonal function in the fetus is limited.

Placental GnRH, hCG, and inhibin

Placental gonadotropin-releasing hormone (GnRH) and inhibin are produced by the cytotrophoblastic cells, whereas human chorionic gonadotropin (hCG) is produced in the syncytiotrophoblast (see Human chorionic gonadotrophin, below). Placental GnRH stimulates the release of hCG which, in turn, influences steroidogenesis. Inhibin may inhibit GnRH release, therefore inhibiting hCG release.

TRH, TSH, and the thyroid

Thyrotropin-releasing hormone (TRH) is detectable by 10 weeks' gestation and the fetal thyroid gland starts producing thyroglobulin by day 29 and thyroxine (T_4) by week 11. Thyroxine-binding globulin (TBG) increases progressively to term, thus increasing the total T_4 count; however, the free T_4 level remains approximately the same. Thyroid hormones are necessary for skeletal, pulmonary, and brain development.

Human chorionic thyrotropin

Human chorionic thyrotropin (hCT) is a product of the cytotrophoblast and is analogous to TRH. However, the hyperstimulation of thyroid tissue that occurs in some women with molar pregnancy is caused by high levels of hCG, not hCT.

Parathyroid hormone and calcium homeostasis

Parathyroid hormone (PTH) appears around the 12–13th gestational week but remains suppressed while calcitonin levels are elevated. High levels of calcium are transported across the placenta for bone formation. Vitamin D metabolism is shared between the fetus and placenta.

Prolactin

Prolactin levels increase until term. Prolactin may play a role in the regulation of normal fetal osmolality, and in bone, adrenal gland, lung, brain, and pancreatic β-cell development.

Growth hormone and somatostatin

Growth hormone (GH) peaks at between 25 and 30 weeks and then decreases in the third trimester. Its role is not entirely clear, but it does stimulate insulin growth factors (IGF)-1 and -2, which are altered in chronic hypoxemia, malnutrition, and steroid hormone biosynthesis. Elevated levels of GH have been identified in premature infants. It is inhibited by somatostatin.

Somatomedin

Somatomedin is a growth-promoting hormone that correlates directly with body weight and appears to be lower in infants with intrauterine growth retardation (IUGR); however, it is not GH dependent.

CRH, ACTH, and the adrenal gland

After the seventh week of gestation, the fetoplacental unit takes over steroidogenesis from the corpus luteum. The fetal adrenal cortex and the placenta rely on each other to complete steroidogenesis pathways.

Placental corticotropin-releasing hormone (CRH) is structurally similar to hypothalamic CRH and is found in the cytotrophoblast. It is highest during the first trimester and diminishes as term approaches. Likewise, placental adrenocorticotropic hormone (ACTH) appears to be structurally similar to pituitary ACTH and has been localized to the syncytiotrophoblast.

The fetal adrenal gland

The fetal adrenal gland is composed of:

1 the outer, or definitive zone (becomes adrenal cortex);
2 the inner, or fetal zone, which involutes after delivery;
3 the fetal adrenal medulla (catecholamine production).

The fetal adrenal cortex is functionally deficient in 3β-hydroxysteroid dehydrogenase, which is abundant in the placenta. It converts pregnenolone to progesterone, which is then returned to the fetus for mineralo- and glucocorticoid synthesis.

The fetal zone produces high levels of dehydroepiandrosterone sulfate (DHEAS), some of which is delivered to the fetal liver, where it is converted to 16α-hydroxy-androstenedione and then further aromatized into estriol. Estrogens are subsequently secreted into the fetal and maternal circulations.

Aldosterone and cortisol are both produced by the definitive zone. Low-density lipoprotein (LDL) cholesterol is used as a substrate for the synthesis of cortisol via the pathways of 17α-, 21-, and 11β-hydroxylation. Progesterone, derived from the placental circulation, can also be used within the definitive zone for the production of cortisol, deoxycorticosterone, corticosterone, and aldosterone. Cortisol stimulates pulmonary surfactant production and is involved in hepatic enzyme development. It is also involved in the development of the hypothalamic–pituitary–adrenal (HPA) axis and may play a role in the initiation of labor.

Renin–angiotensin system

Renin secretion clearly doubles as early as the eighth week of gestation and then increases to 32 weeks when it plateaus. Angiotensin II is formed from angiotensin I by the placenta and reaches higher levels in the mother and fetus than in the nongravid state. Unlike renin, aldosterone continues to increase throughout pregnancy.

Fetoplacental peptides

Human chorionic gonadotropin

The structure of hCG is similar to that of LH, FSH, and thyroid-stimulating hormone (TSH). It is produced by the syncytiotrophoblast and, pathologically, by choriocarcinoma and hydatidiform moles. It is detectable by day 9 at the implantation of the blastocyst, and peaks at 30–60 days. Early on it sustains the corpus luteum; it then stimulates the fetal testes to produce testosterone in the absence of LH. It also regulates DHEAS production and may also be involved in preventing fetal tissue rejection.

Human chorionic somatomammotropin (human placental lactogen)

Human chorionic somatomammotropin (hCS), also known as hPL, is produced by the syncytiotrophoblast layer and is very similar in structure and function to GH. It is also detectable in normal and molar pregnancies, trophoblastic tumors, and in choriocarcinoma of the testes. It ensures the nutritional needs of the fetus by stimulating lipolysis over carbohydrate metabolism.

Further reading

Al-Timim A, Fox H. Immunohistochemical localization of follicle-stimulating hormone, luteinizing hormone, growth hormone, adrenocorticotropic hormone and prolactin in the human placenta. *Placenta* 1986;7:163.

Han. The ontogeny of growth hormone, insulin-like growth factors and sex steroids: molecular aspects. *Horm Res* 1996.

Hosina M, Boime I, Mochizuki. Cytological localization of hPL, hCG, and mRNA in chorionic tissue using in situ hybridization. *Acta Obstet Gynaecol Jpn* 1984;36:397.

Kenimer JG, Herschman JN, Higgins HP. The thyrotropin in hydatidiform moles is human chorionic gonadotropin. *J Clin Endocrinol Metab* 1975;40:482.

Koch C, Platt J. Natural mechanisms for evading graft rejection: the fetus as an allograft. *Springer Semin Immunopathol* 2003;25:95.

Kurman RJ, Young RH, Norris JH, et al. Immunocytochemical localization of placental lactogen and chorionic gonadotropin in the normal placenta and trophoblastic tumors, with emphasis on intermediate trophoblast and the placental site trophoblastic tumor. *Int J Gynecol Pathol* 1984;3:101.

Linné, Y. Effects of obesity on women's reproduction and complications during pregnancy. *Obes Rev* 2004;5:137.

Page, NM. The endocrinology of pre-eclampsia. *Clin Endocrinol* 2002;57:413.

Sheng H, Westphal, H. Early steps in pituitary organogenesis. *Trends Genet* 1999;15:236.

Wilson M, Morganti AG, Zervoudakis I, et al. Blood pressure, the renin aldosterone system and sex steroids throughout normal pregnancy. *Am J Med* 1980;68:97.

Part III Fetal Developmental Biology

6 Fetal lung development and amniotic fluid analysis

Ian Gross and Mathew J. Bizzarro

Fetal lung development

Respiratory distress syndrome (RDS) is a developmental disorder of prematurely born infants characterized by progressive atelectasis and respiratory insufficiency. It is caused, in part, by a developmental deficiency of pulmonary surfactant, a mixture of phospholipids and proteins that acts to reduce the surface tension at the air–alveolar interface and prevent alveolar collapse. The incidence of RDS varies inversely with gestational age.

Clinical conditions that accelerate fetal lung maturation include pregnancy-induced hypertension and chronic maternal disease, for example hypertension and classes D, F, and R diabetes. Lung maturation is delayed in classes A–C diabetes.

Evaluation of fetal lung maturity

The lecithin–sphingomyelin ratio

Assessment of fetal lung maturity by analysis of phospholipids in amniotic fluid began in 1971, when Gluck and coauthors reported gestational changes in amniotic fluid phospholipid concentrations. Total phospholipids in amniotic fluid increase throughout gestation, with a sharp increase in the lecithin (phosphatidylcholine, PC) concentration at approximately 35 weeks (Fig. 6.1). Because sphingomyelin remains fairly constant while lecithin increases, a ratio between the two is used to correct for changes in amniotic fluid volume. The lecithin–sphingomyelin (L/S) ratio reaches

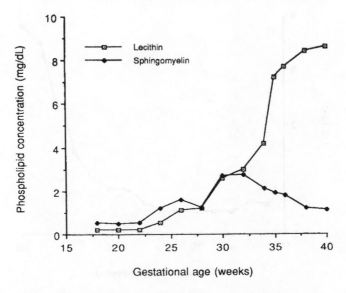

Figure 6.1 Amniotic fluid phospholipid concentration vs. gestational age.

2 : 1, the value usually associated with lung maturity, at approximately 35 weeks (Fig. 6.2). As is shown in Table 6.1, the L/S ratio is very accurate at predicting lung maturity (negative predictive value, negative test = no RDS), but less reliable at predicting immaturity (positive predictive value, positive test = lung immaturity).

Phosphatidylglycerol

Phosphatidylglycerol (PG) appears at 34–35 weeks and increases thereafter. The appearance of PG as 3% or more of the total phospholipids is predictive of lung maturity. In classes A–C diabetes, the appearance of PG is delayed until 37–39 weeks.

The negative predictive value of the L/S–PG test is close to 100%, but the positive predictive value is much lower. The addition of a test for surfactant protein A (SP-A) further improves the predictive value. A variety of other tests using simpler methodologies have also been developed, but their positive predictive values are considered to be unsatisfactory when they are used alone.

Use of antenatal steroids

Glucocorticoids accelerate anatomical, biochemical, and physiological maturation of the lung. Antenatal glucocorticoid therapy reduces the overall incidence of RDS by approximately 50%. The major benefit of glucocorticoid therapy is observed in infants who deliver from 1 to 7 days after the initiation of maternal treatment.

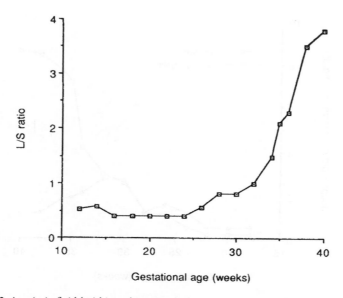

Figure 6.2 Amniotic fluid lecithin–sphingomyelin (L/S) ratio vs. gestational age.

Table 6.1 Predictive value of prenatal tests for lung maturity.

Test	Positive accuracy	Negative accuracy
L/S	0.54	0.98
L/S–PG	0.47	0.99
Shake test	0.12	1.0
A_{650}	0.13	0.99
SP-A	0.32	1.0
L/S–PG + SP-A	0.71	1.0
FELMA	0.33	1.0
TDx-FLM	0.31	0.97

FELMA, microviscosity by fluorescence polarization; L/S, lecithin–sphingomyelin ratio; PG, phosphatidylglycerol; SP-A, surfactant protein A; TDx-FLM, fluorescence polarization, Abbot Laboratories.
Negative test, maturity; *positive test*, immaturity; *negative predictive accuracy*, accuracy with which a mature test predicts no RDS; *positive predictive accuracy*, the accuracy with which an immature test predicts RDS.

However, there is a trend toward decreased RDS in infants who are born less than 24 h or more than 7 days after the initiation of steroid treatment. Other benefits of antenatal steroid administration include a reduction in the incidence of intraventricular hemorrhage (IVH), necrotizing enterocolitis (NEC), and mortality.

Table 6.2 NIH Consensus Development Conference: recommendations for use of antenatal glucocorticoids.

The benefits of antenatal corticosteroids "vastly" outweigh the risks

All fetuses at risk for preterm delivery between 24 and 34 weeks of gestation are candidates for treatment

This decision should not be altered by race, gender, or availability of surfactant therapy

Patients who are eligible for tocolytic therapy are also eligible for steroid therapy

Treatment should be given unless immediate delivery is expected; treatment for less than 24 h is associated with decreased mortality, RDS, and intraventricular hemorrhage

In cases of PROM at less than 30–32 weeks of gestation, treatment is recommended in the absence of clinical chorioamnionitis

In complicated pregnancies in which delivery before 34 weeks is expected, treatment is recommended unless there is evidence that it will have an adverse effect on the mother

Dosing: betamethasone, 12 mg i.m. q24 h × 2 (or dexamethasone, 6 mg i.m. q12 h × 4)

Betamethasone is the steroid of choice as neurotoxicity has been reported with the use of antenatal dexamethasone.

If premature delivery does not occur after a course of glucocorticoid has been given, the American College of Obstetricians and Gynecologists (ACOG) recommends that subsequent repeat courses should not be administered routinely.

Antenatal glucocorticoid therapy is synergistic with postnatal surfactant therapy. Recommendations for the use of antenatal glucocorticoids were published by a National Institutes of Health (NIH) Consensus Development Conference and are listed in Table 6.2. Optimal management of prematurity now includes antenatal assessment of fetal lung maturity, antenatal glucocorticoid administration, and post-natal surfactant therapy if needed.

Further reading

American College of Obstetricians and Gynecologists. Antenatal corticosteroid therapy for fetal maturation. *Committee Opin* 2002;273:9–11.

Ballard PL, Ballard RA. Scientific basis and therapeutic regimens for use of antenatal gluco-corticoids. *Am J Obstet Gynecol* 1995;173:254–262.

Crowley P. Antenatal corticosteroid therapy: a meta-analysis of the randomized trials, 1972 to 1994. *Am J Obstet Gynecol* 1995;173:322–335.

Crowther CA, Harding J. Repeat doses of prenatal corticosteroids for women at risk of preterm birth for preventing neonatal respiratory disease. *Cochrane Database Syst Rev* 2004;2.

Gluck L, Kulovich MV, Borer, RC, et al. Diagnosis of the respiratory distress syndrome by amniocentesis. *Am J Obstet Gynecol* 1971;109:440–445.

Gross I, Ballard PL. Hormonal therapy for prevention of respiratory distress syndrome. In: Polin RA, Fox WW, Abman SH, eds. *Fetal and neonatal physiology*, 3rd edn. Philadelphia, PA: Elsevier; 2003:1069–1074.

Hobbins JC, Brock W, Speroff L, et al. L/S ratio in predicting pulmonary maturity *in utero*. *Obstet Gynecol* 1972;39:660–664.

Kulovich M, Gluck L. The lung profile. II: complicated pregnancy. *Am J Obstet Gynecol* 1979;135:64–70.

Kulovich M, Hallman M, Gluck L. The lung profile. I: normal pregnancy. *Am J Obstet Gynecol* 1979;135:57–63.

National Institutes of Health Consensus Development Panel. The effect of corticosteroids for fetal maturation on perinatal outcomes. *JAMA* 1995;273:413–418.

7 Fetal cardiovascular physiology and response to stress conditions

Jean-Claude Fouron and Amanda Skoll

Maturational changes in the myocardium include:[1] the reorganization and longitudinal orientation of myofibrils; the enhancement of storage and release of calcium by the sarcoplasmic reticulum;[2,3] and the shift toward relatively more efficient isozymes of cardiac myosin.[4,5] Fetal muscle strips exhibit higher resting tension but decreased active tension that can be generated upon stimulation.[6] These differences are due to a greater proportion of noncontractile proteins and differences in activity of adenosine triphosphatase (ATPase) in fetal tissue.[6]

The fetal heart is relatively "stiff" when compared with the adult heart, although it does respond to the Frank–Starling mechanism (Fig. 7.1), albeit in a rather limited way.[6] Factors affecting ventricular preload are different *in utero* for each side of the heart. Left ventricular (LV) preload is determined by the size of the foramen ovale, by inferior vena caval flow, by pulmonary venous return (a more significant contribution as gestation advances),[7,8] and by right ventricular (RV) diastolic function, as pressure differences may be transmitted across the foramen ovale.

RV preload *in utero* is composed of superior vena caval flow and the fraction of inferior vena caval flow that does not cross the foramen ovale. Thus, factors that influence the degree of right to left shunting may significantly impact RV preload (size of the foramen ovale, left ventricular diastolic function).

The greatest influence on LV afterload is the vascular resistance in the upper body,[9] whereas the primary determinant of RV afterload is placental resistance. Combined ventricular output at term has been calculated as approximately 450 mL/kg/min,[10,11] with RV stroke volume being approximately 20% greater than that of the LV. Pressure development in the fetal ventricle appears to be similar to that in the adult. However, in the fetus, acceleration time is shorter in the pulmonary artery than in the aorta.[12] Maturational changes lead to more efficient ventricular

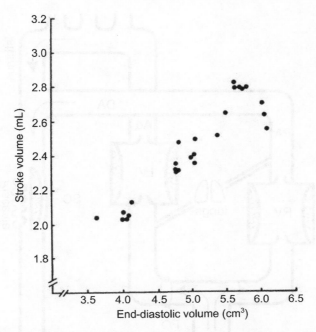

Figure 7.1 Relationship between end-diastolic volume (LVEDV) and stroke volume (SV) of the left ventricle in the fetal lamb (reprinted with permission from ref. 1).

relaxation during diastole. Therefore, ventricular filling is due more and more to active ventricular relaxation as gestation progresses, and relatively less to atrial contraction.

Fetal circulatory dynamics

The parallel arrangement of the fetal ventricles is depicted in Fig. 7.2, and the hemodynamic implications are shown in Table 7.1.

The fetal pulmonary arteries offer a high resistance to flow. This feature is related to a low total cross-sectional pulmonary vascular area in the first half of gestation. However, a progressive increase in cross-sectional area occurs in the latter half of gestation and in the first year of life.[13,14] Down to the level of the terminal bronchioles, the pulmonary vessels are characterized by the presence of a thick muscular layer. Oxygen is a prime factor in determining pulmonary vascular tone, with reduction in O_2 tension causing vasoconstriction.[15,16]

The placenta is a very high-flow, low-resistance vascular bed. Thus, Doppler velocimetry of the umbilical arteries in the setting of normal placental function

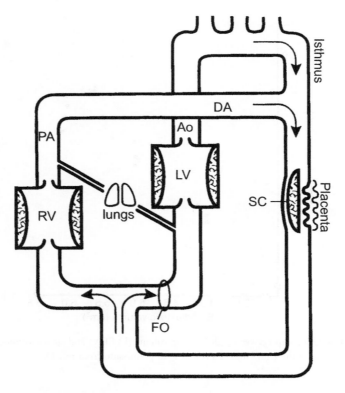

Figure 7.2 Schematic representation of the fetal circulatory dynamic. The right (RV) and left (LV) ventricles are perfusing in parallel the systemic circulation (SC). The upper part of the body receives blood exclusively from the LV. In addition to the lungs, RV perfuses the subdiaphragmatic part of SC via the ductus arteriosus (DA). The parallel disposition of the pulmonary (PA) and the aortic (Ao) arches is well illustrated. The isthmus represents a vascular segment connecting these two parallel systems. FO, foramen ovale.

Table 7.1 Hemodynamic implications of the parallel arrangement of the two ventricles.

Inequality of ventricular outputs
Similarity of systolic pressures
Reciprocal influence of ventricular diastolic functions
Possibility of adequate perfusion by a single ventricle
Special status of the aortic isthmus

shows significant diastolic forward flow, increasing as gestation advances.[17] Mechanisms responsible for the regulation of placental blood flow have not, as yet, been clearly delineated.

Three shunts are classically described in the fetal circulation. The ductus venosus normally allows part of umbilical venous return to flow directly into the inferior vena cava. The foramen ovale allows the shunting of blood from the right to the left atrium. Finally, the ductus arteriosus "shunts" blood from the pulmonary artery into the descending aorta. The ductus arteriosus is increasingly sensitive to the vasoconstrictive effects of oxygen as gestation progresses.[18,19] Conversely, prostaglandins (E_1 and E_2) are important determinants in maintaining ductal patency.[20–23]

Although the ductus arteriosus is indeed a vascular shunt after birth, during fetal life, it more accurately channels the major portion of RV output to the descending aorta and the placenta (Fig. 7.2). Because of the parallel arrangement of the ventricles, the only arterial segment that actually corresponds to the definition of a shunt would be the aortic isthmus. Basically, the direction of blood flow in the isthmus is a result of individual ventricular function and relative resistances in the downstream vascular beds.[24] Specifically, as placental resistance increases, forward diastolic flow in the isthmus decreases.

Fetal cardiocirculatory adjustments to stress

Abnormal loading conditions

Abnormal loading conditions in the fetal circulation can be observed in a variety of disorders, such as arteriovenous malformation, anemia, or twin–twin transfusion syndrome (TTTS). The arteriovenous shunts (sacrococcygeal teratomas, placental chorioangiomas, or cerebral vascular malformation, etc.) are characterized by both elevated preload because of increased venous return from the shunts and reduced afterload due to arteriovenous runoff. In fetuses with arteriovenous malformations in the upper part of the body, only overload of right ventricle is observed; retrograde diastolic flow is also recorded in the aortic isthmus. In contrast, when the arteriovenous malformation is in the lower body, both ventricles share the volume load, and antegrade flow through the aortic isthmus is then increased.

In fetal anemia resulting from isoimmunization, a rise in cardiac output is observed, related to both higher preload (decreased blood viscosity leading to increased venous return) and lower afterload (diminished blood viscosity and peripheral vasodilation due to reduced O_2 content). Peak velocities tend to increase in both parallel circulatory systems.

In twin–twin transfusion syndrome, the hemodynamic picture of the donor twin is mainly influenced by the consequences of his/her volume depletion. Reports of elevated blood levels of endothelin[25] and evidence of renin–angiotensin system stimulation[26] suggest chronic hypotension and peripheral hypoperfusion in these fetuses. In the recipient twin, hypertrophic cardiomyopathy is typically described.[27]

Hypoxic stress

Hypoxemia with normal placental vascular resistances

In these cases, which usually result from maternal pulmonary disease or fetal anemia, placental vascular resistance is generally normal. Therefore, despite a low

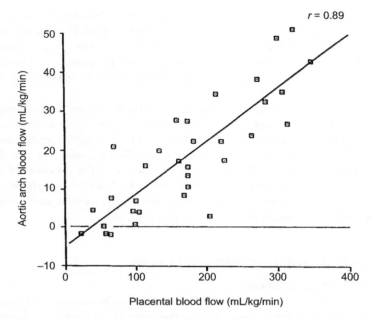

Figure 7.3 Relationship between aortic arch and placental flows in fetal lambs whose resistance to placental perfusion is increased by stepwise compression of the umbilical veins. A strong linear correlation is observed. (In the ovine, the aortic arch is the equivalent of the aortic isthmus in the human.) (Adapted from ref. 45, with permission.)

P_{O_2} in the umbilical vein, buildup of acid metabolites is unlikely. Likewise, fetal P_{CO_2} is unlikely to be elevated if maternal P_{CO_2} is normal.

Acute hypoxic hypoxemia leads to increased blood pressure, decreased heart rate, and redistribution of blood flow to brain, heart, and adrenals.[28,29] These changes are due to adrenal secretion of norepinephrine as well as other neural and humoral mechanisms.[30–32] There is little change in either placental blood flow or combined cardiac output until severe hypoxia leads to acidosis and decreased myocardial contractility.[28,33]

A similar redistribution is seen in the chronic state,[34,35] although long-term hypoxia does not lead to increases in cerebral blood flow.[36] As in the acute state, umbilical blood flow is maintained until severe acidemia leads to a drop in combined cardiac output.

The fetus has the unique ability to selectively adjust arterial O_2 content by the effect of shunts. During hypoxemia, a greater proportion of blood flows directly through the ductus venosus to the inferior vena cava and directly on to the left atrium via the foramen ovale,[37–39] resulting in a higher P_{O_2} in the cerebral blood flow.

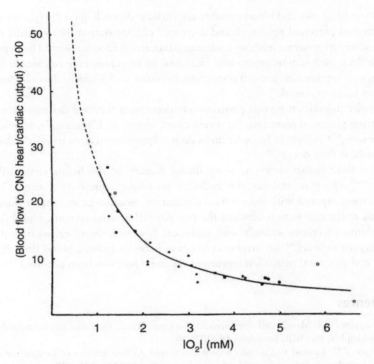

Figure 7.4 Variation in the proportion of the combined ventricular output flowing to the heart and brain of fetal lambs according to arterial O_2 content. This proportion increases by 25% with a reduction from 6 to 1 mM (reprinted with permission from ref. 29).

Doppler studies in the umbilical artery are generally unchanged during periods of hypoxic hypoxemia because of the preservation of low placental resistance.[40–42]

Hypoxemia with elevated placental vascular resistances

In this situation, an increase in placental vascular impedance causes decreased umbilical blood flow, leading to decreased PO_2 in the blood returning to the heart via the IVC. PCO_2 rises and acid metabolites accumulate. Thus, acidemia, with its deleterious effect on O_2 extraction and myocardial contractility, occurs relatively early.

Experimental increases in placental resistance by umbilical venous compression mimics the Doppler velocimetric pattern seen in growth-restricted fetuses (Fig. 7.3).[43–45] This situation is associated with a decrease in combined cardiac output.

Redistribution of blood flow favors the brain, heart, and adrenals (Fig. 7.4).

Effects on heart rate and blood pressure are variable depending on the relative effects of increased placental resistance and decreased cardiac output. Bradycardia occurs when severe hypoxemia leads to acidemia. Myocardial function would be depressed by the decreased venous return and increased by catecholamine release. In fetuses with severe intrauterine growth restriction, hypoxia, and acidosis, diastolic function appears to be impaired.[46]

Doppler insonation reveals progressively decreasing forward diastolic flow with increasing placental resistance. In severe cases, absent and, eventually, reverse flow can be seen.[47] Changes in Doppler flows do not appear until close to a 50% decrease in umbilical flow occurs.[48]

Blood flow redistribution is a significant feature of the hemodynamic disturbance.[49-53] The placental vascular bed may no longer represent the site of lowest resistance compared with the cerebral circulation. Because of the site of the aortic isthmus as the connection between the two parallel arterial systems, blood flow in the isthmus correlates strongly with umbilical flow and, therefore, with fetal cerebral oxygen delivery.[45] An inverse correlation between isthmic blood flow velocity index and postnatal neurodevelopmental outcome has also been reported.[54]

References

1 Anderson PAW. Myocardial development. In: Long W, ed. *Fetal and neonatal cardiology.* Philadelphia, PA: W.B. Saunders; 1990:17–38.
2 Nayler WG, Fassold E. Calcium accumulating and ATPase activity of cardiac sarcoplasmic reticulum before and after birth. *Cardiovasc Res* 1977;11:231–237.
3 Nakanishi T, Jarmakani JM. Developmental changes in myocardial mechanical function and subcellular organelles. *Am J Physiol* 1984;246:H615–625.
4 Lompre AM, Mercadier JJ, Wisnewsky C, et al. Species and age-dependent changes in the relative amounts of cardiac myosin isoenzymes in mammals. *Dev Biol* 1981;84:286–290.
5 Sweeney LJ, Nag AC, Eisenberg B, et al. Developmental aspects of cardiac contractile protein. *Basic Res Cardiol* 1985;80(Suppl. 2):123–127.
6 Friedman WF. The intrinsic physiologic properties of the developing heart. *Prog Cardiovasc Dis* 1972;15:87–111.
7 St John Sutton M, Groves A, MacNeil A, et al. Assessment of changes in blood flow through the lungs and foramen ovale in the normal human fetus with gestational age: a prospective Doppler echocardiographic study. *Br Heart J* 1994;71:232–237.
8 Rasanen J, Wood DC, Weiner S, et al. Role of the pulmonary circulation in the distribution of human fetal cardiac output during the second half of pregnancy. *Circulation* 1996;94:1068–1073.
9 Rudolph AM. Distribution and regulation of blood flow in the fetal and neonatal lamb. *Circ Res* 1985;57:811–20.
10 Kenny JF, Plappert E, Doubilet P, et al. Changes in intracardiac blood flow velocities and right and left ventricular stroke volumes with gestational age in the normal human fetus: a prospective Doppler echocardiographic study. *Circulation* 1986;74:1208–1216.
11 St-John Sutton MG, Gewitz MH, Shah B, et al. Quantitative assessment of growth and function of the cardiac chamber in the normal human fetus: a prospective longitudinal study. *Circulation* 1984;69(4):645–654.
12 Machado MVL, Chita SC, Allan LD. Acceleration time in the aorta and pulmonary artery

measured by Doppler echocardiography in the midtrimester normal human fetus. *Br Heart J* 1987;58:15–18.

13 Hislop A, Reid L. Intrapulmonary arterial development during fetal life – branching pattern and structure. *J Anat* 1972;113:35–48.

14 Hislop A, Reid L. Pulmonary arterial development during childhood: Branching pattern and structure. *Thorax* 1973;28:129–135.

15 Cook CD, Drinker PA, Jacobson HN, et al. Control of pulmonary blood flow in the fetal and newly born lamb. *J Physiol* 1963;169:10–29.

16 Campbell AGM, Cockburn F, Dawes GS, Miligan JE. Pulmonary vasoconstriction in asphyxia during cross-circulation between twin foetal lambs. *J Physiol (Lond)* 1967;192:111–121.

17 Sonesson SE, Fouron JC, Tawile C, et al. Reference values for Doppler velocimetric indices from the fetal and placental ends of the umbilical artery during normal pregnancy. *J Clin Ultrasound* 1993;21:317–324.

18 Kennedy JA, Clark SL. Observations on the physiological reactions of the ductus arteriosus. *Am J Physiol* 1942;136:140–147.

19 McMurphy DM, Heymann MA, Rudolph AM, Melmon KL. Developmental changes in constriction of the ductus arteriosus: Responses to oxygen and vasoactive substances in the isolated ductus arteriosus of the fetal lamb. *Pediatr Res* 1972;6:231–238.

20 Mentzer RM, Ely SW, Lasley RD, et al. Hormonal role of adenosine in maintaining patency of the ductus arteriosus in fetal lambs. *Ann Surg* 1985;202:223–230.

21 Coceani F, Olley PM. The response of the ductus arteriosus to prostaglandins. *Can J Physiol Pharmacol* 1973;51:220–225.

22 Sharpe GL, Thalme B, Larsson KS. Studies on closure of the ductus arteriosus. XI. Ductal closure in utero by a prostaglandin synthetase inhibitor. *Prostaglandins* 1974;8:363–368.

23 Clyman RI, Mauray F, Koerper MA, et al. Formation of prostacyclin (PGI$_2$) by the ductus arteriosus of fetal lambs at different stages of gestation. *Prostaglandins* 1978;16:633–642.

24 Fouron JC. The unrecognized physiological and clinical significance of the fetal aortic isthmus. *Ultrasound Obstet Gynecol* 2003;22:441–447.

25 Bajoria R, Sullivan M, Fisk NM. Endothelin concentrations in monochorionic twins with severe twin-twin transfusion syndrome. *Hum Reprod* 1999;14:1614–1618.

26 Mahieu-Caputo D, Muller F, Joly D, et al. Pathogenesis of twin–twin transfusion syndrome: the renin-angiotensin system hypothesis. *Fetal Diagn Ther* 2001;16:241–244.

27 Fesslova V, Villa L, Nava S, et al. Fetal and neonatal echocardiographic findings in twin–twin transfusion syndrome. *Am J Obstet Gynecol* 1998;179:1056–1062.

28 Cohn HE, Sacks EJ, Heymann MA, Rudolph AM. Cardiovascular responses to hypoxemia and acidemia in fetal lambs. *Am J Obstet Gynecol* 1974;120:817–824.

29 Sheldon RE, Peeters LLH, Jones Jr MD, et al. Redistribution of cardiac output and oxygen delivery in the hypoxemic fetal lamb. *Am J Obstet Gynecol* 1979;135:1071–1078.

30 Paulick RP, Meyers RL, Rudolph CD, Rudolph AM. Hemodynamic responses to alpha-adrenergic blockade during hypoxemia in fetal lamb. *J Dev Physiol* 1991;16:63–69.

31 Comline RS, Silver M. Development of activity in the adrenal medulla of the fetus and newborn animal. *Br Med Bull* 1966;22:16–20.

32 Reuss ML, Parer JT, Harris JL, Krueger TR. Hemodynamic effects of alpha-adrenergic blockade during hypoxia in fetal sheep. *Am J Obstet Gynecol* 1982;142:410–415.

33 Fouron JC, Lafond J, Bard H. Effects of hypoxemia with and without acidemia on the isometric contraction time and the electromechanical delay of the fetal myocardium: an experimental study on the ovine fetus. *Am J Obstet Gynecol* 1990;162:262–266.

34 Rurak DW, Richardson BS, Patrick JE, et al. Blood flow and oxygen delivery to fetal organs and tissues during sustained hypoxemia. *Am J Physiol* 1990;258:R1116–1122.

35 Bocking AD, Gagnon R, White SE, et al. Circulatory responses to prolonged hypoxemia in fetal sheep. *Am J Obstet Gynecol* 1988;159:1418–1424.

36 Kitanaka T, Alonso JG, Gilbert RD, et al. Fetal responses to long-term hypoxemia in sheep. *Am J Physiol* 1989;256:R1348–1354.

37 Behrman RE, Lees MH, Peterson EN, et al. Distribution of the circulation in the normal and asphyxiated fetal primate. *Am J Obstet Gynecol* 1970;108:956–969.

38 Reuss ML, Rudolph AM. Distribution and recirculation of umbilical and systemic venous blood flow in fetal lambs during hypoxia. *J Dev Physiol* 1980;2:71.

39 Edelstone DI. Regulation of blood flow through the ductus venosus. *J Dev Physiol* 1980;2:219–238.

40 Morrow RJ, Adamson SL, Bull SB, Knox Ritchie JW. Acute hypoxemia does not affect the umbilical artery flow velocity waveform in fetal sheep. *Obstet Gynecol* 1990;75:590–593.

41 Muijsers GJJM, Hasaart THM, van Huisseling H, de Haan J. The response of the umbilical artery pulsatility index in fetal sheep to acute and prolonged hypoxaemia and acidaemia induced by embolization of the uterine microcirculation. *J Dev Physiol* 1990;13:231–236.

42 Downing GJ, Yarlagadda P, Maulik D. Effects of acute hypoxemia on umbilical arterial Doppler indices in a fetal ovine model. *Early Human Dev* 1991;25:1–10.

43 Fouron JC, Teyssier G, Maroto E, et al. Diastolic circulatory dynamics in the presence of elevated retrograde diastolic flow in the umbilical artery: A Doppler echocardiographic study in lambs. *Am J Obstet Gynecol* 1991;164:195–203.

44 Sonesson SE, Fouron JC, Teyssier G, Bonnin P. Effects of increased resistance to umbilical blood flow on fetal hemodynamic changes induced by maternal oxygen administration: a Doppler velocimetric study on the sheep. *Pediatr Res* 1993;34:796–800.

45 Bonnin P, Fouron JC, Teyssier G, et al. Quantitative assessment of circulatory changes in the fetal aortic isthmus during progressive increase of resistance to umbilical blood flow. *Circulation* 1993;88:216–222.

46 Kiserud T, Eik-Nes SH, Blaas HG, et al. Ductus venosus blood velocity and the umbilical circulation in the seriously growth-retarded fetus. *Ultrasound Obstet Gynecol* 1994;4:109.

47 Farine D, Kelly EN, Ryan G, et al. Absent and reversed umbilical artery end-diastolic velocity. In: Copel JA, Reed KL, eds. *Doppler ultrasound in obstetrics and gynecology.* New York: Raven Press; 1995:187–197.

48 Schmidt KG, Di Tommaso M, Silverman NH, Rudolph AM. Evaluation of changes in umbilical blood flow in the fetal lamb by Doppler waveform analysis. *Am J Obstet Gynecol* 1991;164:1118–1126.

49 Vyas S, Nicolaides KH, Campbell S. Renal flow-velocity waveforms in normal and hypoxemic fetuses. *Am J Obstet Gynecol* 1989;16:1168–1172.

50 Mari G, Abuhamad AZ, Verpairojkit B, et al. Blood flow velocity waveforms of the abdominal arteries in appropriate and small for gestational age fetuses. *Ultrasound Obstet Gynecol* 1995;6:15–18.

51 Sepulveda W, Bower S, Nicolaides P, et al. Discordant blood flow velocity waveforms in left and right brachial arteries in growth-retarded fetuses. *Obstet Gynecol* 1995;86:734–738.

52 Gembruck U, Baschat AA. Demonstration of fetal coronary blood flow by color-coded and pulsed wave Doppler sonography: a possible indicator of severe compromise and impending demise in intrauterine growth retardation. *Ultrasound Obstet Gynecol* 1996;7:10–16.

53 Mari G, Verpairojkit B, Abuhamad AZ, Copel JA. Adrenal artery velocity waveforms in the appropriate and small for gestational age fetus. *Ultrasound Obstet Gynecol* 1996;8:82–86.

54 Fouron JC, Gosselin J, Raboisson MJ, et al. The relationship between an aortic isthmus blood flow velocity index and the postnatal neurodevelopment status of fetuses with placental circulatory insufficiency. *Am J Obstet Gynecol* 2005;192:497–503.

Further reading

Dawes GS. The fetal circulation. In: Dawes GS, ed. *Fetal and neonatal physiology*. Chicago, IL: Year Book Medical Publishers; 1968:91–105.

Fouron JC. The unrecognized physiological and clinical significance of the fetal aortic isthmus. *Ultrasound Obstet Gynecol* 2003;22:441–447.

Fouron JC, Drblik SP. Fetal cardiovascular dynamics in intrauterine growth retardation. In: Copel JA, Reed KL, eds. *Doppler ultrasound in obstetrics and gynecology*. New York: Raven Press; 1995:281–290.

Long WA. Developmental pulmonary circulatory physiology. In: Long WA, ed. *Fetal and neonatal cardiology*. Philadelphia, PA: W.B. Saunders; 1990:76–96.

Rychik J. Fetal cardiovascular physiology. *Pediatr Cardiol* 2004;25:201–209.

Trudinger BJ, Stevens D, Connely A. Umbilical artery flow velocity waveforms and placental resistance: the effects of embolization of the umbilical circulation. *Am J Obstet Gynecol* 1987;157:1443–1448.

8 Fetal endocrinology

Charles E. Wood and Maureen Keller-Wood

The endocrine systems of the fetus are modulators of the classical physiological organ systems. For example, the basic components of the cardiovascular system work together to transport nutrients and waste products, and to perfuse the tissues with blood. However, the blood volume and osmolality are controlled via the actions of endocrine feedback mechanisms, and the distribution of combined ventricular output is affected by several hormones that are released after fetal stress. The fetal lung makes lung liquid prior to birth and serves as an organ of gas exchange after birth. However, the reabsorption of lung liquid is likely to be coordinated by several hormones that are secreted at the time of birth. This chapter will focus on the endocrinology of the developing fetus. Because of the inherent difficulty in studying developing human fetuses, much of what we know about the developing human has its origins in the study of animal models, mostly fetal sheep. Although more pertinent to the human being, less information has been obtained from primate models of fetal development. Rodents are altricial species (relatively immature at birth); however, useful information about endocrine development (especially relating to first- and second-trimester fetuses) has been obtained from developing rats and mice. However, there are notable exceptions: for example the biosynthesis of estrogen in humans and primates involves a "fetoplacental unit," whereas the biosynthesis of estrogen in sheep is more straightforward. It is, perhaps, the differences among the species that allow us to identify the truly basic principles of endocrine control in fetuses.

Hypothalamus–pituitary–gonadal axis

Gonadotropin-releasing hormone (GnRH) is released into the hypophyseal–portal blood at the median eminence and stimulates the release of both luteinizing hormone (LH) and follicle-stimulating hormone (FSH) from gonadotropes in the anterior pituitary. In the sheep fetus at mid-gestation or before, LH and FSH are present in gonadotropes and GnRH is present in the hypothalamus at both the mRNA and the protein level. Before the maturation of the fetal pituitary, chorionic gonadotropin (CG) from the placenta stimulates fetal gonadal growth, differentiation, and secretory activity. The overall activity of the hypothalamus–pituitary–gonadal (HPG) axis reaches a peak at approximately 30–40% gestation in the sheep fetus, decreasing until birth. The major source of androgens and estrogens in the late-gestation fetus is the placenta. In primate species, including humans, the biosynthesis of androgens and estrogens depends upon an intact fetoplacental unit. The placenta lacks cytochrome $P450_{c17\alpha}$ (CYP17) and therefore 17α-hydroxylase and 17,20-lyase activities. Nevertheless, the placenta synthesizes large amounts of estrogens because it receives a supply of estrogen biosynthetic precursors from the fetal adrenal cortex.

Hypothalamus–pituitary–adrenal axis

The endocrine hierarchy within the fetal hypothalamus–pituitary–adrenal (HPA) axis is similar to that of the adult. Adrenocorticotropic hormone (ACTH) is synthesized and secreted by the corticotropes of the anterior pituitary in response to two hypothalamic-releasing factors: arginine vasopressin (AVP) and corticotropin-releasing hormone (CRH). The two releasing hormones work in concert: each increases the sensitivity of the corticotrope to the other. ACTH stimulates the release of glucocorticoid hormones (i.e., cortisol in the human, primate, and sheep, and corticosterone in rodents) from the *definitive zone* and the estrogen precursors, dehydroepiandrosterone (DHEA) and dehydroepiandrosterone sulfate (DHAS) from the *fetal zone*. The fetal HPA axis is activated progressively throughout the later part of gestation as a normal consequence of ontogenetic development. This has been well documented in fetal sheep and there is good evidence that this is also true in primate fetuses. The activation of the fetal HPA axis can seen as a semilogarithmic increase in circulating concentrations of ACTH and cortisol in nonhuman fetal blood, and DHEA, DHAS, and estrogens in human fetal blood. The cells of the neurointermediate lobe of the pituitary synthesize and contain proopiomelanocortin

(POMC). The major processing products of the POMC-synthesizing cells are α-melanocyte-stimulating hormone (α-MSH) and γ-MSH.

Adrenal medulla

The adrenal medulla becomes innervated by sympathetic preganglionic nerves at approximately 80% gestation (in sheep), and secretes the catecholamines epinephrine and norepinephrine, whereas prior to innervation, the fetal adrenal is directly responsive to hypoxia. The adrenal medullary biosynthesis of epinephrine is dependent upon the expression of phenylethanolamine-N-methyltransferase (PNMT) which is induced, in turn, by cortisol. For this reason, the secretory capacity of the adrenal medulla for epinephrine increases late in gestation.

The adrenal medulla responds to various stresses, such as hypoxia and hypotension, with increased secretion of catecholamines. The increase in response to hypoxia is important for redistributing fetal combined ventricular output away from somatic tissues and towards the umbilical–placental circulation. The adrenal medulla also plays an important role in fetal glucose homeostasis; an increase in fetal epinephrine secretion elevates the fetal plasma glucose level, which is seen, for example, following periods of fetal distress.

Hypothalamus–pituitary–thyroid axis

In the human, the fetal thyroid develops sufficiently to support thyroglobulin biosynthesis by approximately 25% gestation. Thyrotropin (TSH) is present in the fetal pituitary and in fetal plasma at the beginning of the second trimester, at approximately the time of hypothalamo–hypophyseal portal system development. Thyrotropin and thyroxine (T_4) circulate in fetal plasma in increasing concentrations, starting early in the second trimester. Type 3 monodeiodinase, which converts T_4 to reverse triiodothyronine (rT_3), is expressed, leading to an abundance of rT_3 circulating in fetal plasma throughout the second and third trimesters. Circulating concentrations of T_3, however, increase only in the final stages of fetal development, suggesting late development of types 1 and 2 deiodinases (D1 and D2 respectively) in liver and other tissues. Development of the hypothalamus–pituitary–thyroid (HPT) axis of the fetus is critically important for differentiation of the nervous system, but also plays a role in the adaptation to extrauterine life. Congenital hypothyroidism causes mental retardation in human infants. Although the infant can be treated with some success after birth, the infant will tend to be less responsive if the mother also suffered from hypothyroidism during the pregnancy.

Posterior pituitary

Both AVP and oxytocin are synthesized by magnocellular neurons in the supraoptic and paraventricular nuclei. Axons from these neurons terminate in the posterior pituitary. AVP is a hormone with at least three biological activities.

The vasopressor action of this hormone is mediated by V_{1a} vasopressin receptors on vascular smooth muscle cells in the peripheral vasculature. Corticotropin-releasing activity is mediated by the V_{1b} vasopressin receptor (AVP acting as a corticotropin-releasing factor is derived from parvocellular neurons and released into the hypothalamo–hypophyseal portal blood at the median eminence). The antidiuretic activity is mediated by the V_2 vasopressin receptor.

Further reading

Albrecht ED, Pepe GJ. Placental steroid hormone biosynthesis in primate pregnancy. *Endocr Rev* 1990;11:124–150.

Challis JR, Lye SJ, Gibb W. Prostaglandins and parturition. *Ann NY Acad Sci* 1997;828:254–267.

Gunn TR, Gluckman PD. Perinatal thermogenesis. *Early Hum Dev* 1995;42:169–183.

Jenkin G, Young IR. Mechanisms responsible for parturition; the use of experimental models. *Anim Reprod Sci* 2004;82–83:567–581.

McGrath W, Smith R. Corticotrophin-releasing hormone and parturition. *Clin Endocrinol* 2002;55:593–595.

McMillen IC, Phillips ID, Ross JT, et al. Chronic stress: the key to parturition? *Reprod Fertil Dev* 1995;7:499–507.

Pepe GJ, Albrecht ED. Regulation of the primate fetal adrenal cortex. *Endocr Rev* 1990;11:151–176.

Pepe GJ, Albrecht ED. Actions of placental and fetal adrenal steroid hormones in primate pregnancy. *Endocr Rev* 1995;16:608–648.

Polk DH. Thyroid hormone metabolism during development. *Reprod Fertil Dev* 1995;7:469–477.

Thorburn GD, Hollingworth SA, Hooper SB. The trigger for parturition in sheep: fetal hypothalamus or placenta? *J Dev Physiol* 1991;2:71–79.

Wood CE. Baroreflex and chemoreflex control of fetal hormone secretion. *Reprod Fertil Dev* 1995;7:479–489.

Wood CE, Cudd TA. Development of the hypothalamus-pituitary-adrenal axis of the equine fetus: a comparative review. *Equine Vet J* 1997;24(Suppl.):74–82.

9 Sporadic and recurrent pregnancy loss

Robert M. Silver and D. Ware Branch

Pregnancy loss is one of the most common medical problems in reproductive-aged couples, with as many as 25% of all women attempting pregnancy experiencing at least one spontaneous abortion. An estimated 0.5–1.0% of couples attempting pregnancy suffer three or more consecutive losses (recurrent pregnancy loss, RPL), and an even higher proportion have two or more consecutive losses.

In total, 50% or more of human pregnancies are lost before term.[1] The majority are unrecognized pregnancy losses occurring before or with the expected next menses.[2] Approximately 10–12% of all clinically recognized pregnancies are lost as first-trimester or early second-trimester spontaneous abortions. Both spontaneous abortion and fetal death are more likely to occur in older women and those with prior pregnancy losses.

The vast majority of pregnancy losses are *sporadic* in nature (i.e., they occur as an isolated event in a woman whose other pregnancies are successful). The most common apparent cause of spontaneous abortions is genetic abnormalities (Table 9.1). Overall, approximately 50% of sporadic spontaneous abortions are cytogenetically abnormal.[4] Chromosome abnormalities are present in more than 90% of anembryonic abortus tissues, two-thirds of malformed or growth-disorganized embryos, and one-third of malformed fetuses. Approximately 60% of karyotypic abnormalities in early pregnancy losses are autosomal trisomies, 20% are polyploid, and 20% are monosomy X.

Other causes of sporadic pregnancy loss are less certain. Diabetes and thyroid abnormalities have been associated with sporadic miscarriage. However, only poorly controlled disease that is usually clinically apparent is associated with first-trimester or early second-trimester pregnancy loss. A variety of infectious organisms including bacteria, viruses, and spirochetes have been linked to sporadic pregnancy loss, especially after 20 weeks' gestation. Nonetheless, they are rarely associated with early spontaneous abortion and routine assessment is not recommended. Certain drugs and chemical agents, ethanol, coffee, and cigarette smoking have been associated with an increased risk for early pregnancy loss but their contribution to individual losses is unclear.

Symptoms of miscarriage are nonspecific and a definitive diagnosis of pregnancy loss is usually made by ultrasound. Sonographic criteria for the definitive diagnosis

Table 9.1 Potential causes of sporadic pregnancy loss.

Morphologic abnormalities/birth defects

Genetic abnormalities

Medical and hormonal disorders
Diabetes mellitus
Thyroid disease
Luteal phase defect

Infections
Treponema pallidum
Borrelia burgdorferi
Listeria monocytogenes
Ureaplasma urealyticum
Viral infections (e.g., parvovirus; herpes simplex)
Bacterial infections (e.g., group B streptococcus)

Other causes
Tobacco
Drugs and chemicals
Ethanol

Table 9.2 Sonographic criteria for pregnancy loss.

Criteria diagnostic of pregnancy loss
MSD ≥8 mm without yolk sac*
MSD ≥16 mm without an embryo*
Embryo without cardiac activity

Findings associated with poor prognosis
MSD minus CRL ≤5 mm before 9 weeks' gestation
Yolk sac diameter ≥6 mm
Embryonic heart rate ≤80 b.p.m.
Subchorionic hemorrhage ≥40% sac volume

B.p.m., beats per min; CRL, crown–rump length; MSD, mean gestational sac diameter.
*High-resolution endovaginal ultrasound (6.25 MHz or greater probe).

of pregnancy loss are shown in Table 9.2. No specific evaluation of the mother or abortus tissue is indicated in the case of a single pre-embryonic or embryonic loss occurring in an otherwise healthy woman. The clinician should also apprise the patient of the high pregnancy success rate (80–90%) after a single spontaneous abortion, taking the maternal age and past obstetric history into account.

Up to 1% of couples experience three consecutive pregnancy losses. Among the

Table 9.3 Proposed causes of recurrent pregnancy loss.

Genetic abnormalities
Parental structural chromosome abnormalities
Numerical chromosome abnormalities of the conceptus
Molecular genetic abnormalities of the conceptus or placenta

Hormonal and metabolic disorders
Luteal phase defects
Diabetes
Thyroid disease

Uterine anatomical abnormalities
Congenital uterine malformations
Uterine synechiae
Uterine fibroids

Autoimmune causes
Antiphospholipid syndrome

Infections

Thrombophilia
Factor V resistance to activated protein C (factor V Leiden)
Prothrombin gene G20210A mutation
Deficiencies of antithrombin III, protein C, or protein S

numerous proposed causes of RPL, only parental karyotype abnormalities, antiphospholipid syndrome, and uterine malformations are universally accepted. Table 9.3 presents causes of RPL.

In approximately 3–5% of couples with two or more spontaneous losses, one of the partners has a genetically balanced structural chromosome rearrangement.[4] The recurrence risk for spontaneous abortion in cases of parental structural chromosome abnormality is related to many variables, the most important of which is the specific type of abnormality.

Luteal phase defect (LPD) is reported in 25–40% of cases of RPL. However, properly controlled trials proving that LPD is a cause of RPL are lacking and LPD is common in healthy women with normal pregnancies. Diagnosis is made by late-luteal phase endometrial biopsy or serum progesterone determination. There are no convincing studies to show that treatment of LPD improves pregnancy outcome in women with RPL.[5] Nonetheless, treatment is common and usually consists of 25 mg of progesterone twice per day, administered by vaginal suppository, beginning on the third day after ovulation. A reasonable alternative is 200–400 mg per day of oral micronized progesterone, in divided doses.

A total of 10–15% of women with recurrent first-trimester abortions have congenital uterine abnormalities, most commonly uterine septa. Importantly, however,

Table 9.4 International consensus statement on preliminary criteria for the classification of antiphospholipid syndrome.*

Clinical criteria
  Pregnancy complications
    Three or more unexplained early spontaneous abortions
    Premature birth before 34 weeks' gestation (placental insufficiency)
    Unexplained fetal death
  Vascular thrombosis
    Venous thrombosis
    Arterial thrombosis
    Small vessel thrombosis

Laboratory criteria
  Lupus anticoagulant
  Anticardiolipin antibodies (IgG or IgM)
  Medium–high levels (antibodies must be present on two or more occasions at least 6
    weeks apart)

From Wilson WA, Gharavi AE, Koike T, et al. International consensus statement on preliminary classification criteria for definite antiphospholipid syndrome: report of an international workshop. *Arthritis Rheum* 1999;42:1309.
*A diagnosis of definite antiphospholipid syndrome requires the presence of at least one of the clinical criteria and one of the laboratory criteria. No limits are placed on the interval between the clinical event and the positive laboratory findings.

most individuals with uterine abnormalities have normal obstetric outcomes. Although of unproven efficacy, good results have been reported after hysteroscopic resection of uterine septa. Metroplasty is rarely performed to treat RPL.

Antiphospholipid syndrome (APS) is an autoimmune disorder characterized by the presence of specified levels of antiphospholipid antibodies and one or more clinical features including pregnancy loss, thrombosis, or autoimmune thrombocytopenia (Table 9.4). The two most well-characterized antiphospholipid antibodies are lupus anticoagulant and anticardiolipin antibodies. Antiphospholipid syndrome is identified as the cause of pregnancy loss in 5–10% of women with recurrent miscarriage. Treatment with thromboprophylactic doses of heparin (7500 units twice daily) and low-dose aspirin improves obstetric outcome in women with APS.[6] Even treated pregnancies, however, require close surveillance for the development of placental insufficiency.

Heritable thrombophilias (Table 9.5) have also been associated with RPL. The association is stronger for fetal death as opposed to early miscarriage. It is noteworthy that many heritable thrombophilias are common in normal individuals without a history of thrombosis or pregnancy loss[7] and most women with thrombophilias have normal obstetric outcomes. Although of unproven efficacy, taking thromboprophylactic doses of low-molecular-weight heparin has

Table 9.5 Thrombophilic disorders and risk of pregnancy loss.

Thrombophilic disorder	Prevalence in women with pregnancy loss (%)*	Prevalence in control subjects (%)	Risk of pregnancy loss (OR)
Factor V Leiden	8–32	1–10	2–5
Acquired APC resistance (without factor V Leiden)	9–38	0–3	3–4
Prothrombin gene mutation	4–13	1–3	2–9
Antithrombin deficiency	0–2	0–1.4	2–5
Protein C deficiency	6	0–2.5	2–3
Protein S deficiency	5–8	0–0.2	3–40
Hyperhomocysteinemia	17–27	5–16	3–7
Homozygous MTHFR C677T†	5–21	4–20	0.4–3‡
Combined thrombophilia	8–25	1–5	5–14

From Kujovich JL. Thrombophilia and pregnancy complications. *Am J Obstet Gynecol* 2004;191:412–424, with permission.
*Variably defined as first or recurrent early and/or late pregnancy loss.
†5,10-methylenetetrahydrofolate reductase (MTHFR).
‡No significant difference in prevalence or risk in the majority of studies.

Table 9.6 Suggested routine evaluation for recurrent early pregnancy loss.

History
Pattern and trimester of pregnancy losses and whether a live embryo or fetus was present
Exposure to environmental toxins or drugs
Known gynecologic or obstetric infections
Clinical features associated with antiphospholipid syndrome
Genetic relationship between reproductive partners (consanguinity)
Family history of recurrent miscarriage or syndrome associated with embryonic or fetal loss
Previous diagnostic tests and treatments

Physical
General physical examination
Examination of vagina, cervix, and uterus

Tests
Hysterosalpingogram or sonohysterogram
Luteal phase endometrial biopsy; repeat in the next cycle if abnormal
Parental karyotypes
Lupus anticoagulant and anticardiolipin antibodies
Factor V Leiden mutation
Prothrombin G20210A mutation
Other laboratory tests suggested by history and physical examination

resulted in improved outcome in subsequent pregnancies in women with thrombophilias.[7,8]

Other proposed causes of RPL include infection and alloimmune factors. Although microorganisms may cause sporadic pregnancy loss, no infectious agent has been clearly proven to be a cause of RPL. Treatment for allogeneic pregnancy loss includes leukocyte immunization and intravenous immunoglobulin (IVIG). However, these treatments are expensive, are of unproven efficacy, and are not recommended.[9,10]

In as many as 55% of couples with RPL, a complete evaluation is negative. Informative and sympathetic counseling appears to serve an important role in this frustrating situation. Livebirth rates ranging from 35% to 85% are commonly reported in couples with unexplained RPL who undertake an untreated subsequent pregnancy, figures that many couples view as optimistic. A suggested routine for the evaluation of recurrent early pregnancy loss is shown in Table 9.6.

References

1 Boklage CE. Survival probability of human conceptions from fertilization to term. *Int J Fertil* 1990;35:75–93.
2 Wilcox AI, Weinberg CR, O'Connor JF, et al. Incidence of early loss of pregnancy. *N Engl J Med* 1988;319:189–194.
3 Kline J, Stein Z. Epidemiology of chromosomal anomalies in spontaneous abortion: prevalence, manifestation and determinants. In: Bennett MI, Edmonds DK, eds. *Spontaneous and recurrent abortion.* Oxford, UK: Blackwell Scientific Publications; 1987:29–50.
4 DeBrackeller M, Dao TN. Cytogenetic studies in couples experiencing repeated pregnancy losses. *Hum Reprod* 1990;5:519–528.
5 Goldstein P, Berrier J, Rosen S, et al. A meta-analysis of randomized control trials of progestational agents in pregnancy. *Br J Obstet Gynaecol* 1989;96:265–274.
6 Branch DW, Silver RM, Blackwell JL, et al. Outcome of treated pregnancies in women with antiphospholipid syndrome: an update of the Utah experience. *Obstet Gynecol* 1992;80:614–620.
7 Kujovich JL. Thrombophilia and pregnancy complications. *Am J Obstet Gynecol* 2004;191:412–424.
8 Gris JC, Mercier E, Quere I, et al. Low-molecular-weight heparin versus low-dose aspirin in women with one fetal loss and a constitutional thrombophilic disorder. *Blood* 2004;103:3695–3699.
9 Ober C, Karrison T, Odem RR, et al. Mononuclear-cell immunization in prevention of recurrent miscarriages: a randomized trial. *Lancet* 1999;354:365–369.
10 Scott JR. Immunotherapy for recurrent miscarriage. *Cochrane Database Syst Rev* 2003;1: CD000112. DOI: 10.1002/14651858.

10 Ectopic and heterotopic pregnancies

Arnon Wiznitzer and Eyal Sheiner

Incidence

Ectopic pregnancy, i.e., implantation of a fertilized ovum outside the uterus, is a major health problem for women of reproductive age and is the leading cause of pregnancy-related death during the first 20 weeks of pregnancy. Accurate diagnosis and treatment of ectopic pregnancy decreases the risk of death and optimizes subsequent fertility. A significant increase in the number of ectopic pregnancies has occurred in the USA during the past two decades. Importantly, ectopic pregnancy accounted for approximately 9% of all pregnancy-related deaths. The incidence of ectopic pregnancy is higher for nonwhite women, and this discrepancy increases with age. The most common site of ectopic pregnancy implantation is the fallopian tubes, accounting for around 98% of all ectopic pregnancies. The majority of ectopic pregnancies are in the ampullary part of the fallopian tube (79.6%), 12.3% in the isthmus, 6.2% in the fimbria, and 1.9% in the interstitial part. However, in rare cases, implantation can occur in other ectopic sites including the ovary, uterine cervix, and abdomen.

Etiology

The most common denominator is tubal obstruction and injury. Previous pelvic inflammatory disease, especially when caused by *Chlamydia trachomatis*, is a major risk factor for ectopic pregnancy. Other factors associated with an increased risk of ectopic pregnancy include prior ectopic pregnancy, a history of infertility (and specifically *in vitro* fertilization), cigarette smoking (causing alterations in tubal motility and ciliary activity), prior tubal surgery, diethylstilbestrol exposure (which alters fallopian tube morphology), and advanced maternal age. Intrauterine contraceptive devices (IUDs), progesterone-only contraceptives, and sterilization protect women against developing an ectopic pregnancy. Nevertheless, if a woman who has been sterilized or is a current user of an IUD or progesterone-only contraceptives becomes pregnant, her risk for an ectopic pregnancy is increased six- to 10-fold as these methods of contraception provide greater protection against intrauterine pregnancies than for ectopic pregnancy.

Signs and symptoms

Clinical manifestations of ectopic pregnancy are varied and depend on whether rupture has occurred. The classic symptom triad of ectopic pregnancy includes amenorrhea, irregular bleeding, and lower abdominal pain. However, it is present in only one-half of patients and most commonly when rupture has occurred. The most common complaint is sudden severe abdominal pain which is present in over 90% of patients.

Any physical examination should include measurements of vital signs. Abdominal and pelvic tenderness, especially cervical motion tenderness, is common when rupture has occurred (and present in around 75% of patients). However, pelvic examination before rupture is usually nonspecific and a palpable pelvic mass on bimanual examination is established in less than one-half of cases. The accuracy of the initial clinical evaluation before rupture is less than 50% and additional tests are required in order to differentiate ectopic pregnancy from early intrauterine pregnancy.

Laboratory assessment

β-Human chorionic gonadotropin measurements

The first stage in the evaluation of women with suspected ectopic pregnancy is to determine if the patient is pregnant. The β-human chorionic gonadotropin (β-hCG) enzyme immunoassay is positive in virtually all cases of ectopic pregnancy. The levels of β-hCG increase during gestation and reach a peak of approximately 100 000 mIU/mL at 6–10 weeks; they then decrease and remain stable at approximately 20 000 mIU/mL. A 66% rise in the β-hCG level over 48 h represents the lower normal limit for a viable intrauterine pregnancy. Indeed, there is a consensus that the predictable rise in serial β-hCG values is different from the slow rise or plateau of an ectopic pregnancy. Limitations of serial β-hCG testing include its inability to distinguish a failing intrauterine pregnancy from an ectopic pregnancy and the inherent 48-h delay. Serial β-hCG levels are usually required when the initial ultrasound performed fails to demonstrate either intra- or extrauterine pregnancy. At β-hCG levels of approximately 2000 mIU/mL, a viable intrauterine pregnancy should be seen by vaginal ultrasound.

Serum progesterone

A baseline serum progesterone level of <20 nmol/L can be used to identify abnormal pregnancy (either intra- or extrauterine) with a positive predictive value (PPV) of ≥95%. Of pregnant patients with serum progesterone values of less than 5 nmol/L, 85% have spontaneous abortions, 0.16% have viable intrauterine pregnancies, and 14% have ectopic pregnancies. However, serum progesterone levels cannot distinguish ectopic pregnancy from spontaneous abortion. Thus, progesterone levels at defined times can be used to predict the immediate viability of a pregnancy, but cannot be used reliably to predict its location.

Ultrasonography

The best diagnosis of ectopic pregnancy is based on the positive visualization of an extrauterine pregnancy, but it is not seen in all cases. Approximately 90% of ectopic pregnancies may be visualized using transvaginal sonography within 5 weeks of the last menstrual period. When the β-hCG level exceeds the transvaginal discriminatory zone (1000–2000 mIU/mL of β-hCG), the absence of an intrauterine gestational sac is suggestive of ectopic pregnancy, but the differential diagnosis includes failed intrauterine pregnancy. The combination of positive β-hCG and transvaginal ultrasound has a PPV of 95% for an ectopic pregnancy. If an intrauterine pregnancy is detected, this is taken to exclude a diagnosis of ectopic pregnancy because coexistent intra- and extrauterine pregnancies (heterotopic) following spontaneous cycles are rare, with an estimated incidence of 1 in 30 000 normal pregnancies.

The early sonographic appearance of a normal gestational sac is characterized by the double decidual sac sign, i.e., two concentric echogenic rings separated by a hypoechogenic space. The double decidual sign may help guide the physician for early diagnosis of intrauterine pregnancy and for the exclusion of ectopic pregnancy. However, the appearance of an intrauterine sac can be seen in some cases of ectopic pregnancy owing to intrauterine fluid or blood collection, i.e., pseudosac. A pseudosac is a uterine sac without a double decidual ring or a yolk sac.

Dilation and curettage

When serial β-hCG values do not rise or fall appropriately, an abnormal gestation exists. When the pregnancy has been confirmed to be nonviable and when ultrasound is not sufficient, a uterine dilation and curettage can be performed to distinguish an ectopic pregnancy from a miscarriage. Once tissue is obtained by curettage it can be added to saline in order to determine if it floats. Because floating of the material is not 100% accurate, histological verification or serial β-hCG measurements are needed. Visualization of villi in the tissue obtained indicates the occurrence of a spontaneous intrauterine abortion. The absence of chorionic villi in the curettage specimen indicates the possibility of an ectopic pregnancy.

Treatment of ectopic pregnancy

The minority of patients with ectopic pregnancy (less than 10%) present with a surgical abdomen and signs of hypovolemia and shock. They present no diagnostic problem and require no specific intervention besides fluid and blood resuscitation, and immediate operation. Delayed hospital admission and treatment leads to maternal mortality. Cases of ectopic pregnancy can be treated by medical (methotrexate), surgical (laparoscopy or laparotomy), or even expectant management alone. The choice depends on the medical presentation, available resources, and the site of ectopic pregnancy.

Surgical treatment
Laparoscopy versus laparotomy
The standard operative procedure for the treatment of ectopic pregnancy in the developed world is laparoscopy. Almost all tubal pregnancies in hemodynamically

stable women can be removed laparoscopically without the need for laparotomy. The excellent benefits of laparoscopic treatment include less blood loss, less analgesia, less postoperative pain, shorter recovery period, and decreased hospital costs. Because of lower peri- and postoperative morbidity, lower cost, and equivalent efficacy, laparoscopy is preferred to laparotomy for the treatment of ectopic pregnancy. The only absolute contraindication for laparoscopy is shock or hemodynamic instability.

Salpingectomy, salpingotomy, salpingostomy, and milking

The most commonly performed procedures are radical salpingectomy (removal of the affected tube), or salpingotomy (tubotomy that is closed) and salpingostomy (tubotomy that is left open) that preserve the tube. Salpingectomy is preferred in cases of ruptured ectopic pregnancy with uncontrolled bleeding, extensive tubal damage, recurrent ectopic pregnancy in the same tube, and sterilization. Salpingectomy is rarely performed for an unruptured ectopic pregnancy and linear salpingostomy is the procedure of choice. The ectopic pregnancy is removed through a linear incision of 10–15 mm, which is made into the tube on its antimesenteric border. The products will extrude from the incision and can be flushed out and evacuated. Both livebirth rates and recurrent ectopic pregnancy rates after a tubotomy were similar regardless of whether the incision was closed (salpingotomy) or left open to heal by secondary intension (salpingostomy) and, therefore, laparoscopic salpingostomy is the preferred surgical procedure for an unruptured ectopic pregnancy.

Manual expression or milking of the tube in order to effect a tubal abortion is possible only in cases of fimbrial pregnancy. The present consensus among tubal surgeons is that milking should be abandoned as it is associated with an inordinately high rate of recurrent ectopic pregnancies regardless of whether the procedure is performed by laparoscopy or laparotomy.

Medical treatment with methotrexate

Methotrexate is a folinic acid antagonist that inactivates dihydrofolate reductase resulting in the depletion of tetrahydrofolate, a cofactor essential for deoxyribonucleic acid and ribonucleic acid synthesis. It thus interferes with DNA synthesis, repair, and cellular replication. Actively proliferating tissue such as trophoblast cells of an ectopic pregnancy are generally more sensitive to these effects of methotrexate. Methotrexate treatment does not subject patients to surgical intervention and the possible associated complications. Thus, at present, methotrexate is considered to be the treatment of choice for ectopic pregnancy.

Candidates for medical therapy

Hemodynamically stable patients without active bleeding or signs of hemoperitoneum are candidates for medical therapy and these patients should comply with follow-up care. Absolute contraindications to medical therapy include breastfeeding, immunodeficiency, alcoholism, hepatic, pulmonary, renal, or hematological dysfunction, known sensitivity to methotrexate, blood dyscrasias, or peptic ulcer disease. Relative contraindications for methotrexate treatments include embryonic cardiac activity and a gestational sac of 3.5 cm or more.

Because of its potential toxicity, patients receiving methotrexate should be followed up carefully. Patients using this drug should be aware of the potential side-effects and signs of toxicity. During treatment, patients should be counseled to promptly report signs and symptoms associated with tubal rupture such as abdominal pain, dizziness, weakness, and syncope. Sexual intercourse, alcohol use, and nonsteroidal anti-inflammatory drugs, as well as folic acid supplements and prenatal vitamins, are prohibited until serum β-hCG is undetectable. It is clear that the main criteria for successful medical treatment is rigorous patient selection. Several parameters aimed at the suitable choice of patients have already been assessed, such as the presence of fetal cardiac activity, size of the ectopic pregnancy, initial levels of β-hCG, and endometrial thickness.

Treatment protocols

Most commonly, methotrexate is administered using a single-dose method based on 50 mg/m^2 of body surface area, without the need for leucovorin rescue. Otherwise, methotrexate can be given using a multidose regimen of 1 mg/kg intramuscularly, alternating with 0.1 mg/kg of leucovorin intramuscularly, for up to four daily doses of each drug. Both protocols have been demonstrated to have good success rates in the treatment of ectopic pregnancy. The single-dose protocol is easier to administer and monitor, and results in fewer side-effects. However, the single protocol is associated with a higher failure rate. Direct injection of methotrexate has lower efficacy than systemic administration and is not considered as a therapeutic alternative for ectopic pregnancy.

Monitoring efficacy of therapy

The overall success rate of methotrexate treatments is almost 90%. Before treatment with methotrexate, blood analysis is required to establish baseline laboratory values for β-hCG levels and for renal, liver, and bone marrow function. Blood type should be determined as all patients with ectopic pregnancy who are Rh negative require 50 μg of Rh(D) immunoglobulin. Outpatient observation is preferred for its cost-effectiveness and patient convenience. Patient monitoring continues until β-hCG levels are nondetectable. It usually takes a month or longer for β-hCG levels to disappear from plasma. With the single-dose treatment, levels of β-hCG generally increase during the first week subsequent to the treatment and peak 4 days following injection. If a response is observed and the fall in β-hCG levels is greater than 15%, weekly serum β-hCG determinations should be measured until undetectable β-hCG levels are documented. Failure of the β-hCG level to decline requires a second dose of methotrexate. An additional dose of methotrexate may also be given if β-hCG levels plateau or increase in 1 week. Persistent ectopic mass or hemoperitoneum may lead to surgery.

Side-effects

Methotrexate has the potential for serious toxicity and, indeed, high doses can cause bone marrow suppression, hepatotoxicity, stomatitis, pulmonary fibrosis, alopecia, and photosensitivity. Toxic effects are usually related to the amount and duration of therapy. Nevertheless, most side-effects during regular treatment for ectopic pregnancy are minor and self-limited, and generally limited to an increase in hepatic transaminases, mild stomatitis, and gastrointestinal disturbance. Reproductive outcome after methotrexate treatment is generally favorable, and it seems that fertility depends more on the patients' previous medical history (i.e., a history of infertility) than on her treatment for ectopic pregnancy.

Expectant management

For years, gynecologists have stressed the need for early diagnosis and treatment of ectopic pregnancy in order to reduce morbidity and mortality. However, some patients experience spontaneous resolution of their ectopic pregnancy and, in such patients, expectant management is optional in order to avoid unnecessary treatment. After clear demonstrations that select cases of ectopic pregnancy resolve without therapy, several studies of patients with ectopic pregnancy have been conducted with consistent, reassuring results. Candidates for successful expectant management must be asymptomatic with a clear indication of resolution (generally manifested by declining levels of β-hCG). In addition, they should be willing to accept the potential risks of tubal rupture and hemorrhage. Patients with early, small tubal gestations with lower (β-hCG $< 200\,\text{mIU/mL}$) and falling β-hCG levels are the best candidates for expectant management.

Heterotopic pregnancy

Coexistent intrauterine and extrauterine pregnancies are referred to as heterotopic pregnancy. The occurrence of a heterotopic pregnancy following spontaneous cycles is rare, with an estimated incidence of 1 in 30 000 normal pregnancies. However, the incidence increases to around 1% after the use of assisted reproductive technology. It is particularly high among women who are undergoing ovulation induction with gonadotropins, and among women undergoing *in vitro* fertilization, as it has become standard practice to transfer at least two embryos.

Heterotopic pregnancy poses a diagnostic dilemma. Serial β-hCG levels are not helpful because they are increased owing to the intrauterine pregnancy. Routine ultrasound detects only one-half of cases; it is more likely that in cases of a viable intrauterine pregnancy, the intrauterine pregnancy will be detected in the course of workup and the ectopic pregnancy missed. Also, in cases of nonviable intrauterine pregnancy, the presence of chorionic villi in the curettage specimen consistently serves to delay the correct diagnosis. Indeed, 50% of patients suffer from late diagnosis and arrive at the hospital after rupture. There are no specific features to guide the physician to make an accurate, early diagnosis of heterotopic pregnancy other than a general awareness of such a possibility. This is particularly important in cases of abdominal pain and tenderness accompanying normal intrauterine pregnancy, or following uterine curettage for a nonviable intrauterine pregnancy among patients who conceived following assisted reproductive technology. Also, in cases of persistent or rising β-hCG levels following uterine curettage for a nonviable intrauterine pregnancy, the possibility of heterotopic pregnancy should be considered.

Treatment consists of removal of the ectopic pregnancy by surgery and avoidance of intrauterine instrumentation and systemic methotrexate treatment in cases when the pregnancy is desirable (especially following assisted reproductive technology). In hemodynamically unstable patients, an explorative laparotomy is necessary. Expectant management is problematic as β-hCG levels cannot be monitored effectively due to the intrauterine pregnancy. The prognosis for the intrauterine pregnancy is excellent, and the majority are carried to term.

Further reading

ACOG Practice Bulletin. Clinical management guidelines for obstetrician–gynecologists: medical management of tubal pregnancy, no. 3, December 1998.

Ankum WM, Mol BWJ, Van der Veen F, et al. Risk factors for ectopic pregnancy: a meta-analysis. *JAMA* 1996;65:1093–1099.

Barnhart KT, Katz I, Hummel A, et al. Presumed diagnosis of ectopic pregnancy. *Obstet Gynecol* 2002;100:505–510.

Brumsted J, Kessler C, Gibson C, et al. A comparison of laparoscopy and laparotomy for the treatment of ectopic pregnancy. *Obstet Gynecol* 1988;71:889–892.

Carson SA, Buster JE. Ectopic pregnancy. *N Engl J Med* 1993;329:1174–1181.

Hajenius P, Engelsbel S, Mol B, et al. Randomised trial of systemic methotrexate versus laparoscopic salpingostomy in tubal pregnancy. *Lancet* 1997;350:774–779.

Kadar N, Caldwell BV, Romero R. A method of screening for ectopic pregnancy and its indications. *Obstet Gynecol* 1981;58:162–166.

Lipscomb G, McCord M, Stovall T, et al. Predictors of success of methotrexate treatment in women with tubal ectopic pregnancies. *N Engl J Med* 1999;341:1974–1978.

Reece EA, Petrie RH, Sirmans MF, et al. Combined intrauterine and extrauterine gestations: a review. *Am J Obstet Gynecol* 1983;146:323–330.

Stovall TG, Ling FW, Gray LA, et al. Methotrexate treatment of unruptured ectopic pregnancy: a report of 100 cases. *Obstet Gynecol* 1991;77:749–753.

11 Multifetal pregnancies: epidemiology, clinical characteristics, and management

Michelle Smith-Levitin, Daniel W. Skupski, and Frank A. Chervenak

Incidence and embryology

In the USA, the number of twin births has increased by over 60% since 1980, and higher order births increased by 500%. More than 90% of the increase is due to widespread use of assisted reproductive technologies (ART). Placentation for monozygous gestations can be diamnionic–dichorionic (DC), diamnionic–monochorionic (MC), or monoamnionic–monochorionic (MA) (Fig. 11.1). DC placentation occurs in about 30% of monozygotic (MZ) twins, MC placentation in 70%, and MA in less than 1%.

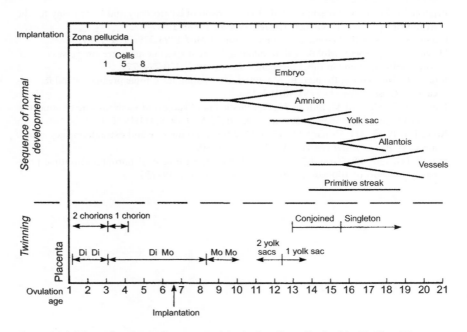

Figure 11.1 The embryology of monozygotic twinning. From Benirschke K, Kim CK. Multiple pregnancy. *N Engl J Med* 1973;288:1276.

Diagnosis

Ultrasound is indispensable (Table 11.1). The most accurate time to determine placentation is in the late first or early second trimester. The visualization of a dividing membrane excludes a diagnosis of an MA pair, but it may be difficult to see until 10–12 weeks in MC multiples. Separate placental disks or fetuses of opposite gender or a "twin peak" sign (Fig. 11.2A) equals a DC placenta. A MC membrane will be thin and wispy with only two layers, and a T-shaped junction will be present (Fig. 11.2B). Assessment of the Y-shaped ipsilon zone helps to establish chorionicity in triplets (Fig. 11.2C).

Fetal complications

Perinatal morbidity and mortality

Twins account for 12.6% of perinatal mortality, although they account for only 3%

Table 11.1 The use of ultrasound in multiple gestations.

First trimester
Diagnosis of multifetal pregnancy
Determination of chorionicity and amnionicity
Accurate pregnancy dating (crown–rump length)
Screening for some anomalies (nuchal translucencies)
Guidance for chorionic villus sampling and multifetal pregnancy reduction

Second trimester
Screening for fetal anomalies
Guidance for amniocentesis
Determination of chorionicity and amnionicity
Determination of placental cord insertion
Biometry to screen for early fetal growth restriction or discordance
Assessment of cervical length

Third trimester
Biometry to screen for fetal growth restriction or discordance
Assessment of cervical length
Fetal status assessment
   Amniotic fluid volume
   Biophysical profile
   Doppler flow studies
Fetal presentation

Intrapartum
Fetal presentation
Guidance for external cephalic version of the second twin

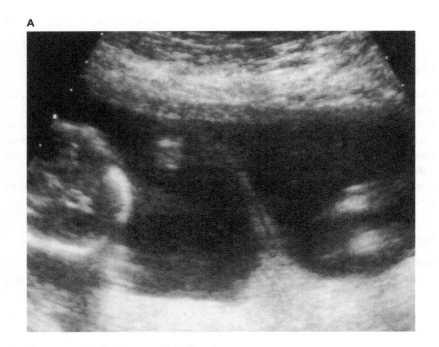

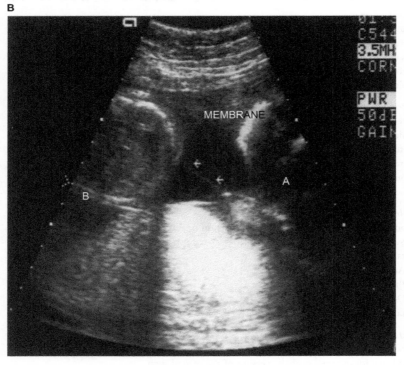

Figure 11.2

of live births. Twenty percent of triplets have a major handicap, and a triplet is 17 times more likely to have cerebral palsy than a singleton.

Prematurity

Fifty-eight percent of twins and 92% of triplets are born prior to 37 weeks (Table 11.2). Twelve percent of twins, 36% of triplets, and 60% of quadruplets are born prior to 32 weeks. Twenty-five percent of twins, 75% of triplets, and all quadruplets are admitted to the neonatal intensive care unit.

Fetal growth

Fetal growth restriction (FGR) complicates up to 60% of multiple gestations. Discordant growth between the fetuses complicates at least 15% of twins and up to 54% of triplets (Fig. 11.3). A combination of some or all of the indices listed in Table 11.3 identifies discordant sets.

Congenital anomalies

The incidence of congenital anomalies in multiple gestations is 1.5 to 3 times higher than in singletons. There is a higher incidence of chromosomal abnormalities, which is related to the increased probability that a woman carrying more than one fetus

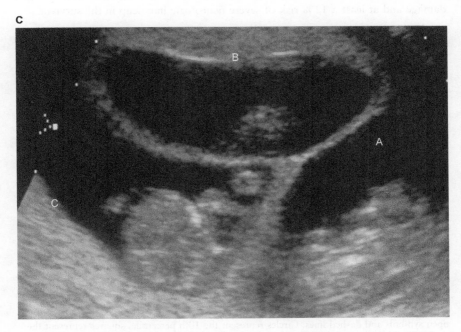

Figure 11.2 *Continued* (A) The twin peak sign and a thick dichorionic membrane. (B) The T-shaped junction of a monochorionic placenta. (C) The Y-shaped ipsilon zone of a trichorionic triplet gestation.

will have at least one that is aneuploid at a younger maternal age than if she were carrying a singleton. Conjoined twins are rare. The most severe form of vascular interchange anomaly is twin reversed arterial perfusion (TRAP). The "pump" twin becomes hydropic, and the "recipient" twin has multiple anomalies. A less severe form of vascular interchange between fetuses is the twin–twin transfusion syndrome (TTTS) occurring in 10–15% of MC twins. It is likely caused by uncompensated deep arterial–venous connections leading to a one-way shunt between the fetuses (Fig. 11.4). The recipient twin becomes hypervolemic and polycythemic, which leads to polyhydramnios, congestive heart failure, and hydrops. The donor becomes hypovolemic and anemic, which leads to decreased renal perfusion, oligohydramnios, and FGR. The criteria for diagnosis include monochorionicity, oligohydramnios around the smaller twin with a small or absent urinary bladder on serial scans, and polyhydramnios around the larger twin with a distended urinary bladder. MA gestations are associated with a high perinatal mortality due to cord entanglement. Single umbilical artery and velamentous cord insertions are more common.

Intrauterine fetal demise

Death of one fetus in the second half of gestation complicates 4–8% of twins and 11–17% of triplets. There is an increased risk of preterm delivery, FGR, and perinatal mortality in the survivors. In MC pregnancies, there is a 20% risk of organ damage and at least a 12% risk of severe neurologic handicap in the survivor.

Table 11.2 Gestational age and birthweight in multiple gestations.

	Twins	Triplets	Quadruplets
Average gestational age (weeks)	35.3	32.2	29.9
Average birthweight (g)	2347	1687	1309

Adapted from Martin JA, Hamilton BE, Sutton PD, et al. Births: final data for 2002. *Natl Vital Stat Rep* 2003;52(10):1–102.

Figure 11.3 (A) Growth rates in twins versus singletons. Twins are represented by open symbols and solid lines. Singletons are represented by solid symbols and dashed lines. Triangles represent the 10th percentiles, squares represent the 50th percentiles, and circles represent the 90th percentiles. From Min SJ, Luke B, Gillespie B, et al. Birth weight references for twins. *Am J Obstet Gynecol* 2000;182:1250–1257, with permission. (B and C) Growth rates in triplets compared with singletons and twins. Singletons and twins are represented by closed symbols and solid lines, respectively, and triplets are represented by open symbols and dashed lines. Circles represent the 10th percentile, squares represent the 50th percentile, and triangles represent the 90th percentile. From Min SJ, Luke B, Min L, et al. Birth weight references for triplets. *Am J Obstet Gynecol* 2004;191:809–814, with permission.

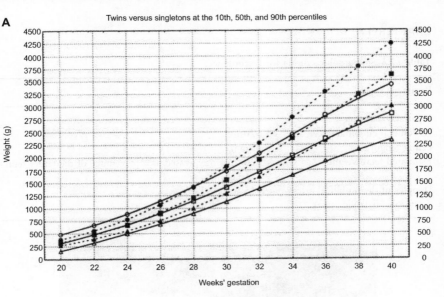

A Twins versus singletons at the 10th, 50th, and 90th percentiles

Weight (g)

Weeks' gestation

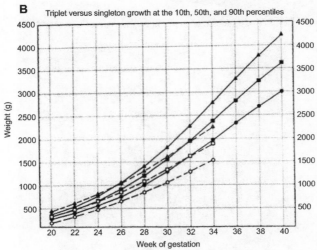

B Triplet versus singleton growth at the 10th, 50th, and 90th percentiles

Weight (g)

Week of gestation

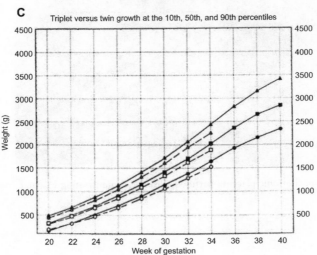

C Triplet versus twin growth at the 10th, 50th, and 90th percentiles

Weight (g)

Week of gestation

Table 11.3 Sonographic criteria for discordance.

Parameter	
Biparietal diameter	≥6 mm
Abdominal circumference	>20 mm
Femur length	≥5 mm
Estimated fetal weight	>20–25% (expressed as a percentage of the larger fetal weight)
Doppler of the umbilical artery (systolic/diastolic ratio)	>15% (or >0.4)

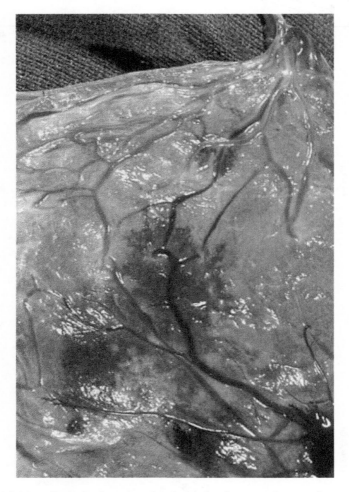

Figure 11.4 Monochorionic placenta perfused with dye demonstrating vascular anastomoses.

Table 11.4 Maternal complications of multiple gestation.

Gastrointestinal Hyperemesis gravidarum Cholestasis of pregnancy Acute fatty liver of pregnancy	*Economic* *Psychologic morbidity* (see Tables 11.5 and 11.6)
Hematologic Anemia Thromboembolism	*Obstetric* Preterm labor (20–90%) Preterm premature rupture of membranes (14–20%)
Dermatologic Pruritic urticaric papules of pregnancy	Antepartum hemorrhage (twofold increase) Abruptio placentae (threefold increase) Postpartum hemorrhage (twofold increase)
Metabolic Gestational diabetes	Increased incidence of Cesarean delivery and subsequent complications
Infectious Urinary tract infections Puerperal infections	Increased hospitalization
Cardiovascular Pregnancy-induced hypertension Preeclampsia (~17% of twins, ~25% of triplets) Increased susceptibility to pulmonary edema Complications of tocolysis	

Maternal medical complications

Women carrying multiple fetuses are at greater risk of medical complications (Table 11.4). Complex ethical and bereavement issues commonly arise (Tables 11.5 and 11.6).

Obstetric complications

Women carrying multiple fetuses are at greater risk of obstetrical complications (Table 11.4).

Cesarean delivery

More than 50% of twins, 75% of triplets, and almost all higher order multiple gestations are delivered by Cesarean section. A trial of labor is justifiable for patients with twins who would like a vaginal delivery after Cesarean section due to low reported uterine rupture rates.

Table 11.5 Loss scenarios in multiple gestations.

First- and second-trimester miscarriage of all fetuses
First-trimester loss of some fetuses (vanishing twin/triplet)
Multifetal pregnancy reduction (MFPR)
Later intrauterine demise of some or all fetuses
Selective or complete termination for anomalies
Expectant management with one or more anomalous fetuses
Complications of monochorionic twins
Intrapartum demise
Delivery at limits of viability
Sudden infant death syndrome (SIDS) (twice as common in twins as in singletons)
Accidental death (more common in multiples)

Adapted from Pector EA, Smith-Levitin M. Bereavement: grief and psychological aspects of multiple birth loss. In: Blickstein I, Keith L, eds. *Multiple pregnancy: epidemiology, gestation, and perinatal outcome.* Abingdon: Taylor and Francis; 2005:862–873.

Table 11.6 A few management pearls for perinatal bereavement after multiple pregnancy loss.

Offer private experiences such as viewing, holding, bathing, and dressing with multiples individually and together (including deceased with survivors)
Offer prenatal mementos (i.e., ultrasound pictures) and matching mementos for each neonate
Offer photos of multiples alone, together, and with parents or other family members: color, black-and-white, digital, or 35 mm
Suggest computer-manipulated photos, sketches, or pastels
Clarify parent preferences for the survivor's crib label (i.e., "twin A" or just "baby Jones")
Clarify parent desires to refer to survivors by the original or the remaining number of babies
Offer multiple-specific grief information and support resources (i.e., Center for Loss in Multiple Birth – www.climb-support.org)

Adapted from Pector EA, Smith-Levitin M. Bereavement: grief and psychological aspects of multiple birth loss. In: Blickstein I, Keith L, eds. *Multiple pregnancy: epidemiology, gestation, and perinatal outcome.* Abingdon: Taylor and Francis; 2005:862–873.

Antepartum management

Multifetal pregnancy reduction (MFPR)
MPFR is a safe and effective procedure reducing the maternal and perinatal morbidity and mortality associated with high-order multiple gestations. MFPR is performed by transabdominal or transvaginal injection of potassium chloride or digoxin into the fetal thorax late in the first trimester. Pregnancy loss rates after

MFPR are 3.3–11.7%, depending on the starting and finishing number. The background loss rates for high-order multiple gestations prior to viability are 8–20%. All mothers discovered to have more than two fetuses should be offered MFPR.

Prenatal diagnosis

Nuchal translucency thickness greater than 2.5 mm in the first trimester is present in a large number of trisomic twin fetuses. Nuchal translucency is currently the single best method for screening in the first trimester for aneuploidy in multiple gestations. Biochemical markers, as a screen for aneuploidy, have unproven validity in the setting of multiple gestations. Maternal serum alpha fetoprotein (MSAFP) greater than 4 MOM in a twin gestation in the second trimester should prompt further evaluation. The three invasive methods available for prenatal diagnosis in multiple gestations are chorionic villus sampling (CVS), amniocentesis, and percutaneous umbilical blood sampling (PUBS). CVS loss rates (2–3%) are similar to those with amniocentesis. CVS can be used in high-order multiples prior to MFPR procedures without increasing loss rates. Standard amniocentesis for analysis of karyotype and AFP can be done in multiple gestations with loss rates prior to 28 weeks of 2.8%.

Selective termination

Selective termination of the abnormal fetus may be performed by injecting potassium chloride or digoxin directly into the affected fetus's heart in the second trimester. Pregnancy loss occurs in 5–6% prior to 13 weeks and in 7–9% after 13 weeks. The injection procedure is not safe in MC gestations. Umbilical cord ligation should be used.

Antenatal care

Supplemental iron (60–80 mg/day) and folate (1 mg/day) should be given in addition to standard prenatal vitamins. Calcium, zinc, and magnesium supplementation may be beneficial. Increased fluid intake (at least 2 L/day) is necessary. A diet that is rich in protein (300–400 g/day) and calories (at least 1000 kcal/day over the requirements for a singleton) is necessary. Women with twins should gain 35–45 pounds (16–20 kg).

Prevention of prematurity

Education and interventions must begin early as most of the mortality (50–80%) occurs before 32 weeks. Cervical length of < 25 mm at 24 weeks is strongly predictive of preterm delivery. Cervical lengths of at least 3.5 cm at 24 weeks in twins are associated with less than a 5% risk of delivery at less than 34 weeks. Cervical length assessments can be made at least every 2 weeks starting in the second trimester. The detection of fetal fibronectin (FfN) is a strong predictor of preterm delivery within 2 weeks. The best positive predictor in twins is a serially positive FfN and a short cervix. FfN has a high negative predictive value in both singletons and multiple gestations. Unnecessary interventions may be avoided in a patient with increased uterine activity but no cervical change and a negative FfN. Prophylactic

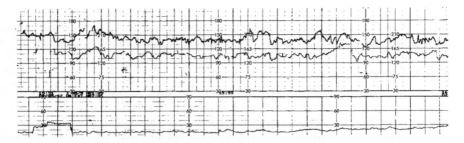

Figure 11.5 A simultaneously reactive twin nonstress test.

cerclage provides no benefit in the absence of cervical incompetence by history. Modification of normal activity and increased rest periods throughout the day may prolong gestation and decrease the incidence of complications such as hypertension and FGR in multiple gestations.

Treatment of preterm labor

Tocolytic agents prolong gestation by at least 24–48 hours in multiple pregnancies. Tocolytics must be used with extra caution and monitoring in women with multiple gestations because of the increased risk of pulmonary edema, volume overload, and cardiac arrhythmias. Antenatal steroids should be used in multifetal pregnancies for the same indications as in singletons.

Fetal surveillance

Sonograms (Table 11.1) should be performed every 3–4 weeks in an uncomplicated multiple gestation to assess fetal growth, amniotic fluid volume, and cervical length. All multiple gestations should undergo antepartum fetal testing. Nonstress test (NST) is the primary method, performed at least weekly beginning at 36 weeks (Fig. 11.5). Biophysical profile (BPP) is also a reliable method of fetal surveillance in multiples, even in those of high order. MC multiple gestations, women with additional risk factors for uteroplacental insufficiency, and fetuses who are already known to have a growth problem should have at least an amniotic fluid volume assessment weekly.

Timing of delivery

Uncomplicated twins should not be electively delivered prior to 38 weeks. Twins have higher stillbirth rates and higher than expected rates of FGR after 38 weeks. Elective delivery of higher order pregnancies can be justified at 36–37 weeks. Earlier delivery may be necessary when there are complications. Confirmation of fetal lung maturity should occur, unless there is an absolute fetal or maternal indication for delivery. Intersac discordance in lung maturity occurs in at least 50% of twins, so both sacs should be sampled.

Antepartum management of fetal complications
Monoamnionic gestations
- Early diagnosis;
- Serial evaluation of fetal growth;
- Frequent antepartum fetal testing with nonstress tests;
- Continuous fetal monitoring when frequent variable decelerations are seen;
- Delivery by Cesarean section for nonreassuring testing.

Mortality with the above management scheme has decreased to 20%. Most experts advocate delivery by Cesarean section around 32–34 weeks.

Conjoined twins
Serial ultrasound, echocardiography, and magnetic resonance imaging (MRI) should be performed. If conjoined twins have a possibility of survival, the patient should be delivered by Cesarean section at a specialized tertiary care center.

Acardiac twins
Mortality for the pump twin is greater than 50% and universally lethal for the recipient. *In utero* treatment is best attempted by umbilical cord ligation.

Twin–twin transfusion syndrome
Isolated "stuck twin" or isolated polyhydramnios is often a sign of a fetal anomaly. TTTS is diagnosed by an MC placenta, severe oligo- and polyhydramnios, and small/absent bladder in one twin with large bladder in the other twin. Treatment options include amniodrainage, septostomy, and fetoscopic laser ablation of anastomotic placental vessels. Fetoscopic laser ablation can achieve a 60% survival rate with a 10% rate of neurologic morbidity in the survivors.

Fetal growth restriction of one or more fetuses
Early detection of FGR requires careful sonography to rule out anomalies and a karyotype analysis.
- Ultrasound for fetal growth every 2 weeks;
- Frequent (weekly or twice-weekly) nonstress and biophysical profile testing and Doppler velocimetry;
- Delivery of the growth-restricted fetus should await fetal lung maturity of all the fetuses unless the testing is nonreassuring or the affected fetus fails to demonstrate any growth over time.

Growth discordance
Severe growth discordance (25–30%) is associated with increased morbidity and mortality. Discordant growth requires more frequent ultrasound examinations and more frequent and earlier fetal testing. There is no indication for early delivery as long as each fetus follows its own growth curve and testing is reassuring. Early intervention should be undertaken if there is progressive growth discordance or signs suggestive of immediate fetal danger.

Single fetal death *in utero*

If the demise is caused by a pregnancy complication that is likely to affect the survivor, delivery should be strongly considered even if the fetus will be premature. If the demise is caused by a problem that is unlikely to affect the survivor, such as a known fetal anomaly, expectant management with close surveillance is warranted. With MC gestations, there is a significant risk to the survivor, but even immediate delivery may not prevent neurologic deficits.

Intrapartum management

Asynchronous birth

Criteria for attempting expectant management of the remaining fetuses after the birth of one or more include: reasonable evidence of fetal well-being, absence of signs of abruption or chorioamnionitis, and DC placentation. Indocin works well as a tocolytic in this setting

Mode of delivery

The authors' management plan is illustrated in Figure 11.6.

Twin A vertex, twin B vertex

Vaginal delivery should be attempted for vertex–vertex twins, even if low or very low birthweight. The time interval between delivery of twins is not critical as long

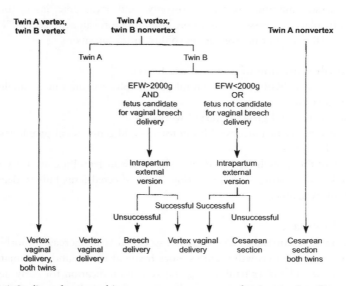

Figure 11.6 Outline of proposed intrapartum management of twin gestation. From Chervenak FA, Johnson RE, Youcha S, et al. Intrapartum management of twin gestation. *Obstet Gynecol* 1985;65:119–112, with permission.

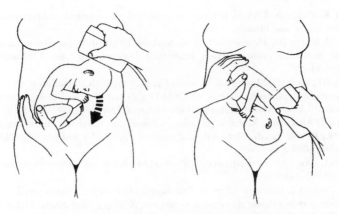

Figure 11.7 The maneuver of external version. From Chervenak FA, Johnson RE, Berkowitz RL, et al. Intrapartum external version of the second twin. *Obstet Gynecol* 1983;62:160.

as the well-being of the second twin is continuously assessed. Cesarean delivery of either or both twins should be undertaken for the same indications as in singletons.

Twin A vertex, twin B nonvertex
One option is elective Cesarean delivery. The preponderance of evidence indicates that Cesarean delivery is not necessary. Another option is external cephalic version with subsequent vaginal delivery from the vertex presentation (Fig. 11.7). There is a 70% success of external cephalic version for the second twin. Another option is total or assisted breech extraction. There is a 95% success rate for breech delivery of the second twin. Vaginal breech delivery criteria include an adequate maternal pelvis, a flexed fetal head, an estimated fetal weight of 1500–3500 g, and size that is not significantly larger than twin A.

Twin A nonvertex
Cesarean delivery is usually recommended.

Higher order births
Most experts recommend Cesarean delivery for all high-order multiple gestations. Vaginal delivery is not contraindicated for select patients.

Further reading

ACOG. Multiple gestation: complicated twin, triplet, and high-order multifetal pregnancy. *ACOG Pract Bull* 2004;56:869–883.
Adams DM, Sholl JS, Haney EL, et al. Perinatal outcome associated with outpatient management of triplet pregnancy. *Am J Obstet Gynecol* 1998;178:843–847.

Blickstein I, Keith L, eds. *Multiple pregnancy: epidemiology, gestation, and perinatal outcome.* Abingdon: Taylor and Francis, 2005.

Evans MI, Goldberg JD, Horenstein J, et al. Selective termination for structural, chromosomal, and mendelian abnormalities: international experience. *Am J Obstet Gynecol* 1999;181:893–897.

Goldenberg RL, Iams JD, Miodovnik M, et al. The preterm birth prediction study: risk factors in twin gestations. National Institute of Child Health and Human Development Maternal-Fetal Medicine Units Network. *Am J Obstet Gynecol* 1996;175:1047–1053.

Malone FD, D'Alton ME. Multiple gestation. Clinical characteristics and management. In: Creasy RK, Resnik R, eds. *Maternal–fetal medicine: principles and practice.* Philadelphia, PA: Elsevier; 2004:513–536.

Pharoah PO, Adi Y. Consequences of in-utero death in twin pregnancy. *Lancet* 2000;335:1597–1602.

Senat MV, Deprest J, Boulvain M, et al. Endoscopic laser surgery versus serial amnioreduction for severe twin-to-twin transfusion syndrome. *N Engl J Med* 2004;351:136–144.

Sibai BM, Hauth J, Caritis S, et al. Hypertensive disorders in twin versus singleton gestations. National Institute of Child Health and Human Development Network of Maternal–Fetal Medicine Units. *Am J Obstet Gynecol* 2000;182:938–942.

Winn HN, Cimino J, Powers J. Intrapartum management of nonvertex second-born twins: a critical analysis. *Am J Obstet Gynecol* 2001;185:1204–1208.

12 Biology of normal and deviant fetal growth

Andrée Gruslin and the late Carl A. Nimrod

Genetic influences

Elements from both the maternal and the paternal genome are required for normal fetal growth and development. Recent data have demonstrated that, for certain genes, only one allele is functional. This is referred to as genetic imprinting, an epigenetic mechanism by which one of the two alleles of a gene is expressed according to its parental origin. The allele that is silenced is called imprinted. In fact, recent human studies have demonstrated that most maternally imprinted genes act as growth suppressors (e.g., H19, p57), whereas paternal ones act as growth promoters (e.g., insulin-like growth factor 2, IGF-2). One of the most striking examples of the importance of this mechanism lies in the influence of IGF-2 imprinting and its disorder on human fetal growth (Fig. 12.1). It has been shown that biallelic expression of IGF-2 leads to overgrowth of the fetus that is recognized clinically as Beckwith–Wiedemann syndrome, characterized by large birthweight, organomegaly, macroglossia, and neonatal hypoglycemia. Conversely, in the mouse, deletion of the paternal IGF-2 allele has been shown to cause fetal growth restriction. The mechanisms by which imprinting is altered include chromosomal deletion/duplication,

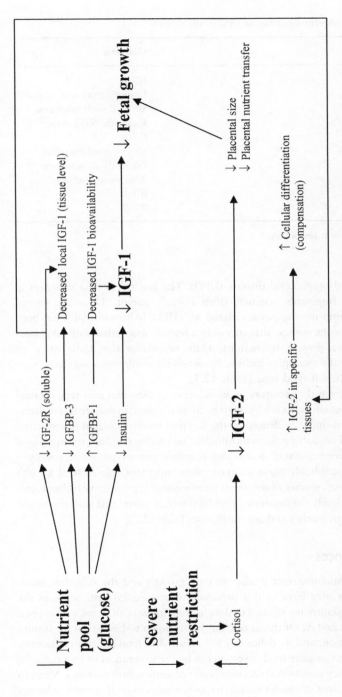

Figure 12.1 Simplified mechanism involving the IGF system in the induction of fetal growth restriction following decreased nutrient and oxygen supply. The lower glucose concentration results in several alterations including ↓ insulin with modulation in receptor concentration and binding proteins status, which all lead to decreased IGF-1 and therefore decreased fetal growth. With ongoing severe nutrient restriction and associated hypoxemia, cortisol concentration increases and IGF-2 decreases, which leads to a decrease in placental growth and function, further impeding fetal growth. Note that the decrease in IGF-2 receptor (IGF-2R; soluble form) results in an increase in IGF-2 concentration locally, in specific tissues. This is believed to promote cellular differentiation and provide some positive stimulus for fetal growth in order to attempt to compensate for the above changes.

Table 12.1 Clinically relevant outcomes of UPD in the human.

UPD	Outcome
Maternal UPD2	IUGR
Paternal UPD6q24	Diabetes (transient neonatal)
Maternal UPD7	Silver–Russell syndrome
Paternal UPD11p15	Beckwith–Wiedemann
Maternal UPD14	IUGR
Paternal UPD14	Short-limbed dwarfism
Maternal UPD15	Prader–Willi syndrome
Paternal UPD15	Angelman syndrome
Maternal UPD16	IUGR
Maternal UPD20	IUGR

IUGR, intrauterine growth restriction.

point mutations, and uniparental disomy (UPD). The last refers to a situation in which chromosome fragments originate from a single parent. There are several examples of human imprinted genes associated with UPD. In humans, UPD has been observed for most chromosomes, although only a few are associated with an abnormal phenotype (often growth restriction), again suggesting that these carry an imprinted gene. Specific examples include Prader–Willi syndrome, Angelman syndrome, and Silver–Russell syndrome (Table 12.1).

There is evidence from the literature of an influence of maternal genotype on fetal growth. These genetic influences are likely to be those involved in maternal size determination and metabolism, as evidenced by the fact that maternal height is correlated with birthweight and probably reflects its influence on uterine size and perhaps blood flow. What is, however, becoming clear is that maternal phenotype, which results in physical constraints, probably plays an even more important role in fetal growth regulation. For instance, studies of outcomes from assisted reproductive technologies using ova donation clearly demonstrated that birthweight correlated with the height and weight of the birth mother and not the donor (Table 12.2).

Nutritional influences

The importance of micronutrient intake on fetal growth and the role that nutrient–gene interactions may have in this process is becoming evident. Some of the more important micronutrients studied to date include folate, zinc, iron, and copper, as well as vitamins E and A. Of these, zinc has been shown to be critical for insulin packaging and secretion, and its deficiency has resulted in fetal growth restriction. Both copper and iron can alter fetal development by the generation of free radicals, whereas their deficiency results in an accumulation of antioxidant enzymes. Vitamin E, an important regulator of insulin sensitivity, contributes to fetal growth, whereas

Table 12.2 Evidence of a role for the IGF system in human fetal growth.

Homozygous deletion of exons 4 and 5 in the IGF-1 gene results in severe IUGR and
postnatal growth failure
Biallelic expression of the IGF-2 gene leads to Beckwith–Wiedemann syndrome
Both IGFs are present in the fetal circulation very early and expressed in the placenta
Positive correlation between cord serum IGF-1 concentration and fetal size
Birthweight positively correlated with IGFBP-3 and negatively with IGFBP-1
Human IUGR associated with increased IGFBP-1 and -2 and decreased IGFBP-3
↑ IGFBP-1 at decidual–placental interface in severe preeclampsia/IUGR
↑ Circulatory levels of IGFBP-1 up to six times in severe preeclampsia
↑ IGFBP-1 in IUGR at term and antenatally (cordocentesis)
↓ PAPP-A →↓ birthweight (PAPP-A protease of IGFBPs)

IGFBP, insulin-like growth factor binding protein; PAPP-A, pregnancy associated plasma
protein A.

vitamin A's role is through the stimulation of growth hormone postnatally and possibly of placental growth hormone prenatally.

More evidence is accumulating to suggest an interaction between gene expression during fetal growth and nutrient availability. For instance, folate deficiency leads to a decrease in remethylation of homocysteine to methionine. As S-adenosylmethionine is a methyl donor, its absence or decrease results in dysregulation of important developmental genes (imprinting defects) and in defective DNA synthesis. This is further supported by animal studies in which methyl-supplemented diets fed to pregnant mice altered the expression of an imprinted gene specific to the coat color of their offspring. As DNA methylation is important in the regulation of gene imprinting, it is likely that folic acid is involved in fetal growth determination through this process.

Nutrient transport

Fetal growth relies on glucose as a major fuel and, as there is no significant gluconeogenesis in the fetus, it must be obtained directly from maternal blood. Placental transfer of glucose depends on the total surface area of the syncytium available for exchange, the thickness of the placental barrier, the placenta's own metabolic needs, the concentration gradient of glucose between maternal and fetal blood, maternal blood supply and, finally, the presence of transporters. Of these, GLUT3 is likely to be the major functional transporter in early pregnancy, whereas GLUT1 is more important near term. The fetus also requires amino acids for protein synthesis, interconversion to other substrates, and oxidation. The transfer of amino acids is also a complex process and involves significant placental metabolism, as the placenta can use, produce, and interconvert several amino acids.

Further reading

Ashworth CJ, Antipatis C. Micronutrient programming of development throughout gestation. *Reproduction* 2001;122:527–535.

Barker DJP. In utero programming of chronic disease. *Clin Sci* 1998;95:115–128.

Boyne MS, Thame M, Bennett FI, et al. The relationship among circulating insulin-like growth factor (IGF)-I, IFG-binding proteins-1 and -2 and birth anthropometry: a prospective study. *J Clin Endocrinol Metab* 2003;88:1687–1691.

Constancia M, Hemberger M, Hughes J, et al. Placental-specific IGF-II is a major modulator of placental and fetal growth. *Nature* 2002;417:945–948.

Devriendt K. Genetic control of intra-uterine growth. *Eur J Obstet Gynecol Reprod Biol* 2000;92:29–34.

Gluckman PD, Pinal CS. Regulation of fetal growth by the somatotropic axis. *J Nutr* 2003;133:1741S–1746S.

Osgerby JC, Wathes DC, Howard D, Gadd TS. The effect of maternal undernutrition on the placental growth trajectory and the uterine insulin-like growth factor axis in the pregnant ewe. *J Endocrinol* 2004;182:89–103.

Reece EA, Wiznitzer A, Le E, et al. The relation between human fetal growth and fetal blood levels of insulin-like growth factors I and II, their binding proteins, and receptors. *Obstet Gynecol* 1994;84:88–95.

Reik W, Constancia M, Dean W, et al. Igf2 imprinting in development and disease. *Int J Dev Biol* 2000;44:145–150.

Roberts CT, Sohlstrom A, Kind KL, et al. Maternal food restriction reduces the exchange surface area and increases the barrier thickness of the placenta in the guinea-pig. *Placenta* 2001;22:177–185.

Sacks D. Determinants of fetal growth. *Curr Diabetes Rep* 2004;4:281–287.

Sibley CP, Coan PM, Ferguson-Smith AC, et al. Placental-specific insulin-like growth factor 2 (Igf2) regulates the diffusional exchange characteristics of the mouse placenta. *Proc Natl Acad Sci USA* 2004;101:8204–8208.

Steegers-Theunissen RPM, Steegers EAP. Nutrient–gene interactions in early pregnancy: a vascular hypothesis. *Eur J Obstet Gynecol Reprod Biol* 2003;106:115–117.

Wutz A, Theussl HC, Dausman J, et al. Non-imprinted Igf2r expression decreases growth and rescues the Tme mutation in mice. *Development* 2001;128:1881–1887.

Part V

Fetal Infections and Teratogenesis

13 Developmental toxicology, drugs, and fetal teratogenesis

Robert L. Brent and Lynda B. Fawcett

Reproductive problems encompass a multiplicity of diseases including sterility, infertility, abortion, stillbirth, congenital malformations, fetal growth retardation, and prematurity. It is estimated that the majority of all conceptions are lost before term, many within the first 3 weeks of development. Severe congenital malformations occur in 3% of births, and include those birth defects that cause death, hospitalization and mental retardation and those that necessitate significant or repeated surgical procedures, are disfiguring, or interfere with physical performance. These clinical problems occur commonly in the general population and, therefore, environmental causes are not always easy to corroborate (Table 13.1).

Basic principles of teratology

To label an environmental exposure as teratogenic, it is necessary to characterize the exposure with regard to the dose, route of exposure, and the stage of pregnancy when the exposure occurred. Labeling an agent as teratogenic indicates only that it may have the potential to produce congenital malformations. When evaluating human and animal studies on the reproductive effects of environmental agents, several important principles should be followed, as outlined in Table 13.2.

The etiology of congenital malformations

The etiology of congenital malformations can be divided into three categories: unknown, genetic, and environmental (Table 13.3). A significant proportion of congenital malformations of unknown etiology are likely to have an important genetic component. Malformations with an increased recurrent risk such as cleft lip and palate, anencephaly, spina bifida, certain congenital heart diseases, pyloric stenosis, hypospadias, inguinal hernia, talipes equinovarus, and congenital dislocation of the hip fit into the category of multifactorial disease as well as the category of polygenic inherited disease.

Table 13.1 Background reproductive risks in pregnancy.

Reproductive risk	Frequency
Immunologically and clinically diagnosed spontaneous abortions per million conceptions	350 000
Clinically recognized spontaneous abortions per million clinically recognized pregnancies	150 000
Genetic diseases per million births:	110 000
Multifactorial or polygenic genetic environmental interactions (i.e., neural tube defects, cleft lip, hypospadias, hyperlipidemia, diabetes)	90 000
Dominantly inherited disease (i.e., achondroplasia, Huntington's chorea, neurofibromatosis)	10 000
Autosomal and sex-linked genetic disease (i.e., cystic fibrosis, hemophilia, sickle-cell disease, thalassemia)	1 200
Cytogenetic (chromosomal abnormalities) (i.e., Down syndrome (trisomy 21), trisomies 13 and 18, Turner syndrome, 22q deletion, etc.)	5 000
New mutations*	3 000
Severe congenital malformations† per million births (resulting from all causes of birth defects: genetic, unknown, environmental)	30 000
Prematurity per million births	40 000
Fetal growth retardation per million births	30 000
Stillbirths (> 20 weeks) per million births	2000–20 900
Infertility	15% of couples

Modified from: Beckman D, Fawcett L, Brent RL. Developmental toxicology. In: Massaro E, ed. *Handbook of human toxicology*. New York: CRC Press; 1997:1007–1084.
*The mutation rate for many genetic diseases can be calculated; this can be readily performed with dominantly inherited diseases when offspring are born with a dominant genetic disease and neither parent has the disease.
†Congenital malformations have multiple etiologies, including a significant proportion that are genetic.

Factors that affect susceptibility to developmental toxicants

A basic tenet of environmentally produced malformations is that teratogens, or a teratogenic milieu, have certain characteristics in common and follow certain basic principles. These principles determine the quantitative and qualitative aspects of environmentally produced malformations.

Stage of exposure

The risk of an exposure to a developmental toxicant resulting in morphological anomalies or intrauterine death varies, depending on the embryonic or fetal stage at which the exposure occurs. The period of sensitivity may be narrow or broad,

Table 13.2 Basic scientific principles of teratology.

Principle	Description
Exposure to teratogens follows a toxicological dose–response curve	There is a threshold below which no teratogenic effect will be observed. As the dose of the teratogen is increased, both the severity and frequency of reproductive effects will increase (Fig. 13.1)
The embryonic stage at which exposure occurs will determine what effects, if any, a teratogen will have	Some teratogens have a broad period of embryonic sensitivity whereas others have a very narrow period of sensitivity
Most teratogens have a confined group of congenital malformations referred to as the syndrome of the agent's effects	Known teratogens may be presumptively implicated by the spectrum of malformations they produce. It is easier to exclude an agent as a cause of a birth defect than to definitively prove it was responsible because of the existence of genocopies of some teratogenic syndromes
No teratogen can produce every type of malformation	The presence of certain malformations can eliminate the possibility that a particular teratogenic agent was responsible because those malformations have not been demonstrated to be part of the syndrome caused by the teratogen, or because production of the malformation is not biologically plausible for that particular alleged teratogen

Based on concepts from: Brent R. Methods of evaluating the alleged teratogenicity of environmental agents. In: Sever J, Brent RL, eds. *Teratogen update: environmentally induced birth defect risks*. New York: Alan R Liss; 1986:199–201.

depending on the environmental agent and the malformation in question. The embryo is most sensitive to the lethal effects of drugs and chemicals during the period of embryonic development from fertilization through the early postimplantation stage. Surviving embryos have malformation rates similar to control subjects because significant cell loss or chromosome abnormalities at these stages have a high likelihood of resulting in embryonic death, not because malformations cannot be produced at this stage.

The period of organogenesis (from day 18 through about day 40 post conception in the human) is the period of greatest sensitivity to teratogens when most gross anatomic malformations can be induced. Most environmentally produced major malformations occur before the 36th day post conception in the human. The exceptions are malformations of the genito-urinary system, the palate, the brain, or deformations resulting from problems of constraint, disruption, or destruction.

Table 13.3 Etiology of human congenital malformations observed during the first year of life.

Suspected cause	Percent of total
Unknown	65–75
Polygenic	
Multifactorial (gene–environment interactions)	
Spontaneous errors of development	
Synergistic interactions of teratogens	
Genetic	15–25
Autosomal and sex-linked inherited genetic disease	
Cytogenetic (chromosomal abnormalities)	
New mutations	
Environmental	10
Maternal conditions: alcoholism, diabetes, endocrinopathies, phenylketonuria, smoking and nicotine, starvation, nutritional deficits	4
Infectious agents: rubella, toxoplasmosis, syphilis, herpes simplex, cytomegalovirus, varicella zoster, Venezuelan equine encephalitis, parvovirus B19	3
Mechanical problems (deformations): amniotic band constrictions, umbilical cord constraint, disparity in uterine size and uterine contents	1–2
Chemicals, prescription drugs, high-dose ionizing radiation, hyperthermia	< 1

Modified from: Brent R. Environmental factors: miscellaneous. In: Brent R, Harris M, eds. *Prevention of embryonic, fetal and perinatal disease.* Bethesda, MD: John E. Fogarty International Center for Advanced Study in the Health Sciences, NIH; 1976:211.

Agents that result in cell depletion, vascular disruption, necrosis, specific tissue or organ pathology, physiological decompensation, or severe growth retardation have the potential to cause deleterious effects throughout gestation.

Dose or magnitude of the exposure and threshold dose

The quantitative correlation between the magnitude of the embryopathic effects and the dose of a drug, chemical, or other agent is referred to as the dose–response relationship. The dose–response relationship of a toxicant should be interpreted carefully. A substance given in large enough amounts to cause maternal toxicity is also likely to have deleterious effects on the embryo such as death, growth retardation, or retarded development. Several considerations affect the interpretation of dose–response relationships (Table 13.4).

The threshold dose is the dosage below which the incidence of death, malformation, growth retardation, or functional deficit is not statistically greater than that

Table 13.4 Considerations that affect the interpretation of dose–response relationships.

Concept	Description	Example
Active metabolites	Metabolites may be the proximate teratogen rather than the administered drug or chemical	The metabolite phosphoramide mustard and acrolein may produce abnormal development resulting from the metabolism of cyclophosphamide
Duration of exposure	A chronic exposure to a prescribed drug can contribute to an increased teratogenic risk	Anticonvulsant therapy; in contrast an acute exposure to the same drug may present little or no teratogenic risk
Fat solubility	Fat-soluble substances can produce fetal malformations for an extended period after the last ingestion or exposure because they have an unusually long half-life	Polychlorinated biphenyls (PCBs). Etretinate may present a similar risk but the data are not conclusive

of control subjects. The threshold level of exposure usually varies between less than one and up to two orders of magnitude below the teratogenic or embryopathic dose of drugs and chemicals that kill or malform one-half of the embryos. An exogenous teratogenic agent, therefore, has a no-effect dose compared with mutagens or carcinogens, which have a stochastic dose–response curve (Table 13.5, Fig. 13.1). The incidence and severity of malformations produced by every exogenous teratogenic agent that has been appropriately studied have exhibited threshold phenomena during organogenesis.

Pharmacokinetics and metabolism of the drug or chemical

Physiological alterations in pregnancy as well as the bioconversion of compounds can significantly influence the teratogenic effects of drugs and chemicals. Tables 13.6 and 13.7 outline the physiological alterations that occur in the mother and the fetus, respectively, during pregnancy and that affect the pharmacokinetics of drugs. Although other organs, including the placenta, can be involved in the metabolism of drugs or chemicals, the major site of bioconversion of chemicals *in vivo* is likely to be the maternal liver. Bioconversion has been shown to be important in the teratogenic activity of several xenobiotics.

Placental transport

It has been alleged that the placental barrier is protective and that harmful substances do not reach the embryo; however, it is now clear that there is no "placental barrier" *per se*, and most drugs and chemicals do cross the placenta. Factors that determine the ability of a drug or chemical to cross the placenta and reach the

Table 13.5 Stochastic and threshold dose–response relationships of diseases produced by environmental agents.

Relationship	Pathology	Site	Diseases	Risk	Definition
Stochastic phenomena	Damage to a single cell may result in disease	DNA	Cancer, mutation	Some risk exists at all dosages; at low exposures the risk is below the spontaneous risk	The incidence of the disease increases with the dose but the severity and nature of the disease remain the same
Threshold phenomena	Multicellular injury	High variation in etiology, affecting many cell and organ processes	Malformation, growth retardation, death, chemical toxicity, etc.	No increased risk below the threshold dose	Both the severity and incidence of the disease increase with dose

From: Brent R. Editorial: definition of a teratogen and the relationship of teratogenicity to carcinogenicity. *Teratology* 1986;34:359.

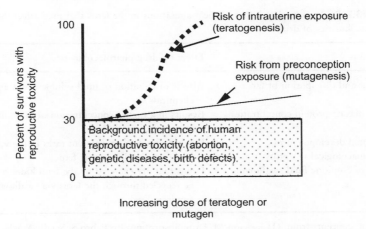

Figure 13.1 Dose–response relationship of reproductive toxins comparing preconception and postconception risks.

Table 13.6 Pregnancy-related physiological alterations in the mother that affect the pharmacokinetics of drugs.

Alteration	Effect on drug pharmacokinetics
Decreased gastrointestinal motility; increased intestinal transit time	Results in delayed absorption of drugs in the small intestine owing to increased stomach retention and enhanced absorption of slowly absorbed drugs
Decreased plasma albumin	Alters the kinetics of compounds normally bound to albumin
Renal elimination	Generally increased but is influenced by body position later in pregnancy
Increased plasma and extracellular fluid volumes	Affects concentration-dependent transfer of compounds
Inhibition of metabolic inactivation in the maternal liver	Increases half-life of drug in plasma
Variation in uterine blood flow	May affect transfer across the placenta (although little is known concerning this)

Based on concepts from: (1) Jackson M. Drug absorption. In: Fabro S, Scialli A, eds. *Drug and chemical action in pregnancy: pharmacological and toxicological principles.* New York: Marcel Dekker; 1986:15; (2) Mattison D. Physiological variations in pharmacokinetics during pregnancy. In: Fabro S, Scialli A, eds. *Drug and chemical action in pregnancy: pharmacological and toxicological principles.* New York: Marcel Dekker; 1986:37–102; and (3) Sonawane B, Yaffe S. Physiologic disposition of drugs in the fetus and newborn. In: Fabro S, Scialli A, eds. *Drug and chemical action in pregnancy: pharmacologic and toxicologic principles.* New York: Marcel Dekker; 1986:103.

Table 13.7 Pregnancy-related physiological alterations in the fetus that may affect the pharmacokinetics of drugs.

Alteration	Effect on drug pharmacokinetics
Amount and distribution of fat	Affects distribution of lipid-soluble drugs and chemicals
Lower plasma protein concentrations	Results in a higher concentration of unbound drug in the fetal circulation
Functional development of pharmacological receptors	Likely to proceed at different rates in the various tissues of the developing fetus
Extent of amniotic fluid swallowing	Drugs that are excreted by the fetal kidneys may be recycled through the fetus via swallowing of amniotic fluid

Based on concepts from: (1) Jackson M. Drug absorption. In: Fabro S, Scialli A, eds. *Drug and chemical action in pregnancy: pharmacological and toxicological principles.* New York: Marcel Dekker; 1986:15; (2) Mattison D. Physiological variations in pharmacokinetics during pregnancy. In: Fabro S, Scialli A, eds. *Drug and chemical action in pregnancy: pharmacological and toxicological principles.* New York: Marcel Dekker; 1986:37–102; and (3) Sonawane B, Yaffe S. Physiologic disposition of drugs in the fetus and newborn. In: Fabro S, Scialli A, eds. *Drug and chemical action in pregnancy: pharmacologic and toxicologic principles.* New York: Marcel Dekker; 1986:103.

embryo include molecular weight, lipid solubility, polarity or degree of ionization, protein binding, and receptor mediation. Compounds with a low molecular weight and lipid affinity, nonpolarity, and without protein-binding properties will easily cross the placenta. In general, compounds with molecular weights of 1000 daltons or more do not readily cross the placenta, whereas those less than 600 daltons usually do; most drugs are 250–400 daltons and therefore cross the placenta.

Environmental agents resulting in reproductive toxicity following exposure during pregnancy

Table 13.8 lists environmental agents that have resulted in reproductive toxicity and/or congenital malformations in human populations. The list should not be used in isolation as many other parameters must be considered when analyzing exposure risks in individual patients. Many of these agents represent a very small risk while others may represent substantial risks; the risks will vary with the magnitude, timing, and length of exposure. Some environmental agents that were thought to show reproductive toxicity have been found, after a careful and complete evaluation, to represent no increased risk; these are listed in Table 13.9.

Table 13.8 Proven human teratogens or embryotoxins: drugs, chemicals, milieu, and physical agents that have resulted in human congenital malformations.

Reproductive toxin	Alleged effects
Aminopterin, methotrexate	Growth retardation, microcephaly, meningomyelocele mental retardation, hydrocephalus, and cleft palate
Androgens	Along with high doses of some male-derived progestins, can cause masculinization of the developing fetus
Angiotensin-converting enzyme (ACE) inhibitors	Fetal hypotension syndrome in second and third trimester resulting in fetal kidney hypoperfusion and anuria, oligohydramnios, pulmonary hypoplasia, and cranial bone hypoplasia. No effect in the first trimester
Antituberculous therapy	The drugs isoniazid (INH) and paraaminosalicylic acid (PAS) have an increased risk for some CNS abnormalities
Caffeine	Moderate exposure not associated with birth defects; high exposures associated with an increased risk of abortion but data are inconsistent
Chorionic villus sampling (CVS)	Vascular disruptive malformations, i.e., limb reduction defects
Cobalt in hematemic multivitamins	Fetal goiter
Cocaine	Very low incidence of vascular disruptive malformations, pregnancy loss
Corticosteroids	High exposures administered systemically have a low risk for cleft palate in some epidemiological studies; however, this is not a consistent finding
Coumarin derivative	Exposure during early pregnancy can result in nasal hypoplasia, stippling of secondary epiphysis, and intrauterine growth retardation. Exposure in late pregnancy can result in CNS malformations as a result of bleeding
Cyclophosphamide and other chemotherapeutic and immunosuppressive agents, e.g., cyclosporine, leflunomide	Many chemotherapeutic agents used to treat cancer have a theoretical risk of producing fetal malformations, as most of these drugs are teratogenic in animals; however, the clinical data are not consistent. Many have not been shown to be teratogenic but the numbers of cases in the studies are small; caution is the byword
Diethylstilbestrol	Genital abnormalities, adenosis, and clear cell adenocarcinoma of the vagina in adolescents. The risk of adenosis can be quite high; the risk of adenocarcinoma is 1:1000 to 1:10 000
Ethyl alcohol	Fetal alcohol syndrome (microcephaly, mental retardation, growth retardation, typical facial dysmorphogenesis, abnormal ears, and small palpebral fissures)

(*Continued*)

Table 13.8 *Continued*

Reproductive toxin	Alleged effects
Ionizing radiation	A threshold greater than 20 rad (0.2 Gy) can increase the risk of some fetal effects such as micocephaly or growth retardation. The threshold for mental retardation is higher
Insulin shock therapy	Microcephaly and mental retardation
Lithium therapy	Chronic use for the treatment of manic depressive illness has an increased risk for Ebstein's anomaly and other malformations, but the risk appears to be very low
Minoxidil	Hirsutism in newborns (led to the discovery of the hair growth-promoting properties of minoxidil)
Methimazole	Aplasia cutis has been reported*
Methylene blue intraamniotic instillation	Fetal intestinal atresia, hemolytic anemia, and jaundice in the neonatal period. This procedure is no longer utilized to identify one twin
Misoprostol	Low incidence of vascular disruptive phenomenon, such as limb reduction defects and Mobius syndrome, has been reported in pregnancies in which this drug was used to induce an abortion
Penicillamine (D-penicillamine)	This drug results in the physical effects referred to as lathyrism, the results of poisoning by the seeds of the genus *Lathyrus*. It causes collagen disruption, cutis laxa, and hyperflexibility of joints. The condition appears to be reversible and the risk is low
Progestin therapy	Very high doses of androgen hormone-derived progestins can produce masculinization. Many drugs with progestational activity do not have masculinizing potential. None of these drugs has the potential for producing congenital malformations
Propylthiouracil	Along with other antithyroid medications can result in an infant born with a goiter
Radioactive isotopes	Tissue- and organ-specific damage is dependent on the radioisotope element and distribution, i.e., high doses of ^{131}I administered to a pregnant woman can cause fetal thyroid hypoplasia after the 8th week of development
Retinoids, systemic	Systemic retinoic acid, isotretinoin, and etretinate can result in an increased risk of CNS, cardio-aortic, ear, and clefting defects, microtia, anotia, thymic aplasia and other branchial arch and aortic arch abnormalities, and certain congenital heart malformations
Retinoids, topical	This is very unlikely to have teratogenic potential because teratogenic serum levels are not achieved from topical exposure

Table 13.8 *Continued*

Reproductive toxin	Alleged effects
Streptomycin	Streptomycin and a group of ototoxic drugs can affect the eighth nerve and interfere with hearing; it is a relatively low-risk phenomenon. Children are even less sensitive to the ototoxic effects of these drugs than adults
Sulfa drug and vitamin K	Hemolysis in some subpopulations of fetuses
Tetracycline	Bone and teeth staining
Thalidomide	Increased incidence of deafness, anotia, preaxial limb reduction defects, phocomelia, ventricular septal defects, and GI atresias during susceptible period from the 22nd to the 36th day post conception
Trimethoprim	This drug was frequently used to treat urinary tract infections and has been linked to an increased incidence of neural tube defects. The risk is not high, but it is biologically plausible because of the drug's lowering effect on folic acid levels. This has also resulted in neurological symptoms in adults taking this drug
Vitamin A (retinol)	Very high doses of vitamin A have been reported to produce the same malformations as reported for the retinoids. Dosages sufficient to produce birth defects would have to be in excess of 25 000 to 50 000 units per day
Vitamin D*	Large doses given in vitamin D prophylaxis are possibly involved in the etiology of supravalvular aortic stenosis, elfin facies, and mental retardation
Warfarin (coumarin)	Exposure during early pregnancy can result in nasal hypoplasia, stippling of secondary epiphysis, and intrauterine growth retardation. Exposure in late pregnancy can result in CNS malformations as a result of bleeding
Anticonvulsants	
Carbamazepine	Used in the reatment of convulsive disorders; increases the risk of facial dysmorphology
Diphenylhydantoin	Used in the treatment of convulsive disorders; increases the risk of fetal hydantoin syndrome, consisting of facial dysmorphology, cleft palate, ventricular septal defect (VSD), and growth and mental retardation
Trimethadione and paramethadione	Used in the treatment of convulsive disorders; increases the risk of characteristic facial dysmorphology, mental retardation, V-shaped eyebrows, low-set ears with anteriorly folded helix, high-arched palate, irregular teeth, CNS anomalies, and severe developmental delay
Valproic acid	Used in the treatment of convulsive disorders; increases the risk of spina bifida, facial dysmorphology, and autism

(*Continued*)

Table 13.8 *Continued*

Reproductive toxin	Alleged effects
Chemicals	
Carbon monoxide poisoning*	CNS damage has been reported with very high exposures, but the risk appears to be low
Gasoline addiction embryopathy	Facial dysmorphology, mental retardation
Lead	Very high exposures can cause pregnancy loss; intrauterine teratogenesis is not established
Methyl mercury	Causes Minamata disease consisting of cerebral palsy, microcephaly, mental retardation, blindness, and cerebellum hypoplasia. Endemics have occurred from adulteration of wheat with mercury-containing chemicals that are used to prevent grain spoilage. Present environmental levels of mercury are unlikely to represent a teratogenic risk, but reducing or limiting the consumption of carnivorous fish has been suggested in order not to exceed the Environmental Protection Agency's (EPA's) maximum permissible exposure (MPE), which is far below the toxic effects of mercury
Polychlorinated biphenyls	Poisoning has occurred from adulteration of food products (cola-colored babies, CNS effects, pigmentation of gums, nails, teeth and groin, hypoplastic deformed nails, intrauterine growth retardation, abnormal skull calcification). The threshold exposure has not been determined, but it is unlikely to be teratogenic at the present environmental exposures
Toluene addiction embryopathy	Facial dysmorphology, mental retardation
Embryonic and fetal infections	
Cytomegalovirus	Retinopathy, CNS calcification, microcephaly, mental retardation
Herpes simplex virus	Fetal infection, liver disease, death
Human immunodeficiency virus (HIV)	Perinatal HIV infection
Parvovirus B19 infection	Stillbirth, hydrops
Rubella virus	Deafness, congenital heart disease, microcephaly, cataracts, mental retardation
Syphilis	Maculopapular rash, hepatosplenomegaly, deformed nails, osteochondritis at joints of extremities, congenital neurosyphilis, abnormal epiphyses, chorioretinitis
Toxoplasmosis	Hydrocephaly, microphthalmia, chorioretinitis, mental retardation

Table 13.8 *Continued*

Reproductive toxin	Alleged effects
Varicella zoster virus	Skin and muscle defects, intrauterine growth retardation, limb reduction defects, CNS damage (very low increased risk)
Venezuelan equine encephalitis	Hydranencephaly, microphthalmia, CNS destructive lesions, luxation of hip
Maternal disease states	
Corticosteroid-secreting endocrinopathy	Mothers with Cushing's disease can have infants with hyperadrenocortism, but anatomical malformations do not appear to be increased
Iodine deficiency	Iodine deficiency can result in embryonic goiter and mental retardation
Intrauterine problems of constraint and vascular disruption	Defects such as club feet, limb reduction, aplasia cutis, cranial asymmetry, external ear malformations, midline closure defects, cleft palate and muscle aplasia, cleft lip, omphalocele, and encephalocele. More common in multiple-birth pregnancies, pregnancies with anatomical defects of the uterus, placental emboli, and amniotic bands
Maternal androgen endocrinopathy (adrenal tumors)	Masculinization
Maternal diabetes	Caudal and femoral hypoplasia, transposition of great vessels
Folic acid insufficiency in the mother	Increased incidence of neural tube defects (NTDs)
Maternal phenylketonuria	Abortion, microcephaly, and mental retardation. Very high risk in untreated patients
Maternal starvation	Intrauterine growth retardation, abortion, NTDs
Tobacco smoking	Abortion, intrauterine growth retardation, and stillbirth
Zinc deficiency*	NTDs

*Controversial.

Table 13.9 Agents erroneously alleged to have caused human malformations.

Agent	Alleged effect
Bendectin	Alleged to cause numerous types of birth defects including limb reduction defects and heart malformations
Diagnostic ultrasonography	No significant hyperthermia, therefore, no reproductive effects
Electromagnetic fields (EMF)	Alleged to cause abortion, cancer, and birth defects
Progestational drugs	Alleged to cause numerous types of nongenital birth defects, including limb reduction defects and heart malformations
Trichloroethylene (TCE)	Alleged to cause cardiac defects

Interpretation of animal study data for assessment of reproductive risks in humans

When a new drug is marketed or a new environmental toxicant is discovered, the only information that is frequently available are the animal data. When using these data to assess the potential risk of adverse effects of human exposure to a drug or chemical, it is important to critically evaluate the studies using the basic principles of teratology guidelines (Table 13.2). As discussed previously, one of the most critical factors for consideration is the dose or magnitude of the exposure and the concept of the threshold dose. A major shortcoming in many studies is the use of weight (mg/kg) as a measure of dose rather than the serum levels of the drug or toxic metabolite that result from such a dose.

The role of the physician in counseling families regarding the etiology of their child's congenital malformations

The clinician must be cognizant of the fact that many patients believe that most congenital malformations are caused by a drug or medication taken during pregnancy. Physicians must also realize that erroneous counseling by inexperienced health professionals may result in nonmeritorious litigation. Unfortunately, it is sometimes assumed that if a drug or chemical has caused birth defects in an animal model or *in vitro* system at a high dose, then it has the potential to produce birth defects at any dose. In fact, the vast majority of consultations involving exposures during pregnancy conclude that the exposure does not change the reproductive risks in that pregnancy.

Before deciding whether a child's malformations are due to a genetic cause or an environmental toxicant or agent, the physician must first carry out a complete examination of the child and a review of the genetic and teratology medical literature. The information that is required for this evaluation is presented in Table 13.10. As well as the usual history and physical evaluation, including descriptive and quantitative information about the physical characteristics of the child, the physician must obtain information about the nature, magnitude, and timing of the exposure. A formal evaluation of the data obtained is then recommended, as described in Table 13.11.

Summary

Approximately 10% of human malformations are due to environmental factors and fewer than 1% of all human malformations are related to chemical agents or prescribed drugs. However, malformations caused by prescription drugs and other therapeutic agents are important because these exposures are preventable. A better understanding of the mechanisms of teratogenesis from all etiologies may improve our ability to predict and test for teratogenicity.

Table 13.10 Information required to analyse the possibility that an environmental agent has altered the risk of congenital malformations in a pregnancy.

What was the nature of the exposure?

Is the exposure agent identifiable? If the agent is identifiable, has it been definitively identified as a reproductive toxin with a recognized constellation of malformations or other reproductive effects?

At what stage did the exposure occur during embryonic and fetal development?

If the agent is known to produce reproductive toxic effects, was the exposure above or below the threshold for these effects?

Were there any other significant environmental exposures or medical problems during the pregnancy?

Is this is a wanted pregnancy or is the family ambivalent about carrying this baby to term?

What is the medical and reproductive history of this mother with regard to prior pregnancies, and the reproductive history of the family lineage?

Table 13.11 Proof of developmental toxicity in humans.

Epidemiological studies
Controlled epidemiological studies consistently demonstrate an increased incidence of a particular spectrum of embryonic and/or fetal effects in exposed human populations

Secular trend data
Secular trends demonstrate a positive relationship between the changing exposures to a common environmental agent in human populations and the incidence of a particular embryonic and/or fetal effect

Animal developmental toxicity studies
An animal model that mimics the human developmental effect at clinically comparable exposures can be developed. Because mimicry may not occur in all animal species, animal models are more likely to be developed once there is good evidence for the embryotoxic effects reported in the human. Developmental toxicity studies in animals are indicative of a potential hazard in general rather than the potential for a specific adverse effect on the fetus when there are no human data on which to base the animal experiments

Dose–response relationship (pharmacokinetics and toxicokinetics)
Developmental toxicity in the human increases with dose (exposure), and the developmental toxicity in animals occurs at a dose that is pharmacokinetically (quantitatively) equivalent to the human exposure

Biological plausibility
The mechanisms of developmental toxicity are understood, and the effects are biologically plausible

---

Modified from: (1) Brent R. Methods of evaluating the alleged teratogenicity of environmental agents. In: Sever J, Brent RL, eds. *Teratogen update: environmentally induced birth defect risks.* New York: Alan R Liss; 1986:199–201; and (2) Brent, R. Method of evaluating alleged human teratogens. *Teratology* 1978;17:83.

Further reading

Brent RL. Bendectin: review of the medical literature of a comprehensively studied human nonteratogen and the most prevalent tortigen-litigen. *Reprod Toxicol* 1995;9:337–349.

Brent RL. Environmental causes of human congenital malformations: the pediatrician's role in dealing with these complex clinical problems caused by a multiplicity of environmental and genetic factors. *Pediatrics* 2004;113:957–968.

Brent RL. Utilization of developmental basic science principles in the evaluation of reproductive risks from pre- and postconception environmental radiation exposures. *Teratology* 1999;59:182–204.

Friedman JM, Polifka JE. *TERIS: The teratogen information system.* Seattle, WA: University of Washington Press, 1999.

Online Mendelian Inheritance in Man, OMIM™. McKusick-Nathans Institute for Genetic Medicine, Johns Hopkins University (Baltimore, MD) and National Center for Biotechnology Information, National Library of Medicine (Bethesda, MD), 2000. World Wide Web URL: http://www.ncbi.nlm.nih.gov/omim/

Schardein JL. *Chemically induced birth defects.* New York: Marcel Dekker; 2002:1109.

Scialli AR, Lione A, Padget GKB. *Reproductive effects of chemical, physical and biologic agents.* Baltimore, MD: Johns Hopkins University Press, 1995.

Sever JL, Brent RL. *Teratogen update: environmentally induced birth defect risks.* New York: Alan R Liss, 1986.

Shepard TH, Lemire RJ. *Catalog of teratogenic agents*, 11th edn. Baltimore, MD: Johns Hopkins University Press, 2004.

Drugs, alcohol abuse, and effects in pregnancy

Stephen R. Carr and Donald R. Coustan

It is daunting to attempt to study the effect of drugs, medications, or substances on developing fetuses. It requires an understanding of embryology, pharmacology, and maternal physiology during pregnancy as well as fetal physiology. Studies of illicit substance use or abuse of licit substances are hampered by inaccurate reporting as well as the problem of multiple substance use. Teasing out the individual effects of a given substance may be challenging indeed. There are numerous compendia available to clinicians describing the effects of marketed pharmaceutical agents.

Alcohol abuse during pregnancy continues to impose a staggering burden on society – upwards of US$40 billion per year (in 1998 dollars) in total, or US$2 million as a lifetime cost per individual affected with fetal alcohol syndrome (FAS).[1] While efforts at establishing a dose–response curve have been stymied by underreporting and multiple substance use, even low and sporadic alcohol ingestion during pregnancy increases the risk of congenital anomalies.[2] The effects of alcohol on the development of the human fetus may result from increased c-myc protein and decreased growth-associated protein 43 levels and their effects on normal neuronal growth and differentiation. As there is no treatment or cure for alcohol-related birth defects, there is no level of alcohol use during pregnancy that can be considered "safe." The "CAGE," "T-ACE," and "TWEAK" questionnaires aid in identifying women at risk for risk drinking, after which counseling interventions will decrease problem drinking by 67%. Drinking cessation at any stage of pregnancy benefits the fetus.

Cocaine is an alkaloid that acts by inhibiting reuptake of norepinephrine and dopamine at presynaptic nerve endings. The elevated dopamine levels are responsible for the euphoria and addictive qualities of cocaine, and the elevated norepinephrine levels are responsible for the hypertension and vasoconstriction seen. Both maternal and fetal effects of cocaine use stem from its vasoconstrictive properties. These include maternal hypertension, increased risk of placental abruption, and increased risk of genitourinary tract anomalies. The increased risk of abruption can persist even if the gravidae stops using cocaine in the first trimester.[3]

Heroin use during pregnancy does not increase structural teratogenesis, but behavioral teratogenesis is likely. Infectious comorbidities including the hepatitides and human immunodeficiency virus (HIV) are substantial. Substitution of methadone for heroin use will decrease the risk of low birthweight babies and premature delivery. The neonatal abstinence syndrome will be minimized with a methadone dose of ≤ 20 mg/day near delivery.

Maternal smoking during pregnancy increases overall perinatal and neonatal mortality by 33%. It is also associated with an increased risk of orofacial clefting anomalies. The "Ask, Advise, Assess, Assist, and Arrange" tool will increase smoking cessation by 30–70% in smoking gravidae, but is most effective in women who smoke ≤ 20 cigarettes per day.

Caffeine is a xanthine and increases intracellular cAMP, altering Ca^{2+} levels and potentiating catecholamine action. Caffeine is teratogenic in rodents, inducing limb and digit anomalies at doses of 50–80 mg/kg. Epidemiologic studies in humans detected no increase in caffeine-associated congenital anomalies. The association between maternal caffeine intake and spontaneous abortion and/or low birthweight is equivocal.

General

Developmental toxicity of drugs or substances depends on:
• dose (total versus chronic infusion versus pulsatile);
• route of administration;
• physiologic handling of the substance by mother/fetus;
• genetic predisposition;
• timing of exposure during pregnancy.

Alcohol use in pregnancy

• FAS seen in 0.3–0.4/1000 live births in the US.

- Effects are secondary to the direct effect of alcohol or its toxic metabolic product acetaldehyde.
- Increased c-myc protein and decreased growth-associated protein 43 levels inhibit normal neuronal growth and differentiation.
- Features of FAS: at least one from each of the following categories:[4]
  - *Growth restriction, either prenatal or postnatal in onset*:
    Small for gestational age (SGA)/intrauterine growth restriction (IUGR);
    Failure to thrive/short stature;
  - *Craniofacial abnormalities*:
    Small eyes;
    Epicanthal folds;
    Long philtrum;
    Midface hypoplasia;
  - *Central nervous system (CNS) abnormalities*:
    Microcephaly;
    Developmental delay;
    Mental retardation;
    Learning disabilities.
  - Alcohol-related birth defects: any of the preceding problems in the offspring of an alcoholic individual.

Categories of alcohol-related birth defects

1 FAS: with confirmed maternal alcohol use and a characteristic pattern of malformations.
2 FAS: without confirmed maternal alcohol use, but with the characteristic pattern of malformations.
3 Partial FAS: with confirmed maternal alcohol use and some components of the characteristic malformations.
4 Alcohol-related birth defects: the presence of congenital anomalies resulting from prenatal alcohol exposure.
5 Alcohol-related neurodevelopmental disorder (ARND): CNS neurodevelopmental abnormalities, neurological hard or soft signs, or behavioral/cognitive abnormalities not consistent with background or environment.

Preventing FAS: CAGE, T-ACE, and TWEAK

CAGE ($\geq$ two positive answers: increased risk for problem drinking).
1 Have you ever felt the need to Cut down drinking?
2 Have you ever felt Annoyed by criticism of your drinking?
3 Have you ever had Guilty feelings about drinking?
4 Have you ever taken a morning "Eye-opener"?

T-ACE (the ability to hold a six-pack of beer or a bottle of wine scores two points on the tolerance question; affirmative answers on the others each score

one point. A cumulative score of more than two points indicates a high probability of being a risk drinker).
1 How many drinks can you hold? (Tolerance)
2 Have you ever felt Annoyed by criticism of your drinking?
3 Have you ever felt the need to Cut down drinking?
4 Have you ever taken a morning "Eye-opener"?

TWEAK (≥ two points on the TWEAK instrument indicates a high probability of problem drinking).[5]
1 Tolerance: how many drinks does it take before you feel the effects of alcohol? (two points for ≥ three drinks)
2 Worry: have close friends or family worried or complained about your drinking in the past year? (two points for yes)
3 Eye-opener: do you sometimes take a drink in the morning when you wake up? (one point for yes)
4 Amnesia: are there times when you drink and afterwards cannot remember what you said or did? (one point for yes)
5 Cut down: do you sometimes feel the need to cut down on your drinking? (one point for yes)

Cocaine use in pregnancy

• Cocaine use seen in 8–24% of pregnant women in various studies.
• Mechanism of action: inhibition of neurotransmitter reuptake at presynaptic nerve terminals.
• Effects of cocaine use in pregnancy:[6]
  – Placental abruption;
  – IUGR;
  – Premature rupture of the membranes;
  – Meconium;
  – Spontaneous abortion;
  – Intrauterine cerebral infarctions;
  – Genitourinary (GU) tract anomalies;
  – Neurobehavioral disorders.
• Increased risk of GU anomalies, with increased trend for other anomalies.
• No such thing as a "crack baby." The effects on neurophysiologic functioning are short-lived and are correlated with other factors such as alcohol, tobacco, and marijuana.[7]

Heroin use in pregnancy

Reported effects of heroin on pregnancy
• Fetal addiction.
• Intrauterine withdrawal/neonatal abstinence syndrome.

- Symptoms of neonatal withdrawal:
  - Tremors;
  - Restlessness;
  - Hyperreflexia;
  - High-pitched cry;
  - Sneezing;
  - Sleeplessness;
  - Tachypnea;
  - Yawning;
  - Sweating;
  - Fever;
  - Convulsions;
  - Vomiting/diarrhea.
- Low birthweight:
  - Relative risk (RR) 4.61 (95% CI, 2.78–7.65) in pregnant heroin users;
  - RR 1.36 (95% CI, 0.83–2.22) in methadone users;
  - RR 3.28 (95% CI, 2.47–4.39) in women who used both.
- Behavioral teratogenesis.
- Sudden infant death syndrome.

Infectious comorbidities associated with drug-seeking behaviors
- HIV;
- Hepatitides.

Tobacco use in pregnancy

- More than 300 substances in tobacco smoke.
- Most effects from nicotine and carbon monoxide.
- Smoking increases perinatal mortality (PNM) by 33%.
- PNM 23.3/1000 births in non-smokers.
- PNM 33.4/1000 births in > 1 pack/day smokers.
- Obstetric morbidities seen in pregnant smokers:
  - Spontaneous abortion;
  - Ectopic pregnancy;
  - Preterm delivery;
  - Placenta previa;
  - IUGR/low birthweight (10–15 g decrease in birthweight per cigarette smoked per day);
  - Placental abruption;
  - Preterm premature rupture of membranes (PPROM);
  - Sudden infant death syndrome.
- Increased risk of orofacial clefts among smokers.
- Prenatal exposure to second-hand smoke manifests as adverse effects on language skills, and visual and spatial abilities.

- Brief interventions increase smoking cessation by 30–70%:
  - *Ask*: ask the patient to chose a statement that best describes her smoking status:
    I've smoked < 100 cigarettes in my lifetime;
    I quit smoking before I found out I was pregnant;
    I quit smoking after I found out I was pregnant;
    I still smoke, but I've cut down;
    I still smoke and I haven't cut down.
  - *Advise*: give clear, firm advice to quit smoking. Stress the benefits to her and the fetus.
  - *Assess*: investigate her willingness to quit.
  - *Assist*: offer and encourage coping mechanisms for quitting smoking (identify trigger situations):
    Provide support as part of the treatment;
    Arrange for social support – involve family and friends;
    Pregnancy-specific smoking cessation programs.
  - *Arrange*: follow-up is essential. Reassess and re-encourage.

Caffeine use in pregnancy

- Caffeine is a xanthine and exerts effects by increasing intracellular cAMP, altering Ca^{2+} levels, and potentiating the effects of catecholamines.
- Caffeine content of drinks:
  - Coffee/tea   100–150 mg/cup;
  - Cola   35–55 mg/12-oz can;
  - Cocoa   200 mg theobromine/cup.
- Increases fetal breathing movements.
- Causes limb defects in rodents given very large doses:
  - Three cases of ectrodactyly in humans associated with 1100–1777 mg daily caffeine intake.
  - No evidence for congenital malformations or other adverse effect on pregnancy for caffeine taken in amounts equivalent to less than 10 cups per day.
- Inconsistent effects of caffeine intake on both birth weight and spontaneous abortion.[10]

References

1 Lupton C, Burd L, Harwood R. Cost of fetal alcohol spectrum disorders. *Am J Med Gen (Part C)* 2004;127C:42.
2 Martinez-Frias ML, Bermejo E, Rodriguez-Pinilla E, et al. Risk for congenital anomalies associated with different sporadic and daily doses of alcohol consumption: a case–control study. *Birth Defects Res (Part A)* 2004;70:194.
3 Chasnoff D, Griggith DR, MacGregor S, et al. Temporal patterns of cocaine use in pregnancy: perinatal outcome. *JAMA* 1989;261:1741.
4 Jones KL, Smith DW. Recognition of the fetal alcohol syndrome in early infancy. *Lancet* 1973;1:999.

5 Russell M, Martier SS, Sokol R. et al. Screening for pregnancy risk drinking. *Alcohol Clin Exp Res* 1994;18:1156.
6 Little BB, Snell LM, Klein VR, et al. Cocaine abuse during pregnancy: maternal and fetal implications. *Obstet Gynecol* 1989;73:157.
7 Frank DA, Augustyn M, Knight WG, et al. Growth, development and behavior in early childhood following prenatal cocaine exposure: a systematic review. *JAMA* 2001;285:1613.
8 Walsh RA. Effects of maternal smoking on adverse pregnancy outcomes: examination of the criteria of causation. *Hum Biol* 1944;66:1059.
9 Meyer KA, Williams P, Hernandez-Diaz S, et al. Smoking and oral clefts: exploring the impact of study design. *Epidemiology* 2004;15:671.
10 Signorello LB, McLaughlin JK. Maternal caffeine consumption and spontaneous abortion: a review of the epidemiologic evidence. *Epidemiology* 2004;15:229.

15 Teratogenic viruses

Antonio V. Sison

There are five known teratogenic viruses: cytomegalovirus (CMV), rubella virus, varicella zoster virus (VZV), herpes simplex virus (HSV), and Venezuelan equine encephalitis (VEE) virus. CMV is the most common cause of congenitally acquired infection; infections with CMV occur at an annual rate of approximately 500–2500 cases per 100 000 newborns worldwide. In comparison, the annual incidence of rubella in the USA in the last few years was approximately 0.05 per 100 000 live births. Table 15.1 provides a summary of birth defects caused by infection with each virus. Recently, the role of parvovirus (Fifth disease) as a teratogenic agent has been questioned. Three of the teratogenic viruses (CMV, VZV, and HSV) are herpesviruses; the fourth member of the herpesvirus group, Epstein–Barr virus, has not been implicated as a teratogen.

All of the teratogenic viruses have a significant effect on the central nervous system (CNS; microcephaly, intracranial calcifications) and the eyes (chorioretinitis, cataracts), and many result in multiorgan damage in the affected newborn. Infants with congenital rubella syndrome (CRS), for example, have findings in many organ systems, such as the CNS, eyes, liver, and lungs. Some viruses cause particular symptoms in the neonate; for example, cicatricial skin scarring and limb hypoplasia is uniquely found in perinatal infection with VZV, whereas oral ulcerations in the neonate are mostly found with herpesvirus infections. Much of the damage caused by teratogenic viruses is subtle and presents only later in life (i.e., learning disabilities, psychomotor retardation, hearing loss, diabetes mellitus, and thyroid disorder).

Diagnosis of congenital infection with teratogenic viruses has generally relied on both clinical manifestations of the disease in the infant and laboratory techniques.

Table 15.1 Birth defects associated with teratogenic viruses.

Cytomegalovirus
Hepatosplenomegaly, jaundice, hepatitis, microcephaly, cerebral calcifications, cerebellar or cortical atrophy, chorioretinitis, optic atrophy, dental defects, microphthalmia, cardiomegaly

Rubella virus
Meningoencephalitis, microcephaly, intracranial calcifications, psychomotor retardation, behavioral disorders, autism, hypotonia, hearing loss, cataracts, retinopathy, glaucoma, cloudy cornea, microphthalmia, subretinal neovascularization, patent ductus arteriosus, pulmonary artery stenosis, pulmonary artery hyperplasia, coarctation of the aorta, ventricular septal defect, atrial septal defect, myocarditis, myocardial necrosis, thrombocytopenia purpura, hepatosplenomegaly, crytorchidism, polycystic kidney

Varicella zoster virus
Cerebral cortical atrophy, microcephaly, encephalitis, intracranial calcifications, bulbar palsy, cerebellar hypolasia, ventriculomegaly, limb paresis, microphthalmia, optic atrophy, cataract, chorioretinitis, anisocoria, corneal opacification, hydrocephalus, meningocele, limb hypoplasia, cicatricial scarring of limb, hypotonia, areflexia, nystagmus, flexion contracture deformities, duodenal stenosis, colon atresia, hydroureter

Herpes simplex virus
Microcephaly, cerebral atrophy, hydrancephaly, intracranial calcifications, encephalitis, learning disability, porencephalic cysts, chorioretinitis, cataracts, retinal dysplasia, keratoconjunctivitis, microphthalmia, hepatosplenomegaly, pneumonitis, oral ulcerations

Venezuelan equine encephalitis
Microphthalmia, microcephaly, absent cerebellum and cerebrum, fluid-filled cranial cavity, CNS necrosis, hydrocephalus, porencephalic cysts, cataracts

The characteristic rashes associated with German measles (rubelliform and macular) and chickenpox (vesicular) have been helpful in differentiating and identifying the cause of infection. Detection of virus-specific IgM in the infant at birth has been used to aid diagnosis; however, infants who acquire an infection during delivery (e.g., HSV) may not show virus-specific IgM at birth. Viral culture has been used in the detection and diagnosis of fetal infection with viruses such as CMV, rubella, and HSV.

The most important milestones in the treatment and prevention of perinatal infection with teratogenic viruses include: (1) the development of vaccines (e.g., rubella and VZV vaccines) to prevent infection and (2) the use of antiviral medication in pregnancy to prevent perinatal transmission. For example, both acyclovir and valaciclovir administered after 35 weeks' gestation have been definitively shown to decrease the symptomatic and asymptomatic viral shedding of herpes simplex virus in the cervix during delivery. This reduction has consequently led to a decrease in Cesarean sections performed solely for active herpes simplex eruptions in labor. For infections such as CMV, when there are no known and definitive treatments, frequent hand washing has been found to be most useful in controlling the spread of the infection.

One of the key challenges in the management of the perinatal transmission of teratogenic viruses is the difficulty of prenatal diagnosis. To date, there are no definitive prenatal diagnostic tests for the teratogenic viruses described in this chapter; most information on prenatal diagnosis comes from samples obtained from amniotic fluid by amniocentesis and from fetal blood by cordocentesis. Detection of virus-specific IgM in these fetal samples has been helpful in prenatal diagnosis, but the specificity and sensitivity of these assays has not been well defined.

Further reading

American College of Obstetricians and Gynecologists Practice Bulletin. Clinical management guidelines for obstetrician-gynecologists, No. 8, 1999. Management of herpes in pregnancy. *Int J Gynecol Obstet* 2000;68:165–173.

American College of Obstetricians and Gynecologists Practice Bulletin. Clinical management guidelines for obstetrician-gynecologists, No. 20, 2000. Perinatal viral and parasitic infections. *Int J Gynecol Obstet* 2002;76:95–107.

Bar-Oz B, Levichek Z, Moretti ME, et al. Pregnancy outcome following rubella vaccination: a prospective controlled study. *Am J Med Genet* 2004;130:52–54.

Castillo-Solorzano C, Carracso P, Tambini G, et al. New horizons in the control of rubella and prevention of congenital rubella syndrome in the Americas. *J Infect Dis* 2003;187(Suppl.1):146–152.

Harger JH, Ernest JM, Thurnau GR, et al. Frequency of congenital varicella syndrome in a prospective cohort of 347 pregnant women. *Obstet Gynecol* 2002;100:260–265.

Jones KL, Johnson KA, Chambers CD. Offspring of women infected with varicella during pregnancy: a prospective study. *Teratology* 1994;49:29–32.

Morris DJ, Sims D, Chiswick M, et al. Symptomatic congenital cytomegalovirus infection after maternal recurrent infection. *Pediatr Infect Dis J* 1994;13:61–64.

Paryani SG, Arvin AM. Intrauterine infection with varicella-zoster virus after maternal rubella. *N Engl J Med* 1986;314:1542–1546.

Revello MG, Gerna G. Pathogenesis and prenatal diagnosis of human cytomegalovirus infection. *J Clin Virol* 2004;29:71–83.

Sheffield JS, Hollier LM, Hill JB, et al. Aciclovir prophylaxis to prevent herpes simplex virus recurrence at delivery: a systematic review. *Obstet Gynecol* 2003;102:1396–1403.

 # Transplacentally acquired microbial infections in the fetus

Santosh Pandipati and Ronald S. Gibbs

Details are provided in Table 16.1.

Table 16.1 Transplacentally acquired microbial infections in the fetus.

Organism /virus	Congenital infection?	Maternal effects	Fetal and neonatal effects	Diagnosis	Treatment
Toxoplasmosis	Yes	Asymptomatic. Malaise, myalgia, fever, painful lymphadenopathy, maculopapular rash, hepatosplenomegaly, lymphocytosis. In immunocompromised patient, pulmonary and central nervous system (CNS) involvement	Intrauterine growth restriction, nonimmune hydrops, hydrocephaly, microcephaly, anencephaly, hydranencephaly, intracranial calcifications, ventricular dilation, hepatomegaly, ascites, placental thickening Neonatal: chorioretinitis, growth restriction, low birthweight, hydrocephalus, microcephaly, intracranial calcifications, jaundice, hepatosplenomegaly, cataracts, microphthalmia, strabismus, blindness, epilepsy, psychomotor or mental retardation,	Maternal: detection of organism-specific IgG and IgM antibodies. Polymerase chain reaction (PCR) utilized in immunocompromised patients Fetal: PCR of amniotic fluid has largely replaced cordocentesis and sampling of fetal blood for detection of organism-specific antibodies	In Europe, treatment of mother aimed at reducing congenital infection. Pyrimethamine (a folic acid antagonist) and sulfa drugs (sulfadiazine or triple sulfonamides), with folinic acid; in Europe, addition of spiramycin Primary prevention is strategy of choice. Pregnant women should wash hands thoroughly after contact with raw meat, cats, and materials potentially contaminated by cat faeces. Meat should be consumed only when it has been cooked to

(Continued)

Table 16.1 *Continued*

Organism /virus	Congenital infection?	Maternal effects	Fetal and neonatal effects	Diagnosis	Treatment
			petechia secondary to thrombocytopenia, anemia, maculopapular rash, pneumonia, vomiting, and diarrhea		hotter than 66°C (about 151°F)
Rubella	Yes	Asymptomatic. Macular rash, malaise, fever, arthralgia, and postauricular and suboccipital adenopathy; arthritis, neuritis, encephalitis, and thrombocytopenia are rare in postnatal infection	Congenital rubella syndrome (CRS): cataracts, cardiac lesions (ventricular septal defect, patent ductus arteriosus, peripheral pulmonic stenosis), retinopathy, thrombocytopenic purpura (blueberry muffin rash), hepatosplenomegaly, osseous lesions, meningoencephalitis, rubelliform rash, developmental delay, hearing loss, growth retardation, pulmonic stenosis, and thrombocytopenia	Maternal: detection of rubella-specific IgM and IgG antibodies. Fetal: cordocentesis to detect rubella-specific IgM in fetal blood at 20–22 weeks' gestation or later. PCR of amniotic fluid possible as well	No specific antiviral therapy for rubella infection. Primary prevention via vaccination is strategy of choice. Administration of vaccine is contraindicated in pregnancy as there is a theoretical risk of acquiring CRS

		Extended CRS: cerebral palsy, mental retardation, developmental and language delay, seizures, cirrhosis, growth retardation, and immunologic disorders (e.g., hypogammaglobulinemia). Delayed CRS: endocrinopathies (diabetes mellitus, thyroid dysfunction, growth hormone deficiency), late-onset deafness and ocular damage, renovascular hypertension, and encephalitis.		
Herpes simplex virus (HSV)	Yes	Systemic symptoms are more common in primary occurrences and can include fever, malaise, myalgia, and headache. Local symptoms include painful vesicles, discharge, adenopathy, Microcephaly, periventricular calcifications, chorioretinitis, intrauterine growth restriction, and vesicular eruptions Neonatal: infection of the skin, eyes,	Viral culture, Pap smear, monoclonal antibody testing, enzyme immunoassay (ELISA), or PCR	Prevention of transmission to fetus and neonate is primary objective. To this end, at term, in cases of active genital lesions or symptoms of vulvar pain or burning, which may indicate an *(Continued)*

Table 16.1 *Continued*

Organism /virus	Congenital infection?	Maternal effects	Fetal and neonatal effects	Diagnosis	Treatment
		dysuria, and urinary retention secondary to pain or local nerve involvement	and mouth, CNS infection (symptoms include seizures, poor feeding, and irritability); disseminated infection, often complicated by encephalitis		impending outbreak, Cesarean delivery is preferable. Minimization of invasive fetal monitoring and avoidance of rupturing membranes more than 4–6h prior to delivery recommended. Among genital HSV patients, prophylactic use of acyclovir starting at 36 weeks' gestation reduces rates of clinical recurrence at delivery, Cesarean delivery for HSV, overall Cesarean delivery, and asymptomatic HSV shedding

| Cytomegalovirus (CMV) | Yes | Usually asymptomatic in immunocompetent host. In some patients, a heterophile-negative mononucleosis-like syndrome may be present; fever, malaise, myalgias, mild pharyngitis, minimal lymphadenopathy, lymphocytosis, and abnormal liver function test results may be present in such cases | Fetal: intrauterine growth retardation, cerebral ventriculomegaly, ascites, microcephaly, hydrocephaly, periventricular calcifications, hepatosplenomegaly, cardiomegaly, hyperechogenic bowel, and oligo- or polyhydramnios, nonimmune hydrops, myocarditis, heart block, and supraventricular tachycardia

Neonatal: hematologic (petechiae/purpura hepatosplenomegaly, jaundice, hemolytic anemia), neurologic (intracranial calcifications, microcephaly, hearing impairment, chorioretinitis, seizures), small for gestational age, pneumonia, and death | Maternal: isolation of the virus from blood, urine, or cervix

Fetal: PCR and/or viral culture of amniotic fluid. Occasionally, cordocentesis to identify virus through CMV-specific IgM antibody, PCR, or viral culture | Symptomatic therapy as necessary for the immunocompetent adult. Currently, no role for antenatal treatment of fetal CMV infection |

(Continued)

Table 16.1 *Continued*

Organism /virus	Congenital infection?	Maternal effects	Fetal and neonatal effects	Diagnosis	Treatment
Parvovirus	Yes	Asymptomatic. Can also include erythema infectiosum, fatigue, fever, adenopathy, arthritis. More serious complications include encephalitis, pneumonia, and hemolytic anemia	Hemolytic anemia, nonimmune hydrops fetalis	Maternal IgM. PCR	Weekly ultrasound evaluation (including monitoring fetal middle cerebral artery peak systolic velocities) for up to 12 weeks following exposure. Intrauterine blood transfusion once there is clinically significant anemia or hydrops fetalis
Varicella	Yes	Fever, malaise, vesicular/pustular rash, pneumonia. Encephalitis, meningitis, myocarditis, glomerulonephritis, and arthritis rare	Fetal: limb hypoplasia, cicatricial skin lesions, atrophic digits, psychomotor retardation, bilateral cortical atrophy, dermatomal skin scarring, ventriculomegaly, microcephaly, gastrointestinal and genitourinary abnormalities	Characteristic clinical presentation. Serologic testing indicated in women with exposure but with a negative or uncertain history of varicella	Vaccination in nonpregnant susceptible women Varicella zoster immune globulin (VZIG) to nonimmune pregnant women with exposure to varicella. Intravenous acyclovir in varicella pneumonia

VZIG for infants at risk

Influenza	No	Abrupt onset of upper respiratory infection, fever, malaise, myalgia, and headache. Pneumonia	None	Isolation of the virus from throat washings during acute illness or by serologic confirmation of a fourfold rise in antibody	Supportive care. Antibiotic therapy for bacterial superinfection
Hepatitis B and C viruses (HBV and HCV)	Yes	Fever, headache, abdominal pain, jaundice, nausea/vomiting, anemia, diabetes. Fulminant hepatitis possible	Not associated with fetal anomalies Congenital infection most often asymptomatic, but can develop jaundice and symptomatic disease by 3–4 months of age	Serologic testing as follows. Acute HBV infection: HBsAg, HBeAg, IgM anti-HBc Chronic HBV infection: HBsAg, ± HBeAg, IgG anti-HBc, anti-HBe Past infection or vaccination: anti-HBs HCV infection: anti-HCV, HCV RNA by RT PCR	Vaccination is mainstay of HBV infection prevention Supportive in cases of acute infection

(Continued)

Table 16.1 *Continued*

Organism/virus	Congenital infection?	Maternal effects	Fetal and neonatal effects	Diagnosis	Treatment
Epstein–Barr virus (EBV)	Rare to have primary infection in pregnancy, even among serosusceptible women; no reported cases of antenatal diagnosis of EBV congenital infection, and only rare case reports of possible association with fetal anomalies	Asymptomatic (>50% of patients) to sore throat, fever, malaise, lymphadenopathy (rare: splenic rupture, meningitis, Guillain–Barré syndrome, death)	Possible association with cardiovascular defects and cataracts, as well as thrombocytopenia, hepatosplenomegaly, seizures, microcephaly, cerebral calcifications in rare case reports only	Maternal: in symptomatic patient, detection of heterophil antibodies or EBV-specific serology Fetal: identification of umbilical cord blood lymphocyte transformation or EBV detection in oropharyngeal secretions	Supportive care in symptomatic patients; in cases with severe complications, corticosteroids and acyclovir have been used
Measles	Rarely causes congenital measles (disease becomes clinically apparent within 10 days of neonatal life)	Fever, cough, coryza, conjunctivitis, maculopapular rash, malaise, Koplik's spots (complications: bacterial pneumonia, otitis media, encephalitis; rare: thrombocytopenic	Increased risk of prematurity, especially with third-trimester disease; no constellation of anomalies	Based on clinical history and clinical presentation	Uncomplicated measles is treated symptomatically; antibiotics for secondary otitis media or pneumonia; susceptible exposed pregnant women, neonates (including

		Clinical manifestations	Effect on fetus/pregnancy	Diagnosis	Treatment
		purpura, myocarditis, subacute sclerosing panencephalitis)			those born to women who have measles in the last week of pregnancy), and contacts should receive passive immunization with immune serum globulin
Mumps	No	Prodrome of fever, malaise, myalgia, anorexia, (bilateral) parotitis (rare: oophoritis, aseptic meningitis, pancreatitis, mastitis, thyroiditis, myocarditis, arthritis, nephritis)	Twofold increase in spontaneous abortion when occurring in the first trimester; possible association with congenital endocardial fibroelastosis	Based on clinical presentation	Symptomatic, supportive treatment; avoid vaccination with MMR vaccine during pregnancy
Listeriosis	Yes	Illness usually in third trimester. May be asymptomatic. Fever, flu-like syndrome, abdominal/back pain, vomiting, diarrhea, headache, myalgia, sore throat. Preterm labor	Fetal and neonatal infection as evidenced by electronic fetal monitoring abnormalities (tachycardia, decreased variability, absence of accelerations); stillbirth; in neonates: respiratory distress, fever, meningismus, seizures, rash, jaundice	Culture and Gram stain of maternal blood, vagina, amniotic fluid (with finding of brown-stained fluid), and neonatal throat, skin, conjunctiva, cerebrospinal fluid	Intravenous antibiotics, usually ampicillin with or without gentamicin

(Continued)

Table 16.1 *Continued*

Organism /virus	Congenital infection?	Maternal effects	Fetal and neonatal effects	Diagnosis	Treatment
Tuberculosis	Yes, most commonly following maternal miliary disease; maternal active pulmonary disease is more likely to lead to postnatal infection	May be asymptomatic. Cough, weight loss, fever, malaise, fatigue, hemoptysis. Increased rate of preeclampsia, placental abruption/ vaginal bleeding	Spontaneous abortion, stillbirth; no increase in anomalies. Neonatal: low birthweight, hepatosplenomegaly, respiratory distress, fever, lymphadenopathy.	Mother and neonate: PPD testing, chest X-ray, possible lumbar puncture, and culture of appropriate sites. Placental examination and culture including acid-fast staining	In pregnant mother: antibiotic therapy for 9 months with rifampin, isoniazid, ethambutol, pyridoxine; pyrazinamide controversial
Group B streptococcus	Yes	Asymptomatic. Chorioamnionitis. Urinary tract infections including pyelonephritis. Rarely causes necrotizing fasciitis and meningitis. Preterm labor. Postpartum endometritis	Neonatal: sepsis, pneumonia, meningitis, possible death Long-term neurologic sequelae possible in cases of meningitis	Rectovaginal culture at 35–37 weeks' gestation, with sensitivities in cases of anaphylactic penicillin allergy	Penicillin. In penicillin-allergic patient without anaphylaxis, treat with cefazolin intrapartum. If history of anaphylaxis, testing for susceptibility to erythromycin and clindamycin; if resistant to either or both, treat with vancomycin intrapartum

Further reading

Brown Z. Preventing herpes simplex virus transmission to the neonate. *Herpes* 2004; 11(Suppl):175A–186A.

Brown ZA, Wald A, Morrow RA, et al. Effect of serologic status and cesarean delivery on transmission rates of herpes simplex virus from infant to mother. *JAMA* 2003; 289(2):203–209.

Centers for Disease Control and Prevention. Prevention of perinatal group B streptococcal disease. *MMWR Morbid Mortal Wkly Rep* 2002:51(RR11).

Centers for Disease Control. Preventing congenital toxoplasmosis. *MMWR Morbid Mortal Wkly Rep* 2000;l49(RR02):57–75.

Cosmi E, Mari G, Delle Chiaie L, et al. Noninvasive diagnosis by Doppler ultrasonography of fetal anemia resulting from parvovirus infection. *Am J Obstet Gynecol* 2002; 187(5):1290–1293.

Poland GA, Jacobson RM. Clinical practice: prevention of hepatitis B with the hepatitis B vaccine. *N Engl J Med* 2004;351(27):2832–2838.

Revello MG, Gerna G. Diagnosis and management of human cytomegalovirus infection in the mother, fetus, and newborn infant. *Clin Microbiol Rev* 2002;15(4):680–715.

Revello MG, Gerna G. Pathogenesis and prenatal diagnosis of human cytomegalovirus infection. *J Clin Virol* 2004;29:71–83.

Sheffield JS, Hollier LM, Hill JB, et al. Acyclovir prophylaxis to prevent herpes simplex virus recurrence at delivery: a systematic review. *Obstet Gynecol* 2003;102:1396–1403.

Viral Hepatitis. Department of Medical Microbiology, University of Cape Town, February 1999. World Wide Web URL: http://web.uct.ac.za/depts/mmi/jmoodie/dihep.html.

17 Antibiotics and other antimicrobial agents in pregnancy and during lactation

Janet I. Andrews and Jennifer R. Niebyl

Most antibiotics are safe to use during pregnancy and lactation. The exceptions are outlined in the following paragraphs.

Amoxicillin/clavulanic acid should be avoided in women at risk for preterm delivery, as it has been shown to increase the risk of necrotizing enterocolitis in the premature infant.[1]

Some reports suggest that certain cephalosporins may increase the risk of birth defects when taken in the first trimester of pregnancy.[2] For this reason, the use of drugs whose actions are better understood, such as erythromycin and ampicillin, is preferred in the first trimester.

Sulfamethoxazole can compete with bilirubin for albumin-binding sites in the newborn and increase the risk of jaundice. These drugs are compatible with pregnancy and lactation unless the infant is ill or premature.[3]

Table 17.1 Teratogenic effects of antibiotics and anti-infective agents.

Drug	First-trimester teratogen	Perinatal effects	Compatible with lactation
Penicillins	No	No	Yes
Amoxicillin/clavulanate	No	Necrotizing enterocolitis in premature infants	Yes
Cephalosporins	Unclear: may be specific to cephalosporin	No	Yes
Sulfamethoxazole	No	Compete with bilirubin for albumin-binding sites; increased risk of jaundice	Yes, except in ill or premature infants
Trimethoprim	Possible	No	Yes
Nitrofurantoin	No	No	Yes
Tetracyclines	No	Tooth discoloration, decreased bone growth	Yes
Aminoglycosides	No	Ototoxicity (deafness)	Yes
Erythromycin	No	No	Yes
Clindamycin	No	No	Yes
Fluoroquinolones	No	Arthropathies in exposed children?	Yes
Metronidazole	No	No	Unknown
Acyclovir	No	No	Yes
Zidovudine	No	No	Yes
Amantidine	Possible	Unknown	Unknown
Isoniazid	No	Maternal hepatitis	Yes

Trimethoprim may be associated with an increased risk of birth defects, particularly cardiovascular defects, when administered during the first trimester of pregnancy.[4] Thus, in combination with sulfa drugs, it should not be used to treat urinary tract infections during this stage of pregnancy.

Tetracyclines given during the second and third trimester of pregnancy can cause tooth discoloration and decreased bone growth.[5] Alternative drugs are therefore preferred.

Aminoglycosides may cause ototoxicity and deafness,[6] and prolonged use during pregnancy should be avoided.

Fluoroquinolones have a high affinity for bone tissue and cartilage and may cause arthropathies in children. No birth defects have been noted;[7] however, the manufacturer recommends against the use of fluoroquinolones in pregnancy and children.

There is no evidence of any teratogenic effect of isoniazid (INH);[8] however, there is a small possibility of liver toxicity. In the treatment of a patient with a positive purified protein derivative (PPD) test with a negative chest radiograph, this therapy should be delayed until after delivery. If the probability of tuberculosis is moderate to high, triple-drug therapy with INH, rifampin, and ethambutol can be given during pregnancy.[9]

The effects of amantadine during pregnancy and lactation are unknown.[10]

References

1 Kenyon SL, Taylor DJ, Tarnow-Mordi W. Broad-spectrum antibiotics for preterm, prelabour rupture of fetal membranes: the ORACLE I randomized trial. ORACLE Collaborative Group. *Lancet* 2001;357:979.

2 Briggs GG, Freeman RK, Yaffe SJ. *Drugs in pregnancy and lactation*, 6th edn. Baltimore, MD: Williams and Wilkins; 2002:222.

3 Harris RC, Lucey JF, MacLean JR. Kernicterus in premature infants associated with low concentration of bilirubin in the plasma. *Pediatrics* 1950;23:878.

4 Briggs GG, Freeman RK, Yaffe SJ. *Drugs in pregnancy and lactation*, 6th edn. Baltimore, MD: Williams and Wilkins; 2002:1393.

5 Cohlan SQ, Bevelander G, Tiamsic T. Growth inhibition of prematures receiving tetracycline. *Am J Dis Child* 1963;105:453.

6 Nishimura H, Tanimura T. *Clinical aspects of the teratogenicity of drugs*. Amsterdam: Excerpta Medica; 1976:131.

7 Pastuszak A, Andreou R, Schick B, et al. New postmarketing surveillance data supports a lack of association between quinolone use in pregnancy and fetal and neonatal complications. *Reprod Toxicol* 1995;9:584.

8 American Thoracic Society. Treatment of tuberculosis and tuberculosis infection in adults and children. *Am J Respir Crit Care Med* 1994;149:1359.

9 Blumberg HM, Burman WJ, Chaisson RE, et al. American Thoracic Society/Centers for Disease Control and Prevention/Infectious Diseases Society of America: treatment of tuberculosis. *Am J Respir Crit Care Med* 2003;167:603.

10 Rosa F. Amantadine pregnancy experience. *Reprod Toxicol* 1994;8:531.

Fetal Diseases

18 Principles of human genetics: chromosomal and single-gene disorders

Joe Leigh Simpson and Maurice J. Mahoney

Introduction

Genetic disorders can result from any one of several mechanisms: numerical or structural alterations in chromosomal constitution, mutation involving a single genetic locus (mendelian), or the cumulative effect of several genes (polygenic), possibly interacting with environmental factors (polygenic–multifactoral). Perturbations of these genetic mechanisms are responsible for most of the anomalies considered in Part VI.

Chromosomal abnormalities

Chromosomal abnormalities represent a common cause of malformations. At birth, 1 in 160 liveborns has a chromosomal abnormality, half of these are due to defects on autosomes and the other half are due to defects on sex chromosomes.[1] Detecting these abnormalities is by far the most common indication for prenatal genetic diagnosis.

Methods of analysis

Chromosomal analyses are usually performed on peripheral blood (lymphocytes) or fibroblasts cultured from skin, gonads, chorionic villi (mesenchyme), or amniotic fluid cells. Very rapidly dividing cells (e.g., bone marrow, chorionic villus trophoblasts, fetal cord blood, newborn cord blood, or cancer cells) may sometimes be analyzed without culturing. Usually, 7–10 days are required to obtain results from cultured villi or amniotic fluid cells. Rapid techniques utilize fluorescence *in situ* hybridization (FISH) in which a single-stranded DNA probe hybridizes to determine whether the complementary sequence is present in (patients') DNA (Fig. 18.1). FISH analysis with chromosome-specific probes can produce results within hours.

Routine cytogenetic analysis usually reveals approximately 450–500 bands per haploid set of chromosomes. At this level, each band consists of approximately 1500–2000 kilobases (kb) of DNA, which are capable of translating perhaps 15–20

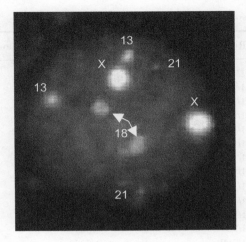

Figure 18.1 Fluorescence *in situ* hybridization (FISH) on a human blastomere biopsied from an eight-cell stage embryo. Fluorescent signals corresponding to specific chromosomes 13, 18, 21, and X are shown, demonstrating detection of a normal female (XX) embryo. Courtesy of Farideh Z. Bischoff. Department of Obstetrics and Gynecology, Baylor College of Medicine, Houston, TX, USA.

genes. Deletions, duplications, and rearrangements involving considerable stretches of DNA can thus pass undetected, even with high-resolution chromosomal analysis.

Numerical chromosomal abnormalities

If a haploid gamete or diploid cell lacks the expected number of chromosomes (n or $2n$), *aneuploidy* exists. If an additional chromosome is present ($2n + 1$), *trisomy* exists.

Trisomy may arise by several cytological mechanisms, but in humans it usually arises *de novo* after meiotic nondisjunction. Nondisjunction may originate after failure of homologous chromosomes to disjoin in meiosis I or failure of sister chromatids to disjoin in either meiosis II or mitosis. In humans, maternal meiosis I is by far the most common cytological origin of autosomal trisomy. In turn, the frequency of trisomy increases with maternal age from at least early in the third decade (Table 18.1).

Structural chromosomal abnormalities

Chromosomal deletion involves the loss of one part of a chromosome. Deficiencies usually result from breakage and loss of an acentric fragment. Autosomal deficiency usually leads to embryonic death or malformation, but deficiency in a sex chromosome is not necessarily as damaging.

111

Table 18.1 Chromosomal abnormalities in liveborns.

Maternal age	Risk of Down syndrome	Total risk of chromosomal abnormalities
20	1/1667	1/526*
21	1/1667	1/526*
22	1/1429	1/500*
23	1/1429	1/500*
24	1/1250	1/476*
25	1/1250	1/476*
26	1/1176	1/476*
27	1/1111	1/455*
28	1/1053	1/435*
29	1/1000	1/417*
30	1/952	1/384*
31	1/909	1/385*
32	1/769	1/322*
33	1/625	1/317
34	1/500	1/260
35	1/385	1/204
36	1/294	1/164
37	1/227	1/130
38	1/175	1/103
39	1/137	1/82
40	1/106	1/65
41	1/82	1/51
42	1/64	1/40
43	1/50	1/32
44	1/38	1/25
45	1/30	1/20
46	1/23	1/15
47	1/18	1/12
48	1/14	1/10
49	1/11	1/7

From ref. 1. Because sample size for some intervals is relatively small, confidence limits are sometimes relatively large. Nonetheless, these figures are suitable for genetic counseling.
*47,XXX excluded for ages 20–32 (data not available).

If, after chromosome breakage or nonhomologous recombination, material is exchanged between two or more chromosomes, a *translocation* is said to have occurred (Fig. 18.2). Rearrangement of genes need not necessarily be deleterious, provided genes are neither lost nor gained. If the individual is phenotypically normal, it is assumed that no genetic material is lost; such a translocation is said to be balanced. If a translocation has led to a deficiency or excess of genetic material, the rearrangement is said to be unbalanced. Even if not evident by karyotype, an

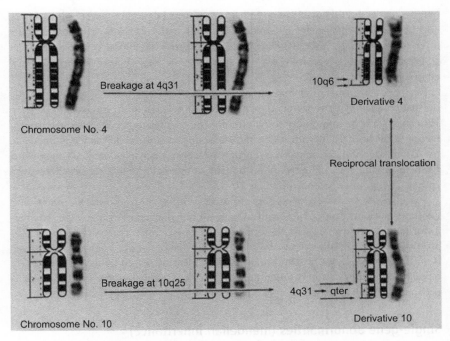

Breakage at 4q31

10q6

Derivative 4

Chromosome No. 4

Reciprocal translocation

Breakage at 10q25

4q31 → qter

Chromosome No. 10

Derivative 10

Figure 18.2 A reciprocal translocation between chromosomes 4 and 10. Origin of derivative chromosomes is shown. From Simpson JL, Tharapel AT. Principles of cytogenetics. In: Phillip E, Barnes J, eds. *Scientific foundations of obstetrics and gynecology*, 4th edn. London: Butterworth-Heinemann; 1991:4;49, with permission.

unbalanced rearrangement can be assumed if the individual is phenotypically abnormal.

Translocations may be either reciprocal or robertsonian. In *reciprocal* translocations, breaks and rearrangements occur in two or more chromosomes but do not involve centromeres. Translocation carriers thus still have 46 chromosomes, although two pairs of homologous chromosomes differ in morphology and composition. In *robertsonian* translocations, acrocentric chromosomes (nos 13, 14, 15, 21, and 22) fuse at their centromere. Because no single acrocentric short arm is essential, heterozygotes are phenotypically normal. These individuals have only 45 chromosomes (centromeres) as a result of the fusion.

Genetic counseling in translocations

Robertsonian translocations involve the acrocentric chromosomes 13, 14, 15, 21, and 22. The most common single translocations involve chromosomes 14 and 21; of those individuals with Down syndrome, 2–3% are affected as a result of this translocation. Although, theoretically, one-third of viable offspring of translocation heterozygotes should have Down syndrome, empirical data reveal that only 10–15% and 2–4% of offspring of female and male heterozygotes, respectively, are affected.[2,3] Liveborn normal offspring have an equal likelihood of showing either translocation heterozygosity ($2n = 45$), like their parents, or normal chromosomal complements ($2n = 46$).

Reciprocal translocation may be ascertained in several ways. A phenotypically normal couple having repeated abortions may show a balanced translocation, or an abnormal fetus or infant may show an unbalanced karyotype. The risk of a parent having a liveborn child with a chromosomal duplication or deficiency is higher in the latter situation, presumably reflecting selection against unbalanced segregants (gametes or embryos.) The risk of both males and females with a reciprocal translocation having an unbalanced fetus is 10–15%.[2,3]

Sometimes a translocation appears to arise *de novo*. In liveborns, an infant with an abnormal phenotype is assumed to have an unbalanced rearrangement, whereas a normal phenotype suggests the opposite. In fetuses, such reasoning is more hazardous because the full extent of a malformation may not yet be manifested. Even if an ultrasound shows no abnormalities, the risk is increased by as much as 7% if a reciprocal translocation is present and by 3–4% if a robertsonian translocation is present.

Single-gene abnormalities (mendelian inheritance)

The familial patterns followed by mendelian traits[4] depend not only on whether the mutant gene is dominant or recessive but also on whether the gene is located on an autosome or a sex chromosome. Potential patterns of transmission include autosomal dominant, autosomal recessive, X-linked dominant, X-linked recessive, and Y-linked.

Autosomal dominant inheritance

An autosomal dominant allele is recognized by its ability to be expressed in more than one generation (Fig. 18.3). In autosomal dominant traits, equal numbers of males and females are usually affected. The likelihood that an individual carrying a mutant autosomal dominant gene (allele) will transmit that allele to any given offspring, male or female, is 50%.

Dominant disorders need not always have been transmitted from an affected parent. The disorder may have arisen *de novo*, as result of a new mutation in a sperm or oocyte. The more severe the trait, the more likely that an affected individual has a new mutation. All individuals with a dominant trait conferring sterility must represent a new mutation.

Autosomal recessive inheritance

An autosomal recessive trait is expressed when an individual is homozygous for a mutant allele. At a given genetic locus, both alleles are abnormal. Alleles can also exist at a single locus (compound heterozygosity) and, for most disorders, this is

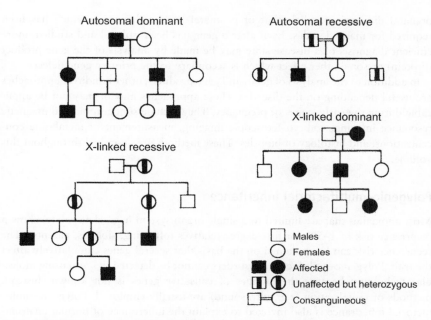

Figure 18.3 Idealized pedigree of common modes of mendelian inheritance. From Simpson JL. Disorders of sexual differentiation: etiology and clinical delineation. New York: Academic Press, 1976;1.

the rule. An individual with a recessive trait is usually the product of a mating between parents who are both heterozygous (carriers) for mutation at the same locus. If two heterozygotes mate, the likelihood that a given offspring will be affected is 25%. Although both alleles must be dysfunctional, the actual mutation present need not necessarily be identical; different nucleotides or other molecular mechanisms may exist.

X-linked recessive inheritance

A mutant recessive gene located on the X chromosome is expressed by all males (46,XY) who carry it; such individuals are said to be hemizygous. X-linked recessive alleles are usually transmitted through phenotypically normal yet actually heterozygous females. Family members at risk include male siblings, maternal uncles, and maternal male first cousins.

Detecting single-gene disorders

The primary abnormality in a single-gene disorder lies in the structure of the gene, or, less often, in a controlling element of that gene. The simplest approach is analysis of the gene *per se*. This has become possible for over 200 genes, but for most mendelian disorders the gene is either not yet known or has not yet been isolated and studied. Thus, other diagnostic strategies are necessary. The situation in prenatal diagnosis parallels that of postnatal genetic diagnosis, which has been required for many decades. Even after a gene has been isolated and studied, more efficient diagnosis of a disease state may be made by analysis of the gene product (protein) or some other effect which is secondary to the primary gene defect.

In addition to the analysis of genes and gene products, other nondirect approaches are useful depending on the disorder. These approaches may or may not be applicable during the early stages of pregnancy. They include sonographic and magnetic resonance imaging, embryo fetoscopic imaging, measurement of metabolite concentrations, and histology of biopsies. These methods are described throughout this volume.

Polygenic–multifactorial inheritance

Most anomalies that are limited to a single organ system (e.g., cleft palate) show a recurrence risk of 1–5% for first-degree relatives (offspring, siblings, parents). The recurrence risk can be explained on the basis that several genes cumulatively affect the trait. Polygenic–multifactoral disorders cannot be detected *in utero* using molecular techniques because the number of causative genes is not known. Instead, methods of visualization (e.g., ultrasound) are usually employed. Polygenic–multifactorial inheritance is also invoked to explain the inheritance of normal anatomical and physiological variables that display *continuous variation*: height, skin color, hair color, blood pressure, age of menarche, and ability to metabolize a given drug or toxin.

References

1 Hook EB. Rates of chromosome abnormalities at different maternal ages. *Obstet Gynecol* 1981;58:282.
2 Boue A, Gallano P. A collaborative study of the segregation of inherited chromosome structural rearrangements in 1356 prenatal diagnoses. *Prenat Diagn* 1984;4:45.
3 Daniel A, Hook EB, Wulf G. Risks of unbalanced progeny at amniocentesis to carriers of chromosome rearrangements: data from European, USA, and Canadian laboratories. *Am J Med Genet* 1989;33:14.
4 Online Mendelian Inheritance in Man, OMIM. McKusick-Nathans Institute for Genetic Medicine, Johns Hopkins University (Baltimore, MD) and National Center for Biotechnology Information, National Library of Medicine (Bethesda, MD), 1998. World Wide Web URL: http://www.ncbi.nlm.nih.gov/omim/.

Further reading

Jorde LB, Carey JC, Bamshad MJ, et al. *Medical genetics*, 3rd edn. St. Louis, MO: Mosby, 2003.
Milunsky A. *Genetic disorders and the fetus: diagnosis, prevention, and treatment*. Baltimore, MD: Johns Hopkins University Press, 2004.
Mueller RF, Young ID. *Emery's elements of medical genetics*, 11th edn. New York: Churchill Livingstone, 2001.

Nussbaum RL, McInnes RR, Willard HF, et al. *Thompson and Thompson genetics in medicine*, 6th edn. Philadelphia, PA: Saunders, 2004.

Simpson JL. Genetic counseling and prenatal diagnosis. In: Gabbe SG, Niebyl JR, Simpson JL, eds. *Obstetrics: normal and problem pregnancies*, 4th edn. New York: Churchill Livingstone; 2002:187–220.

Simpson JL, Elias S. *Genetics in obstetrics and gynecology*, 3rd edn (chapters 1–4). Philadelphia, PA: WB Saunders, 2003.

19 Basic principles of ultrasound

*Mladen Predanic, Frank A. Chervenak, and
E. Albert Reece*

Ultrasound has had a profound influence on the practice of medicine, especially in obstetrics. The latest generation of diagnostic ultrasound machines have superb resolution, three-dimensional capabilities, and various Doppler modalities that are convenient to use and comfortable for the patient.

An *ultrasound* is a sound with frequencies higher than the human ear can detect. The frequency of ultrasound that is used in medicine for fetal imaging is in the range of 3–7.5 million cycles per second (megahertz, MHz). Such high-frequency ultrasound is generated by high mechanical deformation of certain materials (e.g., crystals or ceramics), caused by electrical stimulation, which produces a generation of waves at ultrasound frequencies. This phenomenon is known as the *piezoelectric effect*. Reflected ultrasound "echoes" from the assessed tissue are analyzed by the computer software and converted into an image. Depending on the mode of data analysis, we are able to demonstrate tissue structures as two-, three-, and four-dimensional images, display blood vessels contained in the analyzed tissue or organ in color, or display power and pulsed Doppler images.

Some evidence exists that high-energy ultrasound may produce biological effects in exposed tissues. The most studied effects are the local increase in temperature (thermal changes) and oscillatory and potentially catastrophic motions of bubbles, if present, in the tissues (microcavitation). It is possible that certain stages of embryonic and fetal development may be susceptible to thermal effects, although there appears to be a threshold at which temperature rises of 1.5°C or higher are considered necessary for damage to occur. However, the energy output of the *diagnostic* ultrasound is of such low intensity that it is unlikely to induce a temperature change that is sufficient to produce adverse pregnancy effects. In addition, no recently published study has demonstrated any unequivocal adverse effects of the diagnostic ultrasound. Mechanical effects are described as an interaction of sound with microscopic gas bubbles that pre-exist in tissues which may cause a bioeffect termed *microcavitation* or acoustic cavitation. The succession of positive and negative pressures cause oscillatory motions of bubbles that can produce cell membrane disruption and the release of free radicals that are cell toxic. Although there is no direct evidence to suggest that in humans, under clinical conditions, ultrasound-induced microcavitation produces biological effects, there is consensus that the method of displaying ultrasonic output should control and minimize possible bio-effects in insonated fetal tissues. If an ultrasound machine exceeds predetermined limits for output, either a thermal index or mechanical index must be displayed on the screen. Nevertheless, in general, it is safe to say that, when sonography is performed for a valid medical indication by a well-trained individual who respects the basic rules of time and exposure, the information that can be obtained is of such great value that it clearly overshadows any remote risks that may exist. In contrast to medical indications, performing ultrasound for "keepsake" records of the fetus, especially in the first trimester of the pregnancy, should be discouraged.

The current recommendation of the American College of Obstetricians and Gynecologists (ACOG) is that ultrasound in pregnancy should be performed only when there is a valid medical indication (Table 19.1). Therefore, a physician is not obli-

Table 19.1 Indications for ultrasonography during pregnancy.

Estimation of gestational age
Evaluation of fetal growth
Vaginal bleeding
Abdominal and pelvic pain
Incompetent cervix
Determination of fetal presentation
Suspected multiple gestation
Adjunct to amniocentesis
Significant uterine size and clinical dates discrepancy
Pelvic mass
Suspected hydatidiform mole
Adjunct to cervical cerclage placement
Suspected ectopic pregnancy
Suspected fetal death
Suspected uterine abnormality
Evaluation for fetal well-being
Suspected amniotic fluid abnormalities
Suspected placental abruption
Adjunct to external cephalic version
Premature rupture of membranes and/or premature labor
Abnormal biochemical markers
Follow-up evaluation of a fetal anomaly
Follow-up evaluation of placental location for suspected placenta previa
History of previous congenital anomaly
Evaluation of fetal condition in late registrants for prenatal care

Modified from American Institute of Ultrasound in Medicine (AIUM). Practice guideline for the performance of an antepartum obstetric ultrasound examination. *J Ultrasound Med* 2003; 22: 1116-25.

gated to perform ultrasonography in a patient who is at low risk and has no indications. However, if a patient requests ultrasonography, it is reasonable to honor the request—the final decision to have an ultrasound scan rests with the physician and patient jointly. Regardless of the ultrasound indication, it is our belief that the benefits of routine ultrasound in pregnancy outweigh the risks associated with potential adverse ultrasound effects. An early recognition of fetal anomalies may introduce *in utero* treatment, or at least prepare parents for the emotional ordeal that follows delivery of the fetus with a major malformation. At the present time, three types of ultrasound examinations are performed during the second or third trimester of pregnancy: (1) *standard* examination, which includes an evaluation of fetal presentation, amniotic fluid volume, cardiac activity, placental position, fetal biometry, and an anatomic survey; (2) *limited* examination, which is performed

Table 19.2 Essential elements of the fetal anatomic ultrasound survey.

Head and neck
Cerebellum
Choroid plexus
Cisterna magna
Lateral cerebral ventricles
Midline falx
Cavum septi pellucidi

Chest
The basic cardiac examination includes a four-chamber view of the fetal heart. If technically feasible, an extended basic cardiac examination can also be attempted to evaluate both outflow tracts

Abdomen
Stomach (presence, size, and situs)
Kidneys
Bladder
Umbilical cord insertion site into the fetal abdomen
Umbilical cord vessel number

Spine
Cervical, thoracic, lumbar, and sacral spine

Extremities
Legs and arms (presence or absence)

Gender
Medically indicated in low-risk pregnancies only for evaluation of multifetal gestations

---

Modified from American Institute of Ultrasound in Medicine (AIUM). Practice guidelines for the performance of an antepartum obstetric ultrasound examination. *J Ultrasound Med* 2003; 22: 1116–1125.

Table 19.3 Indications for ultrasound in the first trimester of pregnancy.

To confirm the presence of an intrauterine pregnancy
To evaluate a suspected ectopic pregnancy
To define the cause of vaginal bleeding
To evaluate pelvic pain
To estimate gestational age
To diagnose or evaluate multiple gestations
To confirm cardiac activity
As an adjunct to chorionic villus sampling, embryo transfer, or localization and removal of an intrauterine device
To evaluate maternal pelvic masses or uterine abnormalities
To evaluate suspected hydatidiform mole

Modified from American Institute of Ultrasound in Medicine (AIUM). Practice guideline for the performance of an antepartum obstetric ultrasound examination. *J Ultrasound Med* 2003;22:1116–1125.

when a specific question requires investigation, e.g., it may be employed to verify fetal presentation in a laboring patient, or confirm heart activity in a patient with absent fetal movements; and (3) *specialized* examination, which is a detailed or targeted anatomic examination that is performed when an anomaly is suspected on the basis of the patient's history, biochemical abnormalities, or clinical evaluation (Table 19.2). Other specialized examinations include fetal Doppler studies, biophysical profile, fetal echocardiography or additional biometric studies. In addition to the indications for ultrasound in the second and third trimester of pregnancy, Table 19.3 demonstrates indications for its use in the first trimester of pregnancy.

Further reading

Abramowicz JS, Kossoff G, Marsal K, ter Haar G. International Society of Ultrasound in Obstetrics and Gynecology (ISUOG) Safety and Bioeffects Committee: safety statement. *Ultrasound Obstet Gynecol* 2000;16:594–596.

American College of Obstetricians and Gynecologists. *Clinical management guidelines for obstetrician–gynecologists*, no. 58, December 2004.

American Institute of Ultrasound in Medicine. Mechanical bioeffects from diagnostic ultrasound: AIUM consensus statements. *J Ultrasound Med* 2000; 19:69–168.

American Institute of Ultrasound in Medicine (AIUM). Practice guideline for the performance of an antepartum obstetric ultrasound examination. *J Ultrasound Med* 2003;22:1116–1125.

Barnett SB, Maulik D, International Perinatal Doppler Society. Guidelines and recommendations for safe use of Doppler ultrasound in perinatal applications. *J Maternal Fetal Med* 2001:10:75–84.

Barnett SB, Kossoff G, Edwards MJ. Is diagnostic ultrasound safe? Current international consensus on the thermal mechanism. *Med J Aust* 1994;160:33–37.

Dalecki D. Mechanical bioeffects of ultrasound. *Annu Rev Biomed Eng* 2004;6:229–248.

Duck FA. Is it safe to use diagnostic ultrasound during the first trimester (Editorial)? *Ultrasound Obstet Gynecol* 1999;13:385–388.

Kremkau FW. *Diagnostic ultrasound: principles and instruments*, 6th edn. Philadelphia, PA; WB Saunders, 2002.

Seeds JW. The routine or screening obstetrical ultrasound examination. *Clin Obstet Gynecol* 1996;39:814–830.

20 Prenatal diagnosis of central nervous system malformations

Gianluigi Pilu and Sandro Gabrielli

The incidence of central nervous system malformation is in the range of 1 in 100 births.

Ultrasound allows the diagnosis of many malformations from mid-gestation; the results of the examination partly depend upon the expertise of the sinologist and the time dedicated to the examination; a standard sonogram is performed in low-risk patients by the use of two scanning planes demonstrating the lateral ventricles and posterior fossa. An expert sonogram is performed by using other scanning planes oriented along the sutures and fontanelles of the fetal head that allow the identification of other details; the use of three-dimensional ultrasound facilitates the examination. Magnetic resonance is also frequently used in fetuses at high risk of cerebral malformations, particularly to assess hemorrhage, abnormalities of cortical development, and complex cerebral anomalies.

Measurement of the internal diameter of the lateral ventricular atrium is recommended in any standard examination performed in the second and third trimesters. Under normal conditions, the measurement is less than 10 mm; a value of 10 mm greatly increases the likelihood of a cerebral anomaly; an atrial diameter of more than 15 mm is usually associated with an intracranial malformation. An atrial diameter of 10–15 mm, a condition usually referred to as mild ventriculomegaly, may represent a normal variant, but greatly increases the likelihood of cerebral anomalies and extracerebral anomalies, chromosomal aberrations, and abnormal neurodevelopment (Fig. 20.1).

Anencephaly is easily diagnosed sonographically at mid-gestation and may be identified as early as 12 weeks' gestation; spina bifida is one of the most frequent anomalies of the central nervous system; the most severe type, the open variety, can be identified sonographically by mid-gestation, although the diagnosis is at times difficult; obstetric patients usually undergo screening by assay of maternal serum alpha-fetoprotein; the sonographic diagnosis is assisted by the demonstration of typical cranial alterations, the lemon and banana sign, that are usually easier to identify

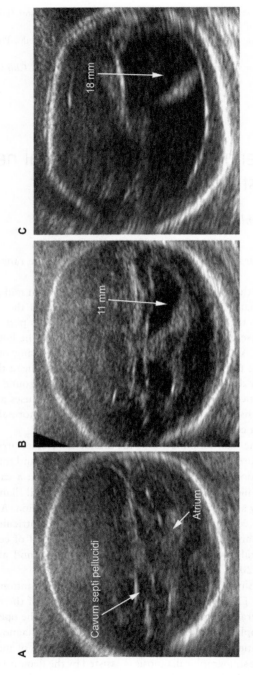

Figure 20.1 (A) Normal transventricular scan demonstrating an atrium of the lateral ventricle of normal size; (B) mild ventriculomegaly; (C) severe ventriculomegaly.

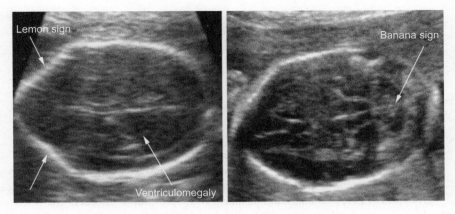

Lemon sign

Banana sign

Ventriculomegaly

Figure 20.2 The cranial signs associated with open spina bifida.

than the spinal defect (Fig. 20.2). Closed spina bifida is usually unpredictable sonographically.

The most severe varieties of holoprosencephaly, the alobar and semilobar forms, are usually recognized by mid-gestation by the demonstration of the absence of the midline echo and the presence of a single rudimentary ventricular cavity; the less severe variety of holoprosencephaly is more difficult to identify and diagnose; the main clue is the absence of the cavum septi pellucidi and the central fusion of the frontal horns. Agenesis of the corpus callosum may be one of the most frequent congenital anomalies; in a standard examination, it may be suspected by indirect findings, such as mild ventriculomegaly and/or the absence of the cavum septi pellucidi; a specific sonographic diagnosis is possible but requires an expert examination; agenesis of the corpus callosum is an important risk factor for mental retardation; infants with isolated agenesis of the corpus callosum may have a normal, albeit frequently low, intellect.

The term Dandy–Walker complex is used to define cases in which the cisterna magna is large (more than 10 mm) and/or there is hypoplasia of the cerebellar vermis; many variations exist, and the prognosis is difficult to predict.

Many congenital anomalies of the cerebrum are not the consequence of an embryogenetic malformative process, but are due to a destructive antenatal event, usually hemorrhagic or ischemic; fetal intracranial hemorrhage may be recognized by sonography, but the findings vary depending upon the time the lesion has occurred and the severity of the hemorrhage; most intracranial bleeding occurs at the level of the ventricles; a recent hemorrhage appears as an echogenic collection that may be associated with ventricular enlargement; in the weeks following the hemorrhage, the blood clot retracts and develops a sonolucent core; severe forms of intraventricular hemorrhage (those associated with either hydrocephalus and/or destruction of the nearby cortex) are associated with an excess of perinatal deaths and neurologic compromise.

Destructive insults to the brain result in cystic cavities (porencephaly) of the cortex; cystic degeneration of the white matter (periventricular leukomalacia) has also been described in the fetus; in some cases, these lesions are the consequence of obstetric complications such as intrauterine hypoxia/ischemia, infections, or congenital coagulopathy.

Microcephaly is associated with an increased risk of neurologic compromise; the fetal head can be effectively measured with sonography, but the diagnosis of microcephaly is hampered by an overlap with normal variations (there is no clear quantitative threshold) and particularly by intrauterine progressive development, which occurs in many cases; when the head is small, a specific antenatal diagnosis may be difficult; as microcephaly is associated with intracranial abnormalities in many cases, a careful inspection of cerebral anatomy may be helpful.

Disorders of neuronal migration include a wide spectrum of disorders characterized by abnormal sulcation of the brain; they may be diagnosed sonographically and/or with magnetic resonance imaging, but usually only in late gestation.

Choroid plexus cysts are small fluid collections within the choroid plexus of lateral ventricles; they are identified in 1% or more of fetuses at mid-gestation, and are transient and benign findings that, however, increase the risk of trisomy 18; as most cases of trisomy 18 are associated with anomalies readily identified by sonography, there is a general consensus that a careful inspection of fetal anatomy is indicated; amniocentesis may not be necessary.

Any time that a sonographic examination is performed in the second or third trimester, a survey of intracranial anatomy should be performed; the sensitivity of antenatal sonography remains uncertain; certainly, many even severe anomalies are associated with subtle antenatal findings or become manifest only in late gestation, and therefore escape antenatal detection.

Further reading

Adamsbaum C, Moutard ML, Andre C, et al. MRI of the fetal posterior fossa. *Pediatr Radiol* 2005;35(2):124–140.

Blaas HG, Eriksson AG, Salvesen KA, et al. Brains and faces in holoprosencephaly: pre- and postnatal description of 30 cases. *Ultrasound Obstet Gynecol* 2002;19(1):24–38.

Filly RA, Cardoza JD, Goldstein RB, Barkovich AJ. Detection of fetal central nervous system anomalies: a practical level of effort for a routine sonogram. *Radiology* 1989;172(2): 403–408.

Filly RA, Callen PW, Goldstein RB. Alpha-fetoprotein screening programs: what every obstetric sonologist should know. *Radiology* 1993;188(1):1–9.

Ghi T, Simonazzi G, Perolo A, et al. Outcome of antenatally diagnosed intracranial hemorrhage: case series and review of the literature. *Ultrasound Obstet Gynecol* 2003;22(2): 121–130.

Johnson SP, Sebire NJ, Snijders RJ, et al. Ultrasound screening for anencephaly at 10–14 weeks of gestation. *Ultrasound Obstet Gynecol* 1997;9(1):14–16.

Malinger G, Lerman-Sagie T, Watemberg N, et al. A normal second-trimester ultrasound does not exclude intracranial structural pathology. *Ultrasound Obstet Gynecol* 2002;20(1): 51–56.

Pilu G, Sandri F, Perolo A, et al. Sonography of fetal agenesis of the corpus callosum: a survey of 35 cases. *Ultrasound Obstet Gynecol* 1993;3(5):318–329.

Pilu G, Falco P, Gabrielli S, et al. The clinical significance of fetal isolated cerebral borderline ventriculomegaly: report of 31 cases and review of the literature. *Ultrasound Obstet Gynecol* 1999;14(5):320–326.

Snijders RJ, Shawa L, Nicolaides KH. Fetal choroid plexus cysts and trisomy 18: assessment of risk based on ultrasound findings and maternal age. *Prenat Diagn* 1994;14(12): 1119–1127.

21 Prenatal diagnosis of thoracic and cardiac abnormalities

Gianluigi Pilu, Philippe Jeanty, and Juliana M.B. Leite

Cardiac anomalies

Abnormalities of the heart and great arteries are among the most common congenital abnormalities, with an estimated incidence of 5 per 1000 births and about 30 per 1000 stillbirths. Fetal echocardiography is the primary diagnostic tool used to assess fetal cardiac structure and function and is usually performed at 18–22 weeks' gestation. A new technique for sonographic evaluation of the fetal heart, based upon the use of three-dimensional ultrasound, has been introduced recently, and is commonly referred to as STIC (spatiotemporal image correlation) technology. There are many potential advantages of this technology both for diagnostic and for screening and teleconsultation.

Septal defects

Defects of the atrial and ventricular septum represent about 10% and 30%, respectively, of all cardiac defects. In general, identification is difficult and is impossible in most cases. Most atrial defects involve the *septum secundum*, which is difficult to analyze owing to the physiologic presence of the foramen ovale. Most ventricular septal defects are small and equally difficult to demonstrate antenatally. As they are usually associated with blood shunting across the septum, color Doppler may aid in the diagnosis.

The core of the heart (the apical portion of the atrial septum), the basal portion of the interventricular septum, and the medial portion of the atrioventricular valves develop from the endocardial cushions. Abnormal development of these structures, commonly referred to as endocardial cushion defects or atrioventricular canal or atrioventricular septal defects, represents about 7% of all cardiac anomalies.

In the complete form, *persistent common atrioventricular canal*, the tricuspid and mitral valve are fused in a large single atrioventricular valve that opens above and bridges the two ventricles. In the partial form, there is a defect in the apical portion of the atrial septum (septum primum defect). There are two separate atrioventricular valves, but they are inserted at the same level on the ventricular septum.

Atrial and ventricular septal defects are not a cause of impairment of cardiac function *in utero*. Most affected infants are asymptomatic even in the neonatal period. When they are not associated with other cardiac anomalies, the prognosis is excellent. Spontaneous closure is frequent.

Univentricular heart
This term defines a group of anomalies characterized by the presence of an atrioventricular junction that is entirely connected to only one chamber in the ventricular mass. Univentricular heart is rare; it represents about 1.5% of all congenital cardiac defects. The 5-year survival after cardiac repair (the Fontan procedure) is about 70%. The long-term outcome is uncertain.

Aortic stenosis
Aortic stenosis represents about 3% of all cardiac defects and is commonly divided into supravalvar, valvar, and subaortic forms. Supravalvar and subaortic are rare and usually cannot be detected antenatally. Most cases of mild to moderate aortic stenosis are probably not amenable to early prenatal diagnosis. In severe valvar aortic stenosis the left ventricle may be either hypertrophic or dilated and hypocontractile. Hyperechogenicity of the aortic valve and pulsed Doppler demonstration of increased peak velocity support the diagnosis. Severe aortic stenosis may result in atrioventricular valve insufficiency and intrauterine heart failure. There have been some attempts at opening the valve prenatally.

Coarctation, tubular hypoplasia, and interruption of the aortic arch
Coarctation is a localized narrowing of the juxtaductal arch, most commonly between the left subclavian artery and the ductus. Cardiac and non-cardiac anomalies are frequently present. Interrupted aortic arch is typically associated with chromosome 22 microdeletion and represents an indication for prenatal diagnosis of this condition.

Coarctation or interruption of the aortic arch should be suspected when the right ventricle is enlarged. The characteristic finding of an ascending aorta that is more vertical than usual, and the impossibility of demonstrating a connection with the descending aorta, suggests the diagnosis of interrupted aortic arch. Critical coarctation and interruption are fatal in the neonatal period after closure of the ductus. Surgery is associated with a mortality of about 10% and the incidence of restenosis in survivors is about 15%.

Hypoplastic left heart syndrome
Hypoplastic left heart syndrome accounts for 4% of all cardiac anomalies at birth, but it is one of the most frequent cardiac malformations diagnosed antenatally. It is a spectrum of anomalies characterized by a very small left

ventricle with mitral and/or aortic atresia or hypoplasia. Prenatal echocardiographic diagnosis of the syndrome depends on the demonstration of a diminutive left ventricle and ascending aorta. Color flow mapping allows the demonstration of retrograde blood flow within the ascending aorta and aortic arch. Hypoplastic left heart is well tolerated *in utero*. The prognosis for infants is extremely poor and this lesion is responsible for 25% of cardiac deaths in the first week of life.

Pulmonary stenosis and pulmonary atresia

Pulmonary stenosis and pulmonary atresia with intact ventricular septum (also known as hypoplastic right ventricle) represent 9% and about 2% of all cardiac anomalies, respectively. The most common form of pulmonary stenosis is the valvar type, owing to the fusion of the pulmonary leaflets. Pulmonary atresia with intact ventricular septum in infants is usually associated with a hypoplastic right ventricle and the prenatal diagnosis relies on the demonstration of a small pulmonary artery with an atretic pulmonary valve.

Patients with mild stenosis are asymptomatic and there is no need for intervention. Patients with severe stenosis and right ventricular overload require balloon valvoplasty in the neonatal period and have excellent survival and a normal long-term prognosis. Fetuses with pulmonary atresia, severe tricuspid insufficiency, and an enlarged right heart have a very high degree of perinatal mortality.

Ebstein's anomaly and tricuspid valve dysplasia

Ebstein's anomaly results from a faulty implantation of the tricuspid valve. The tricuspid valve is usually both incompetent and stenotic. The characteristic echocardiographic finding is that of a massively enlarged right atrium, a small right ventricle, and a small pulmonary artery. Doppler can be used to demonstrate regurgitation in the right atrium. Ebstein's anomalies and tricuspid dysplasia detected prenatally have a dismal prognosis, with a very high perinatal mortality rate.

Conotruncal malformations

Conotruncal malformations are a heterogeneous group of defects that involve two different segments of the heart: the conotruncus and the ventricles.

Conotruncal anomalies account for 20–30% of all cardiac anomalies and are the leading cause of symptomatic cyanotic heart disease in the first year of life. Prenatal diagnosis is of interest for several reasons. Conotruncal anomalies are well tolerated *in utero*.

Transposition of the great arteries is an abnormality in which the aorta arises entirely or in large part from the right ventricle and the pulmonary artery arises from the left ventricle. *Complete transposition* is probably one of the most difficult cardiac lesions to recognize *in utero*. A clue to the diagnosis is the demonstration that the two great vessels do not cross but arise parallel from the base of the heart. *Corrected transposition* is characterized by a double discordance, at the atrioventricular and ventriculoarterial level. Complete transposition is uneventful *in utero*. Surgery is usually carried out within the first 2 weeks of life.

The essential features of *tetralogy of Fallot* are a subaortic ventricular septal defect, aorta overriding the ventricular septal defect, and infundibular stenosis of the aorta. In about 20% of cases there is atresia of the pulmonary valve. Hypertrophy of the right ventricle, one of the classic elements of the tetrad, is always absent in the fetus and only develops after birth. Tetralogy of Fallot does not result in cardiac failure in fetuses. Survival after complete surgical repair is more than 90%, and about 80% of survivors have normal exercise tolerance.

In *double outlet right ventricle* (DORV), most of the aorta and pulmonary valve arise completely or almost completely from the right ventricle. The main echocardiographic features include (1) alignment of the two vessels totally or predominantly from the right ventricle and (2) presence in most cases of bilateral coni (subaortic and subpulmonary). Usually, DORV does not interfere with hemodynamics in fetal life.

A single arterial vessel that originates from the heart overrides the ventricular septum and supplies the systemic, pulmonary, and coronary circulations, characterizing truncus arteriosus. The single arterial trunk is predominantly connected with the right ventricle in about 40% of cases, with the left ventricle in 20%, and is equally shared in 40%. Truncus arteriosus is not associated with alteration of fetal hemodynamics. However, it is frequently a neonatal emergency, with a survival after surgery of about 90%.

Heterotaxy

In heterotaxy, also referred to as cardiosplenic syndromes, the fetus is made of either two left or two right sides. Other terms commonly used include left or right isomerism, asplenia, and polysplenia. Unpaired organs (liver, stomach, and spleen) may be absent, midline, or duplicated. Heterotaxy represents about 2% of all congenital heart defects. The main clue for the diagnosis of fetal heterotaxy is the demonstration of complex cardiac anomalies associated with abnormal disposition of the thoracic and/or abdominal organs. The outcome depends on the number of cardiac anomalies, but it tends to be poor.

Fetal dysrhythmias

Irregular patterns of fetal heart rhythms are a frequent finding and, in the vast majority of cases, have no clinical significance. Short periods of tachycardia, bradycardia, and ectopic beats are also very commonly seen. A sustained bradycardia of less than 100 beats per minute (b.p.m.), a sustained tachycardia of more than 200 b.p.m. and irregular beats occurring more than 1 in 10 should be considered abnormal and require further investigation. At present, M-mode and pulsed Doppler ultrasound are the best available technique for the assessment of irregular fetal heart rhythm.

Premature atrial and ventricular contractions are the most frequent fetal dysrhythmias. They are considered a benign condition but they can give rise to complex rhythm patterns.

Supraventricular tachyarrhythmias include supraventricular paroxysmal tachycardia (SVT), atrial flutter, and atrial fibrillation. SVT is characterized by an atrial frequency of between 200 and 300 bpm and a 1:1 atrioventricular conduction rate. In atrial flutter, the atrial rate ranges from 300 to 400 bpm and the ventricular rate usually ranges from 60 to 200 bpm. In atrial fibrillation, the atrial rate is more than 400 bpm and the ventricular rate ranges from 120 to 200 bpm.

Atrioventricular (AV) block can result from immaturity of the conduction system, absence of connection to the AV node, or abnormal anatomic position of the AV node. AV block is commonly classified into three types. First- and second-degree AV block are not usually associated with any significant hemodynamic perturbance. Third-degree AV block may lead to important bradycardia, determining a decreased cardiac output and congestive heart failure *in utero*. Outcome is poor when there are associated cardiac anomalies and/or hydrops.

Thoracic anomalies

Hyperechogenic and cystic lungs

The typical finding is that of enlarged, brightly echogenic lungs displacing the mediastinum and causing an inversion of the diaphragm. Most frequently, part of one lung or one entire lung is affected. Rarely, both lungs are affected. The pathophysiology is related to obstruction of the respiratory tree, which causes accumulation of fluid and secretions into the lungs that may lead to lung hyperplasia. Early and longstanding obstruction is probably responsible for the histologic alterations that are commonly referred to as *cystic adenomatoid malformation* of the lungs. The etiology is variable. Unilateral echogenic and/or cystic lungs without other anomalies or hydrops have a very good outcome. Dysplastic lung tissue is usually present, however, and must be surgically removed. Conversely, bilateral lesions or those associated with hydrops usually have a poor outcome.

Pleural effusions

Fetal pleural effusions may be an isolated finding or they can occur in association with generalized edema and ascites. Infants usually present in the neonatal period with severe, and often fatal, respiratory insufficiency. Isolated pleural effusions in the fetus may either resolve spontaneously or they can be treated effectively after birth. Attempts at prenatal therapy by repeated thoracocenteses have been generally unsuccessful in reversing the hydropic state. A better approach is chronic drainage by the insertion of thoracoamniotic shunts. Survival after thoracoamniotic shunting is in the range of 50% and is more likely with isolated pleural effusions than with generalized hydrops.

Diaphragmatic hernia

Diaphragmatic hernia is found in about 1 per 4000 births and is usually a sporadic abnormality. However, in about 50% of affected fetuses there are associated chromosomal abnormalities and genetic syndromes. Diaphragmatic hernia is usually diagnosed by the ultrasonographic demonstration of stomach, intestines, or liver in the thorax and the associated mediastinal shift to the opposite side. Antenatal prediction of pulmonary hypoplasia remains one of the challenges of prenatal diagnosis. Poor prognostic signs include herniation of the liver into the fetal chest and a lung–head ratio < 1.0.

Conclusions

Congenital heart defects are among the most common malformations and a major cause of perinatal death. Evaluation of the fetal heart allows a precise diagnosis of most major cardiac anomalies from early in gestation. However, a specific expertise is required. The outcome of some severe cardiac abnormalities may be ameliorated by prenatal diagnosis. Thoracic anomalies are rare. Echogenic lungs and diaphragmatic hernia are the most frequent entities. Diaphragmatic hernia continues to be associated with significant mortality and long-term morbidity. Despite many attempts, the value of antenatal treatment remains highly uncertain.

Further reading

Allan L. Antenatal diagnosis of heart disease. *Heart* 2000;83:367.
Allan LD, Anderson RH, Sullivan ID, Campbell S, et al. Evaluation of fetal arrhythmias by echocardiography. *Br Heart J* 1983;50:240–245.
Allan LD, Crawford DC, Tynan MJ. Pulmonary atresia in prenatal life. *J Am Coll Cardiol* 1986;8:1131–1136.
Estoff JA, Parad RB, Frigoletto FDJ, Benacerraf B. The natural history of isolated fetal hydrothorax. *Ultrasound Obstet Gynecol* 1992;2:162–165.
Hornberger LK, Sahn DJ, Kleinman CS, et al. Tricuspid valve disease with significant tricuspid insufficiency in the fetus: diagnosis and outcome. *J Am Coll Cardiol* 1991; 17(1):167–173.
Lipshutz GS, Albanese CT, Feldstein VA, et al. Prospective analysis of lung-to-head ratio predicts survival for patients with prenatally diagnosed congenital diaphragmatic hernia. *J Pediatr Surg* 1997;32:1634–1636.
Paladini D, Palmieri S, Lamberti A, et al. Characterization and natural history of ventricular septal defects in the fetus. *Ultrasound Obstet Gynecol* 2000;16:118–122.
Perolo A, Prandstraller D, Ghi T, et al. Diagnosis and management of fetal cardiac anomalies: 10 years of experience at a single institution. *Ultrasound Obstet Gynecol* 2001;18:615–618.
Vinals F, Poblete P, Giuliano A. Spatio-temporal image correlation (STIC): a new tool for the prenatal screening of congenital heart defects. *Ultrasound Obstet Gynecol* 2003;22:388–394.

22 Gastrointestinal and genitourinary anomalies

Sandro Gabrielli, Nicola Rizzo, and E. Albert Reece

Structural anomalies of the gastrointestinal (GI) and genitourinary (GU) tract are relatively common. Fetuses with GI or GU anomalies, which often have a good quality of life after postnatal surgical correction, largely benefit from prenatal diagnosis.

Esophageal atresia is a relatively frequent anomaly, occurring in 1 in 3000–3500 live births. It is caused by an impairment in the process of recanalization of the primitive esophagus. Prenatal diagnosis is suspected when, in the presence of polyhydramnios (usually after 25 weeks), serial ultrasound examinations fail to demonstrate the fetal stomach, or the stomach appears permanently small (< 15% of the abdominal circumference) (Fig. 22.1); gastric secretions, however, may be sufficient to distend the stomach and make it visible. Also, in the case of an associated fistula, the stomach may look normal. Prenatal diagnosis can therefore often be missed. Factors such as associated anomalies, respiratory complications at birth, gestational age at delivery, and neonatal weight play the most important prognostic role. Prenatal diagnosis is crucial, as it permits the paediatrician to be alerted, facilitates prompt neonatal diagnostic confirmation, and enables prevention of potentially severe complications, such as aspiration pneumonia.

Duodenal obstruction occurs in approximately 1 in 7500–10 000 live births. It is a sporadic abnormality, although there is an autosomal-recessive pattern of inheritance in some cases. Approximately half the fetuses with duodenal atresia have associated abnormalities, including trisomy 21 in about 40% of cases, and skeletal defects, gastrointestinal abnormalities, and cardiac and renal defects. Detection of two echo-free areas inside the abdomen ("double-bubble" sign), representing the dilated stomach and the first portion of the duodenum, is crucial for prenatal diagnosis (Fig. 22.2). Polyhydramnios is invariably associated. However, obstruction due to a central web may result in only a "single bubble" representing the fluid-filled stomach. Postnatal prognosis of duodenal atresia depends mainly on the following: associated anomalies, birthweight, and prompt confirmation of prenatal diagnosis. Survival rate after surgery in patients with an isolated anomaly is higher than 95%. The most frequent site of small bowel obstruction is the distal ileus, followed by the proximal jejunum. In about 5% of cases, obstructions occur at multiple sites. Although the condition is usually sporadic, in multiple intestinal atresias, familial cases have been described. Associated abnormalities and chromosomal defects are rare. The lumens of the small bowel and colon do not normally exceed 7 mm and 20 mm respectively. Diagnosis of obstruction is usually made late in pregnancy, after 25 weeks, because dilation of the intestinal lumen is slow and progressive. Jejunal

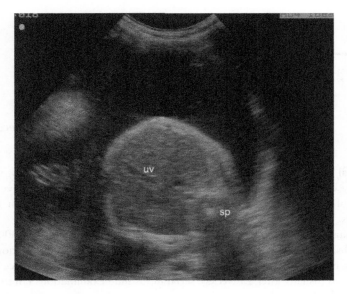

Figure 22.1 Cross-section of the abdomen in a fetus with esophageal atresia. Stomach is not visualized. sp, spine; uv, umbilical vein.

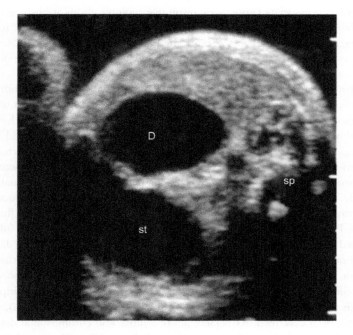

Figure 22.2 Cross-section of the upper fetal abdomen in a case of duodenal atresia, showing the pathognomonic "double-bubble" sign. D, dilated duodenal bulb; sp, spine; st, stomach.

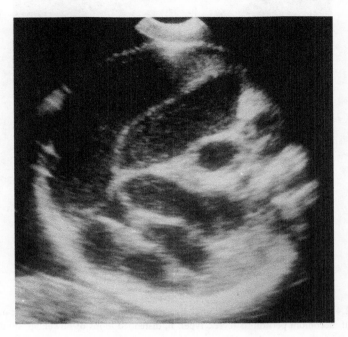

Figure 22.3 Cross-section of the abdomen in a fetus with small bowel atresia. Dilated bowel is visible.

and ileal obstructions are imaged as multiple fluid-filled loops of bowel in the abdomen (Fig. 22.3). The more distal the site of the obstruction, the greater the number of anechoic structures Fetuses with an uncomplicated intestinal obstruction can be delivered vaginally at term. Induction of labor should be considered when perforation with ascites occurs. As meconium begins to accumulate in the fetal bowel at 4 months, any perforation occurring after that time could bring the outflow of meconium into the peritoneal cavity. As a result, an intense reaction occurs, leading to extensive adhesions (Fig. 22.4). Polyhydramnios is a frequent finding; ascites may also be present. Prognosis is usually severe. Omphalocele, or exomphalos, occurs in about 1 in 4000 births, and results from failure of normal embryonic regression of the midgut from the umbilical stalk into the abdominal coeloma. Omphalocele is often associated with other abnormalities, as a result of general interference with embryonic development during early gestation. It is also associated with an increased risk of chromosomal abnormalities. Prenatal diagnosis is based on the demonstration of the midline anterior abdominal wall defect, the herniated sac with its visceral contents, and the umbilical cord insertion at the apex of the sac (Fig. 22.5). Isolated lesions have a good prognosis with a survival rate after surgery of higher than 90%. Maternal transport to a tertiary center and an accurately planned Cesarean delivery would probably avoid the risks of a sudden,

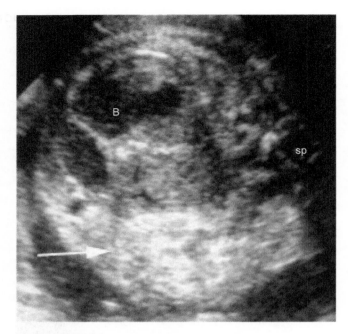

Figure 22.4 Cross-section of the fetal abdomen showing a highly hyperechogenic mass (arrow) of meconium peritonitis (cystic type). B, distended loops of bowel; sp, spine.

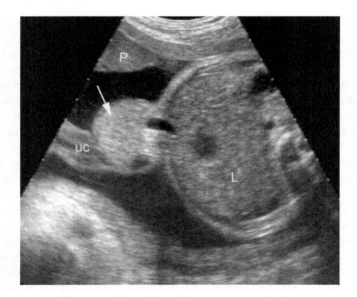

Figure 22.5 Cross-section of a fetus with omphalocele. Note the herniated hyperechogenic mass (arrow) at the level of cord insertion. L, liver; P, placenta; uc, umbilical cord on top of the defect.

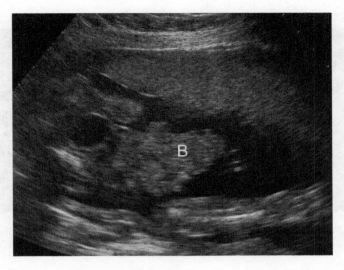

Figure 22.6 A case of gastroschisis diagnosed at 22 weeks' gestation: free-floating loops of bowel (B) herniated through a lateral abdominal wall defect.

unexpected delivery leading to a delay in surgical care. Gastroschisis is found in about 1 in 4000 births. In gastroschisis, the primary body folds and the umbilical ring develop normally, and evisceration of the intestine occurs through a small abdominal wall defect located just lateral and usually to the right of an intact umbilical cord. Associated anomalies are uncommon. Prenatal diagnosis is based on the demonstration of the normally situated umbilicus and the herniated loops of intestine, which are free-floating and widely separated (Fig. 22.6). Prognosis has improved dramatically during the last three decades. It seems crucial, however, that delivery takes place in tertiary-care centers where the neonate can receive intensive care and where neonatal surgical correction is promptly available.

Bilateral renal agenesis is found in 1 in 5000 births, while unilateral disease is found in 1 in 2000 births. Renal agenesis derives from failure of development of the ureteric bud or nephrogenic blastema, because both components occur at the formation of normal kidneys. This abnormality is usually isolated and sporadic. Failed visualization of kidneys and bladder, associated with oligohydramnios, prompts the diagnosis of bilateral renal agenesis (Fig. 22.7). Bilateral renal agenesis is a lethal condition. Unilateral agenesis has a favorable prognosis. Multicystic kidneys are usually unilateral, although bilateral renal involvement has been reported. In the majority of cases, this is a sporadic abnormality, but a few examples of familial cases have been described. Multicystic kidney is often associated with other congenital anomalies, including mainly congenital heart diseases and chromosomal aberrations (mainly trisomy 18), and it is often part of genetic

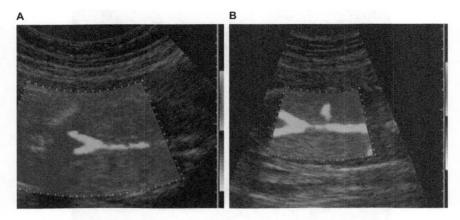

Figure 22.7 Color Doppler failed to demonstrate the renal arteries in a case of bilateral (A) and unilateral (B) renal agenesis.

syndromes. Multicystic kidneys are usually unilateral and appear as a cluster of multiple irregular cysts of variable size with little intervening hyperechogenic stroma (Fig. 22.8). Isolated unilateral multicystic kidneys have a good prognosis. Autosomal-recessive cystic kidneys invariably involves both kidneys, and occurs in of 1 in 20 000 live births. Sonographically, both kidneys usually appear extremely enlarged and hyperechogenic (Fig. 22.9). In severe cases, the bladder is absent and oligohydramnios is extreme. However, these sonographic appearances may be manifest only in late gestation. Prognosis is variable. Autosomal-dominant cystic kidneys almost invariably affects both kidneys, although often symmetrically. It is usually asymptomatic until the third or fourth decade of life. Sonography does not usually demonstrate abnormalities prior to the second or third decade. In a handful of cases, however, affected fetuses have demonstrated findings similar to the autosomalrecessive variety. Kidneys appear grossly enlarged with multiple cysts of variable size intermixed with well-represented, hyperechogenic solid tissue. The experience of prenatal diagnosis is limited. It would not seem that intrauterine presentation is necessarily associated with a poor prognosis. Enlargement of the urinary tract usually occurs, albeit not exclusively as the consequence of obstruction. Mild pyelectasia (anteroposterior diameter between 4 and 10 mm) has recently been suggested as a sonographic marker for chromosomal abnormalities and, in some cases, may reveal vesicoureteric reflux at birth. Hydronephrosis is characterized by dilated renal pelvis and calices (Fig. 22.10).

In cases of megacystis, the bladder is usually greatly enlarged, occupying most of the abdomen and distending it. Urethral obstruction can be caused by urethral agenesis, persistence of the cloaca, urethral stricture, or posterior urethral valves. With posterior urethral valves, there is usually incomplete or intermittent obstruction of

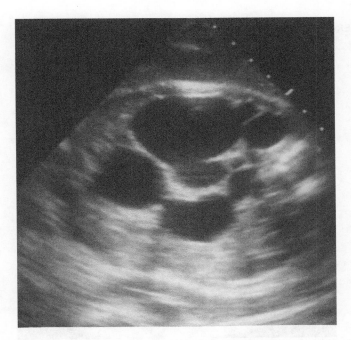

Figure 22.8 Coronal scan of the trunk of a 33-week fetus with unilateral multicystic dysplastic kidney disease. The cysts are clearly separated by echoic tissue.

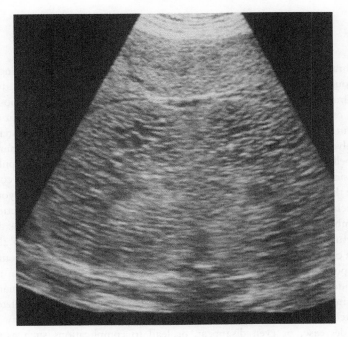

Figure 22.9 Coronal section of a fetus with recessive-type polycystic kidneys. Kidneys appear extremely enlarged and hyperechogenic.

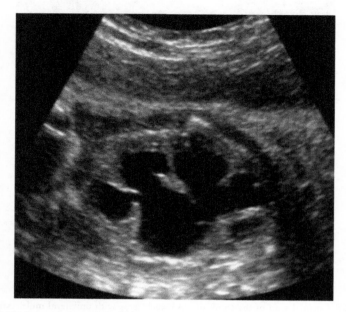

Figure 22.10 Coronal view of the kidney in a case of ureteropelvic junction obstruction. Pelves and calices appear fairly dilated.

the urethra, resulting in an enlarged and hypertrophied bladder with varying degrees of hydroureters, hydronephrosis, a spectrum of renal hypoplasia and dysplasia, oligohydramnios, and pulmonary hypoplasia. The outcome of urethral obstruction depends on how severe it is and how early it occurs. Complete persistent obstruction occurring in the early midtrimester (e.g., urethral atresia, early posterior urethral valves) results in massive distention of the bladder and abdominal wall (prune-belly abdomen), severe oligohydramnios, dysplastic kidneys, and pulmonary hypoplasia. Shunting of the fetal bladder is feasible, although there is no conclusive evidence that such intervention improves renal or pulmonary function beyond what can be achieved by postnatal surgery. Antenatal evaluation of renal function relies on a combination of ultrasonographic findings and analysis of fetal urine obtained by puncture of the bladder or renal pelvis. Ovarian cysts are one of the most common causes of abdominal mass in the female neonate. Prenatal ultrasound diagnosis is possible from the second trimester of pregnancy. Cystic mass in the fetal lower abdomen, integrity of GI and GU tracts, and female sex are the main ultrasound criteria for diagnosis of fetal ovarian cyst. The cyst may be completely fluid or septated and sometimes presents with a fluid-solid level. The cyst may increase in size, decrease, or even disappear, or lead to complications such as torsion, infarction, and rupture. In this light, once prenatal ultrasound diagnosis has been made, serial examinations should be performed throughout gestation to detect any structural changes in the mass. When sudden development of intense hyperechogenicity within the mass followed by a complex, heterogeneous appearance occurs, immediate delivery is recommended. Conversely, small cysts detected *in utero* can subsequently disappear and may not be present on a postnatal ultrasound evaluation.

Further reading

Achiron R, Soriano D, Lipitz S, et al. Fetal midgut herniation into the umbilical cord: improved definition of ventral abdominal anomaly with the use of transvaginal sonography. *Ultrasound Obstet Gynecol* 1995;6:256.

Aubertin G, Cripps S, Coleman G, et al. Prenatal diagnosis of apparently isolated unilateral multicystic kidney: implications for counseling and management. *Prenat Diagn* 2002;22:388.

Baerg J, Kaban G, Tonita J, et al. Gastroschisis: a sixteen-year review. *J Pediatr Surg* 2003;38: 771.

Blazer S, Zimmer EZ, Gover A, et al. Fetal omphalocele detected early in pregnancy: associated anomalies and outcomes. *Radiology* 2004;232:191.

Brantberg A, Blaas HG, Salvesen KA, et al. Surveillance and outcome of fetuses with gastroschisis. *Ultrasound Obstet Gynecol* 2004;23:4.

Haeusler MC, Berghold A, Stoll C, et al. prenatal ultrasonographic detection of gastrointestinal obstruction: results from 18 European congenital anomaly registries. *Prenat Diagn* 2002;22:616.

Jouannic J, Hyett Jon A, Pandya PP, et al. Perinatal outcome in fetuses with megacystis in the first half of pregnancy. *Prenat Diagn* 2003;23:340.

Rizzo N, Gabrielli S, Perolo A, et al. Prenatal diagnosis and management of fetal ovarian cysts. *Prenat Diagn* 1989;9:97.

Romero R, Ghidini A, Gabrielli S, et al. Gastrointestinal tract and abdominal wall defects. In: Brock DJH, Rodeck CH, Ferguson-Smith MA, eds. *Prenatal diagnosis and screening.* Edinburgh: Churchill Livingstone; 1992:227.

Roume J, Ville Y. Prenatal diagnosis of genetic renal diseases: breaking the code. *Ultrasound Obstet Gynecol* 2004;24:10.

23 | Fetal skeletal anomalies

Luís F. Gonçalves, Patricia Devers, Jimmy Espinoza, and Roberto Romero

Skeletal dysplasias are a heterogeneous group of disorders that affect the development of chondro-osseous tissues, resulting in abnormalities in the size and shape of various segments of the skeleton. Estimated prevalences for skeletal dysplasia range from 1.1 to 9.5 per 10 000 births, with higher prevalences observed in populations with a high rate of consanguineous marriage. The four most common skeletal dysplasias are thanatophoric dysplasia, achondroplasia, osteogenesis imperfecta, and achondrogenesis. The most common nonlethal skeletal dysplasia is achondroplasia.

There are two evolving classifications for skeletal dysplasias. The first is the International Nosology and Classification of Constitutional Disorders of Bones (2001), which consists of a combination of morphological and molecular groupings of disorders and genetically determined dysostoses. The second is a classification of skeletal disorders based on the structure and function of implicated genes and proteins (Molecular–Pathogenetic Classification of Genetic Disorders of the Skeleton). The full version of both classifications can be accessed at the website of the International Skeletal Dysplasia Society (http://www.isds.ch/ISDSframes.html, last accessed on 06/11/2005).

Despite the increasing availability of molecular testing, a comprehensive molecular diagnostic search for all skeletal dysplasias is not possible at this time. Indeed, only about one-third of skeletal dysplasias have had their molecular basis defined. Therefore, the roles of diagnostic imaging in the prenatal investigation of skeletal dysplasias are: (1) to narrow the differential diagnosis of skeletal dysplasias so that appropriate confirmatory molecular tests can be selected; (2) to predict lethality; and (3) to identify the fetus with a skeletal dysplasia early enough in pregnancy so that the diagnostic workup can be completed before the limit of fetal viability.

Ultrasound is the primary imaging modality used for the initial diagnostic evaluation of affected fetuses, with an accurate prenatal diagnosis reported in 31–73% of cases. Three-dimensional ultrasound may improve the diagnostic accuracy of skeletal dysplasias by allowing characterization of additional phenotypic features not detectable by two-dimensional ultrasound. Three-dimensional reconstruction of the fetal bones is best performed using the "maximum intensity projection" mode, a rendering algorithm that prioritizes the display of voxels with the highest gray levels contained within a region of interest selected by the user. Case reports and small series of several skeletal dysplasias have been published describing phenotypic characteristics or skeletal features that can be demonstrated by three-dimensional ultrasound (Table 23.1).

A systematic approach to the prenatal diagnosis of skeletal dysplasias is presented in Table 23.2. Several skeletal dysplasias are associated with a narrow thorax and pulmonary hypoplasia (Table 23.3). Prenatal identification of lethal skeletal dysplasias is important, and a number of parameters have been investigated to detect pulmonary hypoplasia *in utero* (Table 23.4 and Figs 23.1 and 23.2). Of particular interest are the measurements of the right lung diameter or the ratio between right lung diameter and bony thoracic circumference, which, in preliminary studies, performed well in diagnosing pulmonary hypoplasia prenatally.

Table 23.1 Additional phenotypic findings and improved visualization in cases of skeletal dysplasias by prenatal three-dimensional ultrasound compared with two-dimensional ultrasound in published reports.

Skeletal dysplasia	Phenotypic characteristics identified better by three- rather than two-dimensional ultrasound
Platylospondylic lethal chondrodysplasia	Enhanced visualization of femoral and tibial bowing, better characterization of the facial soft tissues with surface rendering
Campomelic dysplasia	Micrognathia, flat face, hypoplastic scapulae, bifid foot
Thanatophoric dysplasia	Improved characterization of frontal bossing and depressed nasal bridge, demonstration of redundant skinfolds, low-set dysmorphic ears
Achondroplasia	Improved characterization of frontal bossing and depressed nasal bridge; superior evaluation of the epiphyses and metaphyses of the long bones, with demonstration of a vertical metaphyseal slope; caudal narrowing of the interpedicular distance; clear visualization of trident hand; better visualization of disproportion between limb segments
Chondrodysplasia puntacta, rhizomelic form	Improved characterization of the Binder facies (depressed nasal bridge, midface hypoplasia, small nose with upturned alae); identification of laryngeal stippling
Achondrogenesis	Panoramic demonstration of short neck and severe shortening of all segments of the limbs
Jarcho–Levin syndrome	Vertebral defects with absence of ribs and transverse process
Larsen syndrome	Genu recurvatum, midface hypoplasia, low-set ears

Phenotypic characteristics of osteogenesis imperfecta, short rib–polydactyly syndrome, and Apert syndrome have also been described using three-dimensional ultrasound, although no additional findings with two-dimensional ultrasound were observed.

A careful study of the newborn is always required. The evaluation should include a detailed physical examination performed by a geneticist or an individual with experience in the field of skeletal dysplasias and radiographs of the skeleton. Histologic examination of the chondro-osseous tissue should be performed, and chromosomal studies included. Biochemical studies are helpful in rare instances (e.g., hypophosphatasia). DNA restriction and enzymatic activity assays should be considered in cases in which the phenotype suggests a metabolic disorder such as a mucopolysaccharidosis. DNA should be saved in all cases.

Below, we briefly review the inheritance and ultrasonographic signs associated with the most common osteochondrodysplasias that can be diagnosed *in utero*.

Table 23.2 Steps for examination of the fetus with a suspected skeletal dysplasia by two-
and three-dimensional ultrasound.

1. Measure all long bones

2. Compare with other segments and classify the limb shortening as:
   Rhizomelia
   Mesomelia
   Acromelia
   Severe micromelia

3. Qualitative assessment of long bones:
   Demineralization
   Fractures
   Bowing
   Metaphyseal flaring
   Absence of bones

4. Measure chest dimensions to determine risk of pulmonary hypoplasia

5. Evaluate hands and feet:
   Digits (polydactyly/syndactyly)
   Positional deformities

6. Evaluate the cranium:
   Macrocrania
   Frontal bossing
   Cloverleaf skull
   Hypertelorism/hypotelorism

7. Evaluate for facial clefts

8. Examine the spine:
   Platyspondyly
   Demineralization
   Hemivertebrae
   Coronal clefts
   Vertebral disorganization

9. Evaluate internal organs, including echocardiography

10. Evaluate fetal motion

11. Evaluate amniotic fluid volume

Table 23.3 Nosology of lethal osteochondrodysplasias.

Hypophosphatasia and morphologically similar disorders
Hypophosphatasia
Probable hypophosphatasia
Lethal metaphyseal dysplasia

Chondrodysplasia punctata and similar disorders
Rhizomelic chondrodysplasia punctata
Lethal chondrodysplasia punctata, X-linked dominant
Greenberg dysplasia
Dappled diaphysis dysplasia

Achondrogenesis and similar disorders
Achondrogenesis IA (Houston–Harris)
Achondrogenesis IB (Fraccaro)
New lethal osteochondrodysplasia
Achondrogenesis II (Langer–Saldino)
Hypochondrogenesis

Thanatophoric dysplasia and similar disorders
Thanatophoric dysplasia, type I
Thanatophoric dysplasia, type II
Homozygous achondroplasia
Lethal achondrodysplasia
Glasgow variant

Platyspondylic lethal chondrodysplasias
Platyspondylic chondrodysplasia, Torrance type
Platyspondylic chondrodysplasia, San Diego type
Platyspondylic chondrodysplasia, Luton type
Platyspondylic chondrodysplasia, Shiraz type
Opsismodysplasia
Sixth form of platyspondylic chondrodysplasia
Seventh form of platyspondylic chondrodysplasia

Short rib–polydactyly syndromes
Short rib–polydactyly syndrome, type I (Saldino–Noonan)
Short rib–polydactyly syndrome, type II (Verma–Naumoff)
Short rib–polydactyly syndrome, type III (Le Marec)
Short rib–polydactyly syndrome, type IV (Yang)
Short rib–polydactyly syndromes
Short rib–polydactyly syndrome, type VI (Majewski)
Short rib–polydactyly syndrome, type VII (Beemer)

Lethal metatropic dysplasia and similar disorders
Lethal metatropic dysplasia (hyperchondrogenesis)
Fibrochondrogenesis
Schneckenbecken dysplasia

(Continued)

Table 23.3 *Continued*

Kniest-like disorders
Dyssegmental dysplasia, Silverman type
Dyssegmental dysplasia, Rolland–Desbuquois
Lethal Kniest disease
Chondrodysplasia resembling Kniest dysplasia
Blomstrand chondrodysplasia

Lethal osteochondrodysplasias with pronounced diaphyseal abnormalities
Campomelic syndrome
Stuve–Wiedemann syndrome
Boomerang dysplasia
Atelosteogenesis
Disorder resembling atelosteogenesis
de la Chappelle dysplasia
McAlister dysplasia
Pseudodystrophic dysplasia

Osteogenesis imperfecta and similar disorders
Osteogenesis imperfecta type IIA
Osteogenesis imperfecta type IIB
Osteogenesis imperfecta type IIC
Astley–Kendall dysplasia

Lethal disorders with gracile bones
Fetal hypokinesia phenotype
Lethal osteochondrodysplasia with gracile bones
Lethal osteochondrodysplasia with intrauterine overtubulation

---

Reproduced with permission from Spranger J, Maroteaux P. The lethal osteochondrodysplasias. *Adv Hum Genet* 1990;19:1–2.

Achondroplasia

Nonlethal skeletal dysplasia, with an estimated prevalence of 1/66 000 births, inherited as an autosomal dominant disorder, is caused by mutations in the fibroblast growth factor receptor-3 (*FGFR3*) gene. It is characterized by rhizomelic shortening, limb bowing, lordotic spine, and enlarged head. Flattened nasal bridge, frontal bossing, and broad mandible are frequent features, and trident hand is a specific finding. The major difficulty in the antenatal diagnosis is that the long bone growth in this disease is not recognized in most cases until the third trimester of pregnancy. Heterozygous achondroplasia is compatible with normal life and intellectual development. The disease is lethal in the homozygous state.

Table 23.4 Biometric parameters proposed by different authors for the evaluation of lung hypoplasia.

Author, year	Parameter	Fetuses at risk	Prevalence	Sensitivity (%)	Specificity (%)	Accuracy (%)	Population
Nimrod and colleagues, 1986	TC	45	38	88	96	93	PROM, oligohydramnios, pleural effusion, other conditions affecting lung growth
Fong and colleagues 1988	TC	18	60	60	88	72	Prolonged PROM, oligohydramnios, fetal malformations associated with lung hypoplasia
Songster and colleagues, 1989	FL/TC	26	42	80	92	88	PROM, urinary tract anomalies, fetal skeletal dysplasias, intrauterine growth restriction, twin–twin transfusion syndrome
Vintzileos and colleagues, 1989	TC TA TA-HA (TC × 100)/AC CA/HA (TA-HA) × 100/CA	13	69	33 33 50 33 67 83	57 71 71 86 86 86	46 54 62 62 77 85	Severe oligohydramnios > 5 weeks' duration
Roberts and Mitchell, 1990	LL TC	20	60	92 67	100 100	95 80	PROM < 25 weeks of gestation and > 7 days' duration
D'Alton and colleagues, 1992	TC/AC	16	44	75	100	88	PROM < 26 weeks of gestation
Ohlsson and colleagues, 1992	TC TC/CA TC/FL	58	28	80 80 55	90 97 97	87 91 90	PROM < 30 weeks and 19 cases of congenital anomalies
Maeda and colleagues, 1993	LA	19	79	100	75	95	Non-immune hydrops, polycystic kidneys, PROM, diaphragmatic hernia, immune hydrops, trisomy 18

(Continued)

Table 23.4 *Continued*

Author, year	Parameter	Fetuses at risk	Prevalence	Sensitivity (%)	Specificity (%)	Accuracy (%)	Population
Yoshimura and colleagues, 1996	TC	21*	*	100	83	90	Case–control study: 21 patients at risk for pulmonary hypoplasia (renal anomalies associated with pulmonary hypoplasia; thanatophoric dysplasia; prolonged PROM < 26 weeks of gestation), 30 PROM patients with normal lung function
	TA			100	87	92	
	TC/AC			90	90	90	
	LA	16*		81	100	93	
	TA-HA			100	87	91	
	TA/HA			69	100	89	
	TA-HA/TA			69	97	87	
	LA/TA			31	100	76	
Merz and colleagues, 1999	LD	32	†	100	†	†	Skeletal dysplasias (*n* = 7), renal agenesis (*n* = 11), diaphragmatic hernia (*n* = 7), hydrothorax (*n* = 2)
	TTD			53			
	TSD			47			
	TC			47			
Bahlmann and colleagues, 1999	TC	17	82	14	100	29	Diaphragmatic hernia
	LD			100	100	100	
	LD/TC			100	100	100	
Heling and colleagues, 2001	TTD	29	55	44	50	46	Bilateral renal agenesis, bilateral multicystic kidneys, chronic PROM < 25 weeks of gestation, hydrothorax
	APTD			57	42	52	
	LL			29	66	42	
Laudy and colleagues, 2002	TC	40	43	94	38	61	Prolonged oligohydramnios due to PROM or congenital renal disease
	CC/TC			76	50	61	
	TC/AC			69	71	70	

AC, abdominal circumference; APTD, anteroposterior thoracic diameter; CC, cardiac circumference; FL, femur length; HA, heart area; LA, lung area; LL, lung length; TA, thoracic area; TLD, lung diameter; TSD, thoracic sagittal diameter; TTD, transverse thoracic diameter; TC, thoracic circumference; PROM, premature repture of the membranes.

Only the papers for which data to calculate at least the sensitivity were included.

*Case–control study: all fetuses in the column "Fetuses at risk" had pulmonary hypoplasia; 30 gestational age-matched control fetuses were studied.

†All fetuses had pulmonary hypoplasia.

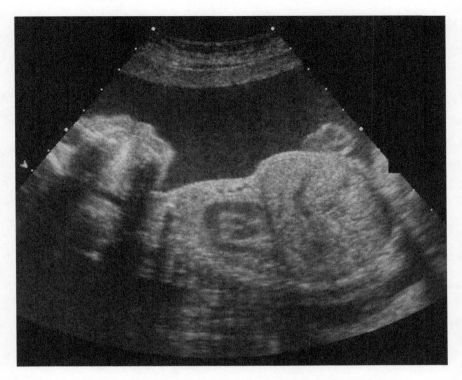

Figure 23.1 Longitudinal section of a fetus with thanatophoric dysplasia. Note the significant disproportion between the chest and abdomen.

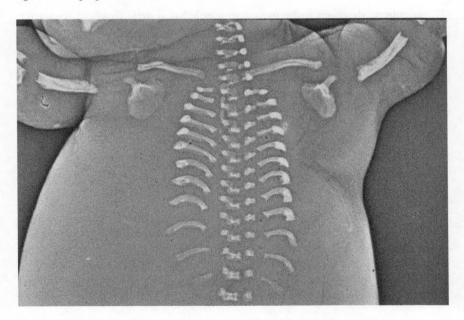

Figure 23.2 Extremely short ribs in a fetus with short rib–polydactyly syndrome.

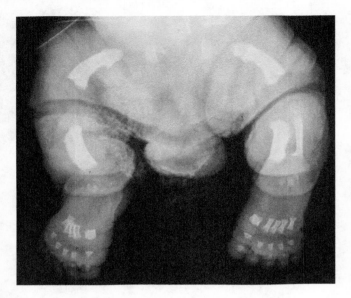

Figure 23.3 Bowed and short femurs in thanatophoric dysplasia.

Thanatophoric dysplasia

Thanatophoric dysplasia is the most common lethal skeletal dysplasia, character-ized by extreme rhizomelia, normal trunk length with a narrow thorax, and large head with a prominent forehead. Platyspondyly is a characteristic finding. There are two subtypes: type 1, with typical bowed "telephone receiver" femurs (Fig. 23.3) and no cloverleaf skull; and type 2, with severe cloverleaf skull (Fig. 23.4) and short, straight long bones. The differential diagnosis between the two types depends on the radiographic findings and histology. Both types of thanatophoric dysplasia are inherited in an autosomal dominant manner. The disease is caused by mutations in the *FGFR3* gene. Thanatophoric dysplasia is a uniformly lethal disorder, although survival of several months has been reported in some isolated cases.

Hypochondroplasia

Hypochondroplasia is an autosomal dominant disorder that resembles achon-droplasia. It can result from mutations in the *FGFR3* gene, although genetic het-erogeneity is suspected. Most cases occur sporadically as a result of a new mutation. The differential diagnosis between this condition and achondroplasia is based on the sparing of the head and lack of tibial bowing in hypochondroplasia. The con-dition is generally first detected during childhood.

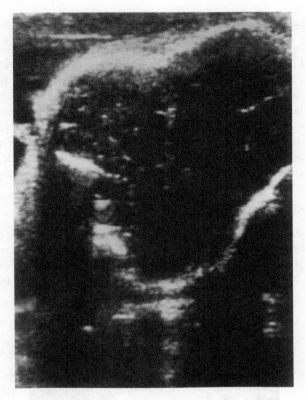

Figure 23.4 Coronal scan of the head of a fetus with thanatophoric dysplasia with a cloverleaf skull.

Fibrochondrogenesis and atelosteogenesis

Fibrochondrogenesis and atelosteogenesis have a clinical presentation similar to that of thanatophoric dysplasia. Fibrochondrogenesis is an autosomal recessive lethal disorder, characterized by micromelia with significant metaphyseal flaring, normal head size, undermineralized skull, platyspondyly, clefting of the vertebral bodies, and a narrow and bell-shaped thorax. The molecular defect involved in fibrochondrogenesis is not known. Atelosteogenesis is a sporadic lethal chondrodysplasia characterized by severe micromelia (with hypoplasia of the distal segments of the humerus and femur), bowing of long bones, narrow chest with short ribs, coronal and sagittal vertebral clefts, and dislocation at the level of the elbow and knee. Clubfoot deformities may also be present.

Achondrogenesis

Achondrogenesis is a lethal chondrodystrophy characterized by extreme micromelia, a short trunk, and macrocrania. Lack of ossification of the vertebral bodies is a characteristic feature. Table 23.5 illustrates the characteristics of the different types of achondrogenesis. Prenatal diagnosis should be suspected on the basis of micromelia, lack of vertebral ossification, and a large head with various degrees of ossification of calvarium. Achondrogenesis types IA and IB are inherited in an autosomal recessive pattern, whereas most cases of achondrogenesis type II and hypochondrogenesis have been sporadic (new autosomal dominant mutations). Some severe cases of type II achondrogenesis follow an autosomal recessive pattern.

Osteogenesis imperfecta

The term "osteogenesis imperfecta" was introduced over a century ago to describe a newborn with extremely brittle bones (Figs 23.5 and 23.6). The most popular classification is that proposed by Sillence and colleagues. A modification of this classification has recently been reported by Rauch and Glorieux and includes three

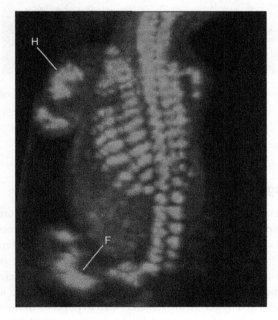

Figure 23.5 Three-dimensional ultrasonography in a case of osteogenesis imperfecta type II. The volume dataset was rendered using the maximum intensity (skeletal) mode. Multiple fractures in the ribs are present. Note the severe bowing and shortening of the left femur (F) and humerus (H).

Table 23.5 Radiologic differences of achondrogenesis types IA/IB, type II, and hypochondrogenesis.

Site	Type IA (Houston–Harris)	Type IB (Fraccaro)	Type II (Langer–Saldino)	Hypochondrogenesis
Skull	Membranous calvarium	All parts of ossified skull well seen	Normal ossification	Normal ossification
Long bones	Extremely shortened with metaphyseal cupping and spurs, "rectangular bones"	Arms and legs shorter than with type IA with minimal ossification; abundant metaphyseal spiking or spurring in lower leg bones, "square or stellate bones"	Short and bowed with metaphyseal flaring and cupping, "mushroom stem bones"	Less bowed and shortened with irregular or smooth metaphyses
Spine	Vertebral bodies unossified, with partly ossified pedicles	Vertebral bodies minimally or not ossified, pedicles ossified	Variable pattern of ossified or unossified vertebral bodies and pedicles	Thoracic and upper lumbar vertebral bodies ossified but still platyspondylic Cervical and lower lumbar bodies unossified
Pelvis	Poorly formed and ossified, with crenated iliac bones, ischial bones poorly ossified, pubic bones unossified	Iliac bones same aspect as in type IA, ischial and pubic bones unossified	Halberd-like iliac bones with unossified ischial and pubic bones	Near normally developed iliac bones with partial ossification of ischial bones and unossified pubic bones
Thorax	Short and barrel shaped, short ribs with cupped metaphyses and multiple fractures	Same as in type IA with unfractured ribs	Short and barrel/bell shaped with short unfractured ribs	Near normal bur shallow cage with short unfractured ribs

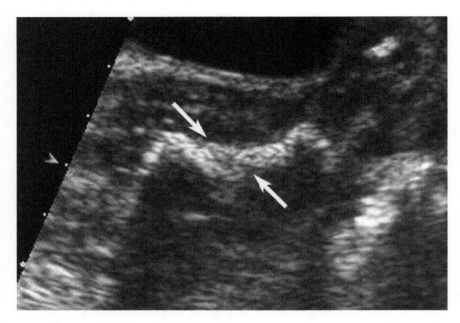

Figure 23.6 *In utero* fracture in a case of osteogenesis imperfecta. The arrows indicate the hypoechogenic fracture line.

additional types (V, VI, and VII—see Table 23.6). Clinically, the most relevant characteristic of osteogenesis imperfecta is bone fragility, with severity increasing in the following order: (1) type I; (2) types IV, V, VI, and VII; (3) type III; and (4) type II. Type II, also known as the perinatal form, is an autosomal dominant lethal condition. There is almost no ossification of the skull, beaded ribs, shortened and crumpled long bones, and multiple fractures *in utero* (Figs 23.5 and 23.6).

Hypophosphatasia

Hypophosphatasia is a rare autosomal recessive disorder characterized by demineralization of bones and low alkaline phosphatase in serum and other tissues. The condition has been subdivided into three clinical types according to the age of onset: congenital/infantile, childhood, and adult. The congenital/infantile and childhood varieties have an autosomal recessive pattern of inheritance, whereas the adult form can be transmitted as either an autosomal dominant or autosomal recessive trait. The congenital (neonatal) form is associated with early neonatal death or stillbirth. Fetuses with congenital hypophosphatasia have generalized demineralization of the skeleton, with shortening and bowing of tubular bones. Multiple fractures are present. The marked demineralization of the cranial vault results in deformation of the skull after external compression.

Table 23.6 Expanded Sillence classification of osteogenesis imperfecta.

Type	Clinical severity	Typical features	Typically associated mutations
I	Mild non-deforming osteogenesis imperfecta	Normal height or mild short stature, blue sclerae, no dentinogenesis imperfecta	Premature stop codon in *COLIAI*
II	Perinatal lethal	Multiple rib and long bone fractures at birth, pronounced deformities, broad long bones, low density of skull bones on radiographs, dark sclerae	Glycine substitutions in *COLIAI* or *COLIA2*
III	Severely deforming	Very short, triangular face, severe scoliosis, grayish sclerae, dentinogenesis imperfecta	Glycine substitutions in *COLIAI* or *COLIA2*
IV	Moderately deforming	Moderately short, mild to moderate scoliosis, grayish or white sclerae, dentinogenesis imperfecta	Glycine substitutions in *COLIAI* or *COLIA2*
V	Moderately deforming	Mild to moderate short stature, dislocation of radial head, mineralized interosseous membrane, hyperplastic callus, white sclerae, no dentinogenesis imperfecta	Unknown
VI	Moderately to severely deforming	Moderately short, scoliosis, accumulation of osteoid in bone tissue, fish-scale pattern of bone lamellation, white sclerae, no dentinogenesis imperfecta	Unknown
VII	Moderately deforming	Mild short stature, short humeri and femora, coxa vara, white sclerae, no dentinogenesis imperfecta	Unknown

Reproduced with permission from Rauch F, Glorieux PF. Osteogenesis imperfecta. *Lancet* 2004;363:1377–1385.

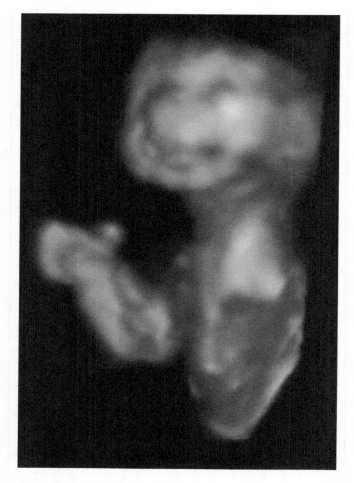

Figure 23.7 Three-dimensional rendered volume of a fetus with diastrophic dysplasia showing a hitchhiker thumb.

Diastrophic dysplasia

Diastrophic dysplasia is characterized by micromelia, clubfoot, hand deformities, multiple joint flexion contractures and scoliosis. Clinical features include rhizomelic-type micromelia, contractures, hand deformities with abducted position of the thumbs ("hitchhiker thumb"—see Figs 23.7 and 23.8) and severe talipes equinovarus. The head is normal, but micrognathia and cleft palate may be associated. This disorder has a wide spectrum, and some cases may not be diagnosable *in utero*. Diastrophic dysplasia is not universally lethal. Intelligence and sexual development

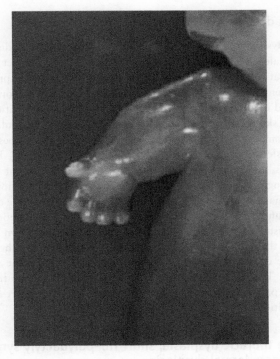

Figure 23.8 Hitchhiker thumb in diastrophic dysplasia.

are unaffected. Death in the neonatal period due to respiratory and spinal abnormalities as well as mental retardation has been reported in some patients.

Kniest syndrome

Kniest syndrome is characterized by involvement of the spine (platyspondyly and coronal clefts) and the tubular bones (shortened and metaphyseal flaring), with a broad and short thorax. There is a wide spectrum of disease and, most commonly, the disorder is compatible with life. However, lethality in the neonatal period has been reported.

Dyssegmental dysplasia

Dyssegmental dysplasia is an autosomal recessive disorder, classified into two types: the mild Rolland–Desbuquois form and the lethal Silverman–Handmaker. The latter is characterized by anarchic ossification of the vertebral bodies, metaphyseal flaring, and severe bowing of the long bones. The Rolland–Desbuquois type has essentially the same features, but the defects are much milder.

Campomelic dysplasia

Campomelic dysplasia is a rare and lethal autosomal dominant disorder with an estimated prevalence of 0.05–1.6 per 10 000 births. A unique aspect of campomelic dysplasia is that 75% of affected infants with a male karyotype present with sex reversal syndrome and have female or ambigous genitalia. Campomelic syndrome is characterized by bowing of the long bones of the lower extremities, an enlarged and elongated skull with a peculiar small facies, hypoplastic scapulae, and several associated anomalies such as micrognathia, cleft palate, talipes equinovarus, congenital dislocation of hip, macrocephaly, micrognathia, hydrocephalus, hydronephrosis, and congenital heart defects. The most important significant features are bowing of the femur and tibia; other tubular bones are normal in length. The thorax is narrow and can be "bell-shaped." Cervical vertebrae are hypoplastic and poorly ossified. There are two "short-bone varieties" of campomelic dysplasia representing distinct syndromes: the normocephalic form is known as kyphomelic dysplasia, and the craniostenotic type appears to be identical to the Antley–Bixler syndrome. The condition is frequently lethal in infancy but some survivors have been reported. The cause of death is respiratory distress due to tracheomalacia. However, cleft palate, micrognathia, hypotonia, and small chest are also associated with this condition.

Asphyxiating thoracic dysplasia, short rib–polydactyly syndromes, and chondroectodermal dysplasia

Table 23.7 illustrates the criteria for the differential diagnoses of asphyxiating thoracic dysplasia, short rib–polydactyly syndromes, and chondroectodermal dysplasia.

Asphyxiating thoracic dysplasia, also known as Jeune syndrome, is a rare autosomal recessive skeletal disorder characterized by a narrow and "bell-shaped" thorax, with short and horizontal ribs. Long bones are normal or mildly shortened. Polydactyly and cleft lip and/or palate can occur in association and the presence of a proximal femoral ossification center at birth is a characteristic finding.

Short rib–polydactyly syndromes are a group of disorders characterized by micromelia, constricted thorax, and postaxial polydactyly (Fig. 23.9). Traditionally, three different types have been recognized (Saldino–Noonan, Majewski, and Naumoff).

Chondroectodermal dysplasia, also known as Ellis–van Creveld syndrome, is inherited with an autosomal recessive pattern. It is characterized by acromesomelia with a normal spine and skull, postaxial polydactyly (Fig. 23.10), long and narrow thorax with short ribs, and congenital heart disease (60% of cases). Polydactyly is a consistent finding; the supernumerary digit usually has well-formed metacarpal and phalangeal bones.

Phocomelia

In phocomelia, the hands and feet are present, but the intervening arms and legs

Table 23.7 Disorders with thoracic dysplasia and polydactyly.

	Asphyxiating thoracic dysplasia (Jeune)	Chondroectodermal dysplasia (Ellis–van Creveld)	Short rib–polydactyly syndrome type I (Saldino–Noonan)	Short rib–polydactyly syndrome type II (Majewski)	Short rib syndrome type III (Naumoff)	Short rib syndrome type IV (Beemer–Langer)
Relative prevalence	Common	Uncommon	Common	Extremely rare	Rare	Rare
Clinical features						
Thoracic constriction	++	+	+++	+++	+++	+++
Polydactyly	+	++	++	++	++	++
Limb shortening	+	+	+++	+	++	++
Congenital heart disease	–	++	++	++	–	–
Other abnormalities	Renal disease	Ectodermal dysplasia	Genitourinary and gastrointestinal anomalies	Cleft lip and palate	Renal abnormality	Cleft lip and palate and genitourinary and gastrointestinal anomalies
Radiographic features						
Tubular bone shortening	+	+	+++	++	+++	++
Distinctive features in femora	–	–	Pointed ends	–	Marginal spurs	–
Short, horizontal ribs	++	++	+++	+++	+++	+++
Vertical shortening of ilia and flat acetabula	++	++	++	–	++	–
Defective ossification of vertebral bodies	–	–	++	–	+	++
Shortening of skull base	–	–	–	–	+	–

+, Not common; ++, common; +++, most common; –, absent.
Reproduced with permission from Cremin BJ. *Bone dysplasias of infancy. A radiological atlas*. Berlin: Springer–Verlag; 1978.

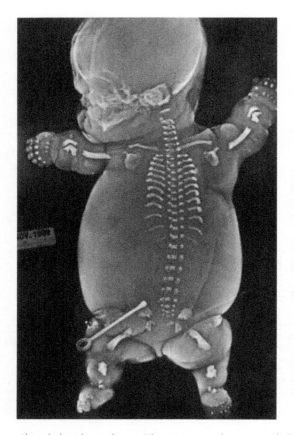

Figure 23.9 Short rib–polydactyly syndrome. There is severe shortening of all long bones, very short and horizontal ribs, and postaxial polydactyly in all four extremities. Note the angulation of the bones in the forearm.

are absent. Hands and feet may be normal or abnormal. Three syndromes must be considered in the differential diagnosis of phocomelia: Roberts syndrome, some varieties of the thrombocytopenia with absent radius (TAR) syndrome, and Grebe syndrome.

Roberts syndrome is an autosomal recessive disorder characterized by the association of tetraphocomelia and facial dysmorphisms (hypertelorism, facial clefting defects, hypoplastic nasal alae). The upper extremities are generally more severely affected than the lower extremities, and the spine is not involved. Polyhydramnios has been noted, and other anomalies associated with the syndrome include horseshoe kidney, hydrocephaly, cephalocele, and spina bifida. Prenatal diagnosis has been reported.

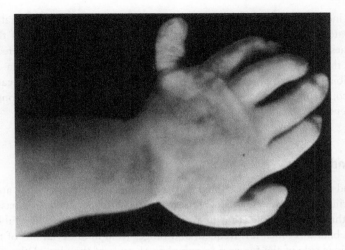

Figure 23.10 Postaxial polydactyly in a fetus with Ellis–van Creveld syndrome.

Grebe syndrome (Grebe–Quelce–Salgado chondrodystrophy) is an autosomal recessive nonlethal disorder of limb development. Affected individuals have normal head, neck, and trunk skeleton, relatively normal humeri and femora, short and deformed radii, ulnae, tibiae, and fibulae, as well as severe abnormalities of hands and feet. Polydactyly is frequent. Digits are very small and have been variously described as "bulbous," "bud-like," "mere knobs," "globular appendages," or "stubby toe-like fingers." The proximal and middle phalanges of the fingers and toes are invariably absent, whereas the distal phalanges are present. Radiographic documentation has provided information on subtle clinical characteristics for obligate heterozygotes: polydactyly, brachydactyly, hallux valgus, and metatarsus adductus. Survivors have normal intelligence and develop normal secondary sexual characteristics. TAR syndrome is discussed in the section on radial clubhand deformities.

Congenital short femur

Proximal femoral focal deficiency, or congenital short femur, refers to a group of disorders encompassing a wide range of congenital developmental anomalies of the femur. The disorder has been classified into five groups: type I, simple hypoplasia of the femur; type II, short femur with angulated shaft; type III, short femur with coxa vara (the most common); type IV, absent or defective proximal femur; and type V, absent or rudimentary femur. One or both femurs may be affected, but the right one is more frequently involved. Anomalies of the upper limbs can also be present and do not exclude the diagnosis. If both femurs are affected, it is important to examine the face carefully, as the disorder may be bilateral femoral hypoplasia and unusual face syndrome, which consists of bilateral femoral hypoplasia and facial defects, including short nose with broad tip, long philtrum, micrognathia, and cleft palate. Long bone abnormalities can extend to other segments of the lower extremities (absent fibula) as well as to the upper extremities. If the defect is unilateral, the differential diagnosis includes either the femur–fibula–ulna or femur–tibia–radius complex. These two syndromes have different implications for genetic counseling: the former is nonfamilial, whereas the latter has a strong genetic component.

Clubhands

Clubhand deformities are classified into two main categories: radial and ulnar. Radial clubhand includes a wide spectrum of disorders that encompass absent thumb, thumb hypoplasia, thin first metacarpal, and absent radius (Table 23.8). Ulnar clubhand is much less frequent and ranges from mild deviations of the hand on the ulnar side of the forearm to complete absence of the ulna. Although radial clubhand is frequently syndromic, ulnar clubhand is usually an isolated anomaly. Table 23.9 shows conditions that present with ulnar ray defects.

Fanconi's anemia (pancytopenia) is an autosomal recessive disease characterized by the association of bone marrow failure (anemia, leukopenia, and thrombocytopenia) and skeletal anomalies, including a radial clubhand with absent thumbs, radial hypoplasia, and a high frequency of chromosomal instability (demonstrated in amniotic fluid cells or fetal lymphocytes as a high frequency of chromosomal breakage after incubation with diepoxy-butane). Approximately 25% of affected individuals do not have limb reduction anomalies. Associated findings include microcephaly, congenital dislocation of the hip, scoliosis, and cardiac, pulmonary, and gastrointestinal anomalies. Intrauterine growth restriction is common. Up to 25% of the patients will show some degree of mental deficiency.

TAR syndrome is an autosomal recessive disorder characterized by thrombocytopenia (platelet count of less than 100 000/mm^3) and bilateral absence of the radius. The thumb and metacarpals are always present. The ulna and humerus may be absent, and clubfoot deformities may be present. Congenital heart disease is present in 33% of the cases (e.g., tetralogy of Fallot and septal defects).

Aase syndrome is an autosomal recessive condition characterized by congenital hypoplastic anemia and a radial clubhand with bilateral triphalangeal thumb and a hypoplastic distal radius. Cardiac defects (ventricular septal defects, coarctation of the aorta) may be present. Triphalangeal thumbs are a feature of several bone dysostoses and malformation syndromes.

Holt–Oram syndrome is an autosomal dominant disorder characterized by congenital heart disease (mainly atrial septal defects, secundum type, and ventricular septal defects), aplasia or hypoplasia of the radius, and triphalangeal or absent thumbs. Limb defects are often asymmetric, with the left side being more affected than the right side. Other findings include hypertelorism, chest wall, and vertebral anomalies.

Table 23.8 Radial ray defects: a differential diagnosis of congenital deficiency of the radius and radial ray.

Isolated: nonsyndromatic

Syndromes with blood dyscrasias
Fanconi's anemia

Thrombocytopenia with absent radii syndrome

Aase syndrome: congenital anemia, nonopposable triphalangeal thumb, scaphoid and distal radius hypoplasia, radioulnar synostosis, short stature with narrow shoulders, autosomal recessive (see Diamond–Blackfan syndrome for a similar, perhaps identical, syndrome)

Syndromes with congenital heart disease
Holt–Oram syndrome

Lewis upper limb–cardiovascular syndrome: more extensive arm malformations and more complex heart anomalies than with Holt–Oram, but probably not a separate syndrome, autosomal dominant

Syndromes with craniofacial abnormalities
Nager acrofacial dysostosis

Radial clubhand and cleft lip and/or cleft palate: sporadic

Juberg–Hayward syndrome: cleft lip and palate, hypoplastic thumbs, short radius, radial head subluxation, autosomal recessive

Baller–Gerold syndrome: craniosynostosis, bilateral radial clubhand, absent/hypoplastic thumb, autosomal recessive

Rothmund–Thomson syndrome: prematurely aged skin changes, juvenile cataract, sparse gray hair, absent thumbs, radial clubhands, occasional knee dysplasia (see progeria syndromes)

Duane radial dysplasia syndrome: abnormal ocular movements, inability to abduct and eyeball retraction with adduction, radius and radial ray hypoplasia, vertebral anomalies, renal malformation, autosomal dominant (see Klippel–Feil variants)

IVIC syndrome (Instituto Venezolano de Investigaciones Cientificas): radial ray deficiency, hypoplastic or absent thumbs and radial clubhands, impaired hearing, abnormal movements of extraocular muscles with strabismus, autosomal dominant

LARD syndrome (lacrimo-auriculo-radial-dental; Levy–Hollister): absent lacrimal structures, protuberant ears, thumb and radial ray hypoplasia, abnormal teeth, autosomal dominant

Radial defects with ear anomalies and cranial nerve VII dysfunction

Radial hypoplasia, triphalangeal thumb, hypospadias, diastema of maxillary central incisors, autosomal dominant

Syndromes with congenital scoliosis
The VATER association
Goldenhar syndrome (oculoauriculovertebral dysplasia)
Kippel–Feil syndrome

Radial aplasia and chromosome aberrations

Syndromes with mental retardation
Seckel syndrome (bird-headed dwarfism): microcephaly, beak-like protrusion of nose, mental retardation, absent/hypoplastic thumbs, bilateral dislocated hips

Thalidomide embryopathy (of historical interest, but some 60% had radial clubhand)

Reproduced with permission from Goldberg MJ. *The dysmorphic child: an orthopedic perspective*. New York: Raven Press, 1987.

Table 23.9 Ulnar ray defects: a differential diagnosis of congenital deficiency of the ulna and ulnar ray.

Isolated: nonsyndromatic absent ulna

Ulna hypoplasia and skeletal deficiency elsewhere
Ulna aplasia with lobster claw deformity of hand and/or foot, autosomal dominant
Femur–fibula–ulna complex

Syndromes with ulna deficiency
Cornelia de Lange syndrome

Miller syndrome (postaxial acrofacial dysostosis): absent ulna and ulnar rays and absent fourth and fifth toes; Treacher–Collins mandibulofacial hypoplasia, autosomal recessive, distinguish from Nagar preaxial acrofacial dysostosis

Pallister ulnar–mammary syndrome: hypoplasia of ulna and ulnar rays, hypoplasia of the breast and absence of apocrine sweat glands, autosomal dominant

Pillay syndrome (ophthalmomandibulomelic dysplasia): absent distal third of ulna, absent olecranon, hypoplastic trochlea and proximal radius, fusion of interphalangeal joints in ulnar fingers, knee dysplasia, corneal opacities, fusion of temporomandibular joint, autosomal dominant

Weyers' oligodactyly syndrome: deficiency of ulna and ulnar rays, antecubital webbing, short sternum, malformed kidney and spleen, cleft lip and palate, sporadic

Schnizel syndrome: absent/hypoplastic fourth, fifth metacarpals and phalanges, hypogenitalism, anal atresia, autosomal dominant

Mesometic dwarfism, Reinhardt–Pfeiffer type (ulno-fibula dysplasia): a generalized bone dysplasia but with a disproportionate hypoplasia of the ulna and fibula, autosomal dominant

Mesomelic dwarfism, Langer's type: a generalized bone dysplasia, but with aplasia of the distal ulna and proximal fibula and hypoplasia of the mandible

---

Reproduced with permission from Goldberg MJ. *The dysmorphic child: an orthopedic perspective.* New York: Raven Press, 1987.

Radial clubhand and scoliosis

When radial clubhand is also associated with scoliosis, three syndromes should be considered: VATER association, Goldenhar syndrome, and Klippel–Feil syndrome.

Typical findings in the VATER association are vertebral segmentation defects (70%), anal atresia (80%), tracheoesophageal fistula (70%), esophageal atresia, and radial and renal defects (65% and 53%, respectively). Other anomalies include a single umbilical artery (35%) and congenital heart disease, occurring in nearly 50% of the patients. The VATER association occurs sporadically, although recurrence within a sibship has been reported.

The Goldenhar syndrome is characterized by hemifacial microsomia, vertebral anomalies, and radial defects. Alterations in the morphogenesis of the first and

Table 23.10 Disorders of the developing motor system on all levels, leading to immobilization.

Disorders of the developing neuromuscular system
Loss of anterior horn cells
Radicular disease with collagen proliferation
Peripheral neuropathy with neurofibromatosis
Congenital myasthenia
Neonatal myasthenia (maternal myasthenia gravis)
Amyoplasia congenita
Congenital muscular dystrophy
Central core disease
Congenital myotonic dystrophy
Glycogen accumulation myopathy
Disorders of developing connective tissue or connective tissue disease
Muscular and articular connective tissue dystrophy
Articular defects by mesenchymal dysplasia
Increased collagen synthesis
Disorders of developing medulla or medullary disease
Congenital spinal epidural hemorrhage
Congenital duplication of the spinal canal
Disorders of brain development (e.g., porencephaly or brain disease)
Congenital encephalopathy

---

second brachial arches result in hypoplasia of the malar, maxillary, or mandibular region, microtia, and ocular and oropharyngeal anomalies.

The Klippel–Feil syndrome is characterized by fusion of any two cervical vertebrae, resulting in a short neck, low posterior hair line, and restricted mobility of the upper spine. Several associated anomalies may be present, including spina bifida, cleft palate, rib abnormalities, lung disorders, congenital heart disease, and limb anomalies.

Arthrogryposis

The term "arthrogryposis multiplex congenita" (AMC) refers to multiple joint contractures present at birth in an intact skeleton. Neurological, muscular, connective tissue, or skeletal abnormalities or intrauterine crowding can lead to impaired fetal motion and AMC. Table 23.10 shows motor systems that can lead to AMC. The deformities are usually symmetric. In most cases of AMC, all four limbs are involved (Fig. 23.11), followed by deformities of the lower extremities only, or bimelic involvement. Many congenital anomalies are associated with AMC. The most

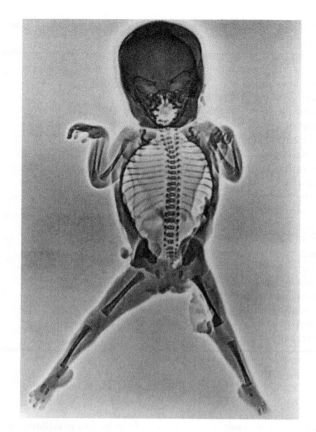

Figure 23.11 Arthrogryposis multiplex congenita. There is flexion of the upper limbs with hyperextension of the lower limbs.

frequent are cleft palate, Klippel–Feil syndrome, meningomyelocele, and congenital heart disease. In total, 10% of patients with AMC have associated anomalies of the central nervous system.

Further reading

Bahlmann F, Merz E, Hallermann C, et al. Congenital diaphragmatic hernia: ultrasonic measurement of fetal lungs to predict pulmonary hypoplasia. *Ultrasound Obstet Gynecol* 1999;14:162–168.

Benoit B. The value of three-dimensional ultrasonography in the screening of the fetal skeleton. *Childs Nerv Syst* 2003;19:403–409.

Doray B, Favre R, Viville B, et al. Prenatal sonographic diagnosis of skeletal dysplasias. A report of 47 cases. *Ann Genet* 2000;43:163–169.

Gaffney G, Manning N, Boyd PA, et al. Prenatal sonographic diagnosis of skeletal dysplasias—a report of the diagnostic and prognostic accuracy in 35 cases. *Prenat Diagn* 1998; 18:357–362.

Gordienko IY, Grechanina EY, Sopko NI, et al. Prenatal diagnosis of osteochondrodysplasias in high risk pregnancy. *Am J Med Genet* 1996;63:90–97.

Hall CM. International nosology and classification of constitutional disorders of bone (2001). *Am J Med Genet* 2002;113:65–77.

Merz E, Miric-Tesanic D, Bahlmann F, et al. Prenatal sonographic chest and lung measurements for predicting severe pulmonary hypoplasia. *Prenat Diagn* 1999;19:614–619.

Parilla BV, Leeth EA, Kambich MP, et al. Antenatal detection of skeletal dysplasias. *J Ultrasound Med* 2003;22:255–258.

Superti-Furga A, Bonafe L, Rimoin DL. Molecular–pathogenetic classification of genetic disorders of the skeleton. *Am J Med Genet* 2001;106:282–293.

Tretter AE, Saunders RC, Meyers CM, et al. Antenatal diagnosis of lethal skeletal dysplasias. *Am J Med Genet* 1998;75:518–522.

Unger S. A genetic approach to the diagnosis of skeletal dysplasia. *Clin Orthop* 2002; 401:32–38.

24 First- and second-trimester prenatal diagnosis

John C. Hobbins

In this chapter, the newest concepts and procedures are outlined to provide the reader with a guide to first- and second-trimester prenatal diagnosis.

Invasive procedures

CVS

The procedure was first described by Brambati and, while commonly utilized in the 1980s, it had a downturn after a report suggested an association between the procedure and transverse limb defects in the fetus. However, data from a large registry negated this correlation when the procedure was done after 9 weeks.

The risk of fetal loss from CVS performed by an experienced operator is about 1%, and there is a suggestion that a transabdominal approach is slightly less risky than the transcervical route.

Early amniocentesis

This procedure initially emerged as an alternative to CVS in the first and early second trimester. However, randomized trials have shown the procedure to be associated with a higher loss rate than with CVS (1.5% versus 0.8%) or with standard amniocentesis (2.5% versus 1.0%). Also, there was an unacceptable rate of club-foot (1.3%), probably resulting from a high rate of amniotic fluid leakage (3.5%).

Second-trimester amniocentesis
The only randomized clinical trial in patients having amniocenteses showed a 1% higher loss rate than in control subjects (1.7% versus 0.7%). A review of the non-randomized trials suggests a procedure-related loss rate of about 0.6%. Although unpublished data from one large trial suggest a lower loss rate from amniocentesis, all other studies in the literature point to a risk of about 1 in 200.

First-trimester prenatal diagnosis—noninvasive

Nuchal translucency (NT)
In 1992, Nicolaides reported on an association between increased NT and chromosome abnormalities. In a large study involving 96 127 patients, 77% of fetuses with Down syndrome (DS) were detected when using an algorithm based on NT, maternal age, and crown–rump length. Other studies have now borne out these results.

Biochemistry
In DS, levels of pregnancy-associated plasma protein A (PAPP-A) are generally low, and levels of human chorionic gonadotropin (hCG) tend to be high [average 0.39 multiples of the median (MoM) and 1.83 MoM respectively]. When used together, they have a sensitivity of 62% at a 5% false-positive rate.

NT and biochemistry in combination ("combined test")
This combination has an 82% detection rate at a screen-positive rate of 5% (Table 24.1).

Table 24.1 Pregnancy loss rate in experienced US centers.

	Continued pregnancy	Spontaneous abortion	Spontaneous abortion (%)
Carolinas Medical Center	3 545	117	2.4
Genetics and IVF	14 116	232	1.6
Illinois Masonic Medical Center	6 580	195	3.0
Thomas Jefferson University	13 629	346	2.5
University of California, San Francisco	10 386	354	3.4
Wayne State University	6 995	143	2.0
Total	55 251	1387	2.5

From Wapner R, Jackson L, Evans MI, et al. *Am J Obstet Gynecol* 1996;174:310.

Second-trimester biochemistry

For the past decade, the triple screen (alpha-fetoprotein, estriol, and hCG) has been widely utilized in screening for DS, trisomy 18, and neural tube defects. Across all maternal ages, the method has a sensitivity for DS of about 62% at a 5% screen-positive rate but, in patients of advanced maternal age (AMA), the detection rate is above 80% (but at a three times higher screen-positive rate). In most laboratories, the quad screen consists of adding inhibin A to the above biochemical triad and enhances the sensitivity by about 5%.

Prenatal diagnosis combinations using ultrasound and biochemistry

Table 24.2 outlines the expected sensitivities with various combinations based on data in the literature with the addition of some mathematical modeling.

Fetuses with increased NT and normal chromosomes have a higher rate of fetal anomalies, especially involving the heart. Anomalies most commonly associated with this finding are holoprosencephaly, diaphragmatic hernias, limb body wall complex, and various skeletal dysplasias. For this reason, patients whose fetuses are in this category should have a detailed second-trimester sonogram and a later fetal echocardiogram (18–22 weeks). If these tests are reassuring, then the likelihood of an adverse outcome drops to at least baseline levels.

Genetic sonogram

This expanded ultrasound examination consists of assessing fetal bone length (often shorter in DS), screening for major anomalies (occurring in 20% of DS fetuses), and searching for ultrasound markers for DS. The various markers that have been commonly evaluated are outlined in Table 24.3.

Table 24.2 Prenatal diagnosis combinations using ultrasound and biochemistry.

Combination type	Sensitivity (%)	FPR (%)
Combined	82	5
NT + first-trimester biochemistry		
Integrated	96	5
NT + first- and second-trimester biochemistry (results only after second blood draw)		
Independent sequential	87	5
Two separate results from combined and standard second-trimester biochemistry	(with triple screen)	
Dependent sequential (also known as "contingency")	95	5
Combined result available to patient, but second-trimester biochemistry calculation is based on result of first-trimester result and not patient's age		

FPR, false-positive rate; NT, nuchal translucency.

Table 24.3 Soft markers.

Nuchal skinfold thickness
Ear length
Frontal lobe length
Nasal bone length
Echogenic focus in the heart
Echogenic bowel
Iliac angle
Iliac bone length
"Sandal gap" feet
Absent or small middle phalanx of the fifth digit
Pyelectasis
Mild ventriculomegaly

Biometry: femur length (vs. biparietal diameter or against expected femur length for gestational age)

Table 24.4 The genetic sonogram experience.

Study	No. of patients	Sensitivity (%)	FPR (%)	LR (+)	LR (−)
Bromley	175	82	14.4	5.7	0.20
Vintzileos	34	82	9.0	9.1	0.20
Bromley	54	75	5.7	13.1	0.27
Benacerraf	45	73	4.4	16.5	0.28
Nyberg	142	74	14.7	5.0	0.30
Bahado-Singh	31	74	15.0	5.0	0.31
Nyberg	186	70	13.3	5.3	0.36
Sohl	55	67	19.4	3.5	0.41
Vergagni	22	59	5.3	11.1	0.43

Each marker found will raise the odds of DS, but it is unclear what risk can be estimated for a given patient when a marker other than the best performers (nuchal skinfold thickness, nasal bone length, and short humerus) is found in isolation. What is clear is that the risk can be adjusted downward from the pre-ultrasound risk when the genetic sonogram is completely "negative." The sensitivity of this method in the literature varies between 59% and 82% (Table 24.4). One can calculate a negative likelihood ratio for a given center based on its own sensitivity and use that figure to re-estimate the risk for a given patient after a reassuring result.

Conclusion

Progress in prenatal diagnosis over the past 10 years has been exponential, and there is every reason to believe that better noninvasive methods will continue to be developed, allowing better informed choices for pregnant patients.

Further reading

Benn PA, Egan JFX, Fang M, et al. Changes in the utilization of prenatal diagnosis. *Obstet Gynecol* 2004;103:1255–1260.

Egan JFX. The genetic sonogram in second trimester Down syndrome screening. *Clin Obstet Gynecol* 2003;46:897–908.

Froster UG, Jackson L. Limb defects and chorionic villus sampling: results from an international registry, 1992–94. *Lancet* 1996;347:484–494.

Malone FD, D'Alton ME. First-trimester sonographic screening for Down syndrome. *Obstet Gynecol* 2003;102:1066–1079.

Nicolaides KH, Azar G, Byrne D, et al. Fetal nuchal translucency: ultrasound screening for chromosomal defects in first trimester of pregnancy. *Br Med J* 1992;304:867–869.

Seeds JW. Diagnostic mid-trimester amniocentesis: how safe? *Am J Obstet Gynecol* 2004; 191:608–616.

Snijders RJ, Nobel P, Sebire N, et al. UK multicentre project on assessment of risk of trisomy 21 by maternal age and fetal nuchal-translucency thickness at 10–14 weeks of gestation. Fetal Medicine Foundation First Trimester Screening Group. *Lancet* 1998;352:343–346.

Sundberg K, Bang J, Smidt-Jensen S, et al. Randomised study of risk of fetal loss related to early amniocentesis versus chorionic villus sampling. *Lancet* 1997;350:697–703.

Wapner R, Thom E, Simpson JL, et al. for the First Trimester Maternal Serum Biochemistry and Fetal Nuchal Translucency Screening (BUN) Study Group. First-trimester screening for trisomies 21 and 18. *N Engl J Med* 2003;349:1405–1413.

25 First- and second-trimester screening for open neural tube defects and Down syndrome

James E. Haddow, Glenn E. Palomaki, and Ronald Wapner

Diagnostic testing for open neural tube defects

Biochemical testing for fetal disorders dates from the discovery that amniotic fluid alpha-fetoprotein (AFP) levels are elevated in the presence of open neural tube defects (NTDs; open spina bifida and anencephaly) during the early second trimester.[1] This discovery led to the availability of diagnostic testing for pregnant women with a previously affected pregnancy. An important limitation of the public-health impact of such testing was that fewer than 5% of the annual births affected by open NTDs occur among women known to be at high risk.

Maternal serum screening for open NTDs

Subsequently, maternal serum levels of AFP were also documented to be sufficiently elevated in the presence of open NTDs that such measurements could be offered to all pregnant women for screening purposes. Women with elevated serum AFP levels would then be offered amniotic fluid AFP measurements as a diagnostic test.[2]

Ultrasound and open NTDs

Ultrasound examination of the fetal spine was initially used diagnostically to help confirm the presence of open spina bifida; however, this examination is technically difficult and was eventually replaced by more reliable ultrasound observations of the fetal cranium and brain (the "lemon" and "banana" signs).

Maternal serum screening for Down syndrome in the second trimester

Data accumulated during the early years of screening for open NTDs set the stage for the discovery that maternal serum AFP levels were lower in the presence of Down syndrome. This allowed an interpretation of Down syndrome risk based on a combination of maternal age and AFP to be added to the existing screening test, with amniotic fluid chromosome analysis offered to women at high risk. The subsequent discovery of other biochemical markers (including unconjugated estriol, uE_3; human chorionic gonadotropin, hCG; and dimeric inhibin-A, DIA) greatly improved the efficiency of second-trimester screening. The "quadruple" second-trimester test, which has a detection rate of 75–80% among ultrasound-dated pregnancies and a corresponding false-positive rate of about 5%, is the present standard of care for millions of women each year.

Maternal serum screening for Down syndrome in the first trimester

A further important breakthrough occurred with the identification of first-trimester maternal serum markers [pregnancy-associated plasma protein-A (PAPP-A) and the free β-subunit of hCG]. The screening performance of these markers varies with gestational age (between 10 and 13 completed weeks' gestation) and does not reach that attained by second-trimester quadruple marker testing.

Role of ultrasound in prenatal genetic screening

Ultrasound is an invaluable complement to AFP testing in the evaluation of NTDs. This diagnosis can require detailed imaging of the fetal spine. The ultrasound diagnosis of NTDs has been greatly enhanced by recognition of associated anomalies of the fetal skull and brain. These findings include ventriculomegaly, microcephaly, frontal bone scalloping ("lemon" sign), and obliteration of the cisterna magna with either an absent or abnormal anterior curvature of the cerebellar hemisphere ("banana" sign). Ultrasound can also detect many other causes of elevated AFP in addition to NTDs, such as omphalocele, gastroschisis, bladder extrophy, and some cases of sacrococcygeal teratoma. Increased AFP levels are also found with other equally severe fetal problems, such as lethal skin disorders and congenital nephrosis, but these may not be detectable using ultrasound.

Ultrasound can be used in the first trimester to evaluate the risk of Down syndrome (trisomy 21). In fetuses with Down syndrome, there is increased fluid in the posterior nuchal area. This is called nuchal translucency (NT), which is defined as the maximum fluid-filled space between the skin of the posterior fetal neck area and the underlying structures. The measurement of NT can be converted to a likelihood ratio and used to predict the risk of Down syndrome.

When used together, biochemistry (PAPP-A and hCG) and ultrasound (NT) will identify over 85% of Down syndrome pregnancies with a 5% false-positive rate. This is more accurate than second-trimester screening, and has the added advantage of early detection.

Individuals with Down syndrome have hypoplasia of the nasal bridge. This finding is present in approximately 65% of fetuses with Down syndrome and can be used as a marker for Down syndrome.

Nasal bone imaging, however, contains some caveats before it can be recommended for routine use: (1) it is difficult to image; (2) visualization is gestational age dependent; and (3) measurements of the nasal bone are not independent of the NT. For these reasons, use of nasal bone imaging is not recommended as part of primary screening in a risk algorithm for Down syndrome.

Fetal aneuploidy other than Down syndrome can also be suspected in the second trimester, based on the finding of specific ultrasound abnormalities.

Combined ultrasound and maternal serum markers in the first trimester

If first-trimester biochemical and NT measurements at 11–13 weeks' gestation are combined, the screening performance is similar to that of the second-trimester quadruple test. Maternal age is always used, in combination with NT and PAPP-A measurements (the two most effective markers). Either the free β-subunit of hCG or total hCG can be used as the fourth marker. Programs can make selections based on other factors, such as availability and cost of reagents.[3]

Integrating first- and second-trimester screening strategies for Down syndrome

Choosing an overall screening strategy for Down syndrome is complicated by the need to consider not only performance but also ancillary issues of program implementation, such as the timing and availability of diagnostic tests, adherence to risk cutoffs, concern about holding first-trimester test results until the second trimester, acceptability to women and health providers, financial costs, medical costs, and second-trimester serum testing for open NTDs. Three screening strategies are considered here: integrated, sequential, and contingent; all include NT measurements.

• In integrated screening, first-trimester information is held until the second-trimester results are also available. A single risk is then provided to the woman and a single risk cutoff level is used to define screen-positive results (e.g., $\geq$ 1:200).

• Sequential screening[4] initially offers counseling and diagnostic testing to all women with a first-trimester risk at or above an initial risk cutoff level (e.g., $\geq$ 1:50); the remaining women are given a quadruple test (AFP, uE$_3$, hCG, and DIA) in the second trimester that is interpreted as an "integrated" test, using information from both trimesters. Women with a Down syndrome risk above a final second-trimester risk cutoff level (e.g., $\geq$ 1:270) are also offered counseling and second-trimester diagnostic testing.

• Contingent screening[5,6] differs from sequential screening by having not only a high-risk cutoff level but also a low-risk level defined in the first trimester (e.g., $\geq$ 1:50 and < 1:1500). Women with Down syndrome risks below the low-risk cutoff level are informed that they do not require further testing as they are unlikely to become screen positive.

Given that integrated screening uses all of the informative markers prior to assigning a risk and determining who should be offered diagnostic testing, the other two strategies will be, of necessity, less efficient, as defined by detection and false-positive rates. This is because both sequential and contingent screening strategies assign an interim risk and make the offer of diagnostic testing in the first trimester based on only a subset of informative markers. Thus, the early detection of some affected pregnancies and the reduced need for second-trimester screening (contingent testing) must logically be "paid for" by having either a somewhat lower detection rate or more false positives. Modeling these three strategies shows that the performance of the two sequential strategies can approach that of the integrated strategy, but only if the proportion of women offered diagnostic testing in the first trimester is kept well below the proportion offered diagnostic testing in the second trimester. All of these strategies perform better than first-trimester combined or second-trimester stand-alone screening.[7]

Speculation

In the near future, Down syndrome screening programs will increasingly combine information from both trimesters as a way of reducing false positives while simultaneously improving detection. Although NT measurements have been shown to be reliable in the research setting, it is not yet clear whether such testing can be reliably offered as a routine screening test.[8] Other improvements, such as repeated measures of biochemical markers[6,9] are being investigated as ways of increasing performance even further, even when NT measurements are not available. Also, methods using multiple contingent policies are being promulgated.[10] Routinely available screening strategies, including those based on maternal serum alone, may soon be able to detect over 90% of Down syndrome pregnancies with only a 1–2% false-positive rate, by combining information from first- and second-trimester screening tests. Research is also continuing in the area of collecting and testing individual fetal cells (or fetal DNA) in the maternal circulation as either a screening or diagnostic test.[11]

References

1 Brock DJ, Sutcliffe RG. Alpha-fetoprotein in the antenatal diagnosis of anencephaly and spina bifida. *Lancet* 1972;2:197.
2 Wald NJ, Cuckle H, Brock JH, et al. Maternal serum-alpha-fetoprotein measurement in antenatal screening for anencephaly and spina bifida in early pregnancy. Report of UK collaborative study on alpha-fetoprotein in relation to neural-tube defects. *Lancet* 1977;1:1323.
3 Reddy UM, Mennuti MT. Incorporating first-trimester Down syndrome studies into prenatal screening: executive summary of the National Institute of Child Health and Human Development workshop. *Obstet Gynecol* 2006;107:167.
4 Wright D, Bradbury I, Benn P, et al. Contingent screening for Down syndrome is an efficient alternative to non-disclosure sequential screening. *Prenat Diagn* 2004;24:762.
5 Benn P, Wright D, Cuckle H. Practical strategies in contingent sequential screening for Down syndrome. *Prenat Diagn* 2005;25:645.
6 Wright DE, Bradbury I. Repeated measures screening for Down's Syndrome. *Br J Obstet Gynaecol* 2005;112:80.
7 Palomaki GE, Steinort K, Knight GJ, Haddow JE. Comparing three screening strategies for combining first- and second-trimester Down syndrome markers. *Obstet Gynecol* 2006;107:367.
8 Malone FD, Canick JA, Ball RH, et al. First-trimester or second-trimester screening, or both, for Down's syndrome. *N Engl J Med* 2005;353:2001.
9 Palomaki GE, Wright DE, Summers AM, et al. Repeated measurement of pregnancy-associated plasma protein-A (PAPP-A) in Down syndrome screening: a validation study. *Prenat Diagn* 2006;DOI:10.1002/pd.1497.
10 Wright D, Bradbury I, Cuckle H, et al. Three-stage contingent screening for Down syndrome. *Prenat Diagn* 2006;26:528.
11 Farina A, LeShane ES, Lambert-Messerlian GM, et al. Evaluation of cell-free fetal DNA as a second-trimester maternal serum marker of Down syndrome pregnancy. *Clin Chem* 2003;49:239.

Further reading

Haddow JE, Palomaki GE, Knight GJ, et al. Reducing the need for amniocentesis in women 35 years of age or older with serum markers for screening. *N Engl J Med* 1994;330:1114.
Palomaki GE, Kloza EM, Haddow JE, et al. Patient and health professional acceptance of integrated serum screening for Down syndrome. *Semin Perinatol* 2005;29:247.
Van den Hof MC, Nicolaides KH, Campbell J, Campbell S. Evaluation of the lemon and banana signs in one hundred thirty fetuses with open spina bifida. *Am J Obstet Gynecol* 1990;162:322.
Wald NJ, Watt HC, Hackshaw AK. Integrated screening for Down's syndrome on the basis of tests performed during the first and second trimesters. *N Engl J Med* 1999;341:461.
Wald NJ, Rodeck C, Hackshaw AK, et al. First and second trimester antenatal screening for Down's syndrome: the results of the Serum, Urine, and Ultrasound Screening Study (SURUSS). *J Med Screen* 2003;10:56.

Part VII

Methods of Evaluation of Fetal Development and Well-being

26   Prenatal diagnosis of deviant fetal growth

E. Albert Reece and Zion J. Hagay

Fetal growth is a fundamental characteristic of the continuity of life and fetal well-being. Cell divisions, cell hyperplasia, and cell hypertrophy are the cornerstones of fetal growth. It has been suggested that, early in pregnancy, growth of fetal organs takes place first by cell hyperplasia or cell division, then by hyperplasia and cell hypertrophy and, finally, by the cessation of hyperplasia, after which growth continues by cellular hypertrophy alone.

In this chapter, we will discuss the two extreme types of deviant fetal growth – diminished [intrauterine growth restriction (IUGR)] and accelerated (macrosomia). In addition, prenatal diagnosis of these conditions will be discussed.

Intrauterine growth restriction

Etiology and definition

IUGR is an abnormality of fetal growth and development that affects 3–7% of all deliveries, depending on the diagnostic criteria used. The growth-restricted fetus is at greater risk for mortality and morbidity. It is estimated that perinatal mortality is 5–10 times higher in the growth-restricted neonate than in the neonate who is sized appropriately for gestational age.

There are several causes of IUGR. These may be conceptually divided into three main categories: maternal, fetal, and uteroplacental (Table 26.1). It should be stressed, however, that in almost half the cases of IUGR, the etiology is unknown. Furthermore, it has been found that the single most important maternal clinical risk factor is a previous history of IUGR. Therefore, suspicion of IUGR should not be based only on the existence of clinical risk factors during the index pregnancy.

One point of confusion and disagreement is the criteria that are used to define IUGR. IUGR has been defined variously as an infant whose birthweight is below the 3rd, 5th, and 10th percentile for gestational age or whose birthweight is more than two standard deviations below the mean for gestational age.

The ponderal index is determined in the neonate by the following formula:

$$\text{Ponderal index} = \text{birthweight (g)} \times 100/(\text{crown–heel length) cm}^3$$

Table 26.1 Risk factors of intrauterine growth retardation.

Maternal risk factors	Fetal risk factors
Alcohol	Genetic disorders (e.g., dwarf syndromes)
Smoking	Chromosomal abnormalities (e.g., trisomies
Drugs	13, 18, and 21)
Corticosteroids	Congenital anomalies (e.g., gastroschisis)
Propranolol	Fetal infection (e.g., viral, protozoan)
Dilantin	*Uterine and placental risk factors*
Coumadin	Müllerian anomalies (e.g., septate uterus)
Heroin	Placental insufficiency due to
Anemia	Infarctions
Malnutrition	Infection
Prepregnancy weight of <50 kg	Chorioangioma
Cyanotic heart disease	Multifetal pregnancy
Chronic hypertension	Circumvallate placenta
Pregnancy-induced hypertension	Previa
Diabetes mellitus (with vasculopathy)	Focal abruption
Connective tissue disease	Marginal insertion of the cord

The ponderal index may identify a neonate who has a small amount of soft tissue clinically evident by loss of subcutaneous tissue and muscle mass, even though the birthweight is normal for gestational age. Neonates with a ponderal index below the 10th percentile for gestational age are probably suffering from malnutrition *in utero*. Unfortunately, there is presently no practical method to evaluate ponderal index *in utero*. Hence, the most commonly used definition of IUGR is a fetal weight below the 10th percentile for gestational age.

Another index, the crown–heel length, has been used to evaluate neonatal size. Prediction from the femur length (FL) measurement, however, has been found to be too imprecise to be useful.

One unresolved problem concerns which growth curve to use. Discrepancies between different birthweight charts from different geographic areas underscore the need for generating birthweight curves from the population to which they will be applied.

Classification of intrauterine growth restriction

Clinically, three categories of IUGR may be recognized. Each reflects the time of onset of the pathologic process.

Type 1, or symmetric, IUGR

Type 1 IUGR refers to the infant with decreased growth potential. This type of IUGR begins early in gestation, and the entire fetus is proportionally small for gestational age (SGA).

Head and abdominal circumferences, length, and weight are all below the 10th percentile for gestational age. However, these infants have a normal ponderal index.

Type 1 IUGR is a result of growth inhibition early in gestation. This early stage of embryonic–fetal development is characterized by active mitosis from 4 to 20 weeks' gestation and is called the hyperplastic stage. Any pathologic process during this stage may lead to a reduced number of cells in the fetus.

Symmetric IUGR accounts for 20–30% of growth-restricted fetuses. This condition may result from the inhibition of mitosis, as is seen in intrauterine infection (e.g., herpes simplex, rubella, cytomegalovirus, toxoplasmosis), chromosomal disorders, and congenital malformations. It should be remembered, however, that symmetrically small fetuses may be constitutionally small and suffer from no abnormality at all.

In general, type 1 IUGR is associated with a poor prognosis: this is in direct relation to the pathologic condition that causes it. Weiner and Robinson (1989) showed that, in the absence of an identifiable maternal factor and sonographically detected abnormality, approximately 25% of fetuses evaluated for severe, early-onset growth restriction have aneuploidy. Therefore, the performance of percutaneous umbilical blood sampling is strongly recommended to search for karyotypic abnormality.

Type 2, or asymmetric, IUGR

Type 2, or asymmetric, IUGR refers to the neonate with restricted growth and is most frequently due to uteroplacental insufficiency.

Type 2 IUGR is a result of a later growth insult than type 1 and usually occurs after 28 weeks' gestation. Normal fetal growth is characterized by a process of hypertrophy. In this hypertrophic stage, there is a rapid increase in cell size and formation of fat, muscle, bone, and other tissues. In this phase, the process of hyperplasia is decreased.

Symmetrically growth-restricted fetuses have a near normal total number of cells, but these cells are decreased in size. Asymmetric IUGR fetuses have low ponderal indices with below average infant weight but normal head circumference (HC) and fetal length. In these cases of asymmetric IUGR, fetal growth is normal until late in the second trimester or early in the third, when head growth remains normal, whereas abdominal growth slows (brain-sparing effect). This asymmetry is a result of a fetal compensatory mechanism that responds to a state of poor placental perfusion. Redistribution of fetal cardiac output occurs with increased flow to the brain, heart, and adrenals and decreased glycogen storage and liver mass. However, if placental insufficiency is aggravated during late pregnancy, the head growth may be flattened, and its size may drop below the normal growth curve.

It is estimated that 70–80% of growth-restricted fetuses are type 2 IUGR. This form of IUGR is frequently associated with maternal diseases such as chronic hypertension, renal disease, diabetes mellitus with vasculopathy, and others (see Table 26.1).

Intermediate IUGR

Intermediate IUGR refers to growth restriction that is a combination of types 1 and 2 IUGR. The insult to fetal growth in intermediate IUGR most probably occurs during the middle phase of fetal growth – that of hyperplasia and hypertrophy – which corresponds to 20 to 28 weeks' gestation. At this stage, there is a decrease in mitotic rate and a progressive overall increase in cell size.

This form of IUGR is estimated as being responsible for 5–10% of all growth-restricted fetuses. Chronic hypertension, lupus nephritis, or other maternal vascular diseases that are severe and begin early in the second trimester may result in an intermediate IUGR with symmetric growth and no significant brain-sparing effect.

Ultrasonic measurements used in the diagnosis of IUGR

The intrauterine detection of restricted fetal growth by clinical means is possible in approximately 30% of affected pregnancies. Ultrasonography offers an objective, reliable, and effective means of identifying restricted intrauterine fetal growth. However, to make a proper diagnosis and appropriately manage the growth-restricted fetus, it is crucial to determine the gestational age as accurately as possible.

Pregnancy dating has traditionally been based on historical and clinical clues. The certain date of a patient's last menstrual period has been regarded as the most reliable method of estimating a fetus' gestational age. However, it has been reported that 20–40% of pregnant women fail to recall the exact date of their last menstrual period.

Therefore, ultrasonography may be of help in dating a pregnancy. In the first trimester, crown–rump length measurement allows for an estimation of gestational age with a range of 4.7 days at the 95% confidence level. Between 12 and 24 weeks' gestation, the biparietal diameter (BPD) measurement provides reliable estimates comparable with those of the crown–rump measurement performed in the first trimester of pregnancy. Beyond 28–30 weeks' gestation, there is a progressive increase in BPD variations, and the establishment of accurate gestational age is less satisfactory.

The FL correlates with gestational age, particularly during 14–22 weeks' gestation, with a range of 6–7 days at the 95% confidence level.

Accurate antenatal diagnosis of IUGR may prevent the high perinatal morbidity and mortality associated with this condition and permit appropriate management and obstetric intervention when fetal compromise is evident. Most authorities believe that, whenever IUGR is diagnosed after 37 weeks' gestation, delivery is indicated to decrease the risk of fetal death. The following sections review several sonographic parameters that may be used in the diagnosis of IUGR.

Biparietal diameter

Nomograms of BPD or HC are available to provide calculated estimates of weekly increments for the size of the fetal head (Tables 26.2 to 26.3). When comparing the observed increase in BPD with the expected rate of growth, the physician should be able to identify growth-restricted fetuses when the head is affected in the growth curtailment. However, single and serial BPD measurements alone are considered to be of poor value by most authors in the detection rates of IUGR, with reported accuracy rates ranging from 43% to 82%.

It seems clear that BPD alone cannot be used as a good predictor of IUGR. This is not surprising, because almost two-thirds of IUGR cases are of the asymmetric or late-flattening type, which have normal growth of the head until late in pregnancy as a consequence of the brain-sparing process. Therefore, BPD in asymmetric IUGR may be normal until late in gestation. In addition, distortion of the fetal head shape (e.g., in dolichocephaly or in breech presentation) may lead to a falsely small BPD. Thus, when utilized singly, BPD determinations fail to identify about 20–50% of IUGR infants and cannot be used as the only parameter in screening for IUGR.

Transverse cerebellar diameter

The cerebellum can easily be visualized as early as the first trimester as a butterfly-shaped figure in the posterior fossa of the fetal head, behind the thalami and in front of the echolucent cisterna magna. The transverse cerebellar diameter (TCD) in millimeters has been shown to correlate with gestational age in weeks up to 24 weeks. Above 24 weeks' gestation, the growth curves turn upward, and this uniform correlation no longer exists. Goldstein and colleagues (1987) have constructed a nomogram of the TCD throughout pregnancy (Table 26.4).

Researchers subsequently evaluated the TCD measurement in IUGR fetuses. They reported that the TCD measurement was not significantly affected by restricted fetal growth and, therefore, the TCD could be used as a reliable predictor of gestational age even in cases of IUGR. This parameter is particularly useful because it is a standard against which other parameters can be compared. Duchatel and colleagues (1989) have corroborated these findings in their report of 12 cases of IUGR below the 3rd percentile in which the TCD remained unaltered. Other investigators have provided additional support for the usefulness of the TCD by constructing a nomogram of the ratio between TCD and abdominal circumference (AC). In a small series, these investigators have shown that this ratio permits the identification of IUGR by demonstrating the fairly consistent growth of the TCD relative to the decrease in AC in cases of IUGR. In yet another study by Hill and colleagues (1990), the TCD was found to be within two standard deviations in only 40% of IUGR cases and, in 60% of cases, the TCD was more than two standard deviations below the mean.

Table 26.2 Gestational age from the biparietal diameter.

BPD (mm)	5th percentile	50th percentile	95th percentile	BPD (mm)	5th percentile	50th percentile	95th percentile
10	7 + 0	10 + 1	13 + 1	39	14 + 0	17 + 1	20 + 1
11	7 + 2	10 + 2	13 + 3	40	14 + 2	17 + 3	20 + 3
12	7 + 3	10 + 4	13 + 4	41	14 + 4	17 + 5	20 + 5
13	7 + 5	10 + 5	13 + 5	42	14 + 6	18 + 0	21 + 0
14	7 + 6	10 + 6	14 + 0	43	15 + 1	18 + 2	21 + 2
15	8 + 1	11 + 1	14 + 1	44	15 + 3	18 + 4	21 + 4
16	8 + 2	11 + 2	14 + 3	45	15 + 6	18 + 6	21 + 6
17	8 + 4	11 + 4	14 + 4	46	16 + 1	19 + 1	22 + 1
18	8 + 5	11 + 5	14 + 6	47	16 + 3	19 + 3	22 + 4
19	9 + 0	12 + 0	15 + 0	48	16 + 5	19 + 5	22 + 6
20	9 + 1	12 + 2	15 + 2	49	17 + 0	20 + 1	23 + 1
21	9 + 3	12 + 3	15 + 3	50	17 + 3	20 + 3	23 + 3
22	9 + 4	12 + 5	15 + 5	51	17 + 5	20 + 5	23 + 6
23	9 + 6	12 + 6	16 + 0	52	18 + 0	21 + 0	24 + 1
24	10 + 1	13 + 1	16 + 1	53	18 + 2	21 + 3	24 + 3
25	10 + 2	13 + 3	16 + 3	54	18 + 5	21 + 5	24 + 5
26	10 + 4	13 + 4	16 + 5	55	19 + 0	22 + 0	25 + 1
27	10 + 6	13 + 6	17 + 0	56	19 + 2	22 + 3	25 + 3
28	11 + 0	14 + 1	17 + 1	57	19 + 5	22 + 5	25 + 6
29	11 + 2	14 + 3	17 + 3	58	20 + 0	23 + 1	26 + 1
30	11 + 4	14 + 4	17 + 5	59	20 + 3	23 + 3	26 + 3
31	11 + 6	14 + 6	18 + 0	60	20 + 5	23 + 6	26 + 6
32	12 + 1	15 + 1	18 + 1	61	21 + 1	24 + 1	27 + 1
33	12 + 3	15 + 3	18 + 3	62	21 + 3	24 + 4	27 + 4
34	12 + 4	15 + 5	18 + 5	63	21 + 6	24 + 6	27 + 6
35	12 + 6	16 + 0	19 + 0	64	22 + 1	25 + 2	28 + 2
36	13 + 1	16 + 2	19 + 2	65	22 + 4	25 + 4	28 + 5
37	13 + 3	16 + 4	19 + 4	66	22 + 6	26 + 0	29 + 0
38	13 + 5	16 + 6	19 + 6	67	23 + 2	26 + 2	29 + 3

Reprinted from Jeanty P, Remero R. *Obstetrical ultrasound*. New York: McGraw-Hill, 1984, with permission.

BPD, biparietal diameter.

The results of this paper are at variance with the three reports discussed earlier. The majority of data available would suggest that the use of the TCD is extremely valuable when gestational age is unknown or IUGR is suspected. The accuracy of the TCD can be enhanced by using biometric ratios, especially FL:AC, as well as amniotic fluid volume and the presence or absence of fetal ossification centers.

Table 26.3 Estimated variability associated with determining menstrual age from biparietal diameter values.

Group (menstrual age)	Hadlock et al.*	Days	Kurtz et al.†	Days
1 (12–18 weeks)	± 0.85 weeks ($r^2 = 90.4\%$)	5.9	± 0.80 weeks	5.6
2 (18–24 weeks)	± 1.29 weeks ($r^2 = 87.6\%$)	9.03	± 1.70 weeks	11.9
3 (24–30 weeks)	± 1.40 weeks ($r^2 = 89.1\%$)	9.8	± 1.34 weeks	9.38
4 (30–36 weeks)	± 1.96 weeks ($r^2 = 76.5\%$)	13.7	± 1.42 weeks	9.94
5 (36–42 weeks)	± 2.06 weeks ($r^2 = 25.6\%$)	14.42	± 1.23 weeks	8.61

Modified from Hadlock FP, Deter R, Harrist R, et al. Fetal biparietal diameter: a critical re-evaluation of the relation to menstrual age by means of real-time ultrasound. *J Ultrasound Med* 1982;1:91; and Kurtz AB, Wapher RJ, Kurtz RJ, et al. Analysis of biparietal diameter as an accurate indicator of gestational age. *J Clin Ultrasound* 1986;8:319.

*Ninety-five percent confidence interval.

†Ninety percent confidence interval (of mean values).

Abdominal circumference

The AC has been reported to be the best fetal biometric parameter that correlates with fetal weight and is the most sensitive parameter for detecting IUGR. Warsof and colleagues (1986) studied the effectiveness of three ultrasonic growth parameters – BPD, HC, and AC – in detecting IUGR in a large group of obstetric populations. They demonstrated that AC measurements are more predictive of IUGR than BPD or HC, singly or in combination. In this study, it was shown that screening for IUGR at 34 weeks' gestation results in a sensitivity of approximately 70% and a positive predictive value of 50%. However, sensitivity was maximized by using the 25th rather than 10th percentile measurement to determine a positive result.

Others have found results that further demonstrate that AC is the single best predictor of IUGR, with an accuracy that may reach 96% of cases. In fact, in contrast to the BPD measurement, AC is smaller in both symmetric and asymmetric types of IUGR, and therefore its measurement has a higher sensitivity. Animal studies have shown that the liver is the most affected organ in IUGR. As the liver is the largest intra-abdominal organ, assessment of the AC at the level of the liver is actually an indirect indication of the nutritional status of the fetus.

Unfortunately, AC has more intraobserver and interobserver variation than either BPD or FL. Furthermore, AC variability may result from fetal breathing movements, compression, or the position of the fetus. To obtain the proper AC, the section should be round and at the level of the fetal stomach and the portal umbilical vein (or the bifurcation of the main portal vein into the right and left branches). Normal values of AC are presented in Table 26.5.

Table 26.4 Nomogram of the transverse cerebellar diameter, biparietal diameter, and head circumference according to percentile distribution.

Gestational age (weeks)	Cerebellum (mm)					Biparietal diameter (mm)					Head circumference (mm)				
	10	25	50	75	90	10	25	50	75	90	10	25	50	75	90
15	10	12	14	15	16	30	31	33	34	35	12	12	126	128	128
16	14	16	16	16	17	34	34	35	36	38	123	125	130	136	141
17	16	17	17	18	18	36	37	38	40	43	134	136	138	149	160
18	17	18	18	19	19	38	40	42	43	44	142	147	154	158	160
19	18	18	19	19	22	42	43	45	46	48	147	154	159	170	178
20	18	19	20	20	22	45	46	47	48	53	146	164	173	190	190
21	19	20	22	23	24	48	49	50	52	57	185	185	191	208	211
22	21	23	23	24	24	50	51	53	54	55	193	193	193	200	203
23	22	23	24	25	26	53	54	56	58	60	203	203	206	222	222
24	22	24	25	27	28	56	59	60	61	64	219	220	224	228	230
25	23	21	28	28	29	61	61	63	66	68	219	224	234	248	251
26	25	28	29	30	32	63	64	65	66	67	235	237	241	246	246
27	26	28	30	31	32	64	67	68	69	70	237	237	243	246	246
28	27	30	31	32	34	68	69	70	71	72	246	247	253	261	264
29	29	32	34	36	38	71	72	74	76	79	254	264	274	288	301
30	31	32	35	37	40	72	74	75	75	79	253	261	277	288	298
31	32	35	38	39	43	75	78	76	81	84	274	277	291	301	303
32	33	36	38	40	42	75	78	80	81	83	275	280	298	307	308
33	32	36	40	43	44	80	80	81	82	87	292	292	297	316	322
34	33	38	40	41	44	81	82	84	86	91	326	326	326	327	327
35	31	37	40	43	47	78	83	87	89	93	300	300	301	303	303
36	36	29	43	52	55	84	85	88	89	91	309	309	313	318	318
37	37	37	45	52	55	87	87	89	92	92	303	303	313	324	324
38	40	40	48	52	55	87	87	90	93	94	–	–	–	–	–
39	52	52	52	55	55	92	92	92	93	92	–	–	–	–	–

Source: from Goldstein et al. 1987.

Table 26.5 Normal values for the abdominal circumference.

Week number	Jeanty			Deter
	5th percentile	50th percentile	95th percentile	50th percentile
12	35	57	80	63
13	45	67	90	74
14	55	77	100	84
15	65	88	110	95
16	76	98	120	106
17	86	109	131	117
18	97	119	142	128
19	108	130	152	139
20	119	141	163	150
21	129	152	174	161
22	140	163	185	172
23	151	173	196	183
24	162	184	206	194
25	172	195	217	205
26	183	205	227	216
27	193	215	238	227
28	206	225	248	238
29	213	235	257	249
30	222	244	267	260
31	231	254	276	271
32	240	262	285	282
33	248	271	293	293
34	256	279	301	304
35	264	286	309	315
36	271	293	316	326
37	278	300	322	337
38	283	306	328	348
39	289	311	333	359
40	294	316	338	370

Reprinted from Geirsson RT, Patel NB, Christie AD. Efficiency of intrauterine volume, fetal abdominal area and biparietal diameter measurements with ultrasound in screening for small-for-dates babies. *Br J Obstet Gynaecol* 1985;92:929.

Long bones

The FL is another important parameter in evaluating fetal growth (Table 26.6). Long bones other than the femur can be equally useful in the assessment of gestational age (Table 26.7). It has been demonstrated by several authors that there is a linear relationship between FL specifically and long bones in general and crown–heel length of a newborn.

Table 26.6 Gestational age estimated from the femur length.

Femur length (mm)	5th percentile	50th percentile	95th percentile	Femur length (mm)	5th percentile	50th percentile	95th percentile
10	10 + 3	12 + 4	14 + 6	46	23 + 1	25 + 3	27 + 4
11	10 + 5	12 + 6	15 + 1	47	23 + 4	25 + 6	28 + 0
12	11 + 1	13 + 2	15 + 4	48	24 + 0	26 + 1	28 + 3
13	11 + 3	13 + 4	15 + 6	49	24 + 3	26 + 4	28 + 6
14	11 + 5	13 + 6	16 + 1	50	24 + 6	27 + 0	29 + 1
15	12 + 0	14 + 1	16 + 3	51	25 + 1	27 + 3	29 + 4
16	12 + 3	14 + 4	16 + 6	52	25 + 4	27 + 6	30 + 0
17	12 + 5	14 + 6	17 + 1	53	26 + 0	28 + 1	30 + 3
18	13 + 0	15 + 1	17 + 3	54	26 + 3	28 + 4	30 + 6
19	13 + 3	15 + 4	17 + 6	55	26 + 6	29 + 1	31 + 2
20	13 + 5	15 + 6	18 + 1	56	27 + 2	29 + 4	31 + 5
21	14 + 1	16 + 2	18 + 4	57	27 + 5	29 + 6	32 + 1
22	14 + 3	16 + 4	18 + 6	58	28 + 1	30 + 2	32 + 4
23	14 + 5	16 + 6	19 + 1	59	28 + 4	30 + 5	32 + 6
24	15 + 1	17 + 2	19 + 4	60	28 + 6	31 + 1	33 + 2
25	15 + 3	17 + 4	19 + 6	61	29 + 3	31 + 4	33 + 6
26	15 + 6	18 + 0	20 + 1	62	29 + 6	32 + 0	34 + 1
27	16 + 1	18 + 2	20 + 4	63	30 + 1	32 + 3	34 + 4
28	16 + 4	18 + 5	20 + 6	64	30 + 5	32 + 6	35 + 1
29	16 + 6	19 + 0	21 + 1	65	31 + 1	33 + 2	35 + 4
30	17 + 1	19 + 3	21 + 4	66	31 + 4	33 + 5	35 + 6
31	17 + 4	19 + 6	22 + 0	67	32 + 0	34 + 1	36 + 3
32	17 + 6	20 + 1	22 + 2	68	32 + 3	34 + 4	36 + 6
33	18 + 2	20 + 4	22 + 5	69	32 + 6	35 + 0	37 + 1
34	18 + 5	20 + 6	23 + 1	70	33 + 2	35 + 4	37 + 5
35	19 + 0	21 + 1	23 + 3	71	33 + 5	35 + 6	38 + 1
36	19 + 3	21 + 4	23 + 6	72	34 + 1	36 + 3	38 + 4
37	19 + 6	22 + 0	24 + 1	73	34 + 3	36 + 6	39 + 0
38	20 + 1	22 + 3	24 + 4	74	35 + 1	37 + 2	39 + 4
39	20 + 4	22 + 5	24 + 6	75	35 + 4	37 + 5	39 + 6
40	20 + 6	23 + 1	25 + 2	76	36 + 0	38 + 1	40 + 3
41	21 + 2	23 + 4	25 + 5	77	36 + 3	38 + 4	40 + 6
42	21 + 5	23 + 6	26 + 1	78	36 + 6	39 + 1	41 + 2
43	22 + 1	24 + 2	26 + 4	79	37 + 2	39 + 4	41 + 5
44	22 + 4	24 + 5	26 + 6	80	37 + 6	40 + 0	42 + 1
45	22 + 6	25 + 0	27 + 1	–	–	–	–

Reprinted from Jeanty P, Romero R. *Obstetrical ultrasound*. New York: McGraw-Hill, 1984, with permission.

Table 26.7 Gestational age in weeks and days as obtained from the long bones.

Bone length (mm)	Humerus percentile			Ulna percentile			Tibia percentile		
	5th	50th	95th	5th	50th	95th	5th	50th	95th
10	9 + 6	12 + 4	15 + 2	10 + 1	13 + 1	16 + 1	10 + 4	13 + 3	16 + 2
11	10 + 1	12 + 6	15 + 4	10 + 4	13 + 4	16 + 4	10 + 6	13 + 5	16 + 4
12	10 + 3	13 + 1	15 + 6	10 + 6	13 + 6	16 + 6	11 + 1	14 + 1	17 + 0
13	10 + 6	13 + 4	16 + 1	11 + 1	14 + 1	17 + 2	11 + 4	14 + 3	17 + 2
14	11 + 1	13 + 6	16 + 4	11 + 4	14 + 4	17 + 5	11 + 6	14 + 6	17 + 5
15	11 + 3	14 + 1	16 + 6	11 + 6	15 + 0	18 + 0	12 + 1	15 + 1	18 + 0
16	11 + 6	14 + 4	17 + 2	12 + 2	15 + 3	18 + 3	12 + 4	15 + 4	18 + 3
17	12 + 1	14 + 6	17 + 4	12 + 5	15 + 5	18 + 6	13 + 0	15 + 6	18 + 6
18	12 + 4	15 + 1	18 + 0	13 + 1	16 + 1	19 + 1	13 + 2	16 + 1	19 + 1
19	12 + 6	15 + 4	18 + 2	13 + 4	16 + 4	19 + 4	13 + 5	16 + 4	19 + 4
20	13 + 1	15 + 6	18 + 5	13 + 6	16 + 6	20 + 0	14 + 1	17 + 0	19 + 6
21	13 + 4	16 + 2	19 + 1	14 + 2	17 + 2	20 + 3	14 + 4	17 + 3	20 + 2
22	13 + 6	16 + 5	19 + 3	14 + 5	17 + 5	20 + 6	14 + 6	17 + 6	20 + 5
23	14 + 2	17 + 1	19 + 6	15 + 1	18 + 1	21 + 1	15 + 1	18 + 1	21 + 1
24	14 + 5	17 + 3	20 + 1	15 + 4	18 + 4	21 + 4	15 + 4	18 + 4	21 + 3
25	15 + 1	17 + 6	20 + 4	16 + 0	19 + 0	22 + 1	16 + 0	18 + 6	21 + 6
26	15 + 4	18 + 1	21 + 0	16 + 3	19 + 3	22 + 4	16 + 3	19 + 2	22 + 1
27	15 + 6	18 + 4	21 + 3	16 + 6	19 + 6	22 + 6	16 + 6	19 + 5	22 + 4
28	16 + 2	19 + 0	21 + 6	17 + 2	20 + 2	23 + 3	17 + 1	20 + 1	23 + 0
29	16 + 5	19 + 3	22 + 1	17 + 5	20 + 6	23 + 6	17 + 4	20 + 4	23 + 4
30	17 + 1	19 + 6	22 + 4	18 + 1	21 + 1	24 + 2	18 + 1	21 + 0	23 + 6
31	17 + 4	20 + 2	23 + 0	18 + 4	21 + 5	24 + 6	18 + 4	21 + 3	24 + 2
32	18 + 0	20 + 5	23 + 4	19 + 1	22 + 1	25 + 1	18 + 6	21 + 6	24 + 5
33	18 + 3	21 + 1	23 + 6	19 + 4	22 + 5	25 + 5	19 + 2	22 + 1	25 + 1
34	18 + 6	21 + 4	24 + 2	20 + 1	23 + 1	26 + 1	19 + 5	22 + 4	25 + 4
35	19 + 2	22 + 0	24 + 6	20 + 4	24 + 4	26 + 5	20 + 1	23 + 1	26 + 0
36	19 + 5	22 + 4	25 + 1	21 + 1	24 + 1	27 + 1	20 + 4	23 + 4	26 + 3
37	20 + 1	22 + 6	25 + 5	21 + 4	24 + 4	27 + 5	21 + 0	23 + 6	26 + 6

38	20 + 4	23 + 3	26 + 1	22 + 1	25 + 1	28 + 1	21 + 4	24 + 3	27 + 2
39	21 + 1	23 + 6	26 + 4	22 + 4	25 + 4	28 + 5	21 + 6	24 + 6	27 + 5
40	21 + 4	24 + 2	27 + 1	23 + 1	26 + 1	29 + 1	22 + 3	25 + 2	28 + 1
41	22 + 0	24 + 6	27 + 4	23 + 4	26 + 5	29 + 5	22 + 6	25 + 5	28 + 4
42	22 + 4	25 + 2	28 + 0	24 + 1	27 + 1	30 + 2	23 + 2	26 + 1	29 + 1
43	23 + 0	25 + 5	28 + 4	24 + 5	27 + 5	30 + 6	23 + 5	26 + 4	29 + 4
44	23 + 4	26 + 1	29 + 0	25 + 1	28 + 2	31 + 2	24 + 1	27 + 1	30 + 0
45	24 + 0	26 + 5	29 + 4	25 + 6	28 + 6	31 + 6	24 + 4	27 + 4	30 + 4
46	24 + 4	27 + 1	30 + 0	26 + 2	29 + 3	32 + 3	25 + 1	28 + 0	30 + 6
47	25 + 0	27 + 5	30 + 4	26 + 6	29 + 6	33 + 0	25 + 4	28 + 4	31 + 3
48	25 + 4	28 + 1	31 + 0	27 + 3	30 + 4	33 + 4	26 + 1	29 + 0	31 + 6
49	26 + 0	28 + 6	31 + 4	28 + 0	31 + 1	34 + 1	26 + 4	29 + 3	32 + 2
50	26 + 4	29 + 2	32 + 0	28 + 4	31 + 4	34 + 5	27 + 0	29 + 6	32 + 6
51	27 + 1	29 + 6	32 + 4	29 + 1	32 + 1	35 + 2	27 + 4	30 + 3	33 + 2
52	27 + 4	30 + 2	33 + 1	29 + 5	32 + 6	35 + 6	28 + 0	30 + 6	33 + 6
53	28 + 1	30 + 6	33 + 4	30 + 2	33 + 3	36 + 3	28 + 4	31 + 3	34 + 2
54	28 + 5	31 + 3	34 + 1	30 + 6	34 + 0	37 + 0	29 + 0	31 + 6	34 + 6
55	29 + 1	32 + 0	34 + 5	31 + 4	34 + 4	37 + 5	29 + 4	32 + 3	35 + 2
56	29 + 6	32 + 4	35 + 2	32 + 1	35 + 1	38 + 2	30 + 0	32 + 6	35 + 6
57	30 + 2	33 + 1	35 + 6	32 + 6	35 + 6	38 + 6	30 + 4	33 + 3	36 + 2
58	30 + 6	33 + 4	36 + 3	33 + 3	36 + 3	39 + 4	31 + 0	33 + 6	36 + 6
59	31 + 1	34 + 1	36 + 6	34 + 0	37 + 1	40 + 1	31 + 4	34 + 3	37 + 2
60	32 + 0	34 + 6	37 + 4	34 + 4	37 + 5	40 + 6	32 + 0	34 + 6	37 + 6
61	32 + 4	35 + 2	38 + 1	35 + 2	38 + 2	41 + 3	32 + 4	35 + 4	38 + 2
62	33 + 1	35 + 6	38 + 5	35 + 6	39 + 0	42 + 0	33 + 0	35 + 6	38 + 6
63	33 + 6	36 + 4	39 + 2	36 + 4	39 + 4	42 + 5	33 + 4	36 + 4	39 + 3
64	34 + 3	37 + 1	39 + 6	37 + 1	40 + 2	43 + 2	34 + 1	37 + 0	39 + 6
65	35 + 0	37 + 5	40 + 4	–	–	–	34 + 4	37 + 4	40 + 3
66	35 + 4	38 + 2	41 + 1	–	–	–	35 + 1	38 + 0	41 + 0
67	36 + 1	38 + 6	41 + 5	–	–	–	35 + 5	38 + 4	41 + 4
68	36 + 6	39 + 4	42 + 4	–	–	–	36 + 1	39 + 1	42 + 0
69	37 + 3	40 + 1	42 + 6	–	–	–	36 + 6	39 + 5	42 + 4

Reprinted from Jeanty P, Rodesch F, Delbeke D, et al. Estimation of gestational age from measurements of fetal long bones. *J Ultrasound Med* 1984;3:75, with permission.

Table 26.8 Head circumference to abdominal circumference ratio compared with gestational age.

Gestational age (weeks)	Head circumference		
	– 2 Standard deviations	Mean	+ 2 Standard deviations
14	1.085	1.230	1.375
15	1.080	1.225	1.365
16	1.075	1.215	1.350
17	1.070	1.205	1.340
18	1.065	1.195	1.330
19	1.060	1.185	1.320
20	1.055	1.178	1.305
21	1.050	1.177	1.295
22	1.045	1.165	1.285
23	1.040	1.155	1.275
24	1.030	1.145	1.265
25	1.025	1.135	1.255
26	1.050	1.125	1.245
27	1.010	1.120	1.235
28	1.000	1.110	1.225
29	0.999	1.095	1.215
30	0.975	1.085	1.200
31	0.965	1.075	1.190
32	0.945	1.060	1.175
33	0.935	1.045	1.163
34	0.925	1.030	1.150
35	0.915	1.020	1.135
36	0.910	1.005	1.120
37	0.905	0.995	1.100
38	0.900	0.980	1.085
39	0.896	0.970	1.065
40	0.895	0.965	1.046
41	0.894	0.960	1.025

Reprinted from Campbell S, Metreweli C, eds. *Practical abdominal ultrasound*. Chicago, IL: Year Book, 1978.

Body proportionality

Indices of body proportionality that have been studied and found clinically useful in the diagnosis of IUGR include the HC/AC ratio (Table 26.8) and the FL/AC ratio.

Head circumference–abdominal circumference ratio

Although the ratio of HC/AC has been shown to have a sensitivity of approximately 70% in detecting asymmetric IUGR, its use is limited by its high false-positive rate in screening a general population.

Further limitations of this technique are its inability to detect asymmetric growth restriction and the need for accurate knowledge of gestational age to make the diagnosis of IUGR. It is therefore believed that the value of the HC/AC ratio lies in the assessment of proportionality, and thus it may assist the clinician to classify IUGR as symmetric or asymmetric. Obviously, an elevated ratio suggests symmetric IUGR.

Femur length–abdominal circumference ratio

The ratio of FL/AC is the equivalent of the postnatal ponderal index and has been proposed as a useful method of detecting asymmetric IUGR. This ratio has the advantage of being age independent, and thus may help in the diagnosis of IUGR when gestational age is unknown. In fact, FL/AC ratios have a constant value of $22 \pm 2\%$ after 21 weeks' gestation.

Estimated fetal weight

Several formulas that use multiple ultrasonic parameters are used to estimate fetal weight. The most widely used formula is that of Shepard and colleagues (1982), in which estimated fetal weight (EFw) is derived from the BPD and AC. This equation predicts fetal weight with an accuracy of 15–20%.

Ott and Doyle (1984) reported accurate predictions of IUGR in 90% of cases in a high-risk population when EFw was determined by BPD and AC. The use of this formula may introduce errors that are related to the variations in BPD that usually occur as a result of changes in head shape in the last weeks of pregnancy, in malpresentation, and in pregnancies complicated by spontaneous rupture of membranes. BPD may be inaccurate if there is dolichocephaly or brachycephaly. We therefore strongly recommend that the physician calculate the cephalic index in each case. If the cephalic index is abnormal (<75% or >80%), one should not rely on estimated weight formulas that include the BPD.

Macrosomia

The etiology of fetal macrosomia is believed to be multifactorial. Although this condition is often associated with diabetes mellitus in pregnancy, especially in women without vasculopathy, macrosomia may also occur in nondiabetics. Fetal macrosomia is defined as either an EFw of more than 4000 g at term or an EFw of more than the 90th percentile for gestational age.

Macrosomic infants and their mothers are at increased risk for intrapartum injury, and perinatal mortality is more common among these fetuses. The principal causes of injury include shoulder dystocia, fractures, and neurologic damage.

Accurate prenatal diagnosis of fetal macrosomia would permit fetuses to be delivered by Cesarean section, thus obviating these complications. On the other hand, liberal Cesarean section may expose the mother to unnecessary operative risks.

Prenatal diagnosis of macrosomic fetuses is often difficult because less than 40% of such infants are born to mothers with identifiable risk factors for macrosomia.

A number of sonographic parameters have been used in an attempt to diagnose altered fetal growth, including the BPD, HC, HC/AC or HC to thoracic circumference ratio, the macrosomic index, and the EFw. Tamura and colleagues (1986) showed that the EFw determined by Shepard and colleagues (1982), when greater than the 90th percentile, correctly predicted macrosomia at birth in 74% of cases. When both the AC and the EFw exceeded the 90th percentiles, macrosomia was correctly diagnosed in 88.8% of pregnant women with diabetes mellitus. The BPD and HC percentiles were significantly less predictive of macrosomia.

Summary

Although the etiology of IUGR is variable, prenatal diagnosis is possible using a variety of biometric parameters. When the gestational age is certain, IUGR is diagnosed if sonographic predictors of gestational age reflect an age significantly reduced from the expected, or an EFw less than the 10th percentile. Adjunctive indices that can enhance the prenatal diagnosis include reduced amniotic fluid volume, early third trimester grade 3 placenta, abnormal Doppler waveform analysis, and abnormal biometric ratios.

When the gestational age is unknown or uncertain, it is necessary to differentiate between the IUGR fetus and the normally grown fetus identified at an inaccurate gestational age. The TCD is a useful parameter for estimating gestational age even in IUGR fetuses, and can be a parameter against which other biometric indices are compared. Biometric ratios, especially FL/AC, may also be useful adjuncts in the prenatal diagnosis of IUGR.

The prenatal diagnosis of macrosomia is best accomplished by the use of EFw. However, a certain amount of caution should be exercised in light of the fact that a margin of error exists with this method of weight estimation. EFw is reported to be accurate to within 10% of the actual birthweight 85% of the time. In the remaining 15% of cases, EFw is less accurate, and the error can range from 15% to 20% of the actual birthweight.

Further reading

Abuhamad AZ. Does Doppler U/S improve outcomes in growth-restricted fetuses? *Contemp Obstet Gynecol* 2003;48:56–73.

ACOG. Intrauterine growth restriction. *ACOG Pract Bull* 2000;12.

Chervenak FA, Skupski DW, Romero R, et al. How accurate is fetal biometry in the assessment of fetal age? *Am J Obstet Gynecol* 1998;178:678–687.

Duchatel F, Mennesson B, Berseneff H, et al. Antenatal echographic measurement of the fetal cerebellum. Significance in the evaluation of fetal development. *J Gynecol Obstet Biol Reprod (Paris)* 1989;18:879.

Goldstein I, Reece EA, Pilu G, et al. Fetal cerebellar growth unaffected by intrauterine growth retardation: a new parameter for prenatal diagnosis. *Am J Obstet Gynecol* 1987;157:632.

Hill LM, Gyzick D, Rivello D, et al. The transverse cerebellar diameter cannot be used to assess gestational age in the small for gestational age fetus. *Obstet Gynecol* 1990;75:329.

Manning FA. Intrauterine growth retardation. Etiology, pathophysiology, diagnosis, and treatment. In: Manning FA, ed. *Fetal medicine: principles and practice*. Norwalk, CT: Appleton & Lange, 1995.

Ott WJ, Doyle S. Ultrasonic diagnosis of altered fetal growth by use of a normal ultrasonic fetal weight curve. *Obstet Gynecol* 1984;63:201.

Resnik R. Intrauterine growth restriction. *Obstet Gynecol* 2002;99:490–496.

Shephard MJ, Richards VA, Verkowitz RL, et al. An evaluation of two equations for predicting fetal weight by ultrasound. *Am J Obstet Gynecol* 1982;142:47.

Tamura RK, Sabbagha RE, Depp R, et al. Diabetic macrosomia: accuracy of third trimester ultrasound. *Obstet Gynecol* 1986;67:828.

Weiner CP, Robinson D. The sonographic diagnosis of intrauterine growth retardation using the postnatal ponderal index and the crown-heel length as standards of diagnosis. *Am J Perinatol* 1989;6:375.

Warsof SL, Cooper DJ, Little D, et al. Routine ultrasound screening for antenatal detection of intrauterine growth retardation. *Obstet Gynecol* 1986;67:33.

Three- and four-dimensional ultrasound and magnetic resonance imaging in pregnancy

Teresita L. Angtuaco

Three-dimensional (3D) and four-dimensional (4D) ultrasound

Three-dimensional ultrasound is a technique that stores complete sets of volume data in a computer memory so that it can be accessed to reconstruct any desired image plane. Four-dimensional (4D) imaging is 3D ultrasound with a dynamic display of rendered images rapidly updated over time (real-time 3D). With these two techniques, an entire sequence of fetal movement can be stored with digital image quality. These volumes can be demonstrated as separate images on the monitor or as animated displays on cine loops. There is enough evidence in the literature regarding the applications of 3D ultrasound in facial and limb deformities. The fetal spine is also among those structures more frequently imaged on 3D ultrasound. Although becoming increasingly popular, applications of 3D ultrasound in the abdomen have had limited success. The most documented application has been in the detection of abdominal wall defects. In the chest, 4D fetal echocardiography in B-mode shows a lot of promise in the detection of cardiac anomalies such as ventricular septal defects, tricuspid atresia, transposition of the great vessels, pulmonary atresia, and interruption of the inferior vena cava with azygous venous return. This provides another dimension in diagnosing complex cardiac defects that are typically difficult to see on conventional 2D ultrasound. The advantages of 3D ultrasound over conventional 2D ultrasound have tremendous implications in terms of time savings because of its ability to increase patient flow through a busy service. Consultations with peers and referring physicians can be conducted at mutually convenient times, and the need for additional images does not necessarily require return clinic visits. Among the disadvantages of 3D ultrasound, imaging of oligohydramnios remains the hardest to resolve, resulting in electronic artifacts. However, with further advances in imaging hardware and software, this may become less and less of a problem in the future.

Magnetic resonance imaging (MRI)

MRI applications in obstetrics are mainly complementary to ultrasound, with MRI serving predominantly as a problem-solving tool when ultrasound is inadequate for diagnosis. Its use has been limited to the late second and third trimesters of pregnancy, mainly because of the uncertainty that bioeffects may eventually be proven in the fetus. Although no untoward sequelae have been reported, it is customary to obtain informed consent prior to the examination. It is best to correlate the images obtained on MRI with a recent ultrasound study to facilitate the interpretation of the MRI examination and direct the conduct of the remainder of the study. Maternal and fetal motion can both compromise the examination because of the artifacts produced. Short scanning sequences and maternal sedation have greatly improved the quality of MRI examinations over the years. An abnormality seen suboptimally on ultrasound should be confirmed with MRI, especially if there is potential for immediate intervention. The strength of MRI has been proven in the diagnoses of central nervous system (CNS) abnormalities, especially in the detection of residual brain mantle in brain anomalies and the determination of the level of obstruction in severe hydrocephalus. The utility of MRI in other areas of the body has not been as successful as in the head or spine. Complicated cases should be interpreted in consultation with a multispecialty team to enhance the diagnostic capability of both imaging techniques.

Further reading

Dyson RL, Pretorius DH, Budorick NE, et al. Three-dimensional ultrasound in the evaluation of fetal anomalies. *Ultrasound Obstet Gynecol* 2000;16:321.

Ertl-Wagner B, Lienemann A, Strauss A, Reiser MF. Fetal magnetic resonance imaging: indications, technique, anatomical considerations, and a review of fetal abnormalities. *Eur Radiol* 2002;12:1931.

Golja AM, Estroff JA, Robertson RL. Fetal imaging of central nervous system abnormalities. *Neuroimag Clin North Am* 2004;14:293.

Goncalves LF, Lee W, Chaiworapongsa T, et al. Four-dimensional ultrasonography of the fetal heart with spatiotemporal image correlation. *Am J Obstet Gynecol* 2003;189:1792.

Krakow D, Williams J, III, Poehl M, et al. Use of three-dimensional ultrasound imaging in the diagnosis of prenatal-onset skeletal dysplasia. *Ultrasound Obstet Gynecol* 2003;21:467.

Levine D, Smith AS, McKenzie C. Tips and tricks of fetal MR imaging. *Radiol Clin North Am* 2003;41:729.

Merz E. 3-D Ultrasound in prenatal diagnosis. In: *Ultrasound in obstetrics and gynecology*, 2nd edn. New York: Thieme; 2005:515–528.

Michailidis GD, Economides DL, Schild RL. The role of three-dimensional ultrasound in obstetrics. *Curr Opin Obstet Gynecol* 2001;13:207.

Nagayama M, Watanabe Y, Okumura A, et al. Fast MR imaging in obstetrics. *Radiographics* 2002;22:563.

Xu HX, Zang QP, Lu MD, Xiao XT. Comparison of two-dimensional and three-dimensional sonography in evaluating fetal malformations. *J Clin Ultrasound* 2002;30:515.

28 Doppler ultrasonography and fetal well-being

Brian J. Trudinger

Doppler ultrasound has provided a noninvasive clinical tool to assess blood flow in pregnancy. The scope of Doppler studies has now extended from the placenta to many fetal vascular beds and a great variety of disorders of pregnancy. Doppler equipment used in obstetric practice ranges from the simplest fetal heart detectors through the fetal heart rate (FHR) monitors to the most sophisticated high-level ultrasound imaging systems. Common to all is the incorporation of the Doppler effect. When there is movement between a wave source and a reflecting target, there is a change in frequency of the reflected wave relative to the transmitted wave, and that change in frequency is proportional to the velocity of the movement. When an ultrasound beam insonnates a blood vessel, the red blood cells act as scatterers, and the difference in frequency between the incident and reflected waves is proportional to the blood flow velocity. This is the Doppler principle.

Two types of Doppler systems are in use: continuous wave and pulsed. Continuous wave systems are continuously emitting from one crystal and receiving through another. In the pulsed system, a short burst of the ultrasound wave is transmitted, and the crystal then acts as a receiver. Integration with an imaging facility provides the ability to steer the ultrasound beam and, for pulsed Doppler systems, to locate the sample volume precisely over the vessel to be studied. With medical equipment (and the commonly used frequencies of 2–10 MHz) and vascular studies, the Doppler shift frequency usually falls in the audible range; therefore, the simplest display is an audio signal. The method of choice is spectral analysis. The frequency spectrum displayed represents all the different velocities across the vessel lumen.

The information made available to the clinician by the Doppler instrumentation is a blood flow velocity waveform (FVW). The envelope of this wave is the maximum flow velocity. Beneath this is a frequency distribution, representing the various velocities of blood flow in the vessel under study. Volume blood flow may be determined as the product of mean velocity and vessel area. In many situations, only the maximum velocity waveform (or the waveform envelope) is used. The shape

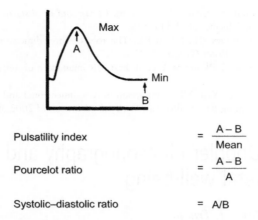

$$\text{Pulsatility index} \quad = \frac{A - B}{\text{Mean}}$$

$$\text{Pourcelot ratio} \quad = \frac{A - B}{A}$$

$$\text{Systolic–diastolic ratio} \quad = A/B$$

Figure 28.1 The three indices of downstream resistance in common clinical use for the analysis of arterial FVWs.

of the waveform envelope can be considered a characteristic of the vascular site. Waveforms recorded from arteries supplying low-impedance vascular beds (e.g., internal carotid, umbilical, and uterine artery in pregnancy) exhibit relatively high forward velocities throughout diastole. A triphasic waveform shape, where there is a period of reverse flow in diastole, is characteristic of sites with high distal impedance. The peripheral impedance, vessel wall elasticity, and the degree and geometry of any proximal stenoses affect the shape of the waveform, and the upstream pump.

The fetal circulation is uniquely suited to Doppler waveform analysis by simple empirical indices. This is because of the absence of degenerative arterial disease. The umbilical circulation was the first studied, and the indices have been directed toward assessing downstream resistance. Three are in common usage (Fig. 28.1). The peak velocity of the FVW envelope has been correlated with volume flow, and this parameter has been used in the cerebral circulation and the aorta. In the central fetal veins (inferior vena cava and ductus venosus), different indices have been used to describe the FVW pattern. Here, the inverse relationship between pressure and flow is important. Changes in the FVW mirror changes in the central venous pressure waveform. In studying the maternal uterine artery FVW, the presence of a dicrotic notch at the end of systole, created by reflected waves when resistance is increased, is relevant.

The umbilical circulation

The umbilical arteries can be readily studied with simple continuous wave Doppler ultrasound systems. The umbilical circulation is a low-resistance vascular bed. Throughout pregnancy, the increase in umbilical blood flow is achieved by a decrease in resistance rather than an increase in pressure. Gestational age is therefore an important influence in determining the pattern of the umbilical FVW in

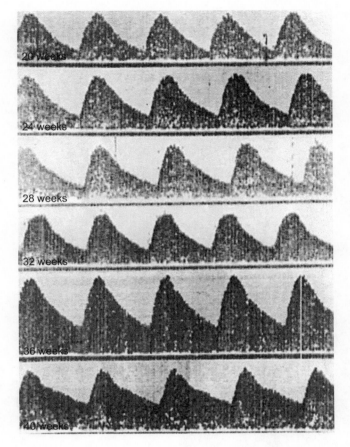

Figure 28.2 The changing form of the umbilical artery FVW recorded from one patient at varying periods of gestation.

normal pregnancy. The pattern of the umbilical artery FVW is one of positive flow velocities throughout the cardiac cycle, and the positive flow in diastole increases relative to the systolic peak as the pregnancy progresses (Fig. 28.2). The indices of resistance therefore decrease as the placenta grows and the umbilical villous vascular bed expands.

In recording the umbilical FVW, it is necessary to review a sequence of 10–20 cycles to confirm that variations due to fetal activity and breathing are absent.

The placental vasculature has been modeled as a lumped electrical circuit equivalent. Using this model, it can be shown that the pulsatility index (PI) of the FVW is proportional to the plasticity of the pressure waveform and the resistance of the umbilical placental villus vascular tree. It is not until some 50–60% of the vessels have been obliterated that the PI is increased beyond the "normal range." In ovine pregnancy, the decreasing vascular resistance has been measured directly. This matches

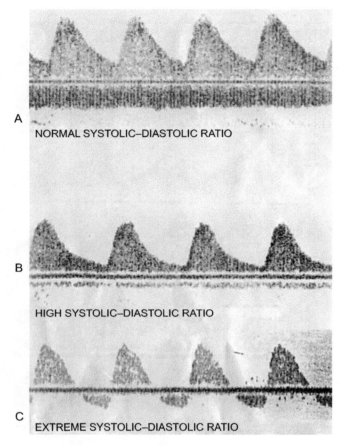

A
NORMAL SYSTOLIC–DIASTOLIC RATIO

B
HIGH SYSTOLIC–DIASTOLIC RATIO

C
EXTREME SYSTOLIC–DIASTOLIC RATIO

Figure 28.3 Examples of (A) a normal umbilical artery waveform, (B) a waveform in which the systolic–diastolic ratio is high, and (C) an extremely abnormal waveform, in which the diastolic flow velocities are reversed.

continuing expansion of the umbilical placental vascular tree. In fetal lambs, embolization of the umbilical cotyledon circulation with microspheres was carried out to increase the resistance of the peripheral vascular bed. This caused a rise in the umbilical systolic:diastolic ratio and a rise in calculated vascular resistance.

The decrease in the umbilical artery FVW indices of resistance seen in normal pregnancy reflects placental growth. This is in contrast to complicated pregnancy. The abnormal umbilical Doppler FVW is characterized by a change in the opposite direction, with decreasing diastolic flow velocities relative to the systolic peak and, in extreme cases, by absent or even reversal of blood flow in diastole (Fig. 28.3). The small arteries and arterioles of the tertiary villi are the "resistance vessels." The modal tertiary villus small arterial vessel count was significantly less in abnormal umbilical artery FVW. A large group of severe placental fetal vascular lesions (fetal thrombotic vasculopathy, chronic villitis with obliterative fetal vasculopathy, chorioamnionitis with severe vasculitis, and meconium-associated fetal vascular necrosis) have been associated with neurological impairment. Avascular villi are a common feature.

Clinical correlates

The abnormal umbilical artery Doppler FVW is characterized by a pattern of reduced, absent, or even reversed diastolic flow velocities relative to the systolic peak velocity (Fig. 28.2). Poor fetal outcome, particularly in terms of birth of an infant small for gestational age (SGA), is the major clinical association reported. Among a group of SGA fetuses, an abnormal Doppler umbilical study predicted those more likely to require early delivery and neonatal intensive care and those with the highest mortality. The trend of umbilical Doppler results proved a very useful measure of neonatal morbidity in those patients with serial studies. An increasing index of resistance suggests a progressive obliteration of arterial vessels in contrast to normal, with a decreasing resistance as the placenta grows.

Tests of fetal welfare exist to identify the potentially compromised fetus (sometimes termed the "at-risk" fetus) and to quantitate fetal condition. Umbilical Doppler study recognizes a vascular pathology in the fetal placenta that may lead to a fetal effect. Umbilical studies better predict the potentially compromised pregnancy. They do not quantify fetal condition.

Fetal arterial Doppler studies

Fetal aorta

The fetal aortic blood FVW (Fig. 28.4) has been analyzed using the same indices of downstream resistance as used for the umbilical circulation. Volume blood flow has been calculated from mean blood flow velocity and vessel area.

The PI of the maximum velocity waveform in the thoracic aorta (1.68 ± 0.28) does not change with gestation in the second half of pregnancy.

Studies of aortic FVW have been used in growth restriction. Downstream resistance has been assessed by measuring the PI and the waveform pattern classified by the presence or absence of forward flow velocities in diastole. Adverse fetal outcome does correlate with an abnormal FVW pattern.

Aortic FVW measurement of the peak mean velocity of the aortic waveform has also been studied. This correlates with hypoxemia, hypercarbia, hyperlactemia, and acidemia as determined from fetal blood obtained at cordocentesis. Indeed, it has been suggested to be the best Doppler predictor of fetal condition.

Fetal cerebral circulation

The fetal intracranial arteries are readily visualized, and Doppler FVW may be recorded using a duplex system. The middle cerebral artery (MCA) has become the standard vessel to image for recording cerebral FVWs.

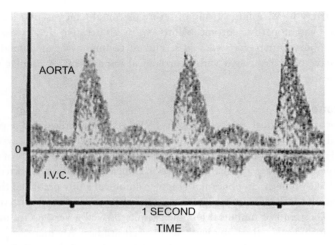

Figure 28.4 The normal FVW recorded from the aorta and inferior vena cava (IVC) in the lower thorax in the third trimester.

The waveform of the fetal internal carotid and MCA is not unlike that of the umbilical artery in shape with forward flow through diastole (Fig. 28.5).

A normal fetal MCA FVW suggests normal cerebral blood flow. Intrauterine fetal growth restriction may be associated with a fetal cerebral artery FVW PI lower than normal. When fetal condition deteriorates with hypoxemia consequent to placental vascular disease, cerebral vasodilation occurs and there is an increase in flow. The cerebral FVW shows a low PI. Whether this effect is adaptive to maintain cerebral oxygen supply or simply a consequence of the occurrence of fetal hypoxia and hypercarbia is not known at present.

The term "centralization of flow" was introduced to describe the situation where there is a low cerebral flow resistance. The suggested explanation was the redistribution of cardiac output to maintain blood flow to vital organs in the profoundly compromised fetus.

The measurement of maximum velocity in the MCA FVW has become the standard method for assessment of fetal anemia in rhesus alloimmunization. The maximum velocity is an index of volume flow.

Fetal venous Doppler studies

The ductus venosus, the inferior vena cava, and the umbilical vein have been the subject of most studies. The FVWs in the central fetal veins are influenced in form by the central venous pressure, and this in turn is a reflection of cardiac function (Fig. 28.6). Venous Doppler studies have become widely incorporated in management protocols to define fetal condition.

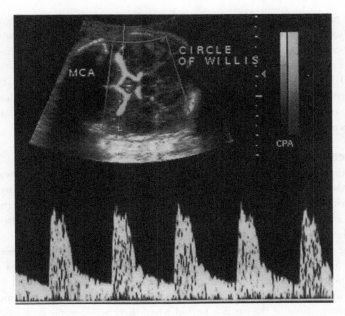

Figure 28.5 Color flow imaging of the circle of Willis of the fetal cerebral circulation. The FVW from the MCA is shown at the bottom.

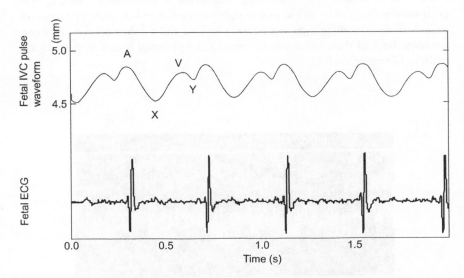

Figure 28.6 A fetal central venous pressure waveform showing the A crest of atrial contraction, the X trough of atrial relaxation in early systole, the V crest as atrial pressure rises with a–v valves closed, and the Y trough when these valves open at the end of systole. ECG, electrocardiogram; IVC, inferior vena cava.

In the presence of vascular disease in the umbilical placental circulation, which receives some 40% of combined ventricular output, there is high resistance in the systemic circulation. This produces a high right ventricular afterload. Resistance in the cerebral circulation is low, reducing the left ventricle afterload in the most compromised fetus. As the fetus becomes significantly hypoxemic, contractility and output from the heart may fall. These are major changes in fetal cardiovascular hemodynamics. A high right ventricular end-diastolic pressure follows, and this in turn affects the central venous pressure.

Fetal ductus venosus and inferior vena cava

The ductus venosus can be identified in a transverse plane directed upwards and backwards to include the region at which the umbilical vein joins the portal sinus. The inferior vena cava is best seen in a sagittal plane, which includes the region where it enters the right atrium. The ductus venosus (Fig. 28.7) may also be seen in this plane, but hepatic veins can confuse.

Among a group of growth-restricted fetuses (ultrasound estimate of weight less than the 5th percentile) with fetal hypoxemia, the dominant feature was a reduction in the velocities during atrial contraction. This can be understood to be the result of an increase in ventricular end-diastolic and atrial pressure. An increase in the percentage time of the cardiac period when there was reverse flow present and an increase in the preload index were noted in studies of the inferior vena cava. For the ductus venosus, the systolic to atrial contraction peak velocity ratio and preload index were increased. The underlying hemodynamic disturbance affecting both great veins is likely to be an increase in right ventricular end-diastolic pressure consequent to an increase in right ventricular afterload and a reduction in cardiac contractility. Both of these are a consequence of the placental lesion (defined by the umbilical Doppler study).

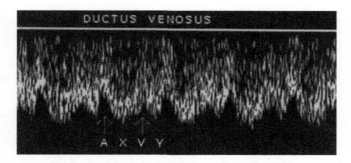

Figure 28.7 The FVW recorded from the fetal ductus venosus in normal pregnancy at 35 weeks. The component A, X, V, and Y waves (see legend of Fig. 28.6) are shown.

Clinical strategies in Doppler and fetal compromise

The approach of the obstetrician to fetal compromise progresses through a sequence of steps, which can be summarized as:

1 Recognition of high-risk pregnancy on the basis of clinical history and examination, supported by the ancillary aids of maternal–fetal movement counting and fundal height measurement. (Is it a high-risk pregnancy?)

2 Confirmation of fetal risk by identifying the placental vascular lesion with Doppler ultrasound studies of the umbilical artery FVW. (Is there a placental pathology threatening the fetus?)

3 Determination of the extent to which the fetus is affected using the direct fetal assessments of biophysical profile, ultrasound growth, and FHR monitoring and direct fetal Doppler studies. This is relevant to the timing of delivery. (How sick is the fetus?)

4 Therapy aimed at improving the intrauterine environment by treating mother or fetus, and delivery if the risks to the fetus of intrauterine death or damage exceed that of delivery.

Included in this approach is the use of Doppler studies at two points. Umbilical Doppler studies are interposed between the clinical identification of the high-risk pregnancy and full fetal surveillance testing to quantitate the degree to which the fetus is affected. Umbilical Doppler is a doorway test confirming the potential for fetal compromise and so leading to intensive fetal testing. Direct fetal Doppler assessments are then used to quantify how sick the fetus is.

The use of umbilical Doppler in clinical practice has been evaluated by several randomized controlled trials. Meta-analysis has established that women with high-fetal-risk pregnancies should have access to Doppler studies of the umbilical artery FVW. Meta-analysis of the umbilical Doppler trials demonstrated a reduction in the odds of a perinatal death by 38% (odds ratio 0.62, 95% confidence interval 0.45–0.85) when umbilical artery Doppler was available.

Maternal uterine circulation

Both pulsed and continuous wave ultrasound have been used to record flow velocity waveforms from the uterine circulation (Fig. 28.8).

The same indices of downstream resistance have been used to assess the FVW of the uterine artery. In addition, the presence or absence of an early diastolic "notch" has been studied. This is attributed to an increased downstream resistance so that reflected waves are present in the uterine circulation producing this sign (Fig. 28.9).

Normal pregnancy

The process of trophoblast invasion of the spiral arteries of the decidual and inner third of the myometrium is believed to lower the resistance to blood flow in the

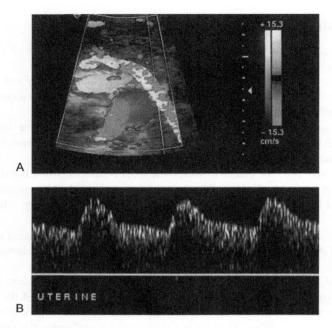

Figure 28.8 The uterine artery can be seen appearing to cross the external iliac vessels in this color Doppler mapping superimposed on a B-mode ultrasound image (A). The FVW in (B) is a normal uterine artery pattern with high diastolic flow velocities.

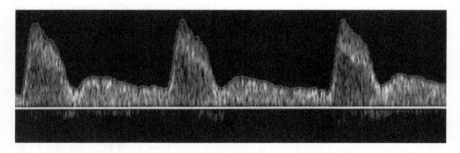

Figure 28.9 A uterine artery flow velocity waveform from a pregnancy with preeclampsia. A dicrotic notch is present. Diastolic flow velocities are low. This is a high-resistance uterine artery pattern.

uterine artery branches opening into the intervillous space. After 20 weeks, the uterine artery systolic–diastolic ratio is less than 2.0 and PI less than 1.5.

Both severe fetal growth restriction and maternal hypertension may be associated with uteroplacental waveforms demonstrating a high systolic–diastolic ratio.

Based on the hypothesis that trophoblast invasion of the spiral arteries causes the change in the uterine waveforms during the first half of pregnancy, and that this invasion is less developed in pregnancy hypertension, uterine waveform studies have also been evaluated for screening in early pregnancy. The test demonstrated a high sensitivity for prediction of preeclampsia and fetal growth restriction, but there was a high false-positive rate.

Further reading

Alfirevic Z, Neilson JP. Doppler ultrasonography in high risk pregnancies: systematic review with meta-analysis. *Am J Obstet Gynecol* 1995;172:1379.

Burke G, Stuart B, Crowley P, et al. Is intrauterine growth retardation with normal umbilical artery blood flow a benign condition? *Br Med J* 1990;300:1044.

Giles WB, Trudinger BJ, Baird P. Fetal umbilical artery flow velocity waveforms and placental resistance: pathological correlation. *Br J Obstet Gynaecol* 1985;92:31.

Gill RW. Doppler ultrasound: physical aspects. *Semin Perinatol* 1987;11:292.

Harrington K, Cooper D, Lees C, et al. Doppler ultrasound of the uterine arteries: the importance of bilateral matching in the prediction of preeclampsia, placental abruption on delivery of a small for gestational age baby. *Ultrasound Obstet Gynecol* 1996;7:182.

Hecher K, Snijders R, Campbell S, Nicolaides S. Fetal venous, intracardiac and arterial blood flow in intrauterine growth retardation. Relationship with blood gases. *Am J Obstet Gynecol* 1995;173:10.

Hecher K, Bilardo CM, Stigter RH, et al. Monitoring of fetuses with intrauterine growth restriction: a longitudinal study. *Ultrasound Obstet Gynecol* 2001;18:564.

Jauniaux E, Jurkovic D, Campbell S. In vivo investigation of the anatomy and the physiology on early human placental circulations. *Ultrasound Obstet Gynecol* 1991;1:435.

Karsdorp VH, van Vugt JM, van Geijn HP, et al. Clinical significance of absent or reversed end-diastolic velocity waveforms in umbilical artery. *Lancet* 1994;344:1664.

Kiserud T, Eik-Nes S, Blaas H, Hellevik LR. Ultrasonographic velocimetry of the fetal ductus venosus. *Lancet* 1991;338:1412.

Soothill PW, Nicolaides KH, Bilardo CM, Campbell S. Relation of fetal hypoxia in growth retardation to mean blood velocity in the fetal aorta. *Lancet* 1986;2:1118.

Trudinger BJ, Cook CM. Umbilical artery flow velocity waveform in high risk pregnancy: randomized controlled trial. *Lancet* 1987;1:188.

Trudinger BJ, Giles WB, Cook CM, et al. Fetal umbilical artery flow velocity waveforms and placental resistance: clinical significance. *Br J Obstet Gynaecol* 1985;92:23.

Antepartum and intrapartum surveillance of the fetus and the amniotic fluid

Lami Yeo, Michael G. Ross, and Anthony M. Vintzileos

Antepartum and intrapartum surveillance of the fetus have the intent of detecting fetal asphyxia so interventions can be made. Testing must be able to survey both acute fetal asphyxia and more chronic disease states. Surveillance of the amniotic fluid volume (AFV) is also crucial.

Antepartum surveillance techniques (fetus and amniotic fluid)

There are multiple maternal and fetal indications for performing antepartum surveillance (Table 29.1), although these are not absolute. The common basis for selecting these patients are those who are at increased risk of perinatal mortality, uteroplacental insufficiency, and fetal asphyxia.

Fetal movement monitoring

Good fetal movement is a sign of fetal well-being. Decreased fetal movements often (but not invariably) precede fetal death. Awareness of fetal movements is affected by maternal, fetal, and uterine factors (Table 29.2). A popular approach is counting 10 movements in a period of up to 2 h (reassuring). If the count is nonreassuring or decreased, further testing is recommended. The relationship between decreased fetal activity and poor perinatal outcome has been well established. While fetal movement monitoring is beneficial in high-risk pregnancies, it may also be useful in low-risk populations in reducing fetal mortality.

Contraction stress test (CST)

An external fetal monitor records the fetal heart rate (FHR) and uterine contractions (20- to 30-min interval). If the patient is contracting spontaneously (frequency is ≥ 3 contractions/10 min, duration of each contraction is ≥ 45 s), uterine stimulation is not required. If these criteria are not met, nipple stimulation or oxytocin is used to elicit contractions. Table 29.3 shows the criteria used by most to interpret CST results. The most common result is a negative CST (indicates adequate fetal oxygenation in the presence of contractions). There is a low incidence ($< 1\%$) of fetal death within 1 week of testing. Fetal outcome is controversial with a negative, nonreactive CST. A positive CST, which implies uteroplacental insufficiency, is associated with adverse perinatal outcome and an increased incidence of intrauterine demise. There is a high incidence of false-positive CSTs (reported to be $> 50\%$),

ANTEPARTUM, INTRAPARTUM SURVEILLANCE & AMNIOTIC FLUID

Table 29.1 Selected indications for antepartum surveillance (fetus and amniotic fluid).

Indications
Diabetes mellitus
Hypertensive disorders (chronic hypertension, preeclampsia)
Renal disease
Collagen vascular disorders
Maternal thyrotoxicosis
Severe anemia or maternal hemoglobinopathies
Isoimmunization
Prior unexplained fetal demise
Third-trimester vaginal bleeding
Premature rupture of membranes
Maternal perception of decreased fetal movements
Postdate pregnancy (>41 weeks)
Elevated maternal serum AFP (normal amniotic fluid AFP)
Abnormal or irregular fetal heart rate on auscultation
Selected fetal anomalies (e.g., gastroschisis)
Multiple gestation
Intrauterine growth restriction
Amniotic fluid abnormalities (oligohydramnios or polyhydramnios)

AFP, alpha-fetoprotein.

Table 29.2 Fetal movement monitoring.

Factors influencing maternally perceived fetal movements
Maternal
Activity
Obesity
Ingestion of medications or drugs that depress (e.g., methadone) or increase (e.g., cocaine) fetal movements
Fetal
Behavioral states
Gestational age
Congenital anomalies (e.g., neuromuscular disorders, fetal akinesia syndrome)
Duration of fetal movements
Uterine
Placental location
Amniotic fluid volume

Table 29.3 Interpretation of the contraction stress test.

Interpretation	Criteria
Nonreactive	No acceleration of at least 15 b.p.m. in amplitude or of 15-s duration during test
Reactive	Any acceleration ≥ 15 b.p.m. for ≥ 15 s during test
Negative	No late deceleration, with at least three contractions/10 min
Positive	Consistent, persistent late decelerations, regardless of contraction frequency, in the absence of uterine hyperstimulation
Equivocal:	
Suspicious	Nonpersistent (< 50% of the contractions) late decelerations
Hyperstimulation	FHR deceleration in the presence of uterine contractions exceeding five/10 min or lasting ≥ 90 s
Unsatisfactory	Insufficient FHR tracing or inability to achieve appropriate uterine contractions

FHR, fetal heart rate; b.p.m., beats per minute.

depending on which perinatal outcome is defined. Patients with a suspicious CST should have a repeat CST within 24 h or be evaluated with another form of antepartum testing. Equivocal tests should be followed up similarly.

Nonstress test (NST)

FHR reactivity depends on normal neurologic development and normal integration of central nervous system (CNS) control of FHR. The most common definition of reactivity is ≥ two FHR accelerations (at least 15 b.p.m. in amplitude above the baseline and lasting 15 s) within a 10- or 20-min period, with or without fetal movement. Many factors can lead to a nonreactive NST. Preterm fetuses are less likely to have FHR accelerations in association with fetal movements. The predictive value of a negative NST (normal outcome with a reactive NST) is very high. Within 1 week of a reactive NST, the perinatal mortality rate is about 3–5/1000. The predictive value of a positive test is low, and the false-positive rate of a nonreactive NST is also very high. With a nonreactive NST, one can either extend the time of the NST or proceed with other forms of testing.

Vibroacoustic stimulation (VAS)

Using an artificial larynx on the maternal abdomen elicits FHR accelerations, is reasonably safe, and safely reduces testing time, without compromising detection of the acidemic fetus. Gestational age affects the FHR response to VAS, with a maturational response as gestation advances.

Biophysical profile (BPP)

BPP assesses both acute (FHR reactivity, fetal breathing movements, fetal movements, fetal tone) and chronic (AFV) markers of fetal condition on ultrasound. The fetus responds to central hypoxemia/acidemia by altering its movement, tone, breathing, and heart rate pattern. A value of 0 or 2 is assigned to each of the biophysical components (Table 29.4). BPP activities developed last *in utero* are also the first to become abnormal in the presence of fetal acidemia or infection. Thus, the presence of reactive NST or fetal breathing in conjunction with normal AFV is considered reassuring. Applying the BPP to high-risk patients results in an improvement in perinatal mortality. The false-negative rate of BPP (fetal death within 1 week of a last normal test result) is 0.645–7.000/1000. Figure 29.1 shows an inverse relationship between last BPP score and perinatal mortality. Figure 29.2 shows an inverse linear correlation between last BPP score and perinatal morbidity. The modified BPP comprises the NST and AFV; perinatal morbidity/mortality using this compares favorably with prior studies (which use the entire BPP). Figure 29.3 shows our suggested protocol for the modified BPP. The BPP is also useful in predicting

Table 29.4 Biophysical profile scoring: technique and interpretation.

Biophysical variable	Normal (score = 2)	Abnormal (score = 0)
Fetal breathing movements	≥ one episode of ≥ 30s in 30min	Absent or no episode of ≥ 30s in 30min
Gross body movements	≥ three discrete body limb movements in 30min (episodes of active continuous movement considered)	≤ two episodes of body limb movements in 30min as single movement
Fetal tone	≥ one episode of active extension with return to flexion of fetal limb(s) or trunk Opening and closing of hand considered normal tone	Either slow extension with return to partial flexion movement of limb in full extension or absent fetal movement
Reactive fetal heart rate	≥ two episodes of acceleration of ≥ 15 b.p.m. and of ≥ 15s associated with fetal movement in 20min	< two episodes of acceleration of fetal heart rate or acceleration of < 15 b.p.m. in 20min
Qualitative amniotic fluid volume	≥ one pocket of fluid measuring 2cm in vertical axis	Either no pockets or largest pocket < 2cm in vertical axis

b.p.m., beats per minute.

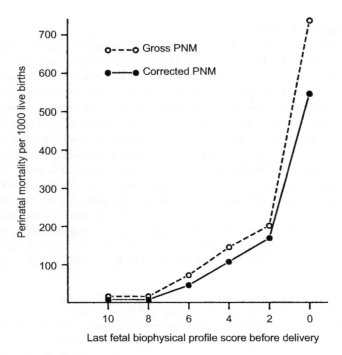

Figure 29.1 The relationship between perinatal mortality (either total or corrected for major anomaly) and the last biophysical profile scoring result. This relationship is exponential, yielding a highly significant inverse correlation using log 10 conversion. PNM, perinatal mortality.

the development of infectious complications in patients with premature rupture of the membranes (PROM).

Amniotic fluid volume (AFV) assessment

AFV is a chronic marker of fetal well-being. Figure 29.4 shows the mean AFV changes during pregnancy. In the second half of pregnancy, the main amniotic fluid (AF) sources include fetal urine excretion (especially) and lung fluid. Various methods of measuring AFV include measuring a vertical single (largest) fluid pocket or the amniotic fluid index (AFI) (Fig. 29.5). Assessment of AF in patients admitted with preterm PROM can also serve as a predictor of amnionitis. Polyhydramnios (AFI > 25 cm) occurs in 0.2–1.6% of the general population and is associated with increased maternal and perinatal morbidity/mortality (Table 29.5). Causes of polyhydramnios include fetal malformations/genetic disorders, diabetes, rhesus (Rh) sensitization, and congenital infections. Oligohydramnios (reduced AFV) occurs in 5.5–37.8% of pregnancies and has an association with adverse pregnancy outcomes (Table 29.6), placental insufficiency, intrauterine growth restriction, urinary tract malformations, postdate pregnancies, and ruptured membranes.

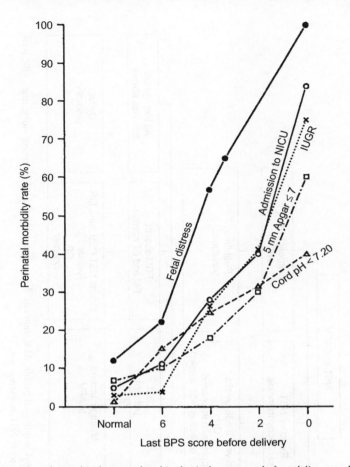

Figure 29.2 The relationship between last biophysical test score before delivery and individual perinatal morbidity variables: presence of fetal distress, admission to neonatal intensive care unit (NICU), intrauterine growth restriction (IUGR), 5-min Apgar score ≤ 7, and umbilical vein pH < 7.20, either alone or in any combination. BPS, biophysical profile score.

Table 29.5 Potential complications associated with polyhydramnios.

Complications	Complications (cont.)
Premature labor	Perinatal mortality
Placental abruption	Maternal respiratory difficulties
Puerperal hemorrhage	

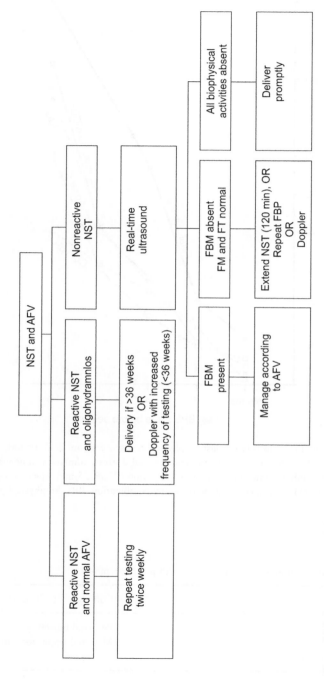

Figure 29.3 Suggested protocol for the modified fetal biophysical profile. AFV, amniotic fluid volume; FBM, fetal breathing movements; FBP, fetal biophysical profile; FM, fetal movements; FT, fetal tone; NST, nonstress test.

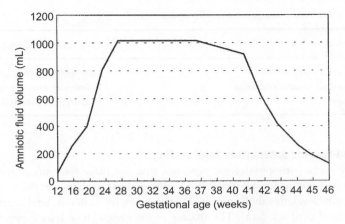

Figure 29.4 Mean amniotic fluid volume (AFV) changes during pregnancy.

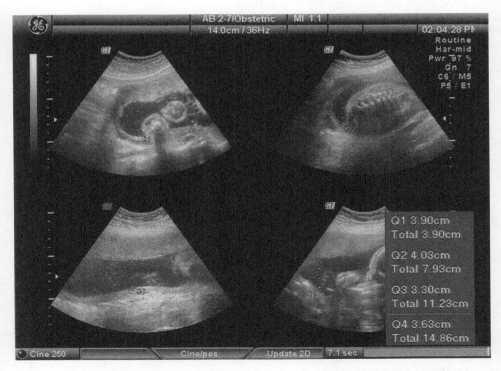

Figure 29.5 Prenatal ultrasound of 30-week fetus depicting vertical measurements (cm) of the amniotic fluid in all four quadrants (Q1–Q4) of the maternal abdomen, comprising the amniotic fluid index (14.86 cm in this case).

Table 29.6 Potential consequences of oligohydramnios.

Consequences	Consequences (cont.)
Umbilical cord compression	Deformation syndrome
Meconium-stained amniotic fluid	Pulmonary hypoplasia
Fetal demise	Maternal or neonatal infection

Condition-specific antepartum fetal testing

There are seven pathophysiologic processes that can place the fetus at risk. These are decreased uteroplacental blood flow, decreased gas exchange at the trophoblastic membrane level, metabolic processes, fetal sepsis, fetal anemia, fetal heart failure, and umbilical cord accidents. The efficacy of the various fetal tests depends on the underlying condition. Table 29.7 shows the various pathophysiologic processes, examples of maternal/fetal conditions, and surveillance tests that may be the most appropriate (condition-specific fetal testing).

Intrapartum fetal surveillance techniques

Fetal heart rate (FHR) monitoring

FHR monitoring can be done either intermittently or continuously. Interpretation of FHR patterns should incorporate knowledge of gestational age, maternal condition, medications, and other factors. The National Institute of Child Health and Human Development (NICHHD) Research Planning Workshop (1997) developed standardized definitions for electronic FHR patterns (Table 29.8) and recommendations for interpreting them. As gestation advances, there is a gradual slowing of the mean baseline FHR. Normal FHR variability is generally described as the most reliable indicator of fetal well-being (reflects intact integration of the CNS and cardiovascular systems). Early decelerations are caused by an increase in vagal tone due to fetal head compression during the contraction. Variable decelerations indicate umbilical cord compression. Late decelerations result from fetal hypoxia, which is often due to decreased placental perfusion; in advanced fetal acidemia, they can also be a result of direct myocardial depression. Figure 29.6 shows a suggested protocol for managing nonreassuring FHR tracings or fetal heart decelerations in labor. The diagnostic accuracy of electronic FHR monitoring (EFM) in predicting fetal compromise is not as good as its accuracy in confirming fetal well-being. While EFM is associated with reductions in neonatal seizures and perinatal deaths due to hypoxia, the price is a small (but significant) increase in operative deliveries.

Fetal acid–base evaluation

Fetal scalp capillary blood sampling is used to improve the positive predictive value of FHR tracings. Figure 29.6 depicts a suggested protocol for managing nonreassuring FHR tracings or fetal heart decelerations in labor, incorporating scalp pH,

Table 29.7 Condition-specific antepartum fetal testing.

Pathophysiologic condition	Maternal/fetal condition	*Appropriate test(s)
Metabolic abnormalities	Type 1 diabetes	NST, CST, BPP, Doppler in class F–R diabetes, maternal blood glucose (goal is normal)
Decreased uteroplacental blood flow	Hypertensive disorders Collagen, renal, vascular disease Most cases IUGR (<32–34 weeks)	NST, CST, BPP, AF assessment, Doppler, EFW by US (growth rate)
Decreased gas exchange	Postdate pregnancy Some cases IUGR (>32–34 weeks)	NST, CST, BPP, AF assessment, first-trimester US (accurate dating), EFW by US
Fetal sepsis	PROM Intra-amniotic infection Maternal fever, primary subclinical intra-amniotic infection	NST, BPP, AF assessment, amniocentesis (rule out infection)
Fetal anemia	Fetomaternal hemorrhage Erythroblastosis fetalis Parvovirus B19 infection	NST (if hydrops present), CST (if hydrops present), BPP (if hydrops present), MCA peak systolic velocity, US to rule out hydrops, fetal liver length, cordocentesis, amniocentesis (>28 weeks)
Fetal heart failure	Cardiac arrhythmia Nonimmune hydrops Chorioangioma placenta Aneurysm of the vein of Galen	NST or CST (if hydrops present/arrhythmia absent), BPP, Doppler (venous circulation), US to rule out hydrops, continuous FHR monitoring (determine time spent in sinus rhythm), M-mode echo (rule out arrhythmias)
Umbilical cord accident	Umbilical cord entanglement (monoamniotic twins) Velamentous cord insertion/funic presentation Noncoiled umbilical cord Oligohydramnios	Frequent NST, umbilical artery Doppler, color Doppler on US (verify diagnosis)

AF, amniotic fluid; BPP, biophysical profile; CST, contraction stress test; EFW, estimated fetal weight; FHR, fetal heart rate; IUGR, intrauterine growth restriction; MCA, middle cerebral artery; NST, nonstress test; PROM, premature rupture of membranes; US, ultrasound.

*Specific surveillance tests that may be the most appropriate and are suggested guidelines.

Table 29.8 Fetal heart rate patterns.

Fetal heart rate pattern	Definition	Comments
Baseline FHR	Approximate mean FHR rounded to increments of 5 b.p.m. during a 10-min segment (excluding periodic/episodic changes, periods of marked FHR variability, segments of the baseline that differ by > 25 b.p.m.)	In any 10-min window, the minimum baseline duration must be ≥ 2 min, or the baseline for that period is indeterminate [one may then need to refer to the previous 10-min segment(s) for determination of the baseline]
Bradycardia	Baseline FHR < 110 b.p.m.	
Tachycardia	Baseline FHR > 160 b.p.m.	
Baseline FHR variability	Fluctuations in the baseline FHR of ≥2 cycles/min	Fluctuations are irregular in amplitude and frequency; visually quantitated as the amplitude of the peak-to-trough (b.p.m.)
Absent FHR variability	Amplitude range undetectable	
Minimal FHR variability	Amplitude range > undetectable and ≤ 5 b.p.m.	
Moderate FHR variability	Amplitude range 6–25 b.p.m.	
Marked FHR variability	Amplitude range > 25 b.p.m.	
Acceleration	Visually apparent abrupt increase (onset of acceleration to peak in < 30 s) in FHR above baseline. Increase is calculated from most recently determined portion of the baseline	Acme is ≥ 15 b.p.m. above baseline, and acceleration lasts ≥ 15 s and < 2 min from onset to return to baseline. Before 32 weeks, defined as acme ≥ 10 b.p.m. above baseline and duration ≥ 10 s
Prolonged acceleration	Duration ≥ 2 min and < 10 min	Acceleration of ≥10 min is a baseline change
Early deceleration	Visually apparent gradual (onset of deceleration to nadir ≥ 30 s) decrease and return to baseline FHR associated with UC	Decrease is calculated from most recently determined portion of baseline. Deceleration is coincident in timing, with nadir occurring at the same time as peak of contraction

(*Continued*)

Table 29.8 *Continued*

Fetal heart rate pattern	Definition	Comments
Variable deceleration	Visually apparent abrupt decrease (onset of deceleration to beginning of nadir < 30 s) in FHR below baseline	Decrease is calculated from most recently determined portion of baseline. Decrease in FHR below baseline is ≥ 15 b.p.m., lasting ≥ 15 s and < 2 min from onset to return to baseline
Late deceleration	Visually apparent gradual (onset of deceleration to nadir ≥ 30 s) decrease and return to baseline FHR associated with UC	Decrease is calculated from most recently determined portion of baseline. Deceleration is delayed in timing, with nadir occurring after peak of contraction
Prolonged deceleration	Visually apparent decrease in FHR below baseline	Decrease is calculated from most recently determined portion of baseline. Decrease from baseline is ≥ 15 b.p.m., lasting ≥ 2 min, but < 10 min from onset to return to baseline Prolonged deceleration of ≥ 10 min is a baseline change
Sinusoidal pattern	Smooth, sine wave-like pattern of regular frequency and amplitude	Excluded in the definition of FHR variability

Adapted from National Institute of Child Health and Human Development Research Planning Workshop. Electronic fetal heart rate monitoring: research guidelines for interpretation. *Am J Obstet Gynecol* 1997;17:1385–1390.

b.p.m., beats per minute; FHR, fetal heart rate; UC, uterine contractions.

fetal pulse oximetry (FPO), or fetal stimulation techniques. A fetal scalp pH ≥ 7.25 is considered normal during the intrapartum period, 7.20–7.24 is preacidemia, while values ≤ 7.19 indicate fetal acidemia. Fetal scalp sampling is now rarely utilized in the United States. Umbilical artery base excess is the most direct measure of fetal metabolic acidosis, and threshold levels of base excess (–12 mmol/L) have been associated with an increased risk of neonatal neurological injury.

Fetal stimulation techniques
VAS or fetal scalp stimulation has been used intrapartum to evoke FHR accelerations and identify the well fetus. Table 29.9 shows that, when data from studies using VAS and studies using scalp stimulation are pooled and compared, the overall efficacy for predicting a scalp pH < 7.20 is similar, regardless of the method of stimulation. Although scalp and acoustic stimulation techniques are simple to perform, they are limited by falsely nonreassuring results.

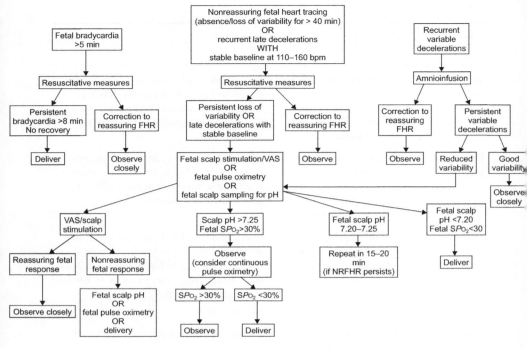

Figure 29.6 Management of nonreassuring fetal heart tracing or fetal heart decelerations in labor. FHR, fetal heart rate; NRFHR, nonreassuring fetal heart rate; SPO_2, arterial oxygen saturation; VAS, vibroacoustic stimulation (from Apuzzio JJ, Vintzileos AM, Iffy L, eds. *Operative obstetrics*, 3rd edn. Abingdon, United Kingdom: Taylor & Francis, 2005, with permission).

Table 29.9 Efficacy of intrapartum fetal stimulation for prediction of a scalp pH of < 7.20.

	VAS (*n* = 405)	Scalp stimulation* (*n* = 488)
Sensitivity	83% (29/35)	98% (43/44)
Specificity	65% (241/370)	67% (298/444)
Positive predictive value	18% (29/158)	23% (43/189)
Negative predictive value	98% (241/247)	99% (298/299)

VAS, vibroacoustic stimulation.

*Scalp stimulation includes scalp puncture, digital pressure, and scalp pinch.

Fetal pulse oximetry (FPO)

FPO measures fetal arterial O_2 saturation during labor and is reserved for use when a nonreassuring FHR has been recorded. The hope is to decrease the Cesarean rate for fetal distress when fetal O_2 saturation is normal. Fetal acidemia is rare when fetal arterial O_2 saturation is continually > 30%. FPO reduces the Cesarean rate for nonreassuring EFM patterns but, as currently used, will not decrease the overall Cesarean rate.

Fetal electrocardiogram (ECG) ST segment automated analysis (STAN)

The fetal ECG can be monitored during labor as an adjunct to continuous EFM, with the aim of improving fetal outcome and minimizing unnecessary obstetric interference. A Cochrane review (2003) assessing the use of fetal ECG as an adjunct to continuous EFM during labor found that using ST waveform analysis was associated with fewer babies with severe metabolic acidosis at birth. Some have found that adding fetal ECG STAN to standard FHR monitoring improved FHR tracing interpretation and observer consistency in both the decision for and the timing of obstetric interventions, and that it may reduce the number of unneeded obstetric interventions when fetal compromise is absent.

Further reading

Chamberlain PF, Manning FA, Morrison I, et al. Ultrasound evaluation of amniotic fluid volume: the relationship of marginal and decreased amniotic fluid volumes to perinatal outcome. *Am J Obstet Gynecol* 1984;150:245–249.

Devoe LD, Castillo RA, Sherline DM. The nonstress test as a diagnostic test: a critical reappraisal. *Am J Obstet Gynecol* 1985;152:1047–1053.

Dildy GA. Fetal pulse oximetry: a critical appraisal. *Best Pract Res Clin Obstet Gynaecol* 2004;18:477–484.

Freeman RK, Anderson G, Dorchester W. A prospective multi-institutional study of antepartum fetal heart rate monitoring: risk of perinatal mortality and morbidity according to antepartum fetal heart rate test results. *Am J Obstet Gynecol* 1982;143:771–777.

Kontopoulos EV, Vintzileos AM. Condition-specific antepartum fetal testing. *Am J Obstet Gynecol* 2004;191:1546–1551.

MacDonald D, Grant A, Sheridan-Pereira M, et al. The Dublin randomized controlled trial of intrapartum fetal heart rate monitoring. *Am J Obstet Gynecol* 1985;152:524–539.

Ross MG, Devoe LD, Rosen KG. ST-segment analysis of the fetal electrocardiogram improves fetal heart rate tracing interpretation and clinical decision making. *J Matern Fetal Neonatal Med* 2004;15;181–185.

Smith CV, Phelan JP, Platt LD, et al. Fetal acoustic stimulation testing. II. A randomized clinical comparison with the non-stress test. *Am J Obstet Gynecol* 1986;155:131–134.

Thacker SB, Stroup D, Chang M. Continuous electronic heart rate monitoring for fetal assessment during labor (Cochrane Review). *The Cochrane Library* Issue 4, 2004.

Vintzileos AM, Campbell WA, Ingardia CJ, Nochimson DJ. The fetal biophysical profile and its predictive value. *Obstet Gynecol* 1983;62:271–278.

30   The fetus at surgery

Robert H. Ball and Michael R. Harrison

The indications for fetal surgical interventions have expanded since the field was founded over two decades ago (Table 30.1). Nevertheless, overall, these procedures remain very limited when compared with the number of pregnancies and even the number of fetuses with malformations.

Open fetal surgery (hysterotomy)

The human experience with open fetal surgery is now quite extensive, from both our own center and others, and is primarily associated with the large numbers of fetal spina bifida repairs. We currently reserve maternal laparotomy/hysterotomy procedures for repair of spina bifida, resection of sacrococcygeal teratoma and other tumors, and lobectomy for cystic adenomatoid malformations.

The risks to the mother are similar to those of any major abdominal surgery, although in this case there is no direct physical benefit to her. In addition, there are the risks associated with aggressive tocolytic therapy and bedrest in a hypercoagulable state. The risks to the fetus are primarily vascular instability and hypoperfusion intraoperatively, leading to injury or death, and prematurity due to postoperative complications. The risks to the pregnancy are primarily preterm labor and premature rupture of membranes (PROM) and preterm delivery. Infectious complications are rare, except when premature rupture leads to prolonged latency. An important additional discussion point is that all subsequent deliveries, including the index pregnancy, must be by Cesarean section. Data regarding future fertility are reassuring, with no increased incidence of infertility in the University College of San Francisco experience in those patients attempting pregnancy. Experience from the Children's Hospital of Pennsylvania suggests a concerning risk of uterine rupture in subsequent pregnancies that may be as high as 18%, which would be considerably higher than the risk after previous low transverse Cesarean section (1% or less) or classical Cesarean section (5–10%). Another potential risk in subsequent pregnancies is placenta accreta. The reason for this is that the site of a hysterotomy performed in the second trimester is never in the same area as a Cesarean section entry. There is an increased risk of placenta accreta in any case in which implantation is in an area of uterine scarring. Multiple incisions will increase the likelihood of

Table 30.1 Fetal conditions that may benefit from treatment before birth.

Fetal condition	Effect on development (rationale for treatment)	Result without treatment	Recommended treatment
Life-threatening defects			
Urinary obstruction (urethral valves)	Hydronephrosis Lung hypoplasia	→Renal failure →Pulmonary failure	Percutaneous vesicoamniotic shunt Fetoscopic ablation of valves Open vesicostomy
Cystic adenomatoid malformation	Lung hypoplasia– hydrops	→Hydrops, death	Open pulmonary lobectomy Ablation (laser/RFA) Steroids Open complete repair
Congenital diaphragmatic hernia	Lung hypoplasia	→Pulmonary failure	Temporary tracheal occlusion Tracheal clip (open and fetoscopic) Fetoscopic balloon (percutaneous/ reversible)
Sacrococcygeal teratoma	High-output failure	→Hydrops, death	Open resection of tumor Vascular occlusion (alcohol/RFA) RFA
Twin–twin transfusion syndrome	Donor–recipient steal through placenta	→Fetal hydrops, death, neurologic damage to survivor	Fetoscopic laser ablation of placental vessels NIH trial Amnioreduction NIH trial Selective reduction NIH trial
Acardiac/anomalous twin (TRAP)	Vascular steal Embolization	→Death/damage to surviving twin	Selective reduction Cord occlusion/ division RFA

(*Continued*)

Table 30.1 *Continued*

	Effect on development (Rationale for treatment)	Result without treatment	Recommended treatment
Aqueductal stenosis	Hydrocephalus	→Brain damage	Ventriculoamniotic shunt
Valvular obstruction	Hypoplastic heart	→Heart failure	Balloon valvuloplasty
Congenital high airway obstruction (CHAOS)	Overdistention by lung fluid	→Hydrops, death	Fetoscopic tracheostomy *Ex utero* intrapartum treatment (EXIT)
Cervical teratoma	Airway obstruction High-output failure	→Hydrops, death	Open resection EXIT Vascular occlusion (alcohol/RFA)
Nonlife-threatening defects			
Myelomeningocle	Spinal cord damage	→Paralysis, neurogenic bladder/bowel, hydrocephalus	Open repair (NIH trial) Fetoscopic coverage
Gastroschisis	Bowel damage	→Malnutrition/ short bowel	Serial amnio-exchange
Cleft lip and palate	Facial defect	→Persistent deformity	Fetoscopic repair* Open repair
Metabolic and cellular defects			
Stem cell–enzyme defects	Hemoglobinopathy Immunodeficiency Storage diseases	→Anemia, hydrops →Infection/death →Retardation/death	Fetal stem cell transplant Fetal gene therapy*
Predictable organ	Agenesis/hypoplasia heart/lung/kidney	→Neonatal heart/lung/ kidney failure	Induce tolerance for postnatal organ transplant* Tissue engineering*

NIH, National Institutes of Health; RFA, radiofrequency ablation.

*Not yet attempted in human fetuses.

implantation in such an area. To our knowledge, there has not been a case of accreta in a fetal surgical patient of ours in a subsequent pregnancy.

Fetoscopic surgery (FETENDO)

With advances in technology and familiarity with endoscopic techniques, the application of this technique to fetal surgery was natural. Common sense would suggest that the smaller the incision in the uterus, the lower the risk of subsequent pregnancy complications. At UCSF, endoscopic approaches were first applied to pregnancies complicated by diaphragmatic hernia, urinary tract obstruction, and twin-to-twin transfusion (Lap-FETENDO).

The initial pioneering approach involved maternal minilaparotomies, with direct exposure of the uterus. Initial caution regarding this approach led to similar perioperative management as that of hysterotomy cases. This included general anesthesia, use of multiple tocolytics, and prolonged hospitalization. One important difference, even initially, was that patients could labor following FETENDO procedures. Since that time, endoscopic procedures have become less invasive with very small instruments passed through 3-mm ports.

Percutaneous FETENDO

Currently, we rarely use the more invasive Lap-FETENDO and have since progressed toward a completely percutaneous approach using a smaller 2 mm endoscope with an operating channel (Micro-FETENDO). We have used this technique for balloon tracheal occlusions, fetal cystoscopies, and for laser ablation in monochorionic twin gestations complicated by severe twin-to-twin transfusion. We anticipate that, based on our early experience and that of others with percutaneous microendoscopy, the risk profile will be similar to that of percutaneous sonoguided procedures (see below). The perioperative management is very different. Patients are treated with prophylactic indomethacin and antibiotics. Postoperative tocolytic therapy is usually based on contraction activity. A 24- to 48-h course of indomethacin or nifedipine is often all that is required.

Fetal intervention guided by sonography (FIGS)

The first fetal procedure, developed in the early 1980s, was percutaneous sonographically guided placement of the Harrison fetal bladder catheter shunt. Many other catheter shunt procedures have been developed and described. More recently, we have developed percutaneous sonographically guided radiofrequency ablation (RFA) procedures for management of anomalous multiple gestations. All these procedures we now group as "fetal intervention guided by sonography" or "FIGS". Very complicated procedures may still require laparotomy (Lap-FIGS).

Percutaneous or Micro-FIGS is used to sample or drain fetal blood, urine, and fluid collection, to sample fetal tissue, to place catheter shunts in the fetal bladder, chest, abdomen, or ventricles, and to do RFA. The most common indication at UCSF is RFA for acardiac twins/TRAP sequence or monochorionic twins for selective reduction. Other operators have used bipolar coagulation or umbilical cord ligation for similar indications. Compared with the 17-gauge RFA needles we use, these techniques are more invasive, using at least 3-mm trocars. Additionally, the length of the cord or its position may preclude the use of these instruments. The perioperative management of these patients is similar to that of current Micro-FETENDO patients. The procedures are performed under spinal anesthesia, with prophylactic antibiotics and indomethacin. Postoperative tocolysis is rarely necessary, and the patients are frequently discharged within hours of the procedure. Ultrasound is critical for both the planning and the execution of the procedure.

Further reading

Callen PW, ed. *Ultrasonography in obstetrics and gynecology*, 4th edn. Philadelphia, PA: W.B. Saunders, 2000.

Harrison MR, Evans MI, Adzick NS, Holzgreve W, eds. *The unborn patient: the art and science of fetal therapy*, 3rd edn. Philadelphia, PA: W.B. Saunders, 2001.

31 Fetal medical treatment

Mark I. Evans, Yuval Yaron, Charles S. Kleinman, and Alan W. Flake

Over the past three decades, numerous methods for the diagnosis of structural and physiologic fetal abnormalities have been developed. Fetal therapy has evolved using three major approaches: surgery, pharmacologic therapy, and stem cell/gene therapy. The prototypes for medical fetal therapy have been neural tube defects (NTDs), congenital adrenal hyperplasia (CAH), and cardiac therapy. Additional disorders that have been treated, but space limitations prohibit their discussion here, include methylmalonic aciduria, multiple carboxylase deficiency, Smith–Lemli–Opitz syndrome, hyperthyroidism, hypothyroidism, and galactosemia. Stem cells represent the first forays into genetic therapies.

Neural tube defects

NTDs result from abnormal closure of the neural tube, which normally occurs between the third and fourth week of gestational age. Socioeconomic status, geographic area, occupational exposure, and maternal use of antiepileptic drugs are also associated with variations in the incidence of NTDs. Preparations containing folate and other vitamins reduce the occurrence of recurrent and first-time NTDs. Since January 1998, the United States Food and Drug Administration mandated supplementation of breads and grains with folic acid. NTD birth prevalence decreased by 19%. Recently, Evans et al. (1997) have shown a nearly 30% drop in high maternal serum alpha-fetoprotein (MSAFP) values in the United States comparing 2000 values with 1997 values, before the introduction of folic acid supplementation.

Congenital adrenal hyperplasia

CAH is actually a group of autosomal recessive metabolic disorders, characterized by enzymatic defects in the steroidogenetic pathway. The most common abnormality, responsible for > 90% of cases of CAH, is caused by a deficiency in the 21-hydroxylase (21-OH) enzyme. This results in increased production of androgens, which produce virilization of the undifferentiated female external genitalia.

We have known for two decades that the fetal adrenal gland can be pharmacologically suppressed by maternal replacement doses of dexamethasone. Hundreds of fetuses have been successfully treated resulting in prevention or amelioration of masculinization.

In utero cardiac therapy

The ability to diagnose structural or functional heart disease prenatally has, predictably, led to a growth of interest in the potential for prenatal therapy. Fetal antiarrhythmic therapy has evolved in a more invasive direction over the past decades, including injection of medication directly into the amniotic fluid, intramuscular administration of medication directly to the fetus, and direct, repetitive administration of intravenous medication through the fetal umbilical vein. Direct instrumentation of the fetal heart was initially attempted in an effort to institute 'transcatheter' pacing of a moribund fetus with congenital complete heart block and hydrops fetalis.

Fetal antiarrhythmic therapy
The fetus with tachycardia

The administration of antiarrhythmic therapy to the mothers of fetuses with sustained supraventricular tachycardia represented the first examples of successful prenatal cardiac therapy that were reported in the medical literature, mostly using digoxin. Many agents are now used.

The fetus with bradycardia

The most important sustained bradyarrhythmia is congenital complete heart block. Such fetuses may develop hydrops fetalis. Many agents have been used – far too numerous for a short summary.

Aortic balloon valvuloplasty

For aortic stenosis, percutaneous cardiac catheterization and aortic balloon valvuloplasty of fetuses have been unsuccessful.

Pulmonary balloon valvuloplasty

Pulmonary balloon valvuloplasty has been performed in two fetuses with severe right ventricular outlet obstruction ("complete" or "almost complete" pulmonary atresia), right ventricular compromise, and "imminent" hydrops fetalis. Both fetuses survived, but it remains to be seen whether such therapy is justified, and whether these fetuses survived "because of," rather than "in spite of" what was done for (to) them.

Prenatal hematopoietic stem cell (HSC) transplantation

The rationale for *in utero* transplantation is to take advantage of the window of opportunity created by normal hematopoietic and immunologic ontogeny. There is a period, prior to population of the bone marrow and thymic processing of self-antigen, when the fetus should theoretically be receptive to engraftment of foreign HSCs without rejection and without the need for myeloablation. In the human fetus, the ideal window would appear to be prior to 14 weeks' gestation, before release of differentiated T lymphocytes into the circulation and while the bone marrow is just beginning to develop sites for hematopoiesis. The ontologic window of opportunity falls well within these diagnostic and technical constraints, making the application of this approach a realistic possibility.

Because of the unique fetal environment, prenatal HSC transplantation could theoretically avoid many of the current limitations of postnatal bone marrow transplantation (BMT). There would be no requirement for human leukocyte antigen (HLA) matching, resulting in expansion of the donor pool. Transplanted cells would not be rejected, and space would be available in the bone marrow, eliminating the need for toxic immunosuppressive and myeloablative drugs.

Diseases amenable to prenatal treatment

Generally speaking, any disease that can be diagnosed early in gestation, that is improved by BMT, and for which postnatal treatment is not entirely satisfactory is a target disease.

The sickle cell anemia and thalassemia syndromes make up the largest patient groups potentially treatable by prenatal stem cell transplantation. Both have been cured by postnatal BMT, but BMT is not recommended routinely because of its prohibitive morbidity and mortality, and the relative success of modern medical management. The development of myeloablation techniques will make it likely that these hemoglobinopathies will be successfully treated by *in utero* transplantation in the future.

Immunodeficiency diseases represent an extremely heterogeneous group of diseases, which differ in their likelihood of cure by their capacity to develop hematopoietic chimerism. Once again, the most likely to benefit from even low levels of donor cell engraftment are those diseases in which a survival advantage exists for normal cells. The best example of this situation is severe combined immunodeficiency (SCID) syndrome. Flake et al. (1996) reported the successful treatment of a fetus with X-linked SCID syndrome in a family in which a previously afflicted child died at 7 months of age. After lengthy informed consent, paternal bone marrow was harvested, T cells depleted, and enriched stem cell populations injected intraperitoneally into the fetus, beginning at about 16 weeks of gestation. The child has achieved normal developmental milestones, and has had no serious infections through

10 years of age. Additional cases have now been reported by Pirovano et al. and Westgren et al. (2002) with similar favorable results.

Inborn errors of metabolism

An even more heterogeneous group of diseases, inborn errors of metabolism, can be caused by a deficiency in a specific lysosomal hydrolase, which results in the accumulation of substrates such as mucopolysaccharide, glycogen, or sphingolipid. Depending on the specific enzyme abnormality and the compounds that accumulate, certain patterns of tissue damage and organ failure occur. These include central nervous system (CNS) deterioration, growth failure, dysostosis multiplex and joint abnormalities, hepatosplenomegaly, myocardial or cardiac disease, upper airway obstruction, pulmonary infiltration, corneal clouding, and hearing loss. The potential efficacy of prenatal HSC transplantation for the treatment of these diseases must be considered on an individual disease basis.

Further reading

Clayton PE, Miller WL, Oberfield SE, et al. ESPE/LWPES CAH Working Group. Consensus statement on 21-hydroxylase deficiency from the European Society for Paediatric Endocrinology and the Lawson Wilkins Pediatric Endocrine Society. *Horm Res* 2002;58:188–195.

Evans MI, Duquette DA, Rinaldo P, et al. Modulation of B12 dosage and response in fetal treatment of methylmalonic aciduria (MMA): titration of treatment dose to serum and urine MMA. *Fetal Diagn Ther* 1997;12:21–23.

Evans MI, Llurba E, Landsberger EJ, et al. Impact of folic acid supplementation in the United States: markedly diminished high maternal serum AFPs. *Obstet Gynecol* 2004;103:474–479.

Flake AW, Roncarolo MG, Puck JM, et al. Treatment of X-linked severe combined immunodeficiency by *in utero* transplantation of paternal bone marrow. *N Engl J Med* 1996;335: 1806–1810.

Harrison MR, Evans MI, Adzick NS, Holzgreve W. *The unborn patient.* Philadelphia, PA: W.B. Saunders, 2002.

Honein MA, Paulozzi LJ, Mathews TJ, et al. Impact of folic acid fortification of the US food supply on the occurrence of neural tube defects. *JAMA* 2001;285:2981–2986.

Kleinman CS, Copel JA, Nehgme RA. The fetus with cardiac arrhythmia. In: Harrison MR, Evans MI, Adzick NS, Holzgreve W, eds. *The unborn patient: the art and science of fetal therapy.* Philadelphia, PA: W.B. Saunders; 2001:417–441.

Pirovano S, Notarangelo LD, Malacarne F, et al. Reconstitution of T-cell compartment after in utero stem cell transplantation: analysis of T-cell repertoire and thymic output. *Haematologica* 2004;89:450–461.

Westgren M, Ringden O, Bartmann P, et al. Prenatal T-cell reconstitution after in utero transplantation with fetal liver cells in a patient with X-linked severe combined immunodeficiency. *Am J Obstet Gynecol* 2002;187:475–482.

Maternal Biological Adaptations to Pregnancy

32 Maternal biological, biomechanical, and biochemical changes in pregnancy

Edward Chien and Helen Feltovich

Pregnancy induces changes in all maternal physiologic systems to accommodate the developing fetus. A thorough understanding of normal adaptations is important in identifying pathologic changes that may adversely affect both fetus and mother.

Cardiovascular system

The cardiovascular system undergoes profound changes during gestation including increased heart rate, increased cardiac output, decreased peripheral vascular resistance, increased oxygen consumption, and decreased blood pressure. The increased demands are met by an increase in both pulse and stroke volume. To accommodate the increased cardiovascular demands, the heart hypertrophies and undergoes anatomic changes, which may lead to misinterpretation of commonly ordered studies including the electrocardiogram (ECG) and chest radiograph. Examination of the heart during pregnancy is also associated with changes in heart sounds, most commonly a split first heart sound and systolic ejection murmurs between the first and second heart sound, which are associated with the increase in blood flow.

Respiratory system

The pulmonary system also adapts to the increase in oxygen consumption. Oxygen consumption throughout gestation increases by 15–20%. The increase in oxygen consumption is met by an increase in ventilation, mainly an increase in tidal volume. The respiratory rate is not elevated during pregnancy. The increased ventilation results in changes in normal blood gas measurements, including an increase in pH and a decrease in $P\text{CO}_2$. Evaluation of pulmonary function by spirometry is unchanged in pregnancy, with normal values for forced expiratory volume in 1 s (FEV_1) and vital capacity.

Hematologic system

Alterations in red blood cell, white blood cell, and clotting factors occur in pregnancy. Plasma volume increases with the onset of pregnancy and continues to expand into the third trimester. Plasma volume expands more rapidly than the increase in red blood cell mass, leading to a dilutional anemia. Overall, blood volume expands by 10–20%. The white blood cell count increases, mainly because of an increase in granulocytes. The lymphocyte population is altered, with a shift in the population of B and T lymphocytes. The coagulation system undergoes marked changes associated with an increased risk of thrombus formation. Although a number of coagulation components may be altered by pregnancy, platelet counts generally remain unchanged.

Urinary tract system

Functional and anatomic changes are seen in both the upper and the lower urinary tract. The kidneys increase in size due to an increase in perfusion that occurs with the onset of pregnancy. The increase in effective renal plasma flow leads to an increase in glomerular filtration rate by at least 30–50%. Tubular absorption is not increased, which can lead to postprandial glycosuria. Increased solute load without an increase in tubular resorption contributes to a fall in serum sodium. Respiratory hyperventilation is associated with increased excretion of bicarbonate. Normal values for serum creatinine and blood urea nitrogen during pregnancy are also lower. High normal values for serum creatinine are suggestive of underlying renal dysfunction. Alterations in the renin–angiotensin–aldosterone system may be associated with the fall in serum osmolality during pregnancy and fluid retention.

Gastrointestinal system

Gastrointestinal complaints are common during pregnancy, occurring in over 50% of patients. One of the most common complaints is gastroesophageal reflux, which is thought to be secondary to decreased esophageal sphincter pressure and increased abdominal pressure due to the expanding uterus. Gastric emptying times are also increased, which contributes to the increased risk of aspiration. Tests of liver function can be altered by pregnancy, and elevations in laboratory values may not reflect dysfunction. Some of the most marked changes are in serum lipid profiles, which are significantly elevated over nonpregnant values. Little is known about changes in exocrine pancreatic function during pregnancy, although serum amylase and lipase levels are not altered.

Endocrine system

Alterations in endocrine function due to pregnancy are widespread and involve the endocrine pancreas, the hypothalamic–pituitary axis, thyroid, and parathyroid systems. Owing to the increased production of binding globulins in the liver, increases in total hormone levels are often common. Unbound hormone levels are generally unchanged. The anterior pituitary increases in size, mainly because of an increased number of prolactin-secreting cells, but also because of an associated rise in serum prolactin levels during gestation. Elevations of corticotropin-releasing hormone (CRH) and adrenocorticotrophic hormone (ACTH) are also seen, especially around the time of delivery, and are due to production by the fetus or fetal membranes and placenta.

Reproductive system

The uterus undergoes marked changes in size and function. The uterine corpus expands over 10-fold in mass, mainly owing to hypertrophy, but also to cellular hyperplasia. Alterations in sensitivity to uterotonic agonists are believed to be due to the expression of proteins associated with increased cell-to-cell communication and contractile-associated proteins. The cervix also undergoes marked changes in structure with changes in overall composition. Changes in cervical composition and structure allow the cervix to remain closed during the majority of pregnancy and then to dilate with the onset of labor. Little is known about decidual function, although it does appear to play a role in prostaglandin metabolism.

Further reading

Baylis C. Glomerular filtration rate in normal and abnormal pregnancies. *Semin Nephrol* 1999;19:133–139.

Carbillon L, Uzan M, Uzan S. Pregnancy, vascular tone, and maternal hemodynamics: a crucial adaptation. *Obstet Gynecol Surv* 2000;55:574–581.

Clark P. Changes of hemostasis variables during pregnancy. *Semin Vasc Med* 2003;3:13–24.

Davison JM. Edema in pregnancy. *Kidney Int* 1997;59(Suppl.):S90–96.

Fantz CR, Dagogo-Jack S, Ladenson JH, Gronowski AM. Thyroid function during pregnancy. *Clin Chem* 1999;45:2250–2258.

Furneaux EC, Langley-Evans AJ, Langley-Evans SC. Nausea and vomiting of pregnancy: endocrine basis and contribution to pregnancy outcome. *Obstet Gynecol Surv* 2001;56: 775–782.

Glinoer D. What happens to the normal thyroid during pregnancy? *Thyroid* 1999;9: 631–635.

Herrera E. Lipid metabolism in pregnancy and its consequences in the fetus and newborn. *Endocrine* 2002;19:43–55.

Hunter S, Robson SC. Adaptation of the maternal heart in pregnancy. *Br Heart J* 1992; 68:540–543.

Mabie WC, DiSessa TG, Crocker LG, et al. A longitudinal study of cardiac output in normal human pregnancy. *Am J Obstet Gynecol* 1994;170:849–856.

Mastorakos G, Ilias I. Maternal and fetal hypothalamic-pituitary-adrenal axes during pregnancy and postpartum. *Ann NY Acad Sci* 2003;997:136–149.

Schwartz KA. Gestational thrombocytopenia and immune thrombocytopenias in pregnancy. *Hematol Oncol Clin North Am* 2000;14:1101–1116.

Maternal nutrition

Barbara Luke

Nutrition in maternity has experienced a renaissance in recent years, with increasing evidence linking alterations in both fetal growth and maternal health with subsequent metabolic and vascular disease. For the developing fetus, altered nutrition *in utero* may result in permanent changes in structure, physiology, and metabolism favoring fetal survival, but with metabolic and vascular disease consequences in adulthood. For the mother, pregnancy complications and subsequent metabolic and vascular disease may share common underlying disease mechanisms. Maternal nutrition, therefore, plays a central role in the immediate and long-term health of the mother and her child.

Diet during pregnancy

Energy and nutrient requirements increase during pregnancy to insure appropriate maternal adaptation to pregnancy and optimal fetal growth. In singleton pregnancies, the daily caloric requirement is approximately 27–30 kcal/kg maternal prepregnancy weight during the first trimester, and 30 kcal/kg maternal prepregnancy weight plus 200–300 kcal during the second and third trimesters. The recommended caloric distribution of macronutrients is 20% of kcal from protein, 30–35% of kcal from fat, and the remainder (45–50% of kcal) from carbohydrates. A summary of recommended dietary allowances (RDAs) and dietary reference intakes from the Food and Nutrition Board, the Institute of Medicine (IOM), is given in Table 33.1.

Use of vitamin–mineral supplements

Ideally, pregnant women should get the level and range of required nutrients through a balanced diet. Adult women in the US generally fail to meet the RDAs for five nutrients: calcium, magnesium, zinc, and vitamins E and B_6. Prenatal use of vitamin–mineral supplements among low-income women has been shown to reduce the risks of preterm delivery and low birthweight (LBW), particularly if initiated during the first trimester. Supplementation in excess of twice the RDA (see Table 33.1) should be avoided, because of the potential for birth defects, including kidney malformations with intakes of 40 000–50 000 IU of vitamin A and aortic stenosis with 4000 IU of vitamin D.

Iron

There are no requirements for routine supplementation, with the possible exception of iron. In instances in which inadequacies cannot be remedied through diet, or if

Table 33.1 Summary of recommended dietary allowances and dietary reference intakes for nonpregnant, pregnant, and lactating women aged 1–50 years.

Nutrient	Nonpregnant (19–30 years)	Nonpregnant (31–50 years)	Pregnancy	Lactation (first 6 months)	Food sources
Folate	400 mcg	400 mcg	600 mcg	500 mcg	Liver, green leafy vegetables, enriched cereals, oranges
Thiamin	1.1 mg	1.1 mg	1.4 mg	1.5 mg	Meats, poultry, pork, beans, enriched cereals and breads
Riboflavin	1.1 mg	1.1 mg	1.4 mg	1.6 mg	Dairy products, meats, liver, eggs, enriched cereals
Niacin	14 mg	14 mg	18 mg	17 mg	Meats, poultry, fish, nuts, legumes, enriched cereals
Vitamin A	800 mcg	800 mcg	800 mcg	1300 mcg	Dark green, yellow, or orange fruits and vegetables, liver
Vitamin B6	1.3 mg	1.3 mg	1.9 mg	2.0 mg	Meats, liver, poultry, fish, nuts, legumes, enriched cereals
Vitamin B12	2.4 mcg	2.4 mcg	2.6 mcg	2.8 mcg	Meats, liver, poultry, eggs, fish, dairy products
Vitamin C	60 mg	60 mg	70 mg	95 mg	Citrus fruits, tomatoes, green leafy vegetables
Vitamin D*	5 mcg	5 mcg	5 mcg	5 mcg	Fortified dairy products
Vitamin E	8 mg α-TE	8 mg α-TE	10 mg α-TE	12 mg α-TE	Vegetable oils, seeds, and cereal grains
Calcium	1000 mg	1000 mg	1000 mg	1000 mg	Dairy products, salmon
Iron	15 mg	15 mg	30 mg	15 mg	Meats, liver, eggs, enriched and whole grains
Magnesium	310 mg	320 mg	350 mg	310 mg	Whole grains, legumes, nuts, green vegetables
Phosphorus	700 mg	700 mg	700 mg	700 mg	Meats, poultry, eggs, pork, fish, dairy products
Zinc	12 mg	12 mg	15 mg	19 mg	Meats, pork, seafood, eggs, legumes
Energy	2200 kcal	2200 kcal	2500 kcal	2700 kcal	Proteins, fats, and carbohydrates
Protein	50 g	50 g	60 g	65 g	Meats, poultry, eggs, fish, and dairy products

Adapted from the National Academy of Sciences, Food and Nutrition Board. Recommended Dietary Allowances, 10th edn, 1989; and Dietary Reference Intakes, 1998.

*As cholecalciferol, 1 mcg = 40 IU of vitamin D.

a woman has unique nutritional requirements, such as multiple gestation, diagnoses of hemoglobinopathies or seizure disorders, or other circumstances, daily supplementation may be the most reasonable alternative.

Mineral intake and supplementation

In addition to being the nutrients most often lacking in women's diets, calcium, magnesium, and zinc have been identified as having the most potential for reducing pregnancy complications and improving outcomes. Prenatal diets low in calcium are associated with increased blood pressure because of heightened smooth muscle reactivity, resulting in an increased risk of pregnancy-induced hypertension and preterm delivery. Nearly all calcium supplementation trials have been shown to lower blood pressure levels. Prenatal calcium supplementation may have more far-reaching effects, beyond pregnancy. Follow-up studies of 7-year-old children whose mothers had received calcium supplementation during pregnancy showed significantly lower systolic blood pressure and lower risk of high systolic blood pressure, particularly among children in the highest quartile of body mass index (BMI). Studies have demonstrated that magnesium is not only effective as therapy for and prophylaxis against preeclampsia, but is safe and potentially beneficial for the neonate in reducing the risk of neurologic damage and cerebral palsy. Magnesium therapy, as prenatal supplementation or as therapy for preeclampsia or preterm labor, may play a neuroprotective role. Plasma zinc concentrations and available zinc intakes are significantly correlated, with zinc supplementation increasing maternal plasma levels. Studies have demonstrated a positive correlation between duration of gestation and zinc concentration at entry to prenatal care. Plasma zinc levels in the lowest quartiles are associated with significantly greater frequency of maternal complications, including infection. Women with premature rupture of membranes (PROM) were found to have significantly lower levels of zinc than women who gave birth at term.

Maternal pregravid weight and gestational weight gain

The factors most strongly correlated with both length of gestation and birthweight are maternal height, pregravid or early pregnancy body weight, maternal fat deposition, and gestational weight gain. Although each factor independently influences birthweight and length of gestation, their effects are neither equal nor additive, but rather: (1) a progressive increase in weight gain was paralleled by an increase in mean birthweight and a decline in the incidence of LBW; (2) increasing pregravid weight diminishes the effect of weight gain on birthweight; (3) there is an inverse relationship between weight gain and perinatal mortality, with gains up to 30 pounds (13.6 kg); and (4) higher gestational weight gains are related to higher birthweights and better growth and development during the first postnatal year. In 1990, the IOM issued pregravid BMI-specific weight gain guidelines for singleton pregnancies (Table 33.2).

Table 33.2 Institute of Medicine (IOM) categories of pregravid body mass index (BMI) and suggested weight gain ranges for singleton pregnancies.

Weight status	BMI range (kg/m²)	Total gain at 40 weeks	Weight gain at trimester 1	Rate of gain at trimesters 2 and 3
Underweight	< 19.8 kg/m²	12.5–18.0 kg (28–40 lb)	2.3 kg (5.1 lb)	0.49 kg/week (1 lb/week)
Normal weight	19.8-26.0 kg/m²	11.5–16.0 kg (25–35 lb)	1.6 kg 0.44 kg/week (3.5 lb)	(1 lb/week)
Overweight	26.1-29.0 kg/m²	7.0–11.5 kg (15–25 lb)	0.9 kg 0.30 kg/week (2.0 lb)	(0.5–0.75 lb/week)
Obese	> 29.0 kg/m²	≥ 6.8 kg (≥ 15 lb)	No recommendation	

Table 33.3 Birthweight and gestation by plurality, USA, 2002.

Plurality	Singletons	Twins	Triplets	Quadruplets	Quintuplets
Number	3 889 191	125 134	6898	434	69
Percent very preterm (< 32 weeks)	1.6%	11.9%	36.1%	59.9%	78.3%
Percent preterm (< 37 weeks)	10.4%	58.2%	92.4%	96.8%	91.3%
Mean gestational age (weeks, SD)	38.8 (2.5)	35.3 (3.7)	32.2 (3.8)	29.9 (4.0)	28.5 (4.7)
Percent very low birthweight (< 1500 g)	1.1%	10.2%	34.5%	61.1%	83.8%
Percent low birthweight (< 2500 g)	6.1%	55.4%	94.4%	98.8%	94.1%
Mean birthweight (g, SD)	3332 (573)	2347 (645)	1687 (561)	1309 (522)	1105 (777)

Adapted from Martin JA, Hamilton BE, Sutton PD, et al. Final data for 2002. National Vital Statistics Reports, vol. 52, no. 10, December 17, 2003.

Table 33.4 BMI-specific dietary recommendations for twin gestations.

| BMI group | Underweight | Normal | Overweight | Obese |
BMI range	< 19.8	19.8–26.0	26.1–29.0	> 29.0
Calories	4000	3500	3250	3000
Protein (20% of calories)	200 g	175 g	163 g	150 g
Carbohydrate (40% of calories)	400 g	350 g	325 g	300 g
Fat (40% of calories)	178 g	156 g	144 g	133 g
Exchanges (servings) per day				
Dairy	10	8	8	8
Grains	12	10	8	8
Meat and meat equivalents	10	10	8	6
Eggs	2	2	2	2
Vegetables	5	4	4	4
Fruits	8	7	6	6
Fats and oils	7	6	5	5

Adapted from Luke B, Brown MB, Misiunas R, et al. Specialized prenatal care and maternal and infant outcomes in twin pregnancy. *Am J Obstet Gynecol* 2003;189:934–938.

Multiple pregnancy

In 2002, in the United States, there were 132 535 infants of multiple births, the highest number ever recorded in the history of the vital statistics system. The incidence of twin births has increased dramatically since 1980. An estimated one-fourth of this rise is due solely to older maternal age, which is associated with a higher natural frequency of multiple births, while three-fourths is due to assisted reproductive technologies. Infants of multiple births are disproportionately represented among the LBW (< 2500 g) and preterm (< 37 weeks) populations (Table 33.3). Specialized prenatal care has been shown to reduce adverse outcomes in these high-risk pregnancies, including targeted diet therapy (Table 33.4) and BMI-specific weight gain recommendations (Table 33.5).

Table 33.5 Optimal rates of maternal weight gain and cumulative gain by pregravid BMI status.

Pregravid BMI	Rates of weight gain (lbs/week)				Cumulative weight gain (lbs)		
	0–20 weeks	20–28 weeks	28 weeks to delivery		to 20 weeks	to 28 weeks	to 36–38 weeks
Underweight (BMI < 19.8)	1.25–1.75	1.50–1.75	1.25		25–35	37–49	50–62
Normal weight (BMI 19.8–26.0)	1.00–1.50	1.25–1.75	1.00		20–30	30–44	40–54
Overweight(BMI 26.1–29.0)	1.00–1.25	1.00–1.50	1.00		20–25	28–37	38–47
Obese (BMI > 29.0)	0.75–1.0	0.75–1.25	0.75		15–20	21–30	29–38

Adapted from Luke B, Hediger ML, Nugent C, et al. Body mass index-specific weight gains associated with optimal birthweights in twin pregnancies. *J Reprod Med* 2003;48:217–224.

Results are from models controlling for diabetes and gestational diabetes, preeclampsia, smoking during pregnancy, parity, placental membranes, and fetal growth before 20 weeks.

BMI, body mass index.

Further reading

Belizàn JM, Vilar J, Bergel E, et al. Long term effect of calcium supplementation during pregnancy on the blood pressure of offspring: follow up of a randomized controlled trial. *Br Med J* 1997;315:281–285.

Gluckman PD, Hanson MA. Living with the past: evolution, development, and patterns of disease. *Science* 2004;305:1733–1736.

Godfrey KM, Barker DJP. Fetal nutrition and adult disease. *Am J Clin Nutr* 2000;7 (Suppl.):1344S–1352S.

Gülmezoglu AM, de Onis M, Villar J. Effectiveness of interventions to prevent or treat impaired fetal growth. *Obstet Gynecol Surv* 1997;6:139–149.

Li R, Haas JD, Habicht J-P. Timing of the influence of maternal nutritional status during pregnancy on fetal growth. *Am J Hum Biol* 1998;10:529–539.

Luke B, Brown MB, Misiunas R, et al. Specialized prenatal care and maternal and infant outcomes in twin pregnancy. *Am J Obstet Gynecol* 2003;189:934–938.

Sattar N, Greer IA. Pregnancy complications and maternal cardiovascular risk: opportunities for intervention and screening? *Br Med J* 2002;325:157–169.

Singer JE, Westphal M, Niswander K. Relationship of weight gain during pregnancy to birth weight and infant growth and development in the first year of life. *Obstet Gynecol* 1968;31:417–423.

World Health Organization. Maternal anthropometry and pregnancy outcomes: a WHO collaborative project. *Bull WHO* 1995;73 (Suppl.).

Wu G, Bazer FW, Cudd TA, et al. Maternal nutrition and fetal development. *J Nutr* 2004;134:2169–2172.

Part X
Maternal Diseases Complicating Pregnancy

34 Trauma, shock, and critical care obstetrics

Erin A.S. Clark, Gary A. Dildy, and Steven L. Clark

Definition of shock

Shock is a condition in which circulation fails to meet the nutritional needs of the cell and remove metabolic wastes. This may result from cardiac dysfunction, hypovolemia (relative or absolute), maldistribution of flow, or intravascular obstruction (Table 34.1). When the circulating blood volume is less than the capacity of its

Table 34.1 Classification scheme for shock.

Type	Physiologic derangement	Examples
Cardiogenic	Diminished cardiac function	Cardiomyopathy, myocardial infarction
Hypovolemic	Decreased intravascular volume	Hemorrhage, dehydration
Distributive	Inappropriate distribution of perfusion	Septic shock, neurogenic shock
Obstructive	Intravascular obstruction	Pulmonary embolus

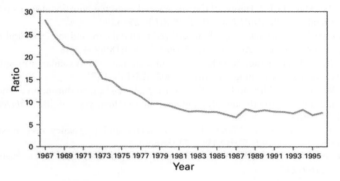

Figure 34.1 Maternal mortality ratio, by year, United States, 1967–1996 (MMWR, 2001).

vascular bed, hypotension with diminished tissue perfusion results, leading to cellular hypoxia and, ultimately, cell death. Depending on the duration and severity of the insult, irreversible organ damage or even death may ensue.

Incidence of shock in the obstetric population

A steady decline in maternal mortality has been noted since 1915, when national vital statistics in the United States were first recorded (Fig. 34.1). Recent statistics for the United States suggest that overall maternal mortality is 11.5 maternal deaths per 100 000 live births during 1991–97 (Table 34.2). The chief cause of a pregnancy-related maternal death depends on whether the pregnancy results in a liveborn, stillbirth, ectopic pregnancy, abortion, or molar gestation (Table 34.3).

General supportive measures

Initial treatment

Several important initial steps should be performed when the diagnosis of shock is made in the obstetric patient. Placement of two large-bore intravenous lines, preferably 16-gauge, for rapid expansion of intravascular volume is the first step. One liter of crystalloid solution should be infused over the first 15 min while other

Table 34.2 Number of pregnancy-related deaths and pregnancy-related mortality ratios (PRMRs)* among Hispanic, Asian/Pacific Islander, American Indian/Alaska Native, non-Hispanic black (black), and non-Hispanic white (white) women, by age group – United States, 1991–1997.

Age group (years)	Hispanic		Asian/ Pacific Islander		American Indian/ Alaska Native		Black		White		Total	
	No.	PRMR	No.	PRMR	No.	PRMR	No.	PRMR	No.	PRMR	No.	PRMR
<20	45	5.5	†		†		160	16.0	96	5.8	306	8.5
20–29	200	7.4	43	8.4	16	11.0‡	590	25.0	35	6.0	1384	9.3
30–34	125	16.0	28	8.7	†		260	38.8	330	7.4	749	11.9
35–39	82	26.0	34	22.7	†		202	70.8	226	12.3	549	21.1
>39	31	48.2	14	42.4§	†		80	151.2	79	25.5	205	44.3
Total	483	10.3	121	11.3	31	12.2	1292	29.6	1266	7.3	3193	11.5
RR§		1.4		1.6		1.7		4.0		(ref)		
95% CI**		(1.3–1.6)		(1.3–1.9)		(1.2–2.4)		(3.8–4.4)				

* Per 100 000 live births.

† Fewer than seven pregnancy-related deaths; considered unreliable (relative standard error [RSE] ≥ 38%).

‡ Point estimates based on 7–19 deaths are highly variable (RSE = 23–38%).

§ Relative ratio of PRMR for each racial/ethnic group divided by PRMR for white women.

** Confidence interval.

Table 34.3 Percentage of pregnancy-related deaths by outcome of pregnancy and cause of death, percentage of all outcomes of pregnancy, and PRMR*, United States, 1987–1990.

Cause of death	Outcome of pregnancy (% distribution)							All outcomes	
	Live birth	Stillbirth	Ectopic	Abortion†	Molar‡	Undelivered	Unknown	Percentage	PRMR
Hemorrhage	21.1	27.2	94.9	18.5	16.7	15.7	20.1	28.8	2.6
Embolism	23.4	10.7	1.3	11.1	0.0	35.2	21.1	19.9	1.8
Pregnancy-induced hypertension	23.8	26.2	0.0	1.2	0.0	4.6	16.3	17.6	1.6
Infection	12.1	19.4	1.3	49.4	0.0	13.0	9.0	13.1	1.2
Cardiomyopathy	6.1	2.9	0.0	0.0	0.0	2.8	13.9	5.7	0.5
Anesthesia complications	2.7	0.0	1.9	8.6	0.0	1.8	1.0	2.5	0.2
Other/unknown	11.1	13.6	0.6	11.1	83.3	27.5	19.3	12.8	1.2
Total§	100.0	100.0	100.0	100.0	100.0	100.0	100.0	100.0	9.2

* Pregnancy-related deaths per 100000 live births.

† Includes spontaneous and induced abortions.

‡ Also known as gestational trophoblastic neoplasia.

§ Percentages may not add to 100.0 due to rounding.

measures are taken. An indwelling bladder catheter is placed for hourly determination of urine output. An arterial line allows continuous measurement of systemic blood pressure, as well as easy access for laboratory investigations. Oxygen should be administered via a facemask at 8–10 L/min and the inspired oxygen concentration adjusted according to arterial blood gas results. Inability to maintain an adequate tidal volume, poor arterial oxygenation, and airway obstruction may require endotracheal intubation with positive pressure ventilation. Initial laboratory investigation should include blood type and cross-match, complete blood count, platelets, fibrinogen, electrolytes, blood urea nitrogen, creatinine, and arterial blood gas. Urine should be sent for analysis and microscopic evaluation. When the patient is stabilized, cultures from blood, urine, sputum, amniotic fluid, endometrial cavity, and stool are taken, as indicated, if sepsis is suspected.

Volume replacement

Whether to give crystalloid or colloid solutions for initial treatment is controversial. In a meta-analysis of several randomized controlled trials, there was no evidence that colloids achieve a superior clinical outcome compared with crystalloid therapy. Crystalloids are reasonable and cost-effective first-line therapy for volume resuscitation. When severe, correction of metabolic acidosis may be aided by adding sodium bicarbonate to intravenous fluids. Lactated solutions should be avoided because aerobic metabolism is required for the conversion of lactate to bicarbonate.

Blood component therapy

In the case of hemorrhagic hypovolemic shock and disseminated intravascular coagulopathy (DIC), blood component therapy is often indicated. Which components should be used is determined largely by laboratory parameters. An obvious exception is profuse hemorrhagic shock, for which immediate blood components, specifically packed red blood cells, are indicated. Table 34.4 demonstrates the therapeutic contents per volume of each blood product.

The use of fresh frozen plasma (FFP) requires specific indications: replacement of isolated or combined factor deficiencies; reversal of warfarin effect in patients actively bleeding or requiring emergency surgery; antithrombin III deficiency; immunodeficiencies; thrombotic thrombocytopenia purpura; and massive blood transfusion in cases in which factor deficiencies are presumed to be the sole or principal derangement. Pathologic hemorrhage in the patient receiving massive transfusion is usually due to thrombocytopenia rather than depletion of coagulation factors. Empiric administration of FFP should therefore be allowed only in those patients in whom factor deficiencies are presumed to be the sole or principal derangement. In massively transfused patients, there is no evidence to support prophylactic transfusion of FFP after transfusion of a certain number of units of packed red blood cells unless coagulation factor defects have been documented. The most useful tests for predicting abnormal bleeding and guiding therapy in massively transfused trauma patients are the platelet count and fibrinogen level. Platelet transfusion should be considered when the platelet count falls to less than 10 000/μL, or

Table 34.4 Summary chart of blood components.

Component	Content	Indications for use	Amount of active substance per unit	Volume (mL)
Red blood cells	Red blood cells, some plasma, some white blood cells and platelets or their degradation products	Increase red blood cell mass for symptomatic anema	200 mL packed red blood cell mass	250–350
Leukocyte-poor red blood cells	Red blood cells, some plasma, few white blood cells	Prevent febrile reactions due to leukocyte antibodies, and increase red blood cells mass	185 mL packed red blood cell mass	200–250
Frozen–thawed washed red blood cells	Red blood cells, no plasma, minimal white blood cells and platelets	Increase red blood cell mass; prevent sensitization to HLAs; prevent febrile or anaphylactic reactions to white blood cells, platelets, and proteins (IgA); provide rare blood cells	170–190 mL packed red blood cells	300
Platelet concentrations	Platelets, few white blood cells, some plasma	Bleeding due to thrombocytopenia or thrombocytopathia	At least 5.5×10^{10} platelets	30–50
Fresh frozen plasma	Plasma, all coagulation factors, no platelets	Treatment of coagulation disorders	0.7–1.0 U factors II, V–VI, VIII-XIII, 500 mg fibrinogen	220–250
Cryoprecipitate	Fibrinogen, factor VIII, factor XIII, von Willebrand's factor	Factor VIII deficiency (hemophilia A) von Willebrand's disease; factor XIII deficiency; fibrinogen deficiency	80 U factor VIII; 200 mg fibrinogen	10–25
Albumin: 5% 25%	Albumin	Plasma volume expansion	12.5 g 12.5 g	250 50

Modified from Borucki 1981.

Blood volume (mL) = weight (kg) × 70 mL/kg

Plasma volume (mL) = Blood volume (mL) × (1.0 − hematocrit)

Fibrinogen requirement (mg) = [Desired fibrinogen level (mg/dL) − initial
  fibrinogen level (mg/dL)] × plasma volume (mL) × 0.01 dL/mL

1 unit cryoprecipitate (22.5 mL) contains 200 mg fibrinogen
1 unit FFP (225 mL) contains 400 mg fibrinogen

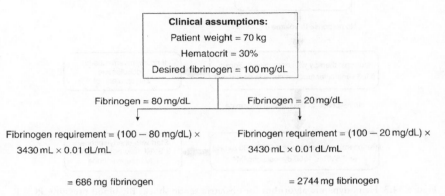

Clinical assumptions:
Patient weight = 70 kg
Hematocrit = 30%
Desired fibrinogen = 100 mg/dL

Fibrinogen = 80 mg/dL	Fibrinogen = 20 mg/dL
Fibrinogen requirement = (100 − 80 mg/dL) × 3430 mL × 0.01 dL/mL	Fibrinogen requirement = (100 − 20 mg/dL) × 3430 mL × 0.01 dL/mL
= 686 mg fibrinogen	= 2744 mg fibrinogen
This patient would require 1.7 units (383 mL) of FFP or 3.4 units (77 mL) of cryoprecipitate	This patient would require 6.9 units (1544 mL) of FFP or 13.7 units (309 mL) of cryoprecipitate
Transfusion of 2 units of FFP would be appropriate if hypervolemia is not a concern	Transfusion of cryoprecipitate is appropriate, as FFP requirements may produce fluid overload

Figure 34.2 Calculation of fibrinogen requirements for obstetric hemorrhage. FFP, fresh frozen plasma.

to less than 35 000/μL in preparation for a surgical procedure or in the face of active bleeding. Cryoprecipitate should be administered instead of FFP when the calculated coagulation factor deficit based on blood fibrinogen levels suggests that FFP will result in inadequate replacement or in volume overload (Fig. 34.2).

Pharmacologic agents
If adequate intravascular volume replacement is not successful in supporting blood pressure (i.e., mean arterial pressure ≥65 mmHg) and other reversible causes of shock are not found (e.g., cardiac arrhythmia, tension pneumothorax), an advanced stage of shock should be suspected (Fig. 34.3). In order to insure tissue perfusion in these refractory cases, cardiac performance should be enhanced through the use of inotropic agents (Table 34.5). Dopamine is considered a first-line inotropic agent.

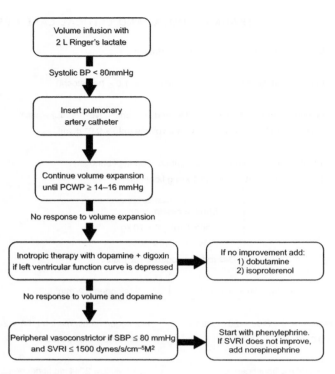

Figure 34.3 Hemodynamic algorithm for obstetric septic shock. BP, blood pressure; PCWP, pulmonary catheter wedge pressure; SBP, systolic blood pressure; SVRI, systemic vascular resistance index (reprinted from Lee et al., 1988, with permission).

Table 34.5 Inotropic agents.

Inotropic agent	Mechanism of action	Dosage
Dopamine	Dopaminergic (0.5–5.0 μg/kg/min) vasodilation of renal and mesenteric vasculature; β_1-adrenergic (5.0–10.0 μg/kg/min) increased myocardial contractility, SV, CO; alpha-adrenergic (15–20 μg/kg/min) increased general vasoconstriction	2–5 μg/kg/min and titrate to BP and CO
Dobutamine	Myocardial β_1-receptor stimulant increased CO, minimal tachycardia	2–10 μg/kg/min
Isoproterenol	β-adrenergic receptors increased contractility and heart rate, but ventricular ectopy, tachycardia, vasodilation	1–20 μg/min
Digoxin	Improved contractility of myocardium	0.5 mg IV push and 0.25 mg q4h × 2, then 0.25–0.37 mg/day

BP, blood pressure; CO, cardiac output; SV, stroke volume.
Modified from Lee et al., 1988.

Table 34.6 Vasopressor agents.

Vasopressor agent	Mechanism of action	Dosage
Phenylephrine (Neo-Synephrine)	Alpha-adrenergic increased systemic vascular resistance	1–5 µg/kg/min
Norepinephrine (Levophed)	Mixed adrenergic alpha and beta generalized vasoconstriction, increased systemic vascular resistance	1–4 µg/min

Modified from Lee et al., 1988.

If satisfactory hemodynamic performance is not achieved and the patient is not profoundly hypotensive, dobutamine or isoproterenol may be added. When blood pressure does not respond to inotropic therapy, a peripheral vasoconstrictor should be considered to maintain appropriate vascular tone (Table 34.6). Although vaso-constrictors are commonly used, there are few data to suggest they improve outcome. Particular caution must be exercised with the use of these agents in gravid patients. Although vasopressors may temporarily correct hypotension, they do so at the expense of uteroplacental perfusion.

Hemodynamic monitoring

The pulmonary artery catheter provides direct measurement of central venous pres-sure, pulmonary artery systolic and diastolic pressure, and pulmonary capillary wedge pressure, whereas thermodilution techniques and physiologic equations allow derivation of cardiac output, systemic vascular resistance, and other hemodynamic parameters. Normal values during pregnancy are summarized in Table 34.7. In select cases, placement of a pulmonary artery catheter should be considered to aid in assessing cardiac function and hemodynamic status. The Swan–Ganz catheter can be used to guide volume resuscitation through the use of the volume challenge (Fig. 34.4). Potential clinical indications for the use of the pulmonary artery catheter in obstetric patients are summarized in Table 34.8.

On insertion of the Swan–Ganz catheter, advancement to the right side of the heart demonstrates characteristic pressure tracings through the right atrium, right ventricle, pulmonary artery, and pulmonary capillary wedge positions (Fig. 34.5). From these waveforms, specific hemodynamic and ventilatory parameters can be determined (Table 34.9). Cardiac output may then be used to construct a ventricu-lar function curve (Fig. 34.6). Hemodynamic subsets of ventricular function can be evaluated by plotting stroke index against left ventricular filling pressure (Fig. 34.7). A knowledge of pulmonary capillary wedge pressure, pulmonary artery diastolic wedge gradient, and the arteriovenous oxygen difference makes it possible to ascer-tain the precise etiology of cardiopulmonary compromise (Fig. 34.8).

Electronic fetal heart rate monitoring

During the development of shock in the pregnant patient, redistribution

Table 34.7 Hemodynamic indices in nonpregnant and normal third-trimester pregnant women measured by pulmonary artery catheter.

Parameter	Normal nonpregnant ($n = 10$)* mean ± SD	Normal third trimester ($n = 10$)* mean ± SD	Severe preeclampsia ($n = 45$)† mean ± SEM	Amniotic fluid embolism ($n = 15$)‡ mean ± SD
Cardiac output (L/min)	4.3 ± 0.9	6.2 ± 1.0	7.5 ± 0.2	–
Heart rate (beats per minute)	71 ± 10	83 ± 10	95 ± 2	–
Systemic vascular resistance (dyne·m·sec^{-5})	1,530 ± 520	1,210 ± 266	1,496 ± 64	–
Pulmonary vascular resistance (dyne·cm·sec^{-5})	119 ± 47	78 ± 22	70 ± 5	176 ± 72
Colloid osmotic pressure (mmHg)	20.8 ± 1.0	18.0 ± 1.5	19.0 ± 0.5	–
Mean arterial pressure (mmHg)	86 ± 8	90 ± 6	138 ± 3	–
Pulmonary capillary wedge pressure (mmHg)	6.3 ± 2.1	7.5 ± 1.8	10 ± 1	18.9 ± 9.2
Central venous pressure (mmHg)	3.7 ± 2.6	3.6 ± 2.5	4 ± 1	–
Left ventricular stroke work index (g·m·m^{-2})	41 ± 8	48 ± 6	81 ± 2	26 ± 19
Mean pulmonary artery pressure (mmHg)	11.9 ± 2.0	12.5 ± 2.0	17 ± 1	26.2 ± 15.7

SD, standard deviation; SEM, standard error of the mean.

Observations in pathophysiologic states (severe preeclampsia and amniotic fluid embolism) are shown for comparison.

Data from *Clark et al. (1988); †Clark et al. (1989); ‡Cotton and Benedetti (1980), and unpublished data from the National Amniotic Fluid Embolism Registry.

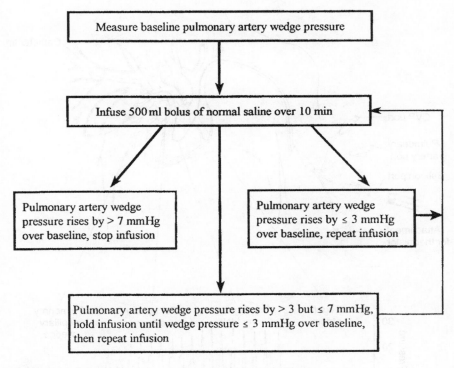

Figure 34.4 Pulmonary artery catheter-guided volume challenge.

Table 34.8 Indications for pulmonary artery catheterization during pregnancy.

1. Massive blood loss with large transfusion requirements, particularly in the face of oliguria or pulmonary edema
2. Septic shock, especially when accompanied by hypotenion or oliguria, required volume resuscitation or vasopressor therapy
3. Cardiac failure or pulmonary edema of uncertain etiology
4. Severe pregnancy-induced hypertension complicated by pulmonary edema, oliguria unresponsive to initial fluid challenge, or severe hypertension refractory to conventional therapy (hydralazine)
5. Labor and delivery in patients with significant cardiovascular disease (New York Heart Association functional class III and IV patients)
6. Intraoperative cardiovascular decompensation (e.g., pulmonary hypertension with shunting secondary to amniotic fluid embolism)
7. During peripartum period in patients with severe preeclampsia and structural cardiac defects
8. Thyroid storm with evidence of high output failure
9. Diabetic ketoacidosis with severe hypovolemia and oliguria

Data from Benedetti et al. (1980); Cotton and Benedetti (1980); Clark et al. (1985); Kirshon and Cotton (1987); Nolan et al. (1992).

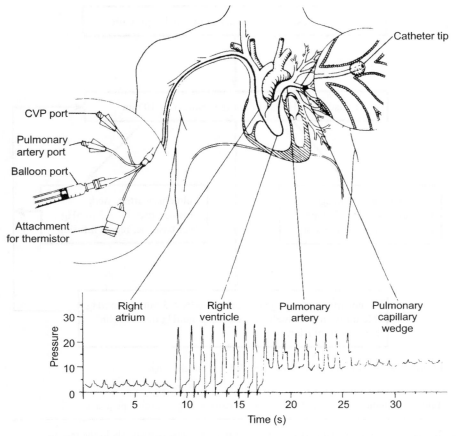

Figure 34.5 Swan–Ganz catheter placement. Swan–Ganz catheter depicting central venous pressure (CVP) port, pulmonary artery and balloon port, and attachment for thermistor. During advancement through the right side of the heart, characteristic pressure tracings are recorded from the right atrial, right ventricular, pulmonary artery, and pulmonary capillary wedge positions (reprinted from Gibson and Kistner, 1982, with permission).

of maternal cardiac output to vital organs may occur at the expense of the utero-placental fetal unit. In the pregnant patient, fetal hypoxia may lead to changes in the heart rate pattern before the mother becomes overtly hypotensive. In the absence of abnormal changes in the fetal heart rate pattern, significant maternal shock is unlikely.

The appropriate duration of electronic fetal monitoring after trauma has been the subject of investigation. The occurrence of adverse outcomes including abruptio placentae is not always predictable on the basis of injury severity. Current evidence suggests that a period of continuous fetal monitoring is prudent in most cases of

Table 34.9 Hemodynamic and ventilatory parameters.

	Nonpregnant	Pregnant
Central venous pressure (mmHg)	1–7	Unchanged
Pulmonary capillary wedge pressure (mmHg)	6–12	Unchanged
Mean pulmonary artery pressure (mmHg)	9–16	Unchanged
Systemic vascular resistance (dyne·cm·sec^{-5})	800–1200	Decreased 25%
Pulmonary vascular resistance (dyne·cm·sec^{-5})	20–120	Decreased 25%
Cardiac output (L/min)	4–7	Increased 30–45%
Arterial po_2 (mmHg)	90–95	104–108
Arterial pco_2 (mmHg)	38–40	27–32
Arterial pH	7.35–7.40	7.40–7.45
Oxygen consumption (mL/min)	173–311	249–331

From ref. 35, with permission.

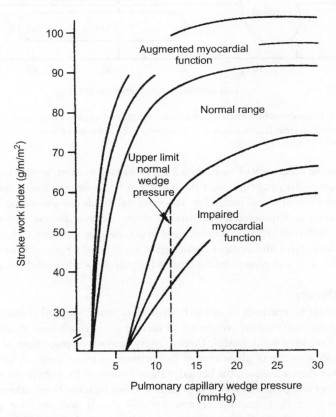

Figure 34.6 Normal ventricular function curve. P, pressure (reprinted from Cotton and Benedetti, 1980, with permission).

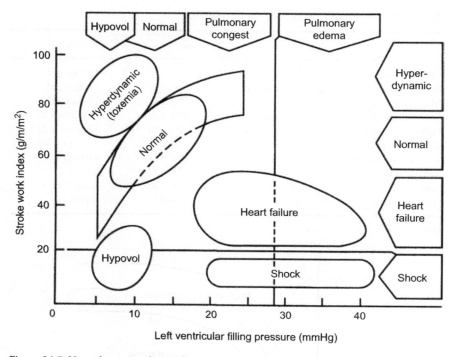

Figure 34.7 Hemodynamic subsets of ventricular function. Congest, congestion; Hypovol, hypovolemic (reprinted from Cotton and Benedetti, 1980, with permission).

trauma during pregnancy of more than 22–24 weeks' gestation. In patients without signs or symptoms of abruption, a period of 2–6 hours of monitoring will suffice. In cases of hemodynamic instability, the maternal condition should be stabilized before delivery is considered for persistent evidence of fetal distress. The fetus may recover as maternal hypoxia, acidosis, and hypotension are corrected. Serial evaluations of fetal status and *in utero* resuscitation are generally preferable to the emergency delivery of a depressed infant from a hemodynamically unstable mother.

Surgical therapy

In postpartum hemorrhage resulting from uterine atony, surgical therapy may be required if the conventional treatments of uterine compression and pharmacologic therapies have been unsuccessful. Uterine artery ligation or placement of a fundus compression suture may abate uterine hemorrhage in many cases. If hemorrhage persists after these measures, the hemodynamic stability of the patient should determine whether one proceeds with a hypogastric artery ligation, transcatheter arterial embolization, or hysterectomy. Hysterectomy is clearly indicated for profound intractable hemorrhage if the patient is unstable or not desirous of future childbearing. After hysterectomy for severe obstetric hemorrhage, diffuse bleeding may

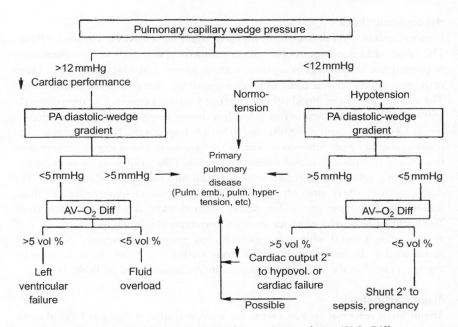

Figure 34.8 Flow diagram for interpretation of Swan–Ganz catheter. AV-O$_2$ Diff, arteriovenous oxygen difference; Emb, embolism; Hypovol., hypovolemia; PA, pulmonary artery; Pulm., pulmonary; Ventr., ventricular (reprinted from Cotton and Benedetti, 1980, with permission).

persist from pelvic surgical sites as a result of associated coagulopathy, and a pelvic pressure pack may be useful.

Cardiopulmonary resuscitation and perimortem Cesarean section

If cardiac or pulmonary arrest occurs in the pregnant woman, cardiopulmonary resuscitation is initiated in the same fashion as for nonpregnant victims. Technical variations specific for pregnancy include lateral uterine displacement to improve venous return and cardiac output, and perimortem Cesarean section if resuscitation is not successful within 4 minutes of the initial event.

Specific etiologies and their management

Shock in the obstetric patient may be categorized as hypovolemic, distributive (sepsis and anaphylaxis), cardiogenic, or obstructive (pulmonary embolism). Although these etiologies are different, they often share common pathophysiologic pathways and ultimately lead to hypoperfusion at the tissue and cellular levels. This decreased perfusion can lead to local tissue hypoxia, organ dysfunction, multiple organ failure, and death. Cardiogenic and obstructive etiologies are discussed elsewhere in this handbook.

Hypovolemic shock

Hypovolemia may result from hemorrhage or solely from loss of intravascular fluids. The causes of hemorrhage in obstetrics are numerous, with the most common cause of postpartum hemorrhage being uterine atony followed by obstetric trauma. Hemorrhage is still the leading cause of pregnancy-related mortality in the United States. The average amount of blood volume expansion during pregnancy is approximately 1500 mL. The average amount of blood lost during a vaginal delivery and elective repeat Cesarean section is 500 mL and 1000 mL respectively. No physiologic compromise should be encountered so long as the volume of blood lost at delivery does not exceed the amount added during pregnancy. When this balance is exceeded, hypovolemia results in decreased venous return and reduced cardiac output. The diagnosis of shock is most often made by the presence of hypotension, oliguria, acidosis, and collapse in the late stage, when therapy is frequently ineffective. Treatment of hemorrhagic shock involves correcting the initiating process as well as instituting general supportive measures, as previously discussed. Uterotonic agents used in the treatment of uterine atony are listed in Table 34.10. Uterorelaxant agents used in the treatment of uterine inversion are listed in Table 34.11.

Anaphylactic shock

Anaphylactic reactions are rare events, but may be fatal in as many as 10% of cases. Antibiotics, nonsteroidal anti-inflammatory drugs, oxytocin, anesthetic agents, blood products, colloid solutions, and latex exposures are some of the more common causes of anaphylaxis in pregnancy. Early recognition and treatment of anaphylactic reactions is essential. Hypotension and tachycardia are universal, and

Table 34.10 Uterotonic agents for uterine atony.

Agent	Administration route	Dose	Comments
Oxytocin (Pitocin)	Intravenous	10–40 U in 1,000 mL of LR or NS	Not to exceed 100 mU/min
Methylergonovine (Methergine)	Intramuscular	0.2 mg q6h	Avoid in hypertensive patients
15-methyl $PGF_{2\alpha}$ (Hemabate)	Intramuscular or intramyometrial	0.25 mg q15–60 min	Side effects include arterial O_2 desaturation, bronchospasm, hypertension
Dinoprostone (Prostin E_2)	Per rectum	20-mg suppository	Use with caution in hypotensive patient because of vasodilation. If available, $PGF_{2\alpha}$ is preferable

LR, lactated Ringer's solution; NS, normal saline; $PGF_{2\alpha}$, prostaglandin F_2 alpha.
From Dildy and Clark (1993).

Table 34.11 Uterorelaxant agents for uterine inversion.

MgSO$_4$	2 g IV over 5–10 min
Terbutaline	0.125–0.250 mg IVP*
Nitroglycerin	100 µg IVP*
Halothane	≥2% general endotracheal

IVP, intravenous push.

*May exacerbate hypotension.

Reprinted from Dildy and Clark (1993), with permission.

rhythm and conduction disturbances are frequently seen. The first priority is removal of the offending antigen, if possible. Further management in severe cases is ventilation, oxygenation, and external cardiac massage, which, in general, is followed by the subcutaneous administration of epinephrine or ephedrine. Aggressive fluid replacement is required.

Septic shock

Septic shock is characterized by hypotension and inadequate tissue perfusion resulting from overwhelming sepsis. Many infections may result in septic shock in obstetric patients, but endometritis, chorioamnionitis, and pyelonephritis are the most common causes. Significant risk factors for septic shock include prolonged rupture of membranes, retained products of conception, and instrumentation of the genitourinary tract. Obstetric infections are usually caused by organisms normally found in the genital tract and thus are often polymicrobial. Most cases of bacterial infection complicated by shock are caused by Gram-negative enteric organisms.

Septic shock has classically been described in three phases that correlate with progressive physiologic derangement: early (warm) shock, late (cold) shock, and secondary (irreversible) shock. Flushed warm skin, fever, chills, diaphoresis, and tachycardia are manifest in the early phase. Pulse pressure and urine output remain stable. The late phase is characterized by cool and clammy skin, a decrease in body temperature, and diminished mental status. Hypotension, tachycardia, and oliguria develop. Myocardial depression becomes a prominent feature of severe septic shock, with marked reductions in cardiac output and systemic vascular resistance. This phase is reversible with treatment. If medical intervention is not begun and cellular hypoxia and anaerobic metabolism continue, the irreversible phase of septic shock develops.

Considerable fluid resuscitation is often necessary secondary to profound vasodilation, increased capillary permeability, and extravasation of fluid into the extravascular space. Blood pressure, heart rate, urine output, and hematocrit may be used initially to guide resuscitation, but a pulmonary artery catheter may ultimately be the best means of guiding optimal fluid and inotrope management in critically ill patients with septic shock and/or multiorgan system dysfunction. Intravenous broad-spectrum antibiotic coverage should be instituted. If response to treatment is not satisfactory, close examination for abscessed or necrotic tissue must be carried out and surgical intervention considered. Timely drainage of abscesses and debridement of necrotic tissue, sometimes via hysterectomy, are required for clinical improvement.

Further reading

American College of Obstetricians and Gynecologists. Hemorrhagic shock. *Tech Bull* 82;1984.

American College of Obstetricians and Gynecologists. Obstetric aspects of trauma management. *Tech Bull* 251;1998.

Ananth CV, Smulian JC. Epidemiology of critical illness and outcomes in pregnancy. In: Dildy GA, Belfort MA, Saade GR, et al, eds. *Critical care obstetrics*, 4th edn. Maldon: Blackwell Science; 2004:3.

Benedetti TJ, Cotton DB, Read JC, et al. Haemodynamic observations in severe preeclampsia with a flow-directed pulmonary artery catheter. *Am J Obstet Gynecol* 1980;136:465.

Borucki DT, ed. *Blood component theraphy: a physician's handbook*, 3rd edn. Washington, DC: American Association of Blood Banks; 1981:25.

Clark SL. Shock in the pregnant patient. *Semin Perinatol* 1990;14:52.

Clark SL, Phelan JP, Montoro M, et al. Transient ventricular dysfunction associated with cesarean section in a patient with hyperthyroidism. *Am J Obstet Gynecol* 1985;151:384.

Clark SL, Cotton DB, Gonik B, et al. Central haemodynamic alterations in amniotic fluid embolism. *Am J Obstet Gynecol* 1988;158:1124.

Clark SL, Cotton DB, Lee W, et al. Central haemodynamic assessment of normal term pregnancy. *Am J Obstet Gynecol* 1989;161:1439.

Cotton DB, Benedetti TJ. Use of the Swan–Ganz catheter in obstetrics and gynecology. *Obstet Gynecol* 1980;56:641.

Dildy GA. Postpartum hemorrhage: new management options. *Clin Obstet Gynecol* 2002;45(2):330.

Dildy GA, Clark SL. Acute puerperal uterine inversion. *Contemp Obstet Gynecol* 1993;38:13.

Dildy GA, Clark SL. Cardiac arrest during pregnancy. *Obstet Gynecol Clin* 1995;22:303.

Gibson RS, Kistner JR. In: Suratt PM, Gibson RS, eds. *Manual of medical procedures*. St Louis, MI: C.V. Mosby; 1982:59.

Gonik B. Intensive care monitoring of the critically ill pregnant patient. In: Creasy RK, Resnik R, eds. *Maternal–fetal medicine: principles and practice*, 2nd edn. Philadelphia, PA: W.B. Saunders; 1989:845.

Katz VL, Dotters DJ, Droegemueller W. Perimortem cesarean delivery. *Obstet Gynecol* 1986;68:571.

Kirshon B, Cotton DB. Invasive hemodynamic monitoring in the obstetric patient. *Clin Obstet Gynecol* 1987;30:579.

Kirshon B, Cotton DB. Fluid replacement in the obstetric patient. In: Sciarra JJ, ed. *Gynecology and obstetrics*, Vol. 3. Hagerstown, MD: Harper & Row; 1989:1.

Lee W, Clark SL, Cotton DB, et al. Septic shock during pregnancy. *Am J Obstet Gynecol* 1988;159:410.

Morbidity and Mortality Weekly Report. Pregnancy-related surveillance – United States, 1987–1990. US Department of Health and Human Services. *Morbidity Mortality Weekly Rep* 1997;46:17.

Morbidity and Mortality Weekly Report. Pregnancy-related deaths among Hispanic, Asian/Pacific Islander, and American Indian/Alaska Native Women – United States, 1991–1997. US Department of Health and Human Services. *Morbidity Mortality Weekly Rep* 2001;50:361.

Nolan TE, Wakefield ML, Devoe LD. Invasive hemodynamic monitoring in obstetrics. A critical review of its indications, benefits, complications and alternatives. *Chest* 1992;101:1429.

35 Hypertensive diseases in pregnancy

Frederick U. Eruo and Baha M. Sibai

Approximately 7–10% of pregnancies are complicated by hypertension. Preeclampsia accounts for 70% of hypertension in pregnancy, and chronic essential hypertension accounts for most of the remaining 30%. The quoted figures may be underestimated as the incidence of hypertension is said to have increased by about 40–50% in the past 10 years. This increase is probably due to the increased incidence of obesity in the United States, delay of pregnancy until later in life (advanced maternal age), and increased rate of multifetal pregnancy.

The American College of Obstetricians and Gynecologists Committee on Terminology defines hypertension in pregnancy as a systolic pressure of ≥ 140 mmHg, a diastolic pressure of ≥ 90 mmHg, or mean arterial blood pressure of 105 mmHg. The blood pressures must be observed on at least two occasions at least 6 hours apart.

Blood pressure is measured with the patient in the sitting position with an appropriately sized blood pressure cuff. The measurement of blood pressure is subject to many inaccuracies. Potential sources of error in blood pressure measurement include faulty equipment, observer bias, improper technique, cuff size, and position of the arm during blood pressure measurement.

Direct intra-arterial blood pressure measurement is the gold standard for blood pressure monitoring and is the preferred method for critically ill patients. However, in clinical practice, the indirect (auscultatory) method is the more convenient and widely accepted technique. Of the indirect methods, the use of a mercury sphygmomanometer is the gold standard in clinical practice. An aneroid sphygmomanometer may be used, but it needs to be validated every 6 months for accuracy.

Classification of hypertensive disease in pregnancy

The normal second-trimester fall in blood pressure may conceal the presence of underlying chronic hypertension (CHTN) and, unless the patient presents in the first trimester or has a well-documented history of chronic hypertension, accurate classification is very difficult. The current classification of hypertensive diseases of pregnancy is as follows:

- gestational hypertension;
- preeclampsia (mild preeclampsia, severe preeclampsia, eclampsia);
- chronic hypertension;
- chronic hypertension with superimposed preeclampsia.

Preeclampsia

Preeclampsia can be classified as mild or severe preeclampsia. Mild preeclampsia is proteinuria with blood pressure (BP) of ≥ 140/90 mmHg on two occasions measured at least 6 hours apart (Table 35.1). The concentration of urinary protein as measured by the dipstick technique is highly variable. It is influenced by several factors, including contamination with vaginal secretions, blood, or bacteria; urine specific gravity and pH; exercise; and posture. Significant proteinuria is defined as ≥ 0.3 g in a 24-h urine collection or 0.1 g/L (≥ 2+ on the dipstick), in at least two random samples collected 6 hours or more apart. The criteria for severe preeclampsia are listed in Table 35.2. Risk factors for preeclampsia are numerous and varied as outlined in Table 35.3.

Eclampsia is defined as the development of convulsions, coma, or both in a patient with signs and symptoms of preeclampsia. Other causes of seizures must be excluded (Table 35.4). Eclampsia may present antepartum, intrapartum, or postpartum.

The HELLP syndrome (hemolysis, elevated liver enzymes and low platelets) (Table 35.5) is a variant of preeclampsia. There is considerable controversy about the definition, diagnosis, incidence, etiology, and management of HELLP syndrome. In terms of diagnosis, the most consistent finding in the literature is thrombocytopenia with a platelet count of ≤100 000/μL.

Table 35.1 Criteria for the diagnosis of mild preeclampsia.

Systolic BP ≥ 140 mmHg or diastolic BP ≥ 90 mmHg on two occasions 6 hours apart after 20 weeks of gestation in a woman known not to have CHTN prior to the pregnancy
Proteinuria ≥0.3 g in a 24-hour urine collection or 2+ proteinuria on qualitative examination or urinalysis
(Edema and excessive weight gain may be present in preeclampsia but are no longer necessary for the diagnosis of preeclampsia)

Table 35.2 Criteria for the diagnosis of severe preeclampsia.

- Systolic BP ≥ 160 mmHg on two occasions at least 6 hours apart
- Diastolic BP ≥ 110 mmHg on two occasions at least 6 hours apart
- Proteinuria ≥ 5 g in a 24-hour urine collection
- Oliguria of ≤ 500 mL in 24 hours
- Cerebral or visual disturbances
- Epigastric pain/right upper quadrant pain
- Pulmonary edema
- Abnormal liver function tests: aspartate transaminase (AST) or alanine transaminase (ALT) more than twice the upper limit for the laboratory
- Thrombocytopenia (platelet count < 100 000/mm^3)

Table 35.3 Risk factors for preeclampsia.

Nulliparity or primiparity
Previous preeclampsia
Family history of preeclampsia
Chronic hypertension
Renal disease
Diabetes mellitus
Morbid obesity/insulin resistance
Age ≥ 35 years
Thrombophilia
Multiple gestation
Unexplained midtrimester elevations of serum AFP, hCG, inhibin A
Abnormal uterine artery Doppler velocimetry
Nonimmune hydrops or hydropic degeneration of placenta

AFP, alpha-fetoprotein; hGG, human chorionic gonadotropin.

Table 35.4 Differential diagnosis of eclampsia.

Cerebrovascular accidents:
   Cerebrovenous thrombosis
   Cerebroarterial embolism
Hypertensive diseases:
   Hypertensive encephalopathy
   Pheochromocytoma
Space-occupying central nervous system lesions:
   Tumor
   Abscess
Infectious diseases:
   Meningitis
   Encephalitis
Metabolic diseases:
   Hypoglycemia
   Hypocalcemia
   Water intoxication
   Epilepsy

Table 35.5 Criteria for the diagnosis of HELLP syndrome*.

Hemolysis
Abnormal peripheral blood smear (burr cells, schistocytes)
Elevated bilirubin ≥ 1.2 mg/dL
Increased LDH more than twice the upper limit of normal for the laboratory
Elevated liver enzymes
Elevated ALT or AST ≥ twice the upper limit of normal for the laboratory
Increased LDH more than twice the upper limit of normal for the laboratory
Low platelet count (< 100 000/mm³)

*Requires at least two of the abnormalities listed.

Gestational hypertension

Mild gestational hypertension is defined as systolic BP ≥ 140 mmHg or diastolic BP ≥ 90 mmHg (without symptoms of proteinuria) measured on two occasions at least 6 hours apart and no more than 7 days apart after 20 weeks of gestation. It is usually mild hypertension, late in onset, often occurs close to term, intrapartum, or within 24 hours of delivery. It often resolves within 10 days of the postpartum period without treatment.

Severe gestational hypertension is defined as sustained systolic BP ≥ 160 mmHg and/or diastolic BP ≥ 110 mmHg measured at least 6 hours apart with no proteinuria. Women with severe gestational hypertension have higher maternal and perinatal morbidities than those with mild gestational hypertension. Women with mild gestational hypertension may progress to severe gestational hypertension or preeclampsia. The rate of progression from gestational hypertension to preeclampsia is dependent on the gestational age at the time of diagnosis; the rate reaches 50% when gestational hypertension develops before 30 weeks of gestation.

Latent or transient hypertension is gestational hypertension in the intrapartum period but becomes transient hypertension (a retrospective diagnosis) if blood pressure returns to normal values and no proteinuria is identified 12 weeks postpartum. If proteinuria occurred before 12 weeks' gestation, then the diagnosis will be gestational hypertension with progression to postpartum preeclampsia. If high blood pressure alone persisted beyond 12 weeks of the postpartum period, then the patient has chronic hypertension.

Chronic hypertension

Chronic hypertension is diagnosed if there is persistent elevation of blood pressure to at least 140/90 mmHg before 20 weeks' gestation on two occasions more than 24 hours apart. It may be difficult to be certain of a diagnosis of chronic hypertension because of the significant changes in blood pressure that occur during mid-pregnancy. Factors that may suggest the presence of chronic hypertension include:
• retinal changes on fundoscopic examination;
• radiologic and electrocardiographic evidence of cardiac enlargement;
• compromised renal function or associated renal disease;
• multiparity with a previous history of hypertensive pregnancies;
• presence of hypertension more than 12 weeks postpartum.

Chronic hypertension occurs in 1–5% of pregnancies. The most common etiology of chronic hypertension is essential or primary hypertension, contributing 90% of cases of chronic hypertension, while secondary hypertension accounts for the rest. Causes of secondary chronic hypertension (Table 35.6) include renal diseases, connective tissue disorders, endocrine disorders, and coarctation of the aorta. Early diagnosis is important because, if untreated, many of these disorders are associated with significant maternal/fetal morbidity and mortality.

Chronic hypertension may be classified as mild or severe hypertension. Mild

Table 35.6 Etiology of chronic hypertension.

Renal factors	Acute and chronic glomerulonephritis
	Acute and chronic pyelonephritis
	Polycystic renal disease
	Renovascular disease
Collagen disease with renal involvement	Lupus erythematosus
	Periarteritis nodosa
	Scleroderma
Endocrine factors	Diabetes with vascular involvement
	Thyrotoxicosis
	Aldosterone-producing tumors
	Pheochromocytoma
Vascular system	Coarctation of the aorta

chronic hypertension implies a systolic BP of less than 160 mmHg and a diastolic BP of less than 110 mmHg. Severe chronic hypertension is diagnosed if blood pressure is ≥ 160/110 mmHg.

Chronic hypertension with superimposed preeclampsia

Chronic hypertension may be complicated by superimposed preeclampsia (or eclampsia), which is diagnosed when there is an exacerbation of hypertension and development of proteinuria that was not present earlier in the pregnancy. Approximately 15–30% of chronic hypertensive women develop superimposed preeclampsia. Conditions necessary for the diagnosis of superimposed preeclampsia on pre-existing chronic hypertension include:
• sudden exacerbation of blood pressure in a woman with previously well-controlled hypertension on antihypertensives;
• new-onset proteinuria (≥ 0.5 g of protein in 24-hour urine collection) in a woman with chronic hypertension but no proteinuria prior to 20 weeks' gestation;
• worsening proteinuria in a woman with chronic hypertension and proteinuria prior to 20 weeks' gestation;
• new-onset elevated AST or ALT;
• new-onset thrombocytopenia with a platelet count of ≤ 100 000/mm^3;
• new onset of symptoms of severe preeclampsia (persistent headache, right upper quadrant pain, epigastric pain, scotomata, nausea, and vomiting).

Management of hypertension in pregnancy

The most effective therapy for preeclampsia, superimposed preeclampsia, eclampsia, or HELLP syndrome is delivery of the fetus and placenta. Mild preeclampsia prior to term may be monitored in hospital or at home with daily fetal kick/movement counts, twice-weekly nonstress test, and amniotic fluid assessment. Indications for hospitalization and/or delivery of a patient with mild preeclampsia include worsening maternal or fetal parameters, a favorable cervix at term, or spontaneous rupture of membranes.

Expectant or conservative management of mild or severe preeclampsia beyond term is not beneficial to the fetus because uteroplacental blood flow may be suboptimal. After 37 weeks' gestation, labor should be induced as soon as the cervix is favorable. Expectant management of preterm patients with severe preeclampsia is an option, as shown in Table 35.7. Severe preeclampsia warrants hospitalization, administration of magnesium sulfate for seizure prophylaxis, whereas antihypertensive medication is instituted for diastolic blood pressure ≥ 110 mmHg or systolic blood pressure ≥ 160 mmHg. The therapeutic objective for the treatment of severe hypertension is to prevent maternal cerebrovascular accidents and congestive heart failure without compromising cerebral perfusion or jeopardizing uteroplacental blood flow.

Parenteral or oral antihypertensive agents (labetalol, hydralazine, nifedipine, sodium nitroprusside, etc.) are used for the acute reduction of blood pressure in women with severe preeclampsia. Oral medications are also used for maintenance

Table 35.7 Guidelines for expectant management of severe preeclampsia remote from term.

Management plan	Clinical findings
Expedited delivery (within 72 h)	One or more of the following: Uncontrolled severe hypertension* Eclampsia Platelet count of < 100 000 cells/mL AST or ALT more than twice upper limit of normal with epigastric pain or right upper quadrant tenderness Pulmonary edema Compromised renal function† Persistent severe headache or visual changes
Expectant management	One or more of the following: Controlled hypertension Urinary protein > 5000 mg/24 h Oliguria (< 0.5 mL/kg/h) that resolves with routine fluid and food intake AST or ALT more than twice upper limit of normal epigastric pain or right upper quadrant tenderness

ALT, alanine aminotransferase; AST, aspartate aminotransferase.
*Blood pressure persistently ≥ 160 mmHg systolic or ≥ 110 mmHg diastolic despite maximum recommended doses of two antihypertensive medications.
†Persistent oliguria (< 0.5 mL/kg/h) or rise in serum creatinine of 1 mg/dL over baseline values.
Reproduced from Schiff et al. (1994).

Table 35.8 Antihypertensive medication in pregnancy.

Class	Medication	Dose	
		Starting dose	Maximum dose
Common drugs for chronic therapy of hypertension			
Central alpha-2 agonist	Methyldopa	250 mg p.o. tid	2 g/day
Calcium channel blocker	Nifedipine	10 mg p.o. qid	120 mg p.o. qid
Alpha- and beta-blocker	Labetalol	100 mg p.o. tid	1200 mg/day
Common drugs for acute therapy of severe hypertension			
Arteriolar dilator	Hydralazine	5–10 mg i.v. every 15–30 min	
Calcium channel blocker	Nifedipine	10–20 mg p.o. every 30 min	
Alpha- and beta-blocker	Labetalol	5–10 mg i.v. per dose, cumulative to 40–80 mg over 20 min (maximum dose is 300 mg)	
Arterial and venous dilator	Nitroprusside	0.2 –0.5 µg/kg/min	

or chronic therapy (Table 35.8). The choice of agents is dependent on the stage of pregnancy (antepartum, intrapartum, or postpartum), the side-effect profile of the agent in question, the presence of other medical problems (renal insufficiency, diabetes mellitus, pulmonary edema, myocardial ischemia, etc.) and, if postpartum, whether the woman is breastfeeding or not.

Delivery is the definitive therapy for HELLP syndrome beyond 34 weeks' gestation or with evidence of fetal lung maturity or fetal or maternal jeopardy. Mode of delivery is dependent on standard obstetric indications. Antihypertensive therapy is as described for women with severe preeclampsia. The use of regional anesthesia is contraindicated because of the risk of bleeding. General anesthesia is the method of choice if Cesarean delivery is indicated in HELLP syndrome.

The protocol used to manage eclampsia is outlined in Table 35.9, and the mode of delivery is dependent on the usual obstetric indications. Parenteral magnesium sulfate ($MgSO_4$) has become the drug of choice for therapy and prophylaxis of eclampsia. Clinical findings associated with elevated serum magnesium levels will help in monitoring therapy (Table 35.10). The first sign of magnesium toxicity is loss of deep tendon reflexes (10–12 mg/dL). Other early signs and symptoms of magnesium toxicity include nausea, feeling of warmth, flushing, slurred speech, and somnolence (9–12 mg/dL).

Mild gestational hypertension is managed essentially as mild preeclampsia. Women with severe gestational hypertension are managed as if they had severe preeclampsia.

Table 35.9 Sibai's protocol for the management of eclampsia.

Convulsions are controlled or prevented with a loading dose of 6 g magnesium sulfate in
  100 mL of 5% dextrose in Ringer's lactated solution, given over 15 min, followed by a
  maintenance dose of 2 g/h. The dose is adjusted according to patellar reflexes and urine
  output in the previous 4-h period
Induction or delivery is initiated within 4 h after maternal stabilization
Magnesium sulfate is continued for 24 h after delivery or, if postpartum, 24 h after the last
  convulsion. In some cases, the infusion may be continued for a longer period
Diuretics, plasma volume expanders, and invasive homodynamic monitoring used only if
  clinically indicated

Table 35.10 Clinical findings associated with increasing maternal serum levels of
magnesium.

Serum magnesium level (mg/dL)	Clinical findings
1.5–2.5	Normal level
4–8	Therapeutic range for seizure prophylaxis
9–12	Loss of patellar reflex
15–17	Muscular paralysis, respiratory arrest
30–35	Cardiac arrest

Management of secondary hypertension is that of the underlying disease; however, most patients with chronic hypertension have essential hypertension. Management of chronic hypertension focuses on the control of blood pressure (Table 35.8) and the assessment of maternal and fetal well-being (Table 35.11). Uncomplicated CHTN in pregnancy is labeled low-risk CHTN, whereas the high-risk group (Table 35.12) includes patients with renal disease, diabetes mellitus, etc. Antihypertensive therapy is restricted to women with severe hypertension. Low-risk CHTN pregnancy is allowed to continue to 40–41 weeks' gestation with close monitoring. High-risk CHTN pregnancies and women receiving antihypertensive drugs are delivered at or before 40 weeks' gestation.

Anesthesia in hypertensive disorders of pregnancy

A sudden increase in blood pressure may occur in general anesthesia during intubation or extubation, leading to a cerebrovascular event. To prevent this hypertensive response, the patient should receive a short-acting antihypertensive agent, such as nitroglycerin, sodium nitroprusside, or labetalol, prior to the induction of anesthesia.

Decreased sympathetic activity due to regional anesthesia leads to dilatation of the capacitance vessels, which causes hypotension. Adequate intravascular volume repletion (fluid preloading) performed before initiating regional anesthesia avoids

Table 35.11 Evaluation of pregnancy complicated by chronic hypertension.

Name:	Date of birth:
Parity: G . . . P . . . :	LMP:
Gestational age:	EDD or EDC:

Ultrasound:
  First trimester ultrasound [for correct dating and nuchal translucence (NT) measurement]:
  Fetal biometry/anatomy ultrasound (at 18–20 weeks):
  Follow-up growth ultrasound at 4-weekly intervals starting in late second trimester

Fetal testing starting in late second or early third trimester (for patients with renal insufficiency):
  Twice-weekly testing or BPP
  Nonstress test (NST) if there is poor growth
  NST and Doppler studies if IUGR (< 10%)

Renal evaluation: 24-h urine protein and creatinine clearance, electrolytes, urea and creatinine levels

ECG: (cardiology consultation if ECG is abnormal)

Maternal cardiac echocardiography:

Comments/comorbid conditions:

Fundoscopy at initial clinic visit:

Table 35.12 High-risk chronic hypertension in pregnancy.

Maternal age greater than 40 years (may consider age ≥ 40 years)
Duration of hypertension more than 5 years
Blood pressure exceeding 160 over 110 mmHg early in pregnancy
Diabetes mellitus (classes B–F)
Cardiomyopathy
Renal disease
Connective tissue disorders
Consider morbid obesity (weight ≥ 300 lb)

---

this relative hypovolemia. This effect is more pronounced if the mother has been in a supine position for a long period or is receiving antihypertensive agents.

Preeclamptic women may have pharyngeal and laryngeal edema rendering intubation and ventilation difficult. Laryngeal mask airway (LMA) may be a useful alternative in cases of difficult airway management and should be anticipated in severe preeclampsia.

Women receiving magnesium sulfate are more sensitive to the depolarizing and nondepolarizing neuromuscular blocking agents; therefore, the dose of muscle relaxant must be adjusted accordingly.

Decreased platelet count and platelet function occur in up to 18% of women with preeclampsia. Epidural anesthesia is safe for women with platelet counts ≥ 100 000/μL.

Postpartum hemorrhage secondary to uterine atony may be due to magnesium sulfate (a tocolytic agent) and/or anesthetic agents (especially the inhalational agents) used in general anesthesia. Platelet dysfunction or thrombocytopenia, as in HELLP syndrome, will increase the risk of bleeding.

Further reading

American College of Obstetricians and Gynecologists. *Chronic hypertension in pregnancy.* ACOG Practice Bulletin no. 29. Washington, DC: American College of Obstetricians and Gynecologists, 2001.

Lindheimer MD, Roberts JM, Cunningham FG, eds. *Chesley's hypertensive disorders in pregnancy,* 2nd edn. Norwalk, CT: Appleton and Lange, 1998.

Magee LA, Schick B, Donnenfeld AF, et al. The safety of calcium channel blockers in human pregnancy: a prospective, multicenter cohort study. *Am J Obstet Gynecol* 1996;174: 823–828.

Magpie Trial Collaboration Group. Do women with pre-eclampsia, and their babies, benefit from magnesium sulphate? The Magpie Trial: a randomized placebo-controlled trial. *Lancet* 2002;359(9321):1877–1890.

National Institute of Health (NIH): National Heart, Lung, and Blood Institute. *National High Blood Pressure Education Program: Working Group Report on high blood pressure in pregnancy.* NIH Publication No. 00-3029, 2000.

Ramanathan J, Bennett K. Pre-eclampsia: fluids, drugs, and anesthetic management. *Anesthesiol Clin North Am* 2003;21(1):145–163.

Schiff E, Friedman SA, Sibai BM. Conservative management of severe preeclampsia remote from term. *Obstet Gynecol* 1994;84:626–630.

Sibai BM. Chronic hypertension in pregnancy. *Obstet Gynecol* 2002;100;369–377.

Sibai BM. Diagnosis and management of gestational hypertension and preeclampsia. *Obstet Gynecol* 2003;102(1):181–192.

Sibai BM. Diagnosis, prevention, and management of eclampsia. *Obstet Gynecol* 2005;102(2): 402–410.

36 | Cardiac diseases in pregnancy

Kjersti Aagaard-Tillery and Steven L. Clark

Pregnancy causes significant alterations in the maternal cardiovascular system. The pregnant patient with normal cardiac function accommodates these physiologic changes without difficulty. In the presence of cardiac disease, however, pregnancy may be extremely hazardous, resulting in decompensation and even death. Despite advances in the diagnosis and treatment of maternal cardiovascular disease, such conditions continue to account for 10–25% of maternal deaths. This summary focuses on the interaction between structural cardiac disease and pregnancy, with an emphasis on means to achieve optimal maternal and perinatal outcome.

Counseling the pregnant cardiac patient

The Criteria Committee of the New York Heart Association (NYHA) has recommended a classification of cardiac disease based on clinical function (classes I–IV). Although such a classification is useful in discussing the pregnant cardiac patient, up to 40% of patients developing congestive heart failure and pulmonary edema during pregnancy are functional class I before pregnancy. In general, however, women who begin pregnancy as functional class I or II have a better outcome than those initially in class III or IV. Counseling the pregnant cardiac patient regarding her prognosis for successful pregnancy is further complicated by recent advances in medical and surgical therapy, fetal surveillance, and neonatal care. Such advances render invalid many older estimates of maternal mortality and fetal wastage.

Table 36.1 represents a synthesis of maternal risk estimates for various types of cardiac disease initially developed by Clark et al. in 1987, and recently revised to account for trends in improving maternal outcomes. It may generally be said that

Table 36.1 Summary of current revised maternal mortality risks associated with selected cardiovascular disorders.

Group	Cardiovascular disorder	Maternal mortality (%)
Group I: Minimal risk of complications	Atrial septal defect	< 1
	Ventricular septal defect, without pulmonary hypertension	< 1
	Patent ductus arteriosus	< 1
	Pulmonic or tricuspid disease	0–0.5
	Corrected tetralogy of Fallot	0.05–1
	Bioprosthetic valve	1
	Mitral stenosis, NYHA classes I and II	0–1.6
	Marfan syndrome with normal aorta*	0–1.1
Group II: Moderate risk of complications	Mitral stenosis with atrial fibrillation	12–17
	Mechanical valve	1–4
	Mitral stenosis, NYHA classes III and IV	5–7
	Aortic stenosis	2–18
	Coarctation of aorta, uncomplicated	2–5
	Uncorrected tetralogy of Fallot	12–15
	Previous myocardial infarction, remote	2–15
Group III: Major risk of complications or death	Primary pulmonary hypertension	35–50
	Coarctation of the aorta, complicated	> 25
	Marfan syndrome with aortic involvement	50
	Previous myocardial infarction, within 2 weeks of delivery	50

The maternal mortality rates represent a compilation from available and identified references. As such, they represent varying degrees of disorder severity, a spectrum of patient ages and ethnic background, and additional associated risk factors. They must thus be regarded as generalizable approximations.

* Normal aorta, defined as aortic root diameter < 4 cm and no evidence of dissection.

maternal mortality is almost exclusively seen in patients with pulmonary hypertension, endocarditis, coronary artery disease, cardiomyopathy, and sudden arrhythmia. Indeed, the most recent recommendations from the American Heart Association and the American College of Cardiology regarding classification of maternal and fetal risk during pregnancy on the basis of the type of valvular abnormality and NYHA functional class (Tables 36.1 and 36.2) note that the absolute risk conferred on a given women by pregnancy is modified by additional clinical factors.

Selective cardiac lesions

Atrial and ventricular septal defect

Atrial septal defect (ASD) is the most common congenital lesion seen during pregnancy and is generally asymptomatic. As a result of the disproportionate number of women with ostium secundum defects being asymptomatic until the reproductive years, it is not unheard of to have women present with a sentinel ASD diagnosis in pregnancy. The two significant potential complications seen with ASD are arrhythmias and ventricular failure.

The hypervolemia and increased cardiac output associated with pregnancy accentuate the left-to-right shunt through the ASD, and thus a significant burden is imposed on the right ventricle. Although this additional burden is tolerated well by most patients, congestive failure and death with ASD have been reported. Thus, peripartum management centers on avoiding vascular resistance changes that increase the degree of the shunt. In contrast to the high-pressure/high-flow state seen with ventricular septal defect (VSD) and patent ductus arteriosus (PDA), ASD is characterized by high pulmonary blood flow associated with normal pulmonary artery pressures. Because pulmonary artery pressures are low, pulmonary hypertension is unusual. The majority of patients with ASD tolerate pregnancy, labor, and delivery without complication. During labor, placement of the patient in the lateral recumbent position, avoidance of fluid overload, oxygen administration, and pain relief with epidural anesthesia, as well judicious use of prophylaxis against bacterial endocarditis, are the most important considerations (Tables 36.3 and 36.4).

VSD may occur as an isolated lesion or in conjunction with other congenital cardiac anomalies, including tetralogy of Fallot, transposition of the great vessels, and coarctation of the aorta. The size of the septal defect is the most important determinant of clinical prognosis during pregnancy. Small defects are tolerated well, whereas larger defects are associated more frequently with congestive heart failure, arrhythmias, or the development of pulmonary hypertension. In addition, a large VSD is often associated with some degree of aortic regurgitation, which then modifies the risk of congestive failure. Pregnancy, labor, and delivery are tolerated well by patients with uncomplicated VSD. Management considerations for patients with uncomplicated VSD are similar to those outlined for ASD.

Eisenmenger's syndrome and pulmonary hypertension

Eisenmenger's syndrome develops when, in the presence of congenital left-to-right

Table 36.2 Valvular heart lesions stratified by maternal and fetal risk derived from ACC/AHA Guidelines.

Maternal risk	Lesion	Description
Low maternal and fetal risk	Asymptomatic aortic stenosis	Low mean outflow gradient (< 50 mmHg)
		Normal LV systolic function (EF > 50%)
	Aortic regurgitation, NYHA I or II	Normal LV systolic function (EF > 50%)
	Mild/moderate mitral stenosis	Mitral valve area > 1.5 cm^2
		Low gradient (< 5 mmHg)
		Absence of severe pulmonary hypertension (severe pulmonary hypertension defined as pulmonary pressure > 75% of systemic pressures)
	Mitral regurgitation, NYHA I or II	Normal LV systolic function (EF > 50%)
	Mitral valve prolapse	Absence of mitral regurgitation OR Mild/moderate mitral regurgitation with normal LV systolic function (EF > 50%)
High maternal and fetal risk	Severe aortic stenosis	Valve area < 1.5 cm^2
	Aortic regurgitation, NYHA III or IV	Symptomatic per NYHA criteria
	Aortic regurgitation in Marfan syndrome	
	Mitral stenosis, NYHA II, III, or IV	Symptomatic per NYHA criteria
	Mitral regurgitation, NYHA III or IV	Symptomatic per NYHA criteria
	Aortic and/or mitral valve disease, with severe pulmonary hypertension	Resultant severe pulmonary hypertension (severe pulmonary hypertension defined as pulmonary pressure > 75% of systemic pressures)
	Aortic and/or mitral valve disease, with left ventricular systolic dysfunction	Abnormal LV systolic function (EF < 40%)
	Maternal cyanosis	

NYHA denotes New York Heart Association classification. By functional status, NYHA I is asymptomatic; NYHA II is symptoms with greater than normal activity; NYHA III is symptoms with normal activity; NYHA IV is symptoms at rest.

LV, left ventricular; EF, ejection fraction.

Table 36.3 Antibiotic prophylaxis for the prevention of bacterial endocarditis.

Cardiac lesion	Prophylaxis for uncomplicated delivery	Prophylaxis for suspected bacteremia (i.e., chorioamnionitis)
Negligible risk category		
Functional heart murmurs	Not recommended	Not recommended
Mitral valve prolapse without regurgitation	Not recommended	Not recommended
Previous rheumatic fever without valve dysfunction	Not recommended	Not recommended
Previous Kawasaki disease without valve dysfunction	Not recommended	Not recommended
Cardiac pacemakers and implanted defibrillators	Not recommended	Not recommended
Prior coronary bypass graft surgery	Not recommended	Not recommended
Moderate-risk category		
Acquired valve dysfunction (rheumatic fever)	Not recommended	Recommended
Congenital cardiac malformations	Not recommended	Recommended
EXCEPT: repaired ASD, VSD, or PDA, or isolated secundum ASD		
Hypertrophic cardiomyopathy	Not recommended	Recommended
Mitral valve prolapse with regurgitation or thickened leaflets	Not recommended	Recommended
High-risk category		
Prosthetic cardiac valves	Optional	Recommended
Prior bacterial endocarditis	Optional	Recommended
Complex cyanotic congenital cardiac malformations	Optional	Recommended
Surgically constructed systemic pulmonary shunts/conduits	Optional	Recommended

Adapted from ACOG Practice Bulletin No. 47 Prophylactic Antibiotics in Labor and Delivery, October 2003. These recommendations are based on ACC/AHA guidelines, which specifically discourage endocarditis prophylaxis for "routine" vaginal or Cesarean delivery. Given a possible increased risk of endocarditis with complicated deliveries such as retained placenta, alongside recommendations to give antibiotics before or within 30 min of starting a "complicated" procedure, the decision to hold or administer subacute bacterial endocarditis (SBE) prophylaxis is not necessarily straightforward. Thus, many obstetricians may elect to administer prophylactic antibiotics to cover unpredictable complicated deliveries.

Table 36.4 Endocarditis prophylaxis regimens for genitourinary/gastrointestinal procedures.

Patient group	Agent	Dosage*
High risk	Ampicillin plus gentamicin	Load: Ampicillin 2 g i.v./i.m. Gentamicin 1.5 mg/kg i.v. to a maximum of 120 mg 6 h later: Ampicillin 1 g i.v./i.m. or amoxicillin 1 g p.o.
Ampicillin-allergic high risk	Vancomycin plus gentamicin	Load: Vancomycin 1 g i.v. over 1–2 h Gentamicin 1.5 mg/kg i.v. to a maximum of 120 mg 6 h later: Ampicillin 1 g i.v./i.m. or amoxicillin 1 g p.o.
Moderate risk	Amoxicillin or ampicillin	Amoxicillin 2 g p.o. 1 h before procedure or ampicillin 2 g i.v./i.m.
Ampicillin-allergic moderate risk	Vancomycin plus gentamicin	Load: Vancomycin 1 g i.v. over 1–2 h

*With respect to i.v.- or i.m.-administered ampicillin, gentamicin, or vancomycin, complete infusion within 30 min of starting the procedure.

shunt, progressive pulmonary hypertension leads to shunt reversal or bidirectional shunting as a result of chronically increased pulmonary vascular blood flow with accompanying pulmonary vascular resistance exceeding systemic vascular resistance. Although this syndrome may rarely occur with ASD, VSD, or PDA, the low-pressure and high-flow shunt seen in ASD is far less likely to result in pulmonary hypertension and shunt reversal than the condition of high-pressure and high-flow symptoms seen with VSD and PDA. Regardless of the etiology, pulmonary hypertension carries a guarded prognosis during pregnancy, although there are published reports suggesting that the greatest risk may be seen in women with Eisenmenger's syndrome. After Eisenmenger's pathophysiology is established, the pulmonary hypertension is permanent, and surgical correction of the defect is unhelpful and may increase mortality.

During the antepartum period, the decreased systemic vascular resistance associated with pregnancy increases both the likelihood as well as the degree of right-to-left shunting. Pulmonary perfusion decreases, with systemic hypotension resulting in hypoxemia and subsequent maternal then fetal deterioration. The peripartum development of systemic hypotension leads to decreased right ventricular filling pressures; in the concomitant presence of a fixed cardiac output state (e.g., pulmonary hypertension), such decreased right heart pressures may be insufficient to perfuse the pulmonary arterial bed, leading to a sudden and profound hypoxemia and death. While there may exist any number of inciting events resulting in systemic hypotension in pregnancy, it most frequently results from hemorrhage or complications of conduction anesthesia. Thus, avoidance of systemic hypotension is the principal clinical concern in the intrapartum management of patients with pulmonary hypertension of any etiology. This fact is punctuated by the longstanding knowledge that the greatest maternal risk occurs in the peripartum period, and most deaths occur between 2 and 9 days postpartum. The precise pathophysiology of such decompensation is unclear, and it is uncertain what, if any, therapeutic maneuvers prevent or ameliorate such deterioration.

Maternal mortality in the presence of Eisenmenger's syndrome ranges from 30% to 60%. Eisenmenger's syndrome associated with VSD appears to carry a higher mortality risk than that associated with PDA or ASD. In addition to the previously discussed problems associated with hemorrhage and hypovolemia, thromboembolic phenomena have been associated with up to 43% of all maternal deaths in Eisenmenger's syndrome. However, other authors have reported that the use of heparin therapy (with bedrest and supplemental oxygen) may modestly positively influence maternal and fetal outcomes; there are no large trials supporting these findings to date. Sudden delayed postpartum death, occurring 4–6 weeks after delivery, has also been reported. Such deaths may involve a rebound worsening of pulmonary hypertension associated with the loss of pregnancy-associated hormones, or thromboembolic events.

Because of the high mortality associated with continuing pregnancy, pregnancy termination should be presented to the patient as the preferred management of choice for the woman with pulmonary hypertension of any etiology. Pregnancy termination in either the first or the second trimester has long been considered the safer alternative over allowing the pregnancy to progress to term. Dilation and curettage in the first trimester or dilation and evacuation in the second trimester is the method of choice. Hypertonic saline and F-series prostaglandins (prostaglandin $F_2\alpha$) are contraindicated, although the careful use of E-series prostaglandins is probably appropriate as long as systemic hypotension is avoided.

For the patient with a continuing gestation, management centers on avoiding increases in pulmonary vascular resistance, maintaining right ventricular preload, left ventricular afterload, and right ventricular contractility. Thus, factors that increase pulmonary vascular resistance should be avoided. In general terms, sympathetic agonists (epinephrine and norepinephrine) and conditions resulting in hypoxia or hypercarbia are associated with a poor outcome. Thus, the mainstays of therapy and management continue to be inpatient care in a tertiary care center with experienced providers, with continuous administration of oxygen, use of pulmonary vasodilators, avoidance of hypotension and anemia, and limited use of operative deliveries.

With respect to pulmonary vasodilators, recent success with inhaled nitric oxide (iNO) alongside prostacyclin and its analogs has been observed. Administration of iNO via a facemask or nasal cannula has been shown to be effective when estimated final alveolar concentrations of 5–40 p.p.m. are reached; great care is taken to avoid accumulation of toxic nitrogen dioxide with the use of continuous monitoring of tidal iNO concentrations using electrochemical monitors (similar to those found in neonatal intensive care unit settings). Given a risk of both maternal and fetal methemoglobinemia, it is also recommended that concentrations should be measured hourly during administration with a goal of < 5 g/dL; in the fetus, postnatal monitoring through the first 48 hours of life is also recommended. High concentrations of methemoglobin can be treated with methylene blue at 2 mg/kg i.v. Prostacylin, a naturally occurring prostaglandin (PGI_2), is a potent vasodilator and inhibitor of platelet aggregation. Infusions of 1–10 ng/kg/min effectively reduce pulmonary vascular resistance, but at the risk of decreasing right ventricular preload.

Anesthesia for patients with pulmonary hypertension is controversial. Theoretically, conduction anesthesia, with its accompanying risk of hypotension, should be avoided. Regional techniques for both vaginal (epidural) and Cesarean (spinal) delivery have been described, and used successfully. In summary of this expanding volume of data, with the concomitant use of systemic vasoconstrictors (ephedrine) and pulmonary vasodilators (iNO and prostacylin analogs), the use of epidural or intrathecal morphine sulfate will be theoretically devoid of any overt effect on systemic blood pressure and thus represents one reasonable approach to anesthetic management of these difficult patients.

Acquired cardiac lesions

By way of introduction, it is often helpful to keep a number of commonly accepted considerations regarding acquired valvular lesions in mind. First, regurgitant lesions are generally better tolerated in pregnancy than stenotic lesions on account of pregnancy-associated systemic vascular resistance improving forward flow, and thus limiting the effects of regurgitation (assuming an absence of left ventricular dysfunction). However, in stenotic lesions, increased cardiac output and tachycardia result in an elevation in left atrial pressure (i.e., mitral stenosis) and thus increased incidence of atrial fibrillation and high-output cardiac failure. Second, maternal and fetal risks of acquired cardiac lesions in pregnancy generally vary with the functional classification at pregnancy onset and term. Thus, the common collective wisdom is that women with functional class I or II heart disease have a favorable prognosis in pregnancy (with the notable exception of mitral stenosis; Table 36.2). Moreover, patients who reach term as class I or II usually tolerate properly managed labor without invasive monitoring. Third, because of increasing cardiovascular demand in the high-output state, functional status will deteriorate during pregnancy among functional class II, III, and IV patients. This is evidenced by the fact that nearly half of all women with acquired valvular lesions will first develop heart failure and pulmonary edema in their third trimester of pregnancy.

Acquired valvular lesions are commonly rheumatic in origin, although endocarditis secondary to intravenous drug use should be considered as an underlying etiology of acquired right heart lesions. During pregnancy, maternal morbidity and mortality with rheumatic lesions result from congestive failure or arrhythmias with a final common sequelae of pulmonary edema, embolic event, or fatal dysrhythmia. Indeed, pulmonary edema is the leading cause of death in rheumatic heart disease patients during pregnancy. The onset of atrial fibrillation during pregnancy carries with it a higher risk of right and left ventricular failure (63%) than fibrillation with onset before gestation. In addition, the risk of systemic embolization after the onset of atrial fibrillation during pregnancy may exceed that associated with onset in the nonpregnant state. In counseling the patient with severe rheumatic cardiac disease on the advisability of initiating or continuing pregnancy, the physician must also consider the long-term prognosis of the underlying disease. In sum of several reports, in the absence of an acute morbid event, pregnancy has no long-term sequelae for patients who survive the pregnancy.

Mitral stenosis

Mitral stenosis is the most common rheumatic valvular lesion encountered during pregnancy. It can occur as an isolated lesion or in conjunction with aortic or right-sided lesions. Severe mitral stenosis (valve area < 1.5 cm^2) carries a maternal mortality recently approximated at 5%. Secondary to a severe stenosis, ventricular diastolic filling obstruction yields elevated left atrial pressure with a relatively fixed cardiac output. Marked increases in cardiac output accompany normal pregnancy, labor, and delivery. When the pregnant patient is unable to accommodate volume fluctuations, right-sided heart failure results in pulmonary edema.

The ability to accommodate an increased cardiac output in patients with mitral stenosis depends largely on two factors. First, these patients depend on adequate diastolic filling time. However, in instances of stenotic mitral lesions, a rapid and dramatic fall in cardiac output and blood pressure in response to tachycardia will compromise this tenuous filling time. Given that an increase in heart rate of approximately 10 bpm is common in normal pregnancy, labor, and delivery, consideration of oral beta-blocker therapy for any patient with severe mitral stenosis who enters labor with even a mild tachycardia ought to be given. Control of acute-onset tachycardia with an intravenous beta-blocking agent may be employed at the following dosages: propranolol 1 mg i.v. every 2 min; metoprolol 5 mg i.v. over 5 min, repeated in 10 min; esmolol drip at 500 μg/kg i.v. over 1 min with an infusion rate of 50–200 μ/kg/min; or labetalol 20–40 mg i.v. followed by 20–80 mg i.v. every 10 min to a maximum dose of 180 mg.

A second important consideration in patients with mitral stenosis centers on left ventricular preload. In the presence of mitral stenosis, pulmonary capillary wedge pressure fails to accurately reflect left ventricular filling pressures. Such patients often require high-normal or elevated pulmonary capillary wedge pressure to maintain adequate ventricular filling pressure and cardiac output. Any preload manipulation (i.e., diuresis) must therefore be undertaken with extreme caution and careful attention to the maintenance of cardiac output. However, it has long been recognized that potentially dangerous intrapartum fluctuations in cardiac output can be minimized by using epidural anesthesia; however, the most hazardous time for these women appears to be the immediate postpartum period. Such patients often enter the postpartum period already operating at maximum cardiac output and cannot accommodate the volume shifts that follow delivery. In our series of patients with severe mitral stenosis, we found that a postpartum rise in wedge pressure of up to 16 mmHg could be expected in the immediate postpartum period. Because frank pulmonary edema generally does not occur with wedge pressures of less than 28–30 mmHg, it follows that the optimal predelivery wedge pressure for such patients is 14 mmHg or lower, as indicated by pulmonary artery catheterization. Such a preload may be approached by cautious intrapartum diuresis with careful attention to the maintenance of adequate cardiac output. Active diuresis is not always necessary in patients who enter with evidence of only mild fluid overload. In such patients, simple fluid restriction alongside sensible and insensible fluid losses endogenous to labor can result in a significant fall in wedge pressure before delivery.

In a patient with hemodynamically significant mitral stenosis, many of the same management considerations apply as those previously discussed under the section dealing with Eisenmenger's syndrome and pulmonary hypertension. Previous recommendations for delivery in patients with cardiac disease have included the liberal use of midforceps to shorten the second stage of labor. In cases of severe disease, Cesarean section with general anesthesia has also been advocated as the preferred mode of delivery. With the aggressive and attentive management scheme presented, we have found that spontaneous vaginal delivery is generally safe and preferable, even in patients with severe disease and pulmonary hypertension.

Aortic stenosis

Aortic stenosis is commonly congenital in origin, secondary to a bicuspid aortic valve, and thus represents 5% of all congenital cardiac anomalies. In several recent series of pregnancies in women with cardiac disease, no maternal deaths due to aortic stenosis were observed. In contrast to mitral valve stenosis, aortic stenosis generally does not become hemodynamically significant until the orifice has diminished to one-third or less of normal. Indeed, severe aortic stenosis is defined as a peak gradient > 50 mmHg with a valve area < 1 cm^2. Given that the major problem experienced by patients with valvular aortic stenosis is maintenance of cardiac output, the relative hypervolemia associated with gestation enables such patients generally to tolerate pregnancy well. With severe disease, however, a fixed cardiac output limits adequate coronary artery or cerebral perfusion under conditions of physical exertion. Inadequate cardiac perfusion subsequently results in angina, myocardial infarction, syncope, or sudden death. Thus, among patients with severe aortic stenosis, limitation of physical activity may be necessary.

Consistent with these recommendations is the longstanding observation that delivery and pregnancy termination are intervals in pregnancy with the greatest risk for inadequate cardiac perfusion. The maintenance of cardiac output is crucial: any factor leading to diminished venous return results in an increase in the valvular gradient with subsequent diminished cardiac output. Indeed, patients with shunt gradients exceeding 100 mmHg are at greatest risk of hemodynamic decompensation. As such, management considerations for the patient with aortic stenosis are similar to those in women with pulmonary hypertension. Of note, because hypovolemia is of greater concern than pulmonary edema, the wedge pressure should be maintained in the range 14–18 mmHg in order to provide a margin of safety against unexpected peripartum blood loss. Hypotension resulting from blood loss, ganglionic blockade from epidural anesthesia, or supine vena caval occlusion by the pregnant uterus may result in sudden death. Pregnancy termination in the midtrimester may be especially hazardous in this regard and has been reported to carry a mortality of up to 40%. Thus, women who have severe stenosis or symptoms are advised to undergo repair prior to attempting pregnancy in an effort to substantially reduce pregnancy-associated morbidity and mortality.

The cardiovascular status of patients with aortic stenosis is occasionally complicated by the frequent coexistence of ischemic heart disease. In these instances, death associated with aortic stenosis may occur secondary to myocardial infarction rather than as a direct complication of the valvular lesion itself.

Peripartum cardiomyopathy

Peripartum cardiomyopathy is defined as cardiomyopathy developing in the last month of pregnancy or the first 6 months postpartum in women without previous cardiac disease and after exclusion of other causes of cardiac failure. It is therefore a diagnosis of exclusion that should not be made without a concerted effort to identify valvular, metabolic, infectious, or toxic causes of cardiomyopathy. Much of the current controversy surrounding this condition is the result of many older reports in which these causes of cardiomyopathy were not investigated adequately. Other peripartum complications, such as amniotic fluid embolism, severe preeclampsia, and corticosteroid- or sympathomimetic-induced pulmonary edema, must also be considered before making the diagnosis of peripartum cardiomyopathy.

The condition is manifest clinically by increasing fatigue, dyspnea, and peripheral or pulmonary edema. As most women in the last trimester of pregnancy manifest these conditions, suspicion for a cardiomyopathy should arise with paroxysmal nocturnal dyspnea, chest pain, nocturnal cough, new regurgitant murmurs, pulmonary crackles, and hepatomegaly. Physical examination reveals classic evidence of congestive heart failure, including elevated jugular venous pressure, rales, and an S3 gallop. Cardiomegaly and pulmonary edema are found on chest radiograph, and the electrocardiogram often demonstrates left ventricular and atrial dilation and diminished ventricular performance, with the reported observance of inverted T waves, Q waves, and nonspecific ST segment changes. In addition, up to 50% of patients with peripartum cardiomyopathy may manifest evidence of pulmonary or systemic embolic phenomena. The diagnosis rests on the echocardiographic finding of new left ventricular systolic dysfunction during a limited period around parturition.

The histologic picture of peripartum cardiomyopathy involves nonspecific cellular hypertrophy, degeneration, fibrosis, and increased lipid deposition. Although some reports have documented the presence of a diffuse myocarditis, the common collective wisdom suggests that peripartum cardiomyopathy may represent a type of myocarditis arising from an infectious (viral), autoimmune, or idiopathic process.

Its existence as a distinct entity is supported primarily by epidemiologic evidence suggesting that 80% of cases of idiopathic cardiomyopathy in women of child-bearing age occur in the peripartum period.

Therapy includes digoxin (dosed to achieve a serum level of 1–2 ng/dL), diuretics (furosemide 20–40 mg orally daily), fluid and sodium restriction (2 L/day and 4 mg/day, maximum, respectively), and prolonged bedrest. In refractory cases or with clear evidence of systolic dysfunction, we employ concomitant afterload reduction with vasodilators (25–100 mg of oral q.i.d. hydralazine being the drug of choice peripartum, with either long-acting nitroglycerin or 5–10 mg of oral daily amlodipine as second-line agents), or use epidural regional analgesia approximating delivery. In general, because of the adverse effects of negative ionotropic agents, other calcium channel blockers should be avoided. In recent years, angiotensin-converting enzyme inhibitors (enalapril 5–20 mg oral twice daily) are the mainstay of treatment postpartum; breastfeeding women should be counseled accordingly. It is of note that patients with poor cardiac function (EF < 40%) are at increased risk of thromboembolism; we recommend anticoagulation with unfractionated heparin (5000–7500 units s.c.) or low-molecular-weight enoxaparin (40 mg s.c. daily) during pregnancy, and consideration of warfarin in the postpartum interval.

When peripartum cardiomyopathy occurs in the last trimester of pregnancy, delivery is indicated. The mode of delivery should be based on obstetric indications. Indeed, the advantages of vaginal delivery over Cesarean section are evident: minimal blood loss, greater hemodynamic stability, and decreased pulmonary and thromboembolic complications. In addition, regional epidural analgesia has the distinct advantage of reducing both preload and afterload, as well as minimizing fluctuations in cardiac output associated with labor. In instances of obstetrically indicated Cesarean delivery, we and others recommend careful monitoring of fluid balance with central monitoring in an effort to clearly define and monitor the central venous pressure.

A notable feature of peripartum cardiomyopathy is its tendency to recur with subsequent pregnancies. Several reports have suggested that prognosis for future pregnancies is related to heart size. Patients whose cardiac size returned to normal within 6–12 months had an 11–14% mortality in subsequent pregnancies; patients with persistent cardiomegaly had a 40–80% mortality. Pregnancy is contraindicated in all patients with persistent cardiomegaly accompanying left ventricular dysfunction; the 11–14% risk of maternal mortality with subsequent pregnancy seen in patients with normal heart size would seem, in most cases, to be unacceptable as well.

Marfan syndrome

Marfan syndrome is an autosomal dominant disorder caused by multiple lineage-specific mutations in the fibrillin gene on chromosome 15; the weakness results in skeletal, ocular, and cardiovascular abnormalities. Among the cardiovascular manifestations, mitral valve prolapse, mitral regurgitation, aortic insufficiency, and aortic root dilation with a marked propensity toward aortic root dissection are common. The most common cause of death among women under 40 years of age with Marfan syndrome is aortic complication, and 50% of aortic aneurysm ruptures in these women occur during pregnancy.

Although some authors believe that pregnancy is contraindicated in any woman with documented Marfan syndrome, prognosis is best individualized and should be based on echocardiographic and computed tomography (CT) assessment of aortic root diameter and postvalvular dilation. It is important to note that enlargement of the aortic root is not demonstrable by chest radiograph until dilation has become pronounced. Women with an abnormal aortic valve or aortic dilation may have up to a 50% pregnancy-associated mortality; women without these changes and an aortic root diameter of less than 40 mm have a mortality of less than 5%. Even in patients meeting these echocardiographic criteria, however, special attention must be given to signs or symptoms of aortic dissection because even serial echocardiographic assessment is not invariably predictive of complications. In counseling women with Marfan syndrome, the genetics of this condition and the shortened maternal lifespan must be considered, in addition to the immediate maternal risk.

Gestational management hinges on aggressive control of hypertension with beta-blocker therapy; utilization of labetalol (an alpha- and beta-antagonist) has the added advantage of controlling mean arterial blood pressure in a rapid fashion, alongside its ability to decrease pulsatile pressure on the aorta. In instances of aortic root dilation approximating 5 cm, we would recommend Cesarean delivery to minimize episodic hypertension that may precipitate aortic root dissection. If Cesarean section is performed, retention sutures should be used because of generalized connective tissue weakness.

Myocardial infarction

Coronary artery disease is uncommon in women of reproductive age; therefore, myocardial infarction in conjunction with pregnancy is rare and occurs in less than 1:10 000 pregnancies. In a review of 68 reported cases, myocardial infarction during pregnancy was associated with a 35% mortality rate, and only 13% of patients were known to have had coronary artery disease before pregnancy. Two-thirds of the women suffered infarction in the third trimester; mortality for these women was 45%, compared with 23% in those suffering infarction in the first or second trimesters. Thus, it appears that the increased hemodynamic burden imposed on the maternal cardiovascular system in late pregnancy may unmask latent coronary artery disease in some women and worsen the prognosis for patients suffering infarction. Fetuses from surviving women appear to have an increased risk of spontaneous abortion and unexplained stillbirth.

Women with class H diabetes mellitus face risks beyond those imposed by their cardiac disease alone. Although successful pregnancy outcome may occur, maternal and fetal risks are considerable. Such considerations, as well as the anticipated shortened lifespan of these patients, make special counseling of such women of major importance.

Antepartum care of women with prior myocardial infarction centers on efforts to minimize myocardial oxygen demands. Diagnostic radionuclide cardiac imaging during pregnancy results in a fetal dose of no more than 0.8 rad and thus does not carry the potential for teratogenesis. If cardiac catheterization becomes necessary, the simultaneous use of contrast echocardiography may reduce the need for cineangiography and thus reduce radiation exposure to the fetus. In women with angina, nitrates have been used without adverse fetal effects. Delivery within 2 weeks of infarction is associated with increased mortality; therefore, if possible, attempts should be made to allow adequate convalescence before delivery. If the cervix is favorable, cautious induction under controlled circumstances after a period of hemodynamic stabilization is optimal. Labor in the lateral recumbent position, the administration of oxygen, pain relief with epidural anesthesia, and shortening of the second stage to reduce myocardial oxygen demands with assisted vaginal delivery are important management considerations; Cesarean delivery is reserved for obstetric indications.

Anticoagulation

Anticoagulation in the patient with an artificial heart valve or atrial fibrillation during pregnancy is controversial and has been the focus of many recent and comprehensive reviews. The key issue involves the lack of consensus on an ideal agent for anticoagulation during pregnancy.

Warfarin (coumadin) is relatively contraindicated at all stages of gestation because of its association with fetal warfarin syndrome (warfarin embryopathy, characterized by nasal hypoplasia and stippled epiphyses) in weeks 6–12, and because of its theoretical relationship to fetal intracranial hemorrhage and secondary brain scarring at later stages. Several series from outside the United States have reported on the use of warfarin in pregnant patients with prosthetic valves, and demonstrated a 2% incidence of embryopathy. Thus, while one can debate the precise risk of embryopathy based on prospective or retrospective acquired data, this risk unequivocally exists.

Balancing the fetal risks with warfarin therapy are the maternal risks with heparin and low-molecular-weight heparin therapy. In sum of a large body of data, there are now multiple series comparing maternal thromboembolic events in patients receiving unfractionated heparin, which demonstrate a two- to fourfold increased risk of treatment failure with maternal mortality from thrombosed valves. In addition, it is suggested that bileaflet valves (St Jude valves) may actually have a lowered thrombogenic potential, albeit one study did not support such findings.

Reported and hypothesized treatment failures with unfractionated heparin led both cardiologists and obstetricians to employ low-molecular-weight heparin (LMWH) for prosthetic valve prophylaxis. However, this too is fraught with controversy and limitations. Both the Food and Drug Administration (FDA) and the American College of Obstetricians and Gynecologists (ACOG) warn against the use of enoxaparin and other LMWHs during pregnancy, citing the risk of thrombosis. The Report and Recommendations of the Anticoagulation in Prosthetic Valves and Pregnancy Consensus Report (APPCR) Panel and Scientific Roundtable has come to the consensus opinion that "There is a substantial body of published, peer-reviewed, trial- and cohort study-based evidence, institutional data sets, and expert clinical experience/opinion to support safe and effective use of enoxaparin for anti-coagulation management of non-pregnant patients with prosthetic mechanical heart valves. There are insufficient data to reliably predict, compare clinical outcomes, or to confirm the safety or effectiveness of enoxaparin, UFH, or warfarin in pregnant patients with mechanical heart valves. In light of the predicatable, published, and problematic aspects encountered with each of the aforementioned anticoagulants currently available in the armamentarium for pregnant patients with mechanical valves, the Panel felt strongly that while concerns about efficacy and safety were justified for all agents (i.e., warfarin, heparin, and LMWH [enoxaparin]), the available literature and index cases did not support selective, asymmetrical warning language in the case of enoxaparin."

In essence, a choice between fetal and maternal risks must be made, and neither choice is considered ideal. That said, two approaches may be termed "acceptable." One involves substitution of heparin or enoxaparin for warfarin from the time pregnancy is diagnosed until 12 weeks' gestation, followed by warfarin until 32 weeks, at which time heparin or enoxaparin is reinstituted until delivery. The

Table 36.5 Treatment approaches for women with mechanical heart valves.

Approach	Dosing regimen	Therapeutic parameters
Adjusted-dose unfractionated heparin throughout pregnancy	Adjusted dosage s.c. every 12 h	Maintain midinterval aPTT at a minimum of twice control OR anti-factor Xa heparin level of 0.3 U/mL
Adjusted-dose LMWH throughout pregnancy	Adjusted dosage s.c. every 12 h	Maintain peak anti-factor Xa heparin levels (4 h post injection) > 0.8 U/mL
Heparin or LMWH in adjusted dose (as above) through the 12th week of gestation, then warfarin until 36 weeks, followed by reinitiation of adjusted-dose heparin or LMWH (as above)	As above, with warfarin after 12 weeks daily	Target INR 2.5–3.5 with warfarin therapy Otherwise as above

INR, international normalized ratio; aPTT, activated partial thromboplastin time.

second approach involves using adjusted-dose subcutaneous heparin or enoxaparin throughout pregnancy. We recommend dosage regimens as outlined in Table 36.5, with acknowledgment of the paucity of data supporting these recommendations. Given the controversies outlined above, with their ensuing medicolegal implications, the patient must be involved in this choice and thoroughly informed of the risks and benefits of either approach.

Further reading

ACC/AHA Guidelines for the Management of Patients with Valvular Heart Disease: a Report of the American College of Cardiology/American Heart Association Task Force on Practice Guidelines (Committee on Management of Patients with Valvular Heart Disease). *J Am Coll Cardiol* 1998;32:1486.

APPCR Panel and Scientific Roundtable. Anticoagulation and enoxaparin use in patients with prosthetic heart valves and/or pregnancy. *Clin Cardiol Consensus Rep* 2002;3(9).

Avila WS, Rossi EG, Ramires JA, et al. Pregnancy in patients with heart disease: experience with 1,000 cases. *Clin Cardiol* 2003;26:135.

Clark SL. Structural cardiac disease in pregnancy. In: Clark SL, Cotton DB, Phelan JP, eds. *Critical care obstetrics*, 3rd edn. Boston: Blackwell Scientific, 1997.

Gei AF, Hankins GD. Cardiac disease and pregnancy. *Obstet Gynecol Clin North Am* 2001;28:465.

Hung L, Rahimtoola SH. Prosthetic heart valves and pregnancy. *Circulation* 2003;107:1240.

Ramsey PS, Ramin KD, Ramin SM. Cardiac disease in pregnancy. *Am J Perinatol* 2001;18:245.

Ray P, Murphy GJ, Shutt LE. Recognition and management of maternal cardiac disease in pregnancy. *Br J Anaesth* 2004;93:428.

Reimold SC, Rutherford JD. Valvular heart disease in pregnancy. *N Engl J Med* 2003;349:52.

Rout CC. Anesthesia and analgesia for the critically ill parturient. *Best Pract Res Clin Obstet Gynecol* 2001;15:507.

37 Maternal pulmonary disorders complicating pregnancy

Steven L. Clark and Calla Holmgren

Pregnant women are afflicted by the same respiratory ailments as nonpregnant women, but these conditions are complicated by the physiologic alterations of pregnancy. Certain lung diseases, such as asthma, are common in women of childbearing age and may often be seen in pregnant women. Asthma and other pulmonary diseases may first manifest during pregnancy or change their course during gestation. Respiratory illness can affect both maternal and fetal outcomes during pregnancy. Pharmacologic treatment of lung disease can be undertaken to minimize adverse effects to both mother and fetus.

Diagnostic techniques

History and physical examination

If the patient has been pregnant in the past, the presence of respiratory symptoms during the previous pregnancy should be noted and compared with the patient's usual respiratory symptoms when not pregnant.

Dyspnea is the most common respiratory complaint during pregnancy, with as many as 60–70% of previously normal women having this symptom at some time during pregnancy. The complaint usually begins in the first or second trimester but is most prevalent at term. It is not usually due to underlying lung disease, but appears to result from the subjective perception of hyperventilation that normally accompanies pregnancy. As the woman acclimatizes to this new sensation, her perception of dyspnea is reduced, and the dyspnea stabilizes as the pregnancy progresses. Unlike pathologic dyspnea, symptoms do not increase with exertion.

Arterial blood gases

In a normal pregnant female, arterial blood gas measurements will usually show a compensated respiratory alkalosis due to maternal hyperventilation. The pH generally ranges from 7.40 to 7.47, and the partial pressure of arterial carbon dioxide is 25–32 mmHg. The partial pressure of arterial oxygen (P_aO_2) may be as high as 106 mmHg in early pregnancy, decreasing during pregnancy but remaining at 100 mmHg, or slightly higher, at term.

Calculating the O_2 content of blood requires a knowledge of the amount of O_2 dissolved in the blood, the maximum amount of O_2 able to be carried per gram of hemoglobin, the hemoglobin concentration, and the O_2 saturation of hemoglobin.

$$O_2 \text{ content} = [(\text{hemoglobin [Hb] (g/dL)} \times 1.39 \text{ mL}$$
$$O_2/\text{g Hb}) \times (O_2 \text{ saturation})] + [(0.003 \text{ mL } O_2/100 \text{ mL of blood})$$
$$\times P_aO_2 \text{ (mmHg)}]$$

Mismatching of ventilation and perfusion is responsible for most of the defective gas exchange in pulmonary diseases. The adequacy of alveolar gas exchange can be assessed by calculating the alveolar–arterial O_2 tension gradient and, if the alveolar O_2 tension (P_AO_2) greatly exceeds the P_aO_2, then alveolar gas exchange is abnormal. Ideal P_aO_2 is calculated as follows:

$$P_aO_2 = F_IO_2 \times (PB - 47) - P_aCO_2/0.8$$

F_IO_2, fractional percentage of inspired O_2; PB, barometric pressure; 47, water vapor pressure; P_aCO_2, arterial blood tension of carbon dioxide; 0.8, respiratory quotient.

Because most acute lung diseases are accompanied by an increased (A–a) O_2 gradient, the gradient should be assessed with the pregnant patient in the upright position and should be considered abnormal if it exceeds 25 mmHg. Blood gas analysis should be accompanied by calculation of the gradient because, given the usual decreased PCO_2 in pregnancy, on casual observation, a "normal" P_aCO_2 can be seen even with an abnormally increased (A–a) O_2 gradient.

Pulmonary function tests

The enlarging fetus and the increased concentration of circulating hormones during pregnancy account for the changes in pulmonary function seen with gestation (Table 37.1). The hyperventilation of pregnancy is characterized by an increased depth of breathing (tidal volume increased from 450 to 600 mL) and not a higher respiratory rate.

A woman with a respiratory disease that is unlikely to deteriorate during pregnancy, an FEV_1 greater than 1 L, and no dyspnea at rest can undertake pregnancy safely.

Radiographic testing

If at any time during pregnancy, the health of the mother or fetus would be compromised by failure to perform a radiologic examination, the examination should be performed. Irradiation *in utero* may increase the risk of childhood

Table 37.1 Pulmonary parameters.

Lung volumes	Description
Tidal volume (TV)	The volume of air inhaled or exhaled with each normal breath
Residual volume (RV)	The volume of air remaining in the lungs after a vital capacity maneuver
Inspiratory reserve volume (IRV)	The maximal additional volume of gas that can be inhaled after a tidal breath is inhaled
Expiratory reserve volume (ERV)	The maximal volume of gas that can be exhaled after a tidal breath is exhaled
Total lung capacity (TLC)	The volume of air in the lungs at maximal inspiration
Vital capacity (VC)	The maximum amount of air that can be exhaled after a maximal inspiration to TLC
Inspiratory capacity (IC)	The maximal volume of gas that can be inspired from the resting expiratory level
Functional residual capacity (FRC)	The volume of air remaining in the lungs after a tidal volume exhalation
Forced vital capacity (FVC)	The volume of air exhaled during a rapid forced expiration starting at full inspiration
Other measurements made by spirometry	
Forced expiratory volume in 1 s (FEV)	The volume of air expelled in 1 s during a forced expiration starting at full inspiration
Minute ventilation (MV)	The amount of air exhaled per minute, measured under resting conditions
Peak expiratory flow rate (PEFR)	The peak rate (L/min) of a forceful expiration of a vital capacity

leukemia and other malignancies by 40–50%. Taking into account the greatest oncogenic risk, the overall risk of any adverse effect from exposure to 1 rad is estimated to be 0.1%, a risk that is thousands of times smaller than the risks of spontaneous abortion, malformation, or genetic disease. Fetal exposure to less than 5 rad is considered to be insufficient reason to recommend the termination of a desired pregnancy.

When chest radiographs are performed in the pregnant patient, normal findings differ from those seen in nonpregnant women of childbearing age. The diaphragm may be elevated 4 cm at term, but there will be a compensatory increase in anteroposterior diameter. There is an increase in the subcostal angle from 68.5° to 103.5° from early to late pregnancy. Also, lung marking may be increased, giving a false impression of mild congestive heart failure. Postpartum pleural effusions may not be a normal occurrence.

Maternal–fetal oxygen exchange

In a woman with no pulmonary disease who is breathing room air, arterial blood typically has a P_aO_2 of 91 mmHg and a PCO_2 of 36 mmHg. In the fetal umbilical vein, a simultaneous blood gas typically shows a PO_2 of 32 mmHg and a PCO_2 of 50 mmHg. Increases in the concentration of inspired O_2 result in the expected rise in O_2 tension in the maternal arteries, but not in large increases in the O_2 tension of the fetal umbilical veins. Nevertheless, even a small increase in the oxygen content can result in a significant increase in oxygen transfer to the fetus. This occurs because of the high maternal perfusion rate of the uterus, the enhanced avidity of fetal hemoglobin for oxygen, and the leftward shift in the fetal oxyhemoglobin dissociation curve. However, the fetus is sensitive to large shifts in oxygen delivery, caused by a fall in cardiac output and, with complete interruption of oxygen supply to the umbilical vein, the fetus has only a 2- to 4-min oxygen reserve.

Maternal alkalosis can result in decreased fetal oxygen tensions because of reduced uterine blood flow due to hypocarbia-induced vasoconstriction of uterine arteries, on account of the mechanical effects of hyperventilation causing decreased maternal venous return, and because of a shift in the maternal oxyhemoglobin dissociation curve to the left, thereby impairing oxygen transfer to the fetus. In the studies by Wulf and colleagues (1972), fetal oxygen delivery was compromised when maternal pH exceeded 7.6 and PCO_2 was 15 mmHg, values unlikely to be reached in acute asthma.

Asthma

Asthma, or reversible narrowing of the large or small airways, is the most common obstructive lung disease affecting women of childbearing age, occurring in 0.4–1.3% of pregnant women.

The effect of asthma on the outcome of pregnancy

Most asthmatics experience pregnancy with few ill effects and, in general, there are no striking differences between the outcome of pregnancy in asthmatics compared with a control population. Nevertheless, severe and inadequately managed asthma can be associated with increased maternal and fetal complications, such as enhanced maternal and fetal mortality, a slight increase in the incidence of premature births, stillbirth, low birthweight babies, and subsequent neurologic abnormalities in the offspring. No differences in the frequency of multiple births or congenital malformations or in the infants' Apgar scores have been seen in the children of asthmatic mothers.

The effect of pregnancy on the course of asthma

Asthma worsens during pregnancy in slightly more than one-third of patients, improves in slightly more than one-third of patients, and remains unchanged in one-third of patients. The change in asthma course associated with pregnancy usually reverts to the prepregnancy course within 3 months after delivery, and the course of asthma tends to be similar in a given woman during subsequent pregnancies.

Clinical presentation

Classically, two clinical patterns of asthma have been recognized. One group, the so-called extrinsic asthmatics, develops asthma at a young age, has a family history of atopy, may have other atopic manifestations (skin and nasal allergies), and has evidence of immunoglobulin (Ig)E-mediated response along with blood and sputum eosinophilia. Attacks are often seasonal and precipitated by well-defined allergens. The second group, the "intrinsic asthmatics," develops asthma later in life, has no family history of asthma or atopy, has no evidence of IgE-mediated bronchospasm, uncommonly has eosinophilia, but may have severe asthma that is difficult to treat. The intrinsic asthmatic is sensitive to environmental irritants, and acute exacerbations are often triggered by viral respiratory illness. Other clinical patterns include the triad of chronic asthma, a history of nasal polyps and pansinusitis, and the development of significant reductions in airflow rates following ingestion of aspirin or nonsteroidal anti-inflammatory drugs. In these patients, bronchospasm develops within minutes to hours, and symptoms may be severe or even life-threatening. Exercise-induced asthma is another common variant and is characterized by the development of bronchospasm following discontinuation of exercise in patients who may or may not have chronic asthmatic symptoms.

An acute attack of asthma is usually heralded by the clinical triad cough, wheezing, and dyspnea. Dyspnea may be interpreted as a tightness in the chest. Attacks often occur at night. Usually, there is a history of exposure to a specific allergen, physical exertion, a viral respiratory tract infection, or emotional excitement preceding the onset of an exacerbation, and the patient will often have a history of similar episodes in the past.

Physical examination during an exacerbation reveals audibly harsh respirations, inspiratory and expiratory wheezing with a prolonged expiratory phase, tachypnea, tachycardia, and mild systolic hypertension. The lungs are overinflated, and the anterior–posterior diameter of the thorax is increased beyond that typically expected in pregnancy. With increased duration and severity of an attack, the accessory respiratory muscles become visibly active, and the patient may develop a paradoxical pulse, both signs of severe respiratory compromise.

The chest radiograph during an acute attack usually shows hyperinflation of the lungs with a small, elongated heart. The chest film may be necessary to exclude complications such as pneumothorax, pneumomediastinum, cardiomegaly, pneumonia, mucoid impaction, or bronchopulmonary aspergillosis, but only when these conditions are suspected on clinical grounds.

Laboratory studies are nonspecific. A complete blood count often displays a mild to moderate eosinophilia that may be reduced or absent if the patient has been taking corticosteroids. Life-threatening risks can be avoided by careful and routine medical attention during pregnancy and by early pharmacologic intervention during an exacerbation. The clinical hallmarks of cough, wheezing, and dyspnea do not correlate in any predictable way with lung function. Thus, if the patient can perform a forced expiration, the FEV_1 or the peak expiratory flow rate (PEFR) should be used to assess the severity and progress of airway obstruction. Carbon dioxide retention begins to occur at an FEV_1 of approximately 750 mL (about 25% of the predicted value), and a PEFR of less than 100 L/min is thought to be associated with an increased risk of a potentially fatal attack. With severe asthma, accessory muscle use and pulsus paradoxicus may be seen, suggesting that the FEV_1 is less than 25% of normal.

Pharmacology of asthma therapy

Because asthma is an airways disease, inhalation therapy is generally preferable to systemic treatment. Aerosolized medications deliver the drug directly to the airways, minimizing systemic side-effects. Inhaled β_2-agonists are usually sufficient therapy for mild, intermittent asthma. If symptoms disappear and pulmonary function normalizes with inhaled β_2-agonists, they can be used indefinitely as needed. However, their use on a daily basis, or even more often than three times a week, usually indicates a need for anti-inflammatory therapy.

Inhaled anti-inflammatory agents are the primary therapy for moderate asthma. Choices include cromolyn sodium or inhaled corticosteroids, which provide effective asthma control with minimal side-effects at the recommended doses. Suppression of symptoms and PEFR improvement are often not maximal until 2–4 weeks of treatment. A spacer, used to bypass the oropharynx during the administration of aerosolized medication, should be considered not only to reduce oropharyngeal candidiasis but also to improve respiratory tract penetration and reduce systemic effects.

A short tapering course of oral corticosteroids is indicated when asthma is not controlled by a combination of bronchodilators, cromolyn sodium, and inhaled corticosteroids. Such deterioration of asthma may be characterized by a reduction in PEFR of 20% or more from normal values that fails to respond to inhaled bronchodilators, by greater intolerance of exercise, or by the development of nocturnal symptoms. At the end of this course, oral corticosteroids can be stopped; if asthma symptoms do not recur and pulmonary functions remain normal, no additional oral steroid therapy is necessary. However, if this "burst" of prednisone does not control symptoms, is effective for fewer than 10 days, or must be repeated frequently, the patient needs additional therapy. Prolonged use of high doses of oral corticosteroids may be associated with increased risk of gestational diabetes and maternal adrenal insufficiency.

Leukotriene modifiers, such as montelukast (Singulair) and zafirlukast (Accolate), are available for the treatment of asthma. The cysteinyl leukotrienes (LTC4, LTD4, and LTE4) are produced by way of arachidonic acid metabolism and are released by mast cells and eosinophils. They then bind to leukotriene receptors in the human airway, causing airway edema, smooth muscle contraction, and altered cellular activity. Leukotriene modifiers bind to these leukotriene receptors, inhibiting the actions of leukotriene at the level of the mast cell and eosinophil. These medications are pregnancy category B and may be continued during pregnancy. Sustained release theophylline or a long-acting oral agonist once a day in the evening may be helpful for the patient with primarily nocturnal symptoms. Otherwise, oral theophylline is generally not used in current clinical practice.

Therapy of acute asthma attacks

Several risk factors for fatal asthma have been identified, and these include the following:
- a history of intubation for asthma;
- two or more hospitalizations for asthma within 1 year;
- three or more emergency room visits for asthma within 1 month;
- recent withdrawal from systemic corticosteroids;
- history of syncope or seizure associated with an asthmatic attack;
- previous admission to a hospital intensive care unit for asthma;
- coexisting psychiatric disease or psychosocial problems.

An acute attack of asthma should be managed aggressively, and the patient should be evaluated carefully for possible hospital admission (Table 37.2). In approximately 10–15% of pregnancies complicated by asthma, the patient may

Table 37.2 Prophylactic evaluation and management of the asthmatic.

Take a careful history, including severity of asthma and identifiable precipitants
Baseline pulmonary function tests and PEFRs
Vaccinate against influenza
Optimize dosage and frequency of medications
Patient counseling
   Appropriate exercise
   Avoidance of precipitants
   Instruction on early recognition of wheezing and need for prompt intervention

require hospitalization for status asthmaticus, a condition characterized by refractory airway obstruction with failure to resolve after appropriate treatment. A quick search for a precipitating event and questioning about prior and current corticosteroid use are part of the initial history. Then examination of pulse, blood pressure, respiratory rate, pulsus paradoxus, and FEV_1 and/or peak expiratory flow is indicated. A pulse of more than 120/min, respiratory rate of more than 30/min, pulsus paradoxus more than 18 mmHg, peak expiratory flow less than 120 L/min, moderate to severe dyspnea, accessory muscle use, and severe wheezing at the time of presentation are all signs of potentially life-threatening disease and probably indicate a need for acute hospitalization.

The emergency management of acute, severe asthma in pregnancy involves several initial steps:

1 Administer O_2 to maintain a P_aO_2 as near normal as possible but at least above 60 mmHg or O_2 of at least 95%.
2 Perform baseline arterial blood gases, continuous pulse oximetry, and intensive fetal monitoring for late second- or third-trimester fetuses.
3 Obtain baseline pulmonary function tests (FEV or PEFR).
4 Administer an inhaled beta-agonist, such as albuterol, 2.5 mg in 2–3 mL of diluent with a pressure-driven nebulizer, every 20 min for up to three doses. Alternatively, terbutaline sulfate, 0.25 mg, is administered subcutaneously every 20–30 min for up to three doses.

In an emergency setting, epinephrine (0.3 mL of 1:1000 dilution) can be given subcutaneously with serial injections leading to cumulative improvements in airway function. This therapy should be avoided in patients with marked hypertension (systolic BP > 200 mmHg) or in those patients with an irregular pulse.

Further management is based on clinical response and improvements in pulmonary function testing. If these maneuvers improve the PEFR to more than 70% of baseline, the patient may be discharged, often with a short course of oral corticosteroids. For a PEFR that is 40–70% of baseline, the beta-agonist therapy is continued (at intervals as frequent as every hour in patients without heart disease) and methylprednisolone, 80 mg every 6 h, is initiated. If the initial response results in a PEFR less than 40% of baseline, the patient should be admitted to the hospital. A PEFR of less than 25% or PCO_2 of more than 35 mmHg suggests imminent respiratory failure. The patient should be admitted to an intensive care unit. Intubation may be necessary if deterioration continues. In a patient with a viable fetus (> 24 weeks), it may be prudent to employ external fetal monitoring to ensure adequate oxygen delivery to the fetus.

Other obstructive lung disorders

Severe emphysema due to α_1-antitrypsin deficiency and cystic fibrosis (CF) can occur in women of childbearing age. Care of these patients is primarily supportive, with attention to the physiologic parameters of lung function and oxygenation discussed earlier.

A National Institutes of Health study followed 129 pregnancies in CF patients and found only 86 viable infants, leading the investigators to conclude that CF patients have greatly increased fetal wastage. In the study, there were six spontaneous abortions, 25 therapeutic abortions, and 11 perinatal deaths. Ten of the perinatal deaths occurred in infants born at less than 37 weeks' gestation. Premature labor occurred in 26 of the 129 pregnancies, and infant mortality was 18% within 24 months of delivery. The authors recommended that pregnancy be avoided unless the potential CF mother was clinically healthy. Published studies relate the severity of maternal disease at the onset of pregnancy more than the effects of CF on pregnancy to outcomes. Factors such as pancreatic insufficiency, nutritional status, and low Taussig score were predictors of poor prognosis in pregnancy. Any woman with pulmonary hypertension should not undertake pregnancy. A reasonable set of guidelines is to advise against pregnancy in any CF patient with a vital capacity of less than 50% of predicted, hypoxemia, pulmonary hypertension, or pancreatic insufficiency. The absence of pancreatic insufficiency may identify a subgroup more able to tolerate pregnancy. A recent study showed that women with CF, after adjusting for demographic differences, who became pregnant did not have worse survival.

Bronchial drainage, antibiotic therapy, prophylactic immunization (including annual influenza vaccine administration), and optimal nutritional and psychosocial care are essential components in the care of the CF patient contemplating pregnancy.

Aspiration of stomach contents

The aspiration of low-pH liquid stomach contents into the tracheobronchial tree, with subsequent chemical pneumonitis, was first described in women undergoing labor and delivery. This syndrome is most likely to develop if aspirated material has a pH of less than 2.5, but some reports suggest that some degree of respiratory dysfunction can occur even if the pH of the aspirate is higher. Other syndromes that can result from aspiration are bronchial obstruction by an aspirated foreign body and bacterial pneumonia from aspiration of oropharyngeal bacteria.

Immediate clinical illness may appear if the aspiration is massive, but typically there is generally a delay of at least 6–8 h before the first appearance of signs and symptoms such as bronchospasm, tachycardia, hypotension, tachypnea, cyanosis, and frothy pink sputum. Diagnosis is facilitated by having a high index of suspicion in the postpartum patient with respiratory distress.

Treatment of acid aspiration is supportive with O_2 and mechanical ventilation if needed. If aspiration is observed, endotracheal suctioning should be performed, but saline lavage is not indicated and may even serve to spread the acid to uninvolved areas. Bronchodilators may be used to control bronchospasm, and the prophylactic use of broad-spectrum antibiotics should be considered. Corticosteroids have been used in the treatment of witnessed gastric aspiration, but are of unproven benefit.

Prophylaxis of aspiration should always be undertaken in the pregnant patient undergoing surgery, with antacids given during labor to raise the gastric pH to more than 2.5 and thus reduce the chance of a dangerous aspiration. Adverse pulmonary reactions may result from aspirating antacid particles; thus, the use of nonparticulate agents is preferred. Various combinations of oral nonparticulate antacids and H_2-receptor blockers have been advocated as a convenient prophylactic regimen for patients about to undergo elective or emergency Cesarean section, but no particular combination appears to be clearly superior. Additional prophylactic measures include limiting oral intake to essential medications once labor is started, nasogastric evacuation of a distended stomach, selection of regional anesthesia when possible, use of a cuffed endotracheal tube, and use of cricoid pressure during intubation.

Respiratory infections

Bacterial pneumonia

Pneumonia of all etiologies is a relatively common cause of maternal mortality. It has been reported in 0.1–0.84% of all pregnancies, with a mortality rate of 3.5–8.6%, although antibiotics and modern obstetric care have improved the prognosis. *Streptococcus pneumoniae* is the most common infectious agent implicated in antepartum pneumonia, and other common bacterial pathogens include *Mycoplasma pneumoniae* and *Haemophilus influenzae*. *Legionella pneumoniae* and *Listeria monocytogenes* have rarely been reported to cause respiratory failure in pregnancy.

Pneumococcal pneumonia classically begins with the abrupt onset of shaking chills, fever, pleuritic chest pain, cough productive of purulent sputum, and shortness of breath. The physical examination often shows signs of consolidation, such as dullness to percussion, tactile fremitus, and egobronchophony. A chest radiograph usually reveals evidence of lobar consolidation, but bronchopneumonia may also occur. Laboratory examination may reveal a polymorphonuclear leukocytosis in the range of 12 000 to 25 000 cells/mL, but a normal white blood cell count can also be seen, especially in patients with overwhelming infection and bacteremia. A sputum specimen for culture and Gram's stain should generally be obtained and may demonstrate Gram-positive encapsulated cocci in pairs and short chains. Blood cultures are positive in approximately 20–30% of patients and should be collected before the administration of antibiotics.

Although penicillin U has long been considered the antibiotic of choice, recent evidence suggests that penicillin nonsusceptibility is found in nearly 40% of strains of *Streptococcus pneumoniae* causing disease in adults. Given this, any gravid patient thought to have bacterial pneumonia should be admitted to hospital and started on a third-generation cephalosporin and a macrolide (e.g., azithromycin) until sputum culture reveals the causal organism and sensitivities. Once established, antibiotic treatment can be tailored to the responsible organism. This will typically lead to defervescence within 48 h. Once the patient is afebrile for 48 h, parenteral antibiotic therapy can be discontinued and oral cephalosporin continued for 10–14 days.

Mycobacterium pneumoniae produces symptoms similar to a viral infection, with a flu-like syndrome, interstitial infiltrates, and alveolar filling. Because tetracycline is relatively contraindicated in pregnancy, erythromycin is the drug of choice. *Haemophilus influenzae* pneumonia may have a gradual rather than an abrupt onset and may be clinically indistinguishable from *S. pneumoniae*. It is infrequently seen in young adults unless the patient has a history of chronic obstructive lung disease or is an alcoholic. The chest radiograph may show either bronchial or lobar consolidation, and pleural effusions are common. Again, because the occurrence of ampicillin resistance may be significant, the patient should be managed as stated above with susceptibility testing performed on all culture isolates and antibiotic therapy tailored appropriately.

Influenza

In a review of all deaths due to influenza from 1957 through 1960, 1–11% occurred in pregnant patients. These deaths were concentrated late in the third trimester and early puerperium and were more likely to occur with increased maternal age. However, because earlier studies were based on the clinical diagnosis of influenza, the conclusion that pregnancy predisposes to infection or to an enhanced severity of illness is controversial.

Influenza usually begins abruptly with systemic symptoms, such as headache, fever, chills, myalgia, and malaise accompanied by an upper respiratory illness. In an uncomplicated case, complaints of a sore throat and cough may persist for a week or more. Physical findings may be minimal, but injection of the mucous membranes and a postnasal discharge can be seen along with mild cervical adenopathy. The chest examination may be normal but can reveal rhonchi, wheezes, and scattered rales. Occasionally, the disease can progress rapidly to fulminant cardiopulmonary failure, or it can be complicated by secondary bacterial or mixed viral–bacterial pneumonia involving *Streptococcus*, *Staphylococcus*, or *H. influenzae*.

Amantadine, an oral antiviral agent active against influenza A, can be used therapeutically and prevents 70–90% of experimentally produced and natural infections. It is not effective in treating infections due to influenza B. If used within 48 h of the onset of symptoms, amantadine shortens the duration of the illness by up to 50%, reduces fever, and hastens the resumption of normal activities. If given concomitantly with an influenza vaccine, it can protect the patient for the 2–3 weeks necessary for immunity to develop during exposure to an epidemic. Other antivirals, zanamivir and osteltamivir, may reduce the duration of uncomplicated influenza A and B. No clinical study has been conducted regarding the safety or efficacy of any of these antiviral medications during pregnancy.

Although influenza virus can cross the placenta, it has not been isolated from fetal blood, and transplacental passage does not appear to cause congenital defects. Fetal abnormalities, such as circulatory defects, central nervous system malformations, cleft lip, and childhood cancer, have been attributed to influenza, but most investigators have concluded that no influenza-induced congenital syndrome exists. Influenza vaccine may be administered appropriately in pregnant women in any trimester with standard indications for such immunization. Because increased mortality from infections usually occurs late in pregnancy, vaccination can often be delayed until the middle of the second trimester if necessary.

Viral pneumonia

Other life-threatening viral pneumonias can develop in the pregnant patient, including varicella pneumonia, which may accompany chickenpox and can range from a mild to a rapidly fatal illness. In pregnancy, varicella is rare, but if pneumonia develops, mortality is high, ranging from 30% to 40% in some series. In addition, varicella pneumonia has been associated with an increased incidence of premature labor. Maternal varicella infection in any trimester of pregnancy can be associated with infrequent, but possibly lethal, congenital anomalies. If the maternal infection occurs within 5 days of delivery, the infant is at risk of fatal disseminated infection. Given the high mortality rate associated with varicella pneumonia occurring in pregnancy and the lack of demonstrated human fetal toxicity, it is recommended that any gravid patient with varicella pneumonia be admitted to hospital for parenteral therapy with acyclovir. The dose is $500\,mg/m^2$ every 8 h and should be continued until the symptoms of the illness resolve. An important consideration of varicella pneumonia during pregnancy is the issue of prevention. Patients considering pregnancy should be questioned regarding their history of varicella and, if unsure, titers should be drawn to confirm immunity. If the patient is not immune, then the varicella vaccine can be given prior to pregnancy. If the patient is not immune, but exposed to varicella peripartum, many authors have recommended the administration of varicella zoster immune globulin.

Fungal pneumonia

Cryptococcus neoformans, *Blastomyces dermatitidis*, and *Sporothrix schenckii* have rarely been reported as causing serious respiratory infection in pregnancy. The clinical course and outcome are generally the same in pregnant and nonpregnant patients. It has been estimated that coccidioidomycosis occurs in less than one of every 1000 pregnancies. However, infection in pregnancy, particularly during the second and third trimesters, increases the rate of disseminated infection from 0.2% to more than 20%. It has been suggested that 17β-estradiol has a stimulatory effect on the fungus and may be responsible for the increased risk of dissemination associated with pregnancy. Maternal mortality rate from disseminated coccidioidomycosis approaches 100%, a rate approximately twice that seen in nonpregnant patients. Dissemination is associated with increased fetal prematurity and mortality.

Amphotericin B has been used to treat cryptococcoses, blastomycosis, and disseminated coccidioidomycosis in pregnancy. It crosses the placenta and can be found in both amniotic fluid and fetal blood. Although use in pregnancy has not been well studied, normal, full-term infants have been born to patients who received amphotericin B in the first trimester. Its use is associated with anemia; thus, serial hematocrits must be followed.

Pneumocystis carinii pneumonia

Pneumocystis carinii pneumonia is the most common opportunistic infection affecting the lungs of patients with acquired immunodeficiency syndrome (AIDS). It can be confused with atypical mycobacterial infection, cryptococcoses, and histoplasmosis.

There are several case reports of *P. carinii* pneumonia (PCP) complicating pregnancy and evidence to suggest that PCP has a more aggressive course during pregnancy, with increased morbidity and mortality. The treatment of choice in pregnant women with AIDS and *P. carinii* pneumonia is trimethoprim-sulfamethoxazole (SXT). Concomitant use of steroids is controversial. Studies of *in utero* exposure to SXT failed to show an increase in prematurity, hyperbilirubinemia, or kernicterus. Patients should be monitored for drug toxicity, such as rash, fever, neutropenia, thrombocytopenia, and hepatitis. Nausea and vomiting may occur and can exacerbate hyperemesis gravidarum.

In patients who cannot tolerate trimethoprim-sulfamethoxazole, pentamidine may be required because of the life-threatening risk of withholding treatment from the mother. If pentamidine is used, the mother should be closely monitored for hypoglycemia. Aerosolized pentamidine, because of poor systemic absorption and decreased systemic side-effects, has been advocated as safe, effective prophylaxis for *P. carinii* pneumonia. Prophylaxis against PCP with trimethoprim-sulfamethoxazole is known to be very effective, with rates of prevention of 90–95%. Given this, in pregnant patients with known human immunodeficiency (HIV)-positive status, prophylaxis should be strongly considered.

Amniotic fluid embolism

Amniotic fluid embolus (AFE) is a devastating, pregnancy-specific condition, in which both maternal and fetal death is the most probable outcome. It is one of the principal causes of maternal death in developed countries. There is direct support for the anaphylactoid nature of this condition, based on marked clinical similarities between a large series of patients with AFE and patients with both septic and anaphylactic shock.

Clinically, AFE manifests by the sudden development of hypoxia, hypotension, or cardiac arrest and disseminated intravascular coagulation (DIC). All components of the full AFE syndrome are not invariably present. AFE occurs as fetal tissue enters the maternal circulation and incites the reaction described above, probably via the release of various endogenous mediators. This most commonly occurs during labor but, in susceptible maternal–infant pairs, it has clinical onset at the time of Cesarean section.

The diagnosis of AFE is a clinical one based on physiologic manifestations and must be made after the exclusion of other conditions, such as myocardial infarction and pulmonary thromboembolism. The presence of a consumptive coagulopathy, although not required for the diagnosis of AFE, supports its diagnosis because acute consumptive coagulopathy in obstetrics is limited to AFE and placental abruption. Because some fetal debris is commonly found in the maternal circulation, the presence or absence of histologic pulmonary findings is not sufficient by itself to make the diagnosis of AFE, nor does its absence rule this syndrome out in the presence of appropriate clinical manifestations.

There is currently no way to predict or prevent AFE. Treatment of the mother is supportive, and involves the administration of O_2 in response to clinical hypoxia, preload and inotropic support of falling blood pressure, and blood component replacement for DIC with clinical hemorrhage. With the development of lethal cardiac dysrhythmia, standard basic and advanced cardiac life support protocols should be instituted.

In the presence of maternal cardiac arrest, maternal survival without profound neurologic impairment is rarely achieved. However, a clear relationship exists between arrest-to-delivery interval and neonatal outcome. Thus, expeditious perimortem Cesarean section should be initiated on the diagnosis of maternal cardiac arrest, regardless of its etiology, assuming the gestation has advanced to the point of fetal viability.

Venous air embolism

Venous air embolism may account for as many as 1% of maternal deaths, with risk factors being the performance of surgery, intravenous infusions, and central venous catheter placement. However, because the venous sinuses of the uterus are particularly susceptible to the entry of air during pregnancy, air embolism can occur during normal labor, delivery of a placenta previa, criminal abortions using air, orogenital sex, and insufflation of the vagina during gynecologic procedures. Maternal mortality associated with a clinically significant event exceeds 90% in untreated cases. The severity of a venous air embolism depends on the amount and rate of air entry. Small amounts of venous air are clinically undetectable, but accidental bolus injections of 100–300 mL^3 of air have been reported to be fatal. However, there are reports of patients surviving infusions of up to 1600 mL^3.

Embolization of a large bolus of venous air to the right ventricle results in mechanical obstruction to the forward flow of blood in the pulmonary artery outflow tract. In addition, the pumping action of the right ventricle acting on blood and air may produce platelet damage and fibrin formation, resulting in fibrin emboli that lodge in the pulmonary vascular bed. Maldistribution of pulmonary blood flow may result in ischemia or hyperperfusion, with the hyperperfused areas being susceptible to developing interstitial and alveolar edema. Areas that are initially ischemic may also become abnormally permeable once perfusion is restored. Paradoxical embolization can occur if there is an atrial septal defect, resulting in arterial ischemia or occlusion.

The patient initially presents with a feeling of faintness, dizziness, fear of impending doom, dyspnea, cough, diaphoresis, and substernal chest pain. Physical examination may reveal a state of altered consciousness, cyanosis, tachypnea, wheezing, tachycardia, hypotension, elevated jugular venous pressure, gallop rhythm, and an evanescent "mill wheel" or "waterwheel" murmur heard over the precordium. Paradoxical embolism may be evidenced by bubbles in the retinal arterioles, marble-like skin (air in the superficial dermal vessels), and possibly stroke or myocardial infarction. A blood gas test characteristically reveals hypoxemia, and there may be an associated metabolic acidosis. Chest radiography may occasionally demonstrate air in the right side of the heart or the main pulmonary artery, and the electrocardiogram may show signs of right heart strain, ischemia, or arrhythmia.

Therapy must be instituted promptly, and the patient should be placed in the left lateral decubitus position to minimize obstruction to the right ventricular outflow tract.

Administration of 100% O_2 promotes removal of nitrogen from the air bubble and results in more rapid absorption of the embolus. Nitrous oxide is highly soluble and, in a patient receiving general anesthesia, it should be discontinued because it can increase the size of the air embolus. In the presence of cardiovascular collapse, closed chest compression and aspiration of air from the right side of the heart via venous catheterization or transthoracic puncture have been suggested, although actual improved survival of pregnant women so treated has not been demonstrated. Hyperbaric O_2 may be useful in the setting of cerebral venous air embolism, and anticoagulation has been suggested to minimize the formation of fibrin microemboli. Mechanical ventilation may be necessary to treat permeability pulmonary edema.

Adult respiratory distress syndrome

Adult respiratory distress syndrome (ARDS) is the final common pathway of pathophysiologic changes occurring in the lungs as a consequence of a variety of acute bodily insults that reach the lung directly or via the vasculature. Clinically, patients present with marked respiratory distress, tachypnea, hypoxemia refractory to O_2 therapy, "stiff' noncompliant lungs that require high pressures to achieve inflation, and diffuse bilateral interstitial and alveolar infiltrates on chest radiograph. The central pathophysiologic event in ARDS is injury to the alveolar–capillary membrane, either directly or via mediators delivered by the pulmonary vasculature, which results in increased vascular permeability and noncardiogenic pulmonary edema. Severe hypoxemia results from both increased shunting of unoxygenated blood and impaired ventilation and perfusion matching in the alveoli, with an arterial PO_2 of typically less than 50–60 mmHg despite an inspired O_2 concentration of 60% or more. To make the diagnosis of ARDS, chronic pulmonary disease and left heart failure (cardiogenic pulmonary edema) must be excluded, and an appropriate precipitating event should be present. Right heart catheterization is often required to demonstrate that the pulmonary capillary hydrostatic pressure is not elevated, but the data thus obtained should be assessed in the light of the expected decrease in colloid oncotic pressure during pregnancy and in the immediate postpartum

Table 37.3 Causes of ARDS in pregnant women.

Abruption	Intra-abdominal abscess
Air embolism	Intrauterine fetal demise
Amniotic fluid embolism	Lung contusion
Aspiration	Nonthoracic trauma
Bacterial pneumonia	Pancreatitis
Blood transfusion	Preeclampsia, eclampsia
Carcinogenesis	Pyelonephritis
Diabetic ketoacidosis	Seizure
Drugs	Septic abortion
Fat embolism	Septicemia
Fractures	Shock
Fungal and *Pneumocystis carinii* pneumonia	Tocolytic therapy
Head trauma	Tuberculosis
Inhaled toxin	Uremia

period. Mortality in patients with ARDS continues to exceed 50%, a figure that has remained fairly constant over the last 20 years.

In the pregnant patient, ARDS can be associated with many of the factors that complicate pregnancy and delivery including septicemia, AFE, aspiration of stomach contents, eclampsia, septic abortion, venous air embolism, abruptio placentae, blood transfusion (with white blood cell agglutination in the pulmonary circulation), dead fetus syndrome (with DIC), drug overdose (narcotics, barbiturates, aspirin), fat embolism (after long bone fracture), hemorrhagic shock, seizures, and overwhelming pneumonia (Table 37.3).

Clinical presentation
Clinically, the patient with ARDS of any etiology may go through four clinical stages:
1 injury;
2 apparent stability;
3 respiratory insufficiency;
4 terminal stage.

The initial injury may occur without outward clinical signs and usually lasts for 6h or more. Next, the patient develops dyspnea associated with rapid shallow breathing and a persistent cough. Approximately 12–24h after injury, the chest radiograph may begin to show bilateral infiltrates that coalesce into a diffuse haze, representing perivascular fluid accumulation, interstitial edema, and alveolar edema.

Therapy of ARDS
Corticosteroids, in doses up to several grams of methylprednisolone over 24h, have been widely used in the treatment of full-blown ARDS without good evidence that

they are effective. However, although corticosteroids have not been shown to be effective in treating "early ARDS," there is some evidence to suggest that their use in the management of "late ARDS" is useful. The use of corticosteroids and mineralocorticoids to treat patients who are in shock that might be caused by or accompanied by adrenal insufficiency is warranted. Surfactant, a complex substance containing phospholipids and apoproteins, is used to treat RDS in premature infants, but there are some data to suggest that, when instilled by way of bronchoscopy, it may be useful in the treatment of ARDS. Efforts to identify pharmacologic agents effective in enhancing lung repair or blocking mediators of lung injury in ARDS have been largely unsuccessful. Nonsteroidal anti-inflammatory drugs, such as ibuprofen, meclofenamate, and indomethacin, have been studied *in vitro* and in animals and have shown some promise.

Reversible causes of ARDS, such as occult intra-abdominal or pelvic abscesses, should be sought because early surgical intervention and antimicrobial therapy may be life-saving. Patients with abruptio placentae, dead fetus syndrome, and septic abortion often have accompanying DIC. These patients should undergo delivery of the fetus or evacuation of the uterus as soon as the coagulopathy has been addressed and the patient is surgically stable.

Mechanical ventilation in ARDS

Ventilator therapy should be instituted when refractory hypoxemia is present and should be considered at the earliest recognition of ARDS-related symptoms to ensure fetal well-being. With correction of hypoxemia and respiratory alkalosis, fetal O_2 delivery can often be maintained at an adequate level. Pregnant patients with ARDS should be placed in the left lateral decubitus position, with the right buttock and hip elevated approximately 15°, or with the uterus manually displaced to the left, to maximize venous return. Continuous external fetal heart monitoring should be instituted when appropriate, and pulse oximetry can permit continuous monitoring of arterial oxygenation. Periodic blood gas determinations should be obtained to check acid–base status.

If the maternal arterial O_2 saturation cannot be maintained at or above 90%, with an F_iO_2 of 0.6 or less, then positive end-expiratory pressure (PEEP) should be added. Despite the lack of any clear evidence that its use improves mortality rates, PEEP is almost universally employed because it improves oxygenation and can reduce O_2 needs below potentially toxic concentrations. PEEP recruits atelectatic areas for gas exchange that would otherwise collapse during expiration and which are difficult to expand due to the loss of surfactant and structural derangements. The result is an increase in systemic arterial O_2 tension and in the lung's FRC and compliance. The use of PEEP is not without pitfalls, however, as it can overdistend alveoli, thereby decreasing compliance and increasing the risk of pneumothorax. The most important adverse effect is to decrease cardiac output by impeding venous return to the right side of the heart, particularly when the blood volume is low. An optimal PEEP has been defined as a level that increases oxygenation without significantly reducing cardiac output and, consequently, O_2 delivery.

Further reading

Ahmad H, Mehta NJ, et al. *Pneumocystis carinii* pneumonia in pregnancy. *Chest* 2001; 120(2):666–671.

Anon. Influenza vaccination and treatment during pregnancy. *ACOG Committee Opin* 2004; 305:1125–1126.

Barth W. Asthma in pregnancy. In: Clark SL, Cotton DB, Hankins GDV, Phenlan J, eds. *Critical care obstetrics*, 3rd edn. Malden, MA: Blackwell Science, 1997.

Benedetti TJ, Valle R, et al. Antepartum pneumonia in pregnancy. *Am J Obstet Gynecol* 1982;144(4):413–417.

Cheek TG, Gutsche BB. Maternal physiologic alterations during pregnancy. In: Shnider SH, Levinson G, eds. *Anesthesia for obstetrics*. Baltimore: Williams & Wilkins; 1984:3.

Clark SL, Hankins GD, et al. Amniotic fluid embolism: analysis of the national registry. *Am J Obstet Gynecol* 1995;172(4 Pt 1):1158–1167; discussion 1167–1169.

Fowler MJ Jr, Thomas CE, et al. Diffuse cerebral air embolism treated with hyperbaric oxygen: a case report. *J Neuroimaging* 2005;15(1):92–96.

Gardner MO, Doyle NM. Asthma in pregnancy. *Obstet Gynecol Clin North Am* 2004;31(2): 385–413, vii.

Mabie WC, Barton JR, et al. Adult respiratory distress syndrome in pregnancy. *Am J Obstet Gynecol* 1992;167(4 Pt 1):950–957.

38 Diabetes mellitus in pregnancy

Carol J. Homko, Zion Hagay, and E. Albert Reece

Diabetes mellitus is a heterogeneous disorder characterized by hyperglycemia, which is a result of relative or absolute insulin deficiency. It is estimated that diabetes mellitus affects approximately 4 million women of childbearing age in the United States.

Classification

Diabetes during pregnancy is still generally classified using the original system proposed by Priscilla White almost 40 years ago. White's classification relates the onset of diabetes, its duration, and the degree of vasculopathy to the outcome of pregnancy. Practically speaking, women with pregnancies complicated by diabetes mellitus may be separated into one of two groups:

1 Gestational diabetes: women with carbohydrate intolerance of variable severity, with onset or first recognition during the present pregnancy.

2 Pregestational diabetes: women known to have diabetes before pregnancy.

Table 38.1 presents the classifications that include these two groups.

Table 38.1 Classification of diabetes in pregnancy.

Pregestational diabetes:

Class	Age of onset (years)	Duration (years)	Vascular disease	Therapy
A	Any	Any	No	Diet only
B	> 20	< 10	No	Insulin
C	10–19	10–19	No	Insulin
D	Before 10	> 20	Benign retinopathy	Insulin
F	Any	Any	Nephropathy	Insulin
R	Any	Any	Proliferative retinopathy	Insulin
H	Any	Any	Heart disease	Insulin

Gestational diabetes:

Class	Fasting glucose level		Postprandial glucose level
A-1	< 105 mg/dL	*and*	< 120 mg/dL
A-2	> 105 mg/dL	*and/or*	> 120 mg/dL

Based on the American College of Obstetricians and Gynecologists (ACOG), Technical Bulletin no. 92 (Chicago), May 1986, with modifications.

Table 38.2 Classification of glucose intolerance.

	Nomenclature	Old name(s)
Type I	Type 1 diabetes	Insulin-dependent diabetes
		Juvenile-onset diabetes
Type II	Type 2 diabetes	Noninsulin-dependent diabetes
		Maturity-onset diabetes
Type III	Other specific types	Secondary diabetes
Type IV	Gestational diabetes mellitus	

From the Report of the Expert Committee on the Diagnosis and Classification of Diabetes Mellitus. *Diabetes Care* 1997;7:1183.

Epidemiology and etiology

As diabetes mellitus is a heterogeneous disorder rather than a single disease, the different types of diabetes should be distinguishable from each other (see Table 38.2).

Ninety percent of all pregnant diabetic patients have gestational diabetes mellitus (GDM), whereas type 1 (insulin-dependent diabetes) and type 2 (noninsulin-dependent diabetes) account for the remaining 10%. In general, type 1 and type 2

Table 38.3 Predominant characteristics of type 1 and type 2 diabetes.

Characteristic	Type 1	Type 2
Prevalence	0.1–0.5%	5–10%*
Weight at onset	Nonobese	Often obese
Age at onset	Usually young, < 30 years	Usually older, > 40 years
Seasonal variations	Yes	No
Insulin level	Low or absent	Variable
Ketosis	Most often	Unusual
MHC gene associations	HLA-DR$_4$, HLA-DR$_3$, HLA-DQ	No
Twin studies	30–50% concordance	80–100% concordance
Anti-islet cell antibodies	Positive in 70% of individuals with new type 1	No

HLA, human leukocyte antigen; MHC, major histocompatibility complex.
*Prevalence in Western countries.

diabetes can be distinguished from each other using clinical criteria and/or islet cell antibody studies (Tables 38.3 and 38.4).

Metabolic changes in normal and diabetic pregnancies

Insulin secretion and insulin resistance in normal pregnancy

Insulin is the major hormonal signal regulating metabolic responses to feeding and tissue use of carbohydrates; it is also the major glucose-lowering hormone. It is produced by the B cells of the pancreas and is secreted into the hepatic portal circulation, from which it reaches and acts on the liver and other peripheral tissues (i.e., muscle and fat). Insulin suppresses endogenous glucose production by inhibiting hepatic glycogenolysis and gluconeogenesis. On the other hand, it stimulates glucose uptake and fuel storage of glycogen and triglyceride in the liver, muscle, and adipose tissue (Table 38.5).

Late pregnancy is characterized by accelerated growth of the fetoplacental unit, rising plasma concentrations of several diabetogenic hormones including human placental lactogen and estrogens, and increasing insulin resistance. Several investigators have demonstrated increased first- and second-phase insulin release during late gestation as well as increased plasma insulin/glucose ratios. Buchanan and colleagues (1990), using the minimal model technique, found that peripheral insulin sensitivity was reduced to approximately one-third of normal during late gestation. Similar findings have been reported by other investigators using the euglycemic–hyperinsulinemic clamp technique. Decreases of 50% and 33% in insulin-stimulated glucose uptake have been reported, indicating peripheral insulin resistance during the third trimester of pregnancy.

Table 38.4 Empiric risk for offspring of parents with type 1 and type 2 diabetes developing diabetes.

Affected parent(s)	Empiric risk estimate of offspring
Type 1 diabetes	
Mother	1%
Father	6%
Parents unaffected, sibling affected	Overall 5–6%
	No. of haplotypes shared:
	1 haplotype = 5%
	2 haplotypes = 13%
	No haplotypes = 2%
Both parents affected	33%
Type 2 diabetes	
MODY	50%
Obese	7%
Nonobese	15%
Both parents affected	60–75%

MODY, maturity-onset diabetes of youth.

Table 38.5 Summary of the metabolic effects of insulin.

Target tissue	Enhances glucose and amino acid uptake
	Increases glycogen synthesis
	Converts glucose into fatty acids
	Inhibits glyconeogenesis
Muscle	Enhances glucose and amino acid uptake
	Increases glycogen synthesis
Adipose tissue	Increases glucose and amino acid transport
	Increases fatty acid synthesis
	Inhibits release of fatty acids from fat stores
	"Fat-sparing effect" is enhanced by glucose utilization in many tissues
Central nervous system	Has little or no effect on uptake or metabolism of glucose
All tissues	Increases protein synthesis
	Inhibits protein catabolism

From Brumfield C, Huddleston JF. The management of diabetic ketoacidosis in pregnancy. *Clin Obstet Gynecol* 1984;27:50.

Gestational diabebes mellitus

Definition and incidence

GDM is defined as carbohydrate intolerance of variable severity with onset or first recognition during the present pregnancy. This means that the glucose intolerance may have antedated the pregnancy but was not recognized by the patient or the physician. The incidence of GDM varies in different study populations and is estimated to occur in 3–5% of pregnant women. The likelihood of developing gestational diabetes is significantly increased among certain subgroups, and these include women with a family history of type 2 diabetes, advancing maternal age, obesity, and nonwhite ethnicity.

Screening for gestational diabetes

In the United States, screening for gestational diabetes mellitus consists of a 50-g oral glucose load, followed 1 h later by a plasma glucose determination. The screen is performed without regard to the time of day or interval since the last meal. It is recommended that screening be carried out at 24–28 weeks' gestation in average-risk women not known to have diabetes mellitus. Women deemed to be at high risk for GDM should be tested as soon as possible. Women possessing all of the following characteristics are considered to be a low risk and may not require testing: < 25 years of age, of normal weight, without a history of abnormal glucose metabolism or poor obstetric outcome, and with no first-degree relative with diabetes.

A value of plasma venous glucose between 130 and 140 mg/dL has been recommended as a threshold to indicate the need for a full diagnostic oral glucose tolerance test (OGTT). When the plasma glucose screening test results are > 185 mg/dL, patients are gestational diabetics and no further testing is required (Table 38.6).

Diagnosis

The diagnosis of GDM is, in most cases, based on an abnormal result of an OGTT during pregnancy. The OGTT is administered under standard conditions: 100 g of glucose is given orally in at least 400 mL of water after an overnight fast of 8–14 h.

Table 38.6 Incidence of a positive glucose tolerance test among 96 gravidas with 50-g, 1-h screening test values > 134 mg/dL (plasma, glucose oxidase).

Screening test result (mg/dL)	Incidence of gestational diabetes (%)
135–144	14.6
145–154	17.4
155–164	28.6
165–174	20.0
175–184	50.0
> 185	100.0

From Carpenter MW, Coustan DR. Criteria for screening tests for gestational diabetes. *Am J Obstet Gynecol* 1982;144:768.

Table 38.7 Oral glucose tolerance test (100-g) values for the diagnosis of gestational diabetes (mg/dL).

	Study: O'Sullivan*	NDDG†	Carpenter and Coustan‡
Fasting	90	105	95
1-h	165	190	180
2-h	145	165	155
3-h	125	145	140

*From O'Sullivan JB, Mahan CM. Criteria for the oral glucose tolerance test in pregnancy. *Diabetes* 1964;13:278.
†From the National Diabetes Data Group. Classification and diagnosis of diabetes mellitus and other categories of glucose intolerance. *Diabetes* 1979;28:1039.
‡From Carpenter and Coustan (1982).

The patient should have at least 3 days of unrestricted diet with more than 150 g of carbohydrates and should be at rest during the study. Diagnosis requires that at least two out of four glucose levels of the OGTT meet or exceed the upper limits of normal values. Whole blood and plasma glucose criteria of the OGTT used for the diagnosis of GDM are presented in Table 38.7.

Pregestational diabetes mellitus

Congenital anomalies in infants of diabetic mothers
The frequency of major congenital anomalies among infants of diabetic mothers has been estimated at 6–10%, which represents a two- to fivefold increase over the frequency observed in the general population. Congenital malformations in fetuses of diabetic patients are now responsible for approximately 40% of all perinatal deaths, replacing respiratory distress syndrome (RDS) as the leading cause of infant death. These malformations usually involve multiple organ systems (Table 38.8), with cardiac anomalies being the most common, followed by central nervous system and skeletal malformations.

Prevention of fetal anomalies
Clinical studies suggest that euglycemia during organogenesis is critical in the prevention of congenital anomalies. Several investigators have recruited diabetic women before pregnancy and attempted to place them under tight glycemic control before conception. These studies are summarized in Table 38.9.

Periconceptional care
Management of the pregnant diabetic woman is a complex task that ideally begins before conception. Prepregnancy clinics for diabetics were initiated in Edinburgh in 1976. In such clinics, physicians have the opportunity to explain to the patient and her partner the practice of diabetes care during pregnancy, in particular the need

Table 38.8 Congenital anomalies of infants of diabetic mothers.

Skeletal and central nervous system
  Caudal regression syndrome
  Neural tube defects excluding anencephaly
  Anencephaly with or without herniation of neural elements
  Microcephaly
Cardiac
  Transposition of the great vessels with or without ventricular septal defect
  Ventricular septal defects
  Coarctation of the aorta with or without ventricular septal defect or patent ductus
    arteriosus
  Atrial septal defects
  Cardiomegaly
Renal
  Hydronephrosis
Renal agenesis
  Ureteral duplication
  Gastrointestinal
  Duodenal atresia
  Anorectal atresia
  Small left colon syndrome
Other
  Single umbilical artery

From Reece EA, Hobbins IC. Diabetes embryopathy, pathogenesis, prenatal diagnosis and prevention. *Obstet Gynecol Surv* 1986;41:325.

for stringent glycemic control. At the initial visit, the patient's general medical status is assessed, and signs of retinopathy, nephropathy, hypertension, and ischemic heart disease are looked for. The patient undergoes ophthalmologic evaluation, electro-cardiography, and kidney function tests. Optimization of blood glucose control should be achieved before a woman is advised to become pregnant. It is generally recommended that women achieve a glycosylated hemoglobin level that is less than 1% above the upper limit of normal. Women should receive appropriate contraceptive therapy while preparing for pregnancy. For women who are not already following an intensive diabetes regimen, an extensive period of education and the institution of self blood glucose monitoring is also necessary.

Diabetes management during pregnancy

Diabetes during pregnancy has been associated with increased perinatal mortality, an increased rate of Cesarean sections, significant risk of macrosomia, and other neonatal morbidities, including serious birth trauma, hypoglycemia, hypocalcemia, polycythemia, and hyperbilirubinemia. Management is therefore directed toward reducing perinatal mortality and morbidity, a goal that may be achieved by maintaining close surveillance of the mother and fetus and stringent glucose control.

Table 38.9 Summary of selected clinical studies using a program of preconceptional metabolic control to prevent diabetes-associated birth defects.

Investigator (year)	No. of patients — Control group	Malformation rate (%)	Glucose control achieved	No. of patients — Study group	Malformation rate (%)	Glucose control achieved
Pedersen et al. (1979)	284	14.1	Inadequate	363	7.4	Improved
Miller et al. (1981)	58	22.4	HbA$_{1c}$ > 8.5%	58	3.4	HbA$_{1c}$ ≤ 8.5%
Fuhrmann et al. (1983)	292	7.5	Mean daily plasma glucose ≥110 mg/dL in 88.3% of patients	128	0.8	Mean daily plasma glucose ≥110 mg/dL in 20.7% of patients
Steel (1988)	65	9.2	–	78	3.9	–
Goldman et al. (1986)	31	9.6	MBG = 163 ± 10.2 mg/dL HbA$_{1c}$ = 10.42 ± 0.47%	44	0	MBG = 110 ± 6.5 mg/dL HbA$_{1c}$ = 7.39 ± 0.34%
Kitzmiller et al. (1986)	53	15.1	HbA$_{1c}$ < 9.0% in 47% of patients	46	2.2	HbA$_{1c}$ < 9.0% in 87% of patients
Mills et al. (1988)	279	9.0	–	397	4.9	–
Damm et al. (1989)	61	8.2	Mean HbA$_{1c}$ 7.3 ± 1.5%	193	1.0	Mean HbA$_{1c}$ 7.1 ± 1.2%
Steel et al. (1990)	143	10.4		96	1.4	
Kitzmiller et al. (1991)	110	25	HbA$_{1c}$ > 10.6%	84	1.7	HbA$_{1c}$ < 7.9%
Wilhoite et al. (1993)	123	6.5	–	62	1.6	–

HbA$_{1c}$, hemoglobin A$_{1c}$; MBG, mean blood glucose.

From Reece EA, Friedman AM, Copel J, Kleinman CS. Prenatal diagnosis and management of deviant fetal growth and congenital malformations. In: *Diabetes mellitus in pregnancy*, 2nd edn. New York: Churchill Livingstone, 1995.

Diet

Diet therapy is considered a standard treatment for diabetes mellitus. The goals of diet therapy are to provide adequate maternal and fetal nutrition, appropriate gestational weight gain, and to minimize glucose excursions. For women with pregestational diabetes, guidelines suggest that diet composition should be based on an individualized nutrition assessment. In GDM, it is generally accepted that carbohydrate levels should not exceed 40–45% of total calories. Restricted saturated fats and cholesterol and increased dietary fiber are suggested. Most patients are instructed on how to maintain a diet that consists of three meals and one to three snacks, the last snack usually being taken at bedtime. The bedtime snack should be composed of complex carbohydrates with proteins to maintain adequate blood glucose levels during the night, thereby avoiding nocturnal hypoglycemia.

Patient weight gains are assessed at each visit to the clinic, and caloric intake is adjusted accordingly. The aim is to prevent weight reduction and its associated ketogenic risk while ensuring optimal weight gain. It is desirable to increase weight by 2–4 lb (0.9–1.7 kg) in the first trimester and 0.5–1.0 lb (200–450 g) per week thereafter until term. A total weight gain of 22–30 lb (10–13 kg) during normal and diabetic pregnancy is recommended.

It is generally agreed that pregnancy is not the time for weight reduction; however, excessive weight gain should be firmly discouraged. Dietary advice to the obese pregnant diabetic patient is a matter of controversy. Several authors have indicated that caloric restriction in obese pregnant patients is contraindicated. However, there are data to show that modest caloric restriction (25–30 kcal/day), especially for the morbidly obese patient, is not associated with ketonuria or elevated plasma ketone concentrations.

Insulin administration

Insulin is the only pharmacologic therapy currently recommended to treat diabetes during pregnancy. The goal of insulin therapy is to achieve blood glucose levels that are nearly identical to those observed in healthy pregnant women. Therefore, multiple injections of insulin are usually required in women with pre-existing diabetes. Human insulin is the least immunogenic of all insulins and is exclusively recommended in pregnancy. The rapid-acting insulin analogs with peak hypoglycemic action 1–2 h after injection offer the potential for improved postprandial glucose control. Studies support their safety during pregnancy and their ability to improve blood glucose control. Insulin requirements may change dramatically throughout the various stages of gestation. In the first trimester, the maternal insulin requirement is approximately 0.7 U/kg of body weight/day. This is increased in the third trimester to 1.0 U/kg/day. There are several different approaches to insulin administration, as outlined in Table 38.10. We prefer to use the three-injection scheme, which permits better control of the fasting blood glucose levels while minimizing the risk of middle-of-the-night hypoglycemia.

In addition, continuous subcutaneous insulin infusion pumps have also been shown to be effective during pregnancy. Insulin therapy delivered by a subcutaneous

Table 38.10 General guidelines for insulin administration.

Regimen no.	Prebreakfast insulin	Prelunch insulin	Predinner insulin	Bedtime insulin	Comments
I. Two-injection scheme	NPH + regular or rapid-acting analog; 2:1	–	NPH + regular or rapid-acting analog	–	Give two-thirds of the total dose as prebreakfast dose and one-third as predinner dose. Disadvantage: predinner NPH may cause nocturnal hypoglycemia (1–3 AM) and may not be effective in controlling the early morning glucose level
II. Three-injection scheme	NPH + regular or rapid-acting analog; 2:1	–	Regular or rapid-acting analog	NPH	This regimen may be more effective than regimen I. By changing the administration of NPH to bedtime, nocturnal hypoglycemia may be prevented and early morning glucose control may be achieved
III. Four-injection scheme	NPH + regular or rapid-acting analog	Regular or rapid-acting analog	Regular or rapid-acting analog	NPH	This is the most effective regimen. We use it as an alternative to regimen II. Here the dose of insulin given at bedtime replaces basal daily insulin requirements. This regimen (with a rapid-acting analog) works especially well for patients with morning sickness or erratic schedules

NPH, neutral protamine Hagedorn.

infusion pump more closely resembles that of physiologic insulin release. Insulin pumps deliver a continuous basal rate of insulin infusion with pulse-dose increments before meals.

Insulin therapy should be initiated in all women with GDM who fail to maintain euglycemia with diet. We start women on a daily insulin dose of 20 U of neutral protamine Hagedorn (NPH) and 10 U of regular insulin daily. Insulin doses are adjusted according to blood glucose levels, and an evening injection is added if fasting hyperglycemia persist. Some investigators have advocated the use of prophylactic insulin in

GDM to reduce the risk of macrosomia. However, the advantages of this therapy must be weighed against the disadvantages of no treatment.

Although the current data demonstrate a relationship between metabolic control and neonatal complications, maternal glycemia may not be the sole parameter of optimal control. In women with gestational diabetes, Buchanan and colleagues (1990) have suggested the use of fetal ultrasound to identify pregnancies at risk of fetal macrosomia and related morbidity. They have found that a fetal abdominal circumference < 75th percentile for gestational age obtained in the late second trimester or early third trimester can distinguish pregnancies at low risk from those at high risk of producing large for gestational age (LGA) infants. Their data suggest that maternal glucose concentrations alone may not accurately predict which fetuses are at high risk of excessive fetal growth and support the use of fetal criteria to direct metabolic therapies in GDM.

Self-monitoring of blood glucose

Self blood glucose monitoring has become the mainstay of management for pregnancies complicated by diabetes mellitus. Blood glucose measurements should be obtained at least four times a day (fasting and 1–2 h after meals) in women with gestational diabetes and five to seven times a day in women with pre-existing diabetes. In addition to this regular monitoring, patients should also test whenever they feel symptoms of either hyperglycemia or hypoglycemia. Detailed record keeping is useful to help identify glucose patterns. Daily urine ketone testing should be performed to insure early identification of the development of starvation ketosis or ketoacidosis. Ketone testing should also be performed any time the blood glucose level exceeds 200 mg/dL, during illness, or when the patient is unable to eat.

Antepartum assessment

Maternal assessment

Ophthalmologic and renal function tests, including creatinine clearance and total urinary protein excretion, are performed in each trimester, or more often if indicated. In patients with vasculopathy, an electrocardiogram is performed at the initial visit and repeated, if clinically indicated. In patients in White's class H, the electrocardiogram is performed routinely in each trimester. The echocardiogram is performed at enrollment and repeated in the pregnancy, depending on the initial findings. It is extremely important to detect early signs of pregnancy-induced hypertension; therefore, an assessment of blood pressure and the signs of proteinuria and edema formation is essential. It is estimated that approximately 25% of all diabetics develop preeclampsia during pregnancy. The highest incidence is seen among patients with vasculopathy.

Fetal surveillance

All pregnancies complicated by diabetes require extra assessment. The use of ultrasonography provides essential information about the fetus. A first-trimester scan is used to date the pregnancy and to establish viability and fluid volume status. A second-trimester scan is repeated at 18–20 weeks' gestation to rule out fetal anomalies. Subsequent ultrasound evaluations are then performed at 4- to 6-week intervals to assess fluid volume and fetal growth. Because diabetic patients are at risk of growth aberrations (intrauterine growth restriction and macrosomia), this frequency is recommended to identify states of altered growth.

Antepartum fetal testing

In pregnant diabetic patients, stillbirth occurs with increased frequency, particularly in the third trimester. Therefore, a program of fetal monitoring should be initiated, usually at 32–33 weeks. Currently, in most medical centers, outpatient protocols for antepartum fetal surveillance include either once- or twice-weekly nonstress tests (NSTs), once-weekly oxytocin challenge tests (OCTs), or biophysical profiles. Which is the best test remains controversial because controlled, prospective randomized studies comparing the various methods of antepartum fetal assessment are lacking. Many investigators have concluded that the NST is simple, inexpensive, and reasonably reliable. Therefore, the NST is most widely used for pregnancies complicated by diabetes mellitus.

Timing and mode of delivery

In recent years, there has been a significant change in the attitude of obstetricians and perinatologists toward the mode and timing of delivery of type 1 and type 2 pregnant patients. It is now recognized worldwide that, if the pregnant diabetic patient and her fetus are under stringent metabolic control and antepartum surveillance, delivery may be safely delayed in most cases until term or the onset of spontaneous labor. During labor and delivery, it is necessary to maintain maternal euglycemia to avoid neonatal hypoglycemia.

Maternal complications

Diabetic women have a markedly higher risk of a number of pregnancy complications. Because of a paucity of data on maternal complications during diabetic pregnancy, the exact relative risk for each complication is not known. Complications that have been reported to be more frequent in diabetic pregnancy include spontaneous abortion, preterm labor, pyelonephritis, polyhydramnios, and hypertensive disorders. Also directly related to metabolic control are hypoglycemia and diabetic ketoacidosis (DKA; Fig. 38.1). These complications, together with the vascular alterations and the higher Cesarean section rate, contribute to the higher maternal morbidity and mortality among diabetic pregnant patients.

Morbidity of the infant of the diabetic mother

In the last decade, the perinatal morbidity rate in pregnancies complicated by diabetes mellitus has been remarkably reduced. However, severe neonatal morbidity in infants

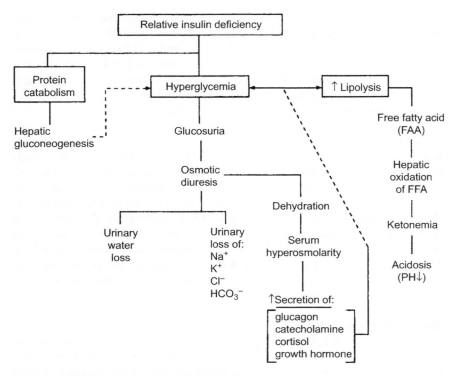

Figure 38.1 Metabolic alterations in diabetic ketoacidosis.

of diabetic mothers is still a problem that may affect even infants delivered at term. The following sections briefly discuss the most common neonatal morbidities.

Hypoglycemia

Hypoglycemia is diagnosed when plasma glucose levels are less than 35 mg/dL and 25 mg/dL in term and preterm infants respectively. Infants of diabetic mothers in unsatisfactory glycemic control often develop hypoglycemia during the first few hours of life. The reported incidence ranges from 25% to 40% of infants of diabetic mothers. Poor glycemic control during pregnancy and high maternal plasma glucose levels at the time of delivery increase the risk of occurrence, particularly if the patients have been delivered by Cesarean section. The most efficient means of therapy for hypoglycemia is continuous dextrose infusion at a rate of 4–6 mg/kg/min. The use of a bolus of a hypertonic glucose infusion should be avoided to prevent later rebound hypoglycemia. Occasionally, hypoglycemia may persist beyond the second day of life and may require the use of glucocorticoids.

Hypocalcemia and hypomagnesemia

There is a significant increase in the incidence of hypocalcemia and hypomagnesemia in infants of diabetic mothers. The incidence of neonatal hypocalcemia, defined as calcium levels at or below 7 mg/dL, has been reported to approach 20% in a group of infants with a mean gestational age at delivery of 38 ± 0.2 weeks.

Polycythemia

Polycythemia is diagnosed when the venous hematocrit exceeds 65%. This condition has been reported to affect one-third of neonates of diabetic mothers in the first few hours of life. The mechanism responsible for polycythemia in these babies may be related to chronic intrauterine hypoxia that leads to an increase in erythropoietin and a consequent increase in red blood cell production.

Respiratory distress syndrome (RDS)

RDS was considered a common neonatal morbidity in the infants of diabetic mothers in the past. However, the incidence has decreased dramatically with the initiation of strict glycemic control. Factors contributing to the development of RDS in these infants are preterm deliveries, delayed fetal lung maturation, and a high rate of elective Cesarean section.

Hyperbilirubinemia

Infants of diabetic mothers have a higher incidence of hyperbilirubinemia than do infants of nondiabetic mothers matched for gestational age. The mechanism of this increased risk of jaundice is not clear. Early treatment of polycythemia may further reduce the risk of hyperbilirubinemia.

Cardiomyopathy

Infants of diabetic mothers have a higher risk of hypertrophic types of cardiomyopathy and congestive heart failure. The characteristic findings in echocardiography are generalized myocardial hypertrophy with disproportionate hypertrophy of the interventricular septum. Infants of diabetic mothers with severe cardiomyopathy may develop left ventricular outflow tract obstruction with reduced cardiac output and congestive heart failure. The natural history of cardiomyopathy in infants of diabetic mothers is different from other types of cardiomyopathy in that there is a complete regression of hypertrophic changes to normal after several months.

Conclusion

The diagnosis of diabetes mellitus during pregnancy has certain implications for the well-being of both the mother and the fetus. Advances in medical and obstetric care have dramatically improved the outlook for women with diabetes and their offspring. However, both mother and child remain at increased risk for a number of complications. Research indicates that the majority of these complications are associated with hyperglycemia. The achievement and maintenance of euglycemia has therefore become the major focus of management.

Further reading

American College of Obstetricians and Gynecologists. Management of diabetes in pregnancy. *ACOG Tech Bull* 1994;200:1–8.

Buchanan TA, Metzger BE, Freinkel N, et al. Insulin sensitivity and B-cell responsiveness to glucose during late pregnancy in lean and moderately obese women with normal glucose tolerance or mild gestational diabetes. *Am J Obstet Gynecol* 1990;162:1008–1014.

Engelgau MM, Herman WH, Smith PJ, et al. The epidemiology of diabetes and pregnancy in the US, 1998. *Diabetes Care* 1995;18:1029–1033.

Homko CJ, Sivan E, Reece EA, Boden G. Fuel metabolism during pregnancy. *Semin Reprod Endocrinol* 199;17:119–125.

Jovanovic-Peterson L, Peterson CM. Exercise and the nutritional management of diabetes during pregnancy. *Obstet Gynecol Clin North Am* 1996;23:75–86.

Kjos SL, Schaefer-Graf U, Sardesi S, et al. A randomized controlled trial using glycemic plus fetal ultrasound parameters versus glycemic parameters to determine insulin therapy in gestational diabetes with fasting hyperglycemia. *Diabetes Care* 2001;24:1904–1910.

Metzger BE, Coustan DR. Summary and recommendations of the Fourth International Workshop Conference on Gestational Diabetes Mellitus. *Diabetes Care* 1998;21(Suppl. 2):B161–167.

Reece EA, Homko CJ. Why do diabetic women deliver malformed infants? *Obstet Gynecol Clin* 2000;43:32–45.

Reece EA, Coustan DR, Gabbe SG, eds. *Diabetes in women: adolescence, pregnancy and menopause*, 3rd edn. Philadelphia, PA: Lippincott Williams & Wilkins, 2004.

Weintrob N, Karp M, Hod M. Short and long-range complications in offspring of diabetic mothers. *J Diabetes Complic* 1996;10:294–301.

White P. Pregnancy complicating diabetes. *Am J Med* 1949;7:609.

39 Endocrine disorders in pregnancy

Fred Faas

Significant endocrine changes occur during normal pregnancy (see Table 39.1). Prolactin levels rise progressively to 100–300 ng/mL by late pregnancy (Fig. 39.1). Twenty-four-hour urine free cortisol, plasma cortisol, and adrenocorticotrophic hormone (ACTH) levels all rise normally during pregnancy as a result of large rises in corticotrophic-releasing hormone (CRH), derived from the fetal–placental unit (Table 39.2). Salt and water metabolism changes during pregnancy with a decrease in plasma osmolality to a level of about 10 mOsmol/kg below normal. Renin and aldosterone levels rise progressively to more than twice the levels in the nonpregnant state (Fig. 39.2). A placental growth hormone variant is secreted into the circulation during pregnancy rising to mean levels of > 20 ng/mL, which results in the doubling of insulin-like growth factor (IGF)-1 levels (Fig. 39.3). Total calcium levels fall during pregnancy as a result of hemodilution, but ionized calcium levels, serum 25(OH)vitamin D, and parathyroid hormone levels are typically normal.

Table 39.1 Significant changes in endocrine hormonal levels during normal pregnancy.

Increase in serum prolactin
Increase in serum ACTH and cortisol
Mild decrease in TSH
Increase in plasma renin activity and serum aldosterone
Increase in serum IGF-1

ACTH, adrenocorticotrophic hormone; IGF-1, insulin-like growth factor-1; TSH, thyroid-stimulating hormone.

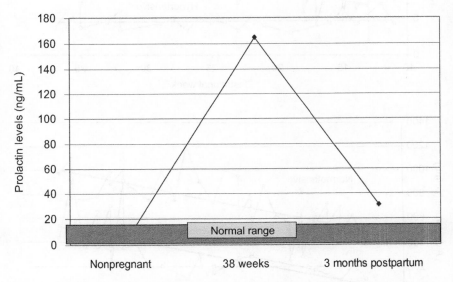

Figure 39.1 Changes in serum prolactin levels during pregnancy and in the postpartum period. Data shown in the figure were derived from the data from O'Leary et al. (1991) and Campino et al. (2001).

Table 39.2 Mean concentrations of CRH, ACTH, cortisol and urine free cortisol in pregnant and non-pregnant women.

Study group	CRH (pg/mL)	ACTH (pg/mL)	Serum cortisol (µg/dL)	Urine free cortisol (µg/24 h)
Non-pregnant	< 41	1.3 ± 0.4	9.2 ± 4.0	29 ± 1
21–24 weeks' gestation	158 ± 5	8.2 ± 1.8	15.4 ± 1.9	–
25–28 weeks' gestation	315 ± 50	11.4 ± 0.9	23.7 ± 3.1	–
29–32 weeks' gestation	705 ± 115	15.0 ± 0.9	31.9 ± 5.0	–
22–34 weeks' gestation	–	–	–	89 ± 14
33–36 weeks' gestation	2060 ± 490	16.4 ± 3.2	36.7 ± 5.4	–
37–40 weeks' gestation	4410 ± 893	13.2 ± 1.8	37.7 ± 4.0	–

Adapted from Goland R, Conwell I, Warren W, et al. Placental corticotropin-releasing hormone and pitultary–adrenal function during pregnancy. *Neuroendocrinology* 1992;56:742.

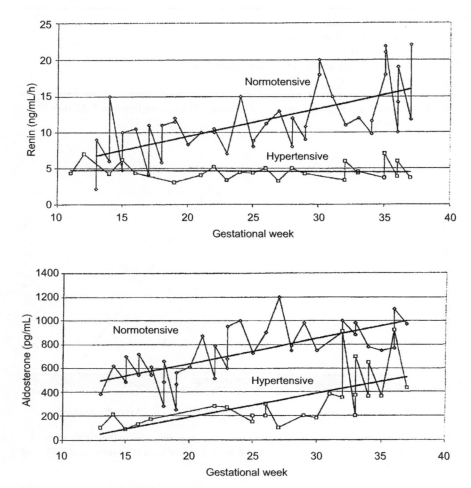

Figure 39.2 Plasma renin activity and aldosterone levels during pregnancy in normotensive and hypertensive women. Reprinted from Elshikh A, Creatsas G, Mastorakos G, et al. The renin–aldosterone system during normal and hypertensive pregnancy. *Arch Gynecol Obstet* 2004;264:182.

Thyroid-binding globulin levels increase during pregnancy as a result of increased estrogen levels, which leads to increases in total thyroxine (T_4) and total tri-iodothyroxine (T_3) levels without changes in free hormone levels. However, because of a thyrotropic effect of the high human chorionic gonadotropin (hCG) levels in pregnancy, a mild decrease in thyroid-stimulating hormone (TSH) occurs. Free T_4 levels may rise slightly but generally remain within the normal range. This requires different normal ranges for TSH during each trimester of pregnancy. An increase in thyroid size may occur during pregnancy, likely due to a relative iodine deficiency.

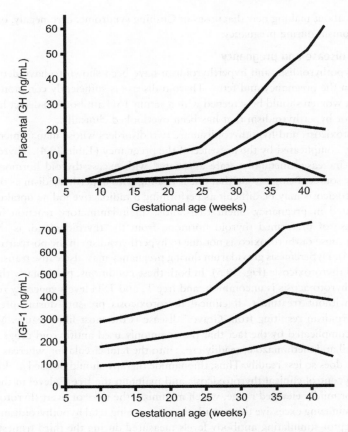

Figure 39.3 Placental growth hormone (GH) and IGF-1 levels during pregnancy. The lines shown represent the mean and 95% confidence interval. Reprinted with minor changes from Chellakooty M, Vangsgaard K, Larsen T, et al. A longitudinal study of intrauterine growth and the placental growth hormone (GH)–insulin-like growth factor 1 axis in maternal circulation: association between placental GH and fetal growth. *J Clin Endocrinol Metab* 2004;89:384.

Table 39.3 Endocrine disorders whose diagnosis is substantially complicated by hormonal changes occurring during normal pregnancy.

Prolactinoma, Cushing syndrome, acromegaly, hyperaldosteronism

Endocrine disorders in pregnancy

As a result of the above changes, diagnostic evaluation of certain endocrine disorders is more difficult (Table 39.3). A new diagnosis of a prolactin-producing tumor is not often a clinical problem as most such patients are infertile. One should be cautious about making new diagnoses of Cushing syndrome, acromegaly, or hyper-aldosteronism during pregnancy.

Thyroid disease and pregnancy

Overt hypothyroidism and hyperthyroidism have been shown to have detrimental effects on the pregnancy and fetus. Thyroid disease is sufficiently common that all pregnant women should be screened with a serum TSH antibody to detect hypothyroidism or hyperthyroidism that has been overlooked clinically.

Thyrotoxicosis and hypothyroidism are two disorders whose management is significantly complicated by the presence of the pregnancy (Table 39.4). Thyrotoxicosis is an increased metabolic state associated with excess thyroid hormone levels from any source. Being certain that one is dealing with hyperthyroidism as the cause of thyrotoxicosis may be difficult as performing a radioactive iodine uptake is contraindicated in pregnancy. Silent thyroiditis, an inflammatory reaction inducing the release of preformed thyroid hormone from the thyroid gland, is the most common cause of thyrotoxicosis not due to hyperthyroidism in the postpartum state (Fig. 39.4). Hyperemesis gravidarum during pregnancy may also cause transient biochemical thyrotoxicosis (Fig. 39.5). In both these conditions, particularly the latter, clinical thyrotoxicosis is uncommon, and free T_4 and TSH levels generally return to normal without treatment. If clinical thyrotoxicosis presents during pregnancy, hyperthyroidism resulting from Graves' disease is the most likely cause. Management is complicated by the fact that the commonly used antithyroid drugs, propylthiouracil and methimazole, readily cross into the fetal circulation whereas thyroid hormone does so less readily. Thus, thionamide therapy should be used at doses sufficient to control clinical thyrotoxicosis and maintain the free T_4 level in the upper normal or mildly elevated range, which minimizes the risks of overt thyrotoxicosis, while minimizing excessive thionamide therapy causing fetal hypothyroidism. Serum TSH receptor-stimulating antibody levels measured during the third trimester may help to predict the risk of transient thyrotoxicosis in the neonate (Fig. 39.6).

Hypothyroidism, even mild, should be treated promptly during pregnancy. Pregnant women with hypothyroidism on L-thyroxine therapy should be monitored frequently during pregnancy as L-thyroxine requirements may increase by as much as 50%.

Pituitary disorders and pregnancy

Pituitary prolactinoma is another endocrine disorder whose management is signifi-

---

Figure 39.4 Clinical pattern of postpartum thyroid dysfunction in three women studied weekly for 30 weeks postpartum. FT3, free T_3; FT4, free T_4; RAIU, percent radioactive iodine uptate at 24 h; TPOAb, thyroid peroxidase antibodies. The top part of the figure shows hormone levels from a patient with transient hyperthyroidism developing 8–9 weeks postpartum; the middle part of the figure is from a patient with transient hyperthyroidism developing 22–24 weeks postpartum; and the lower part of the figure is from a patient developing modest transient hyperthyroidism followed by severe transient hypothyroidism. Note the significant rise in anti-TPO antibody. Reprinted from Lazarus et al. (1996).

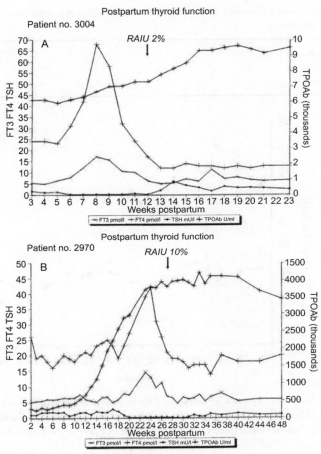

Postpartum thyroid function

Patient no. 3004

A

RAIU 2%

Postpartum thyroid function

Patient no. 2970

B

RAIU 10%

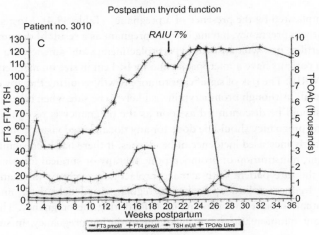

Postpartum thyroid function

Patient no. 3010

C

RAIU 7%

Table 39.4 Endocrine disorders whose management is significantly complicated by the presence of pregnancy.

Thyrotoxicosis
Hypothyroidism
Prolactinoma

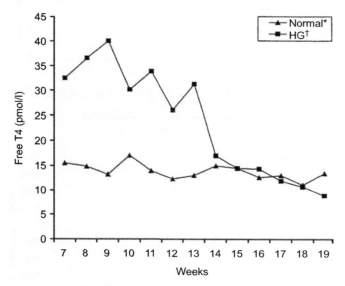

Figure 39.5 Mean free T_4 levels by gestation. *Mean free T_4 levels established in the normal population. †Mean free T_4 levels in women with hyperemesis gravidarum. Reprinted from Tan J, Loh K, Yeo G, et al. Transient hyperthyroidism of hyperemesis gravidarum. *Br J Obstet Gynaecol* 2002;109:683.

cantly complicated by the presence of a pregnancy (Table 39.4). Most such patients present early in pregnancy, having become pregnant as a result of dopamine agonist-induced fertility in a woman with hyperprolactinemia and amenorrhea. The majority of such patients have a microprolactinoma [< 1 cm in size on magnetic resonance imaging (MRI)]. The risk of significant tumor growth requiring therapy during pregnancy is small. Although bromocryptine is likely to be safe when taken during pregnancy, it should be discontinued as soon as the pregnancy is recognized. A repeat MRI during pregnancy should be done for any documented visual field disturbances or significantly increased incidence of headaches. If there has been significant tumor enlargement, reinstitution of bromocryptine therapy or surgical intervention is necessary. In the rare patient with a macroprolactinoma who is pregnant, one must undertake frequent follow-up including regular visual field determinations by a neuro-ophthalmologist and a follow-up MRI during the pregnancy. There is a risk of significant symptomatic tumor enlargement during pregnancy. In such patients,

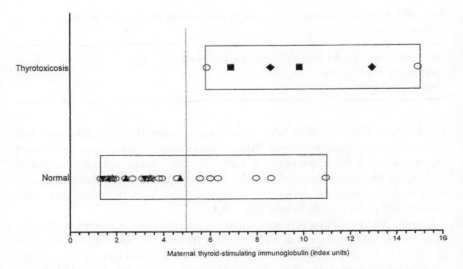

Figure 39.6 Maternal thyroid-stimulating immunoglobulin values and pregnancy outcomes in 35 pregnancies. There are 29 data points in the bar with normal outcomes. Solid figures of similar shape represent different pregnancies from the same mother. Reprinted from Peleg D, Cada S, Peleg A, et al. The relationship between maternal serum thyroid-stimulating immunoglobulin and fetal and neonatal thyrotoxicosis. *Obstet Gynecol* 2002;99:1040.

one must weigh up the advantages and disadvantages of continuing or initiating dopamine agonist therapy against careful follow-up therapy. Both bromocryptine and cabergoline are probably safe when given throughout pregnancy.

Pituitary tumors other than prolactinomas have no particularly association with pregnancy but may coexist with pregnancy. Secretory pituitary tumors such as pituitary Cushing disease and acromegaly have occasionally been seen in pregnancy. Because of the increased levels of ACTH, cortisol, placental growth hormone and IGF-1 that occur during a normal pregnancy, caution should be exercised in making these diagnoses in a pregnant patient (Table 39.3). If a patient with known acromegaly or Cushing diseases becomes pregnant, the best course is to delay treatment of the primary disease until the pregnancy is complete unless there are pressing clinical reasons to do otherwise.

In the unusual patient with partial hypopituitarism who is pregnant, thyroid replacement should be monitored with free T_4 levels, keeping free T_4 in the middle to high normal range. Patients with diabetes insipidus may experience worsening of their condition during pregnancy related to increased clearance of arginine vasopressin. Desmopressin is the preferred therapy in such patients. Cortisol replacement should consist of 30 mg of hydrocortisone daily in divided doses.

Postpartum endocrine disorders

Several endocrine disorders have an increased incidence in the postpartum period

Table 39.5 Endocrine disorders more likely to occur during pregnancy or in the post-partum period.

Silent thyroiditis with thyrotoxicosis and/or hypothyroidism
Lymphocytic hypophysitis
Sheehan syndrome

(Table 39.5). Silent thyroiditis (also known as postpartum thyroiditis) is more likely to occur in the postpartum period than at other times. It may present as transient thyrotoxicosis or hypothyroidism. A low radioactive iodine uptake is helpful in making the diagnosis. It generally resolves without specific therapy, although treatment with beta-blockers during the thyrotoxic phase or L-thyroxine during the hypothyroid phase may be helpful (Fig. 39.4).

Lymphocytic hypophysitis is an uncommon inflammatory autoimmune disorder of unknown etiology occurring with increased frequency in the postpartum period (Table 39.5). It usually presents with symptoms of a mass effect including headaches, visual field disturbances, and a sellar/suprasellar mass visualized on MRI. Partial hypopituitarism and diabetes insipidus are frequently present. Careful observation is appropriate as lymphocytic hypophysitis often improves spontaneously or responds to glucocorticoid therapy.

Sheehan syndrome is another endocrine disorder presenting in the postpartum period. It usually presents as panhypopituitarism, which results from hypotension due to massive vaginal bleeding at or around the time of delivery. Typically, the key to diagnosis is the history of bleeding, the failure to lactate in the postpartum period, and failure of the resumption of menses. Once the diagnosis is suspected, diagnostic evaluation and therapeutic hormonal replacement should be instituted immediately.

Adrenal gland disorders

Congenital adrenal hyperplasia

Pregnancy in a woman with congenital adrenal hyperplasia presents some special issues. Prenatal diagnosis of 21-hydroxylase deficiency in the fetus is now possible, raising the issues of when prenatal diagnosis and possible therapeutic intervention is appropriate. Such decisions must be made after counseling of the parents by someone trained in genetic counseling, and informing them of the potential risks of the procedure, the probability of the fetus being affected, and the risks and benefits of identifying an affected fetus. Optimal treatment to prevent virilization in the affected female fetus requires the administration of glucocorticoids, preferably dexamethasone, prior to the seventh week of gestation followed by chorionic villus sampling at 10 weeks. As the chances of the fetus being an affected female are fairly small, a decision to undergo these procedures should only be made after thoughtful consideration.

Adrenocortical tumors and pheochromocytoma are not increased in prevalence during pregnancy, but they raise special diagnostic or therapeutic considerations because of the pregnancy. In primary hyperaldosteronism, Cushing syndrome due to an adrenal adenoma, or pheochromocytoma, therapeutic decisions must be individualized, always balancing the risk to the fetus and mother of drug therapy or surgical intervention against the risk of nonintervention.

In patients with adrenal insufficiency, management should be the same as in the nonpregnant state except that it may be best to use replacement hydrocortisone doses at the higher end of usual replacement therapy such as 30 mg daily in divided doses.

Disorders of calcium metabolism

Adequate vitamin D intake is important during pregnancy and in the postpartum period while the mother is nursing. Even in the absence of frank vitamin D deficiency, recent studies have indicated that taking 2000–4000 IU of supplemental vitamin D daily while nursing during the first few months after birth may be helpful and is safe.

The diagnosis of hyperparathyroidism is not complicated by pregnancy other than that total calcium levels during pregnancy are a bit lower than in the nonpregnant state. Only in severe hyperparathyroidism with a serum calcium > 12 mg/dL is surgical therapy recommended. Patients with idiopathic or surgical hypoparathyroidism who become pregnant should be managed just as if they were not pregnant with sufficient doses of calcitriol and calcium to keep the serum calcium in the low normal range.

Summary

In this chapter, the endocrine changes that occur during normal pregnancy have been reviewed, emphasizing the impact of these changes on the diagnosis and treatment of various endocrine disorders in pregnancy. It is hoped that this review will make the physician better able to diagnose and treat the pregnant woman with an endocrine disorder.

Further reading

Alexander E, Marqusee E, Lawrence J, et al. Timing and magnitude of increases in levothyroxine requirements during pregnancy in women with hypothyroidism. *N Engl J Med* 2004;351:241.

Campino C, Torres C, Rioseco A, et al. Plasma prolactin/oestradiol ratio at 38 weeks gestation predicts the duration of lactational amenorrhoea. *Hum Reprod* 2001;16:2540.

Garner P. Congenital adrenal hyperplasia in pregnancy. *Semin Perinatol* 1998;22:446.

Gharib H, Tuttle R, Baskin J, et al. Consensus statement. Subclinical thyroid dysfunction: a joint statement on management from the American Association of Clinical Endocrinologists, the American Thyroid Association, and the Endocrine Society. *J Clin Endocrinol Metab* 2005;90:581.

Hollis B, Wagner C. Vitamin D requirements during lactation: high-dose maternal supplementation as therapy to prevent hypovitaminosis D for both the mother and nursing infant. *Am J Clin Nutr* 2004;80(Suppl.):1752S.

Laurberg P, Nygaard B, Glinoer D, et al. Guidelines for TSH-receptor antibody measurements in pregnancy: results of an evidence-based symposium organized by the European Thyroid Association. *Eur J Endocrinol* 1998;139:584.

Lazarus J, Hall R, Othman S, et al. The clinical spectrum of postpartum thyroid disease. *Q J Med* 1996;89:429.

Mastorakos G, Ilias I. Maternal and fetal hypothalamic-pituitary-adrenal axis during pregnancy and postpartum. *Ann NY Acad Sci* 2003;997:136.

Molitch M. Pituitary tumors and pregnancy. *Growth Hormone IGF Res* 2003;13:S38.

Nader S. Thyroid disease and other endocrine disorders in pregnancy. *Obstet Gynecol Clin North Am* 2004;31:257.

O'Leary P, Boyne P, Flett P, et al. Longitudinal assessment of changes in reproductive hormones during normal pregnancy. *Clin Chem* 1991;37:667.

Reis F, Florio P, Cobellis L, et al. Human placenta as a source of neuroendocrine factors. *Biol Neonate* 2001;79:150.

Tan J, Loh K, Yeo G, et al. Transient hyperthyroidism of hyperemesis gravidarum. *Br J Obstet Gynecol* 2002;109:683.

40 Gastrointestinal diseases complicating pregnancy

Washington Clark Hill and Alfred D. Fleming

Pregnancy can complicate almost any gastrointestinal disease. The pregnant woman may enter pregnancy with a gastrointestinal disorder, or it may develop during pregnancy. The physiologic effects of pregnancy may cause gastrointestinal disturbances such as nausea, vomiting, hyperemesis gravidarum, and esophageal reflux. Conversely, gastrointestinal disorders such as ruptured appendix, gallbladder, and inflammatory bowel disease may affect the course of pregnancy. This chapter discusses the various gastrointestinal diseases complicating pregnancy and their effect on the fetus and mother.

Diseases within the gastrointestinal tract

Nausea, vomiting, and hyperemesis gravidarum

Nausea with or without vomiting is an especially common symptom during early pregnancy. It usually occurs during the first trimester of pregnancy and, by midpregnancy, most women no longer complain of these symptoms. In its mildest form, it is referred to as "morning sickness." The cause of nausea and vomiting during pregnancy is unknown. The management of nausea and vomiting during pregnancy is primarily supportive. Therapeutic regimens include reassurance, physical and psychological support, frequent small meals, the avoidance of foods that are unpleasant or that may initiate symptoms, adequate hydration and fluid intake, and selective, occasional use of antiemetics. There is no ideal antiemetic currently available for the treatment of morning sickness. When symptoms require treatment, both pyridoxine and doxylamine are still available over the counter as Unisom (25 mg).

Antiemetic therapy should be used when supportive measures are not effective. Other antiemetics that have also been used successfully in the treatment of nausea and vomiting in pregnancy include the phenothiazines, trimethobenzamide, metoclopramide, and diphenhydramine.

Hyperemesis gravidarum is the abnormal condition of pregnancy associated with pernicious nausea and vomiting. These patients experience persistent intractable nausea and vomiting associated with weight loss, fluid and electrolyte imbalance, ketonuria, and ketonemia. Electrolyte imbalance may include decreased sodium, potassium, and chloride, and metabolic alkalosis. The patient usually becomes clinically dehydrated. Outpatient therapy consisting of intravenous fluid hydration is usually sufficient, along with supportive therapy. Intravenous pyridoxine, 100 mg/L of intravenous fluid, has been included as a part of the therapy. However, when the patient's condition does not improve, hospitalization with appropriate electrolyte, caloric, and fluid management is necessary.

Refractory hyperemesis gravidarum has been successfully treated with corticosteroid therapy. Corticosteroids are effective in suppressing symptoms of intractable hyperemesis, decreasing the length of hospitalization, and allowing normal maternal nutrition. Studies have established the efficacy and safety of corticosteroid therapy for refractory hyperemesis. Methylprednisolone in tapering doses is the drug of choice.

Oral cavity complications of pregnancy

Bleeding from the gingivae, a common complaint of pregnant women, due to pregnancy gingivitis, requires no treatment. Gingivitis that is due to poor dentition and hygiene is treated by good cleaning of the teeth and by meticulous dental care. There is no basis for delaying dental care during pregnancy, and patients who require treatment should obtain it promptly. Pregnancy tumor is a granuloma that forms as a result of exaggerated gingival enlargement during pregnancy.

The treatment of dental problems associated with pregnancy is rarely contraindicated and may be performed safely. If the treatment is necessary but elective, it is best delayed until the second trimester, when there is the least risk of teratogenesis. Emergency treatment should be obtained whenever indicated. There is little or no harm to the fetus when dental radiographs are taken with the necessary precautions, good techniques, and modern equipment. Laboring patients with oral jewelry should remove the hardware before receiving anesthesia for safety reasons. There is now evidence that maternal periodontal disease and incident progression are significant contributors to obstetric risk for preterm delivery.

Reflux esophagitis

Heartburn or pyrosis is really a symptom of reflux esophagitis. Reflux esophagitis is the pathophysiologic process in the esophagus that causes the symptoms of heartburn. Heartburn is a very common, bothersome complaint during pregnancy. Treatment of reflux esophagitis during pregnancy consists primarily of neutralizing the acid material that is being refluxed into the esophagus, thereby decreasing gastro-esophageal reflux. Symptomatic strategies include dietary modification. The avoid-ance of recumbency, particularly immediately after eating a meal, is likewise to be avoided. A variety of antacids have been prescribed for heartburn. All these over-the-counter preparations neutralize gastric acid, which is responsible for the symp-toms. The use of metoclopramide and similar drugs, although safe, should be avoided except in severe cases. The histamine H2 receptor antagonists and/or the proton pump inhibitors can also be prescribed for severe and persistent symptoms. The symptoms of reflux esophagitis can be so severe or difficult to treat that esophagoscopy, parenteral hyperalimentation, and parenteral nutrition are neces-sary. These procedures may be performed safely, when necessary, during pregnancy for this and other gastrointestinal diseases complicating pregnancy.

Peptic ulcer disease

The development of peptic ulcer disease during pregnancy is uncommon and rare. Patients who have peptic ulcers before pregnancy frequently experience fewer symp-toms during pregnancy and may even become totally asymptomatic.

The symptoms of peptic ulcer disease are quite similar to those of reflux esophagi-tis. The most common symptom of peptic ulcer disease is complaints of heartburn or dyspepsia. Peptic ulcer disease is diagnosed by the visualization of the ulcer by radiography or endoscopy. Although the upper gastrointestinal series is sometimes used to diagnose peptic ulcer disease in a nonpregnant patient, esophagoscopy when necessary should be used in the pregnant patient. This is usually not necessary except in the patient who has symptoms that do not respond to antacids. However, patients with persistent and serious gastrointestinal signs and symptoms from peptic ulcer disease or other disorders may require endoscopy during pregnancy.

The treatment of peptic ulcer disease consists primarily of the use of antacids, which are safe to use during pregnancy. A combination of magnesium trisilicate and aluminum hydroxide is found in most antacid preparations. Sodium bicarbonate should not be used as an antacid during pregnancy, because it can lead to the absorp-tion of large amounts of sodium. Patients with peptic ulcer disease should avoid a diet of foods that cause discomfort. Smoking, which should be avoided in both preg-nant and nonpregnant women, and alcohol should certainly be eliminated from the diets of these patients. Aspirin and the nonsteroidal and inflammatory drugs such as indomethacin can produce gastric irritation and, with prolonged use, gastric ulcers. Indomethacin, which is used for tocolysis, should be avoided in patients with active or a history of peptic ulcer disease.

Histamine H2 receptor blockers such as cimetidine and ranitidine are second-line therapy for peptic ulcer disease. They do cross the placenta, but no teratogenic risk has been detected from their use during the first trimester. H2 receptor antagonists decrease the production of histamine. Histamine H2 blockers are a mainstay in the medical therapy of peptic ulcer disease. There are several concerns about the use of cimetidine during pregnancy. It is an antiandrogen and has produced gynecomastia and impotence in a small number of male animals and male users. Cimetidine's use is and should be reserved for those patients who have symptoms refractory to antacid therapy. Ranitidine, famotidine, and nizatidine are other H2 receptor antagonists that have been used for ulcer therapy during pregnancy without maternal or neonatal complications.

The newest antisecretory agents are the proton pump inhibitors: omeprazole, lansoprazole, esomeprazole, pantoprazole, and rabeprazole. These drugs suppress gastric acid secretion by a direct inhibitory effect on the gastric parietal cell. The use of these drugs during pregnancy has been limited. The use of proton pump inhibitors during pregnancy, although limited, does not present a teratogenic risk when used in recommended doses.

Acute intestinal obstruction

Intestinal obstruction is a serious complication of pregnancy that is occurring with increasing frequency. Acute intestinal obstruction is most common in the third trimester, less common in the second, and least likely in the first trimester. The most common cause of intestinal obstruction in the pregnant and nonpregnant woman is adhesions.

The diagnosis of intestinal obstruction in pregnancy is not easy. As with appendicitis, delay in diagnosis is not uncommon. Pain, although usually present, may be constant, colicky, mild, severe, diffuse, or localized. Physical examination may or may not reveal guarding or rebound tenderness. Abdominal distention can easily be missed in late pregnancy because of the normally large uterus and abdomen. Bowel sounds may be normal, absent, or high-pitched with rushes. Physical examination, however, can be completely nondiagnostic. If there is considerable delay in diagnosis and the patient is not appropriately treated, then third spacing of fluids occurs. This results in dehydration, electrolyte imbalance, hypotension, oliguria, fever, tachycardia and, eventually, shock and death.

Diagnosis, once suspected clinically, can be made by limited radiographic studies showing bowel distention, intraluminal fluid levels, and decreased gas in the large bowel. The concern of obtaining radiographic studies during pregnancy should be tempered by the increased maternal and fetal mortality associated with delayed or misdiagnosis. Radiographic or serial studies showing dilated, gas-filled loops of bowel with air–fluid levels is diagnostic.

Treatment of intestinal obstruction during pregnancy is the same as in the nonpregnant patient. Exploratory laparotomy is the treatment of choice. Prior to surgery, close attention must be paid to the correction of fluid and electrolyte imbalance, maintenance of adequate urinary output, administration of blood and blood products, and fetal monitoring.

Inflammatory bowel disease

The term inflammatory bowel disease refers to a group of idiopathic chronic inflammatory diseases of the intestinal tract. The two most commonly seen during pregnancy are ulcerative colitis and Crohn's disease, also called regional enteritis. Both these disorders are not uncommon in women during their reproductive years and are frequently seen either before or during pregnancy.

The pathologic features of these two diseases distinguish and differentiate them. These two disorders share a common cause, clinical findings, and management. Ulcerative colitis and Crohn's disease may be so similar clinically that a specific diagnosis of the type of inflammatory disease present cannot be made. They can be characterized as chronic disorders that go through periods of quiescence and exacerbation, making differentiation even more difficult.

The best prognosis for pregnancy is in those patients who had inactive disease at the time of conception or whose active disease is limited to early pregnancy. Patients with inactive ulcerative colitis that becomes active during early pregnancy do not have an increased risk of spontaneous abortion; patients who develop active disease later in pregnancy or postpartum are at increased risk for spontaneous abortion, stillbirth, and preterm labor. The effect of Crohn's disease on pregnancy is similar. Adverse pregnancy outcome, as reflected by prematurity, stillbirths, spontaneous abortion, or congenital anomalies, does not appear to be increased. The route of delivery may be affected by inflammatory bowel disease. Cesarean section has been recommended if severe perineal fistulas or scarring, which can occur as a complication of Crohn's disease, are present.

Inflammatory bowel disease is treated by both medical and surgical measures during pregnancy. The mainstay of the medical therapy for both ulcerative colitis and Crohn's disease is the use of mesalamine preparations, sulfasalazine, and corticosteroids. Mesalamine is more efficacious in the treatment of ulcerative colitis than in regional enteritis. Mesalamine is now the most commonly used drug in the treatment of inflammatory bowel disease and is safe to use during pregnancy (FDA risk category B; see Tables 40.1 and 40.2).

Corticosteroid therapy has been used in both these diseases to suppress the inflammatory response present in the bowel. It is also frequently used in treating exacerbations of Crohn's disease. The corticosteroids most frequently used are prednisone, hydrocortisone, and prednisolone. There are no adverse effects on the fetus from the use of corticosteroids during pregnancy. Breastfeeding likewise is not contraindicated in the mother on corticosteroid therapy.

Medical management should include nutritional assessment and treatment, as in any patient with a chronic disease. Adequate calories should be provided to help prevent weight loss. General therapeutic measures include antidiarrheal drugs such as codeine, opium, paregoric, and diphenoxylate with atropine (Lomotil). As in the treatment of hyperemesis gravidarum, the patient should have the opportunity to discuss the psychological factors of pregnancy or other aspects of her life, which may be playing a part in the precipitation of inflammatory bowel disease. Inflammatory bowel disease may require surgical treatment.

Appendicitis

Appendicitis remains the most common cause of an acute abdomen during pregnancy. The incidence during pregnancy has been reported to vary from 1 per 1000 to 1 per 2000 pregnancies, with an average incidence of 1 per 1500 deliveries. There

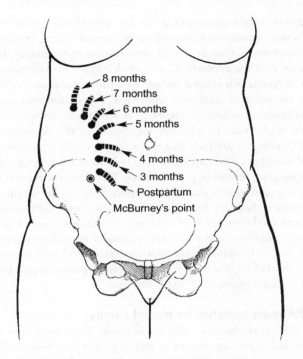

Figure 40.1 Change in the position of the appendix during pregnancy.

appears to be no increased frequency during any particular trimester. Appendicitis occurring postpartum is particularly difficult to diagnose, because peritonitis is a less prominent finding.

The pregnant woman with appendicitis has symptoms and signs similar to those in the nonpregnant patient, but may not experience abdominal rigidity, rebound, or similar signs of peritonitis. Abdominal pain is present, but usually not at McBurney's point. This is due to the change in the position and direction of the appendix during pregnancy (Fig. 40.1). As pregnancy advances, the cecum is displaced toward the iliac crest, thus moving the appendix laterally, superiorly, and posteriorly. The abdominal pain of appendicitis is typically mild at onset. During pregnancy, it is even less severe. It may be intermittent or colicky, due to a fecalith within the appendix. The pain is followed within an hour or two by anorexia, nausea, and vomiting, symptoms frequently seen during a normal pregnancy. The temperature may be normal, or there may be a low-grade fever. An increasing left shift in the differential may be helpful in making the diagnosis. The urinalysis is usually not helpful other than in excluding the diagnosis of urinary tract infection. Both computed tomography (CT) and magnetic resonance imaging (MRI) are helpful and safe during pregnancy in the diagnosis of acute appendicitis.

Appendectomy is the treatment of choice for appendicitis during pregnancy. It is the most frequent nonobstetric procedure performed during pregnancy. Laparoscopic appendectomy is now as safe as open surgery in pregnancy. It is becoming the standard of care for appendicitis and cholelithiasis management during pregnancy. Some surgeons still suggest the use of a transverse muscle-splitting incision directly over the point of maximum tenderness. During the operation, the uterus should be manipulated as little as possible. The left lateral position with uterine displacement should be used to minimize the chance of the development of supine hypotension. Antibiotics are indicated when the appendix is perforated or there is extensive inflammation. There are no data to indicate that tocolysis reduces the incidence of uterine contractions or preterm labor. Therefore, the routine usage of such agents in these circumstances cannot be supported. When the diagnosis is made in the third trimester, there are few, if any, indications for a simultaneous Cesarean delivery, except in the presence of obstetric indications. Vaginal delivery is not precluded, with minilaparotomy and appendectomy immediately postpartum. The complication rate with rupture of the appendix can be very high, including fetal loss and maternal morbidity. When the diagnosis is made promptly and procrastination in treatment does not occur, fetal loss is lowered.

Pregnancy following operation for morbid obesity

Over the past 30 years, patients who are morbidly obese have been undergoing a variety of surgical bypass operations to induce weight loss. Seventy-five percent of these patients are women and therefore may be seen after their bypass pregnant. Most pregnant women with a jejunoileal bypass tolerate pregnancy quite well. It has been recommended that they receive supplemental iron, folic acid, vitamin B12, and a prenatal vitamin–mineral preparation. An occasional patient appears to do poorly, developing intrauterine growth retardation and metabolic disorders. Pregnancy is not contraindicated after jejunoileal bypass, but a 2-year interval before pregnancy is undertaken has been suggested so that the patient will not become pregnant during the highest phase of weight loss and to allow the weight loss to plateau. Because of long-term complications, including persistent electrolyte abnormalities, the jejunoileal bypass procedure is no longer performed. Gastric restrictive operations have now developed as the operations of choice for the patient who is morbidly obese. These include gastroplasty, gastric stapling, and gastric bypass techniques. It has been recommended that a woman undergoing one of these procedures should not become pregnant for at least 1 year.

Constipation

Constipation is a common symptom of pregnancy. The treatment of constipation during pregnancy should consist mainly of nutrition counseling, increased fluid intake, and dietary modification. Constipation may result in the development of hemorrhoids. These can usually be treated by topical ointments or sprays, stool softeners, sitz baths, and over-the-counter preparations. When hemorrhoids develop during the puerperium after vigorous pushing, they may become thrombosed. Incision after local anesthesia may be necessary and beneficial.

Diseases adjacent to the gastrointestinal tract

Gallbladder disease

Classically, the female patient with gallbladder disease has been described as "fair, fat, forty, and fertile." Gallbladder disease is uncommon during pregnancy. It may occur as cholelithiasis or acute cholecystitis.

Cholelithiasis

Pregnancy predisposes to gallstones. Biliary colic or pain, which is due to choledocholithiasis, is a form of chronic cholecystitis in which the gallstones become impacted or pass through the biliary tract, and is the most common symptom that gallstones produce during pregnancy. The pain is due to the passage of the gallstones from the gallbladder into the cystic duct or the common bile duct. This produces a spasm of the gallbladder or the biliary duct involved. Although biliary colic is most frequently present in the right upper quadrant, it may also be epigastric, colicky, or steady in intensity. Unlike appendicitis, the pain of biliary colic is not altered in location or character. The patient may also experience nausea, vomiting, and, if cholangitis is present, fever. Jaundice may be present, although gallstones account for only 5% of the causes of jaundice during pregnancy. Depending on where the stone becomes impacted in the biliary tree, obstructive jaundice (common bile duct) or acute pancreatitis (ampulla of Vater) may occur. The symptoms of cholelithiasis may cease spontaneously once the stone is passed through the biliary tract or may persist, requiring surgical removal.

Laboratory diagnosis of gallstones in pregnancy is the same as in nonpregnant patients. The leukocyte count and differential may be normal or slightly elevated, depending on the degree of cholangitis. Hyperbilirubinemia and elevation in levels of aminotransferases, aspartate aminotransferase (AST; formerly called SGOT) and alanine aminotransferase (ALT; formerly called SGPT) may be present. The serum alkaline phosphatase level is elevated by biliary obstruction. This is not helpful during pregnancy because elevated serum alkaline phosphatase is normal in the pregnant patient as a result of placental production. The presence of acute pancreatitis as a result of common duct stones may cause pancreatitis and elevated serum amylase and lipase levels.

Real-time ultrasound has revolutionized the diagnosis of biliary tract disease during pregnancy. Several studies have shown ultrasound to be 95–98% sensitive in diagnosing both solitary and multiple gallstones in the gallbladder or biliary tract. Cholecystectomy is the second most frequent nonobstetric abdominal surgical procedure performed in pregnancy. Nonoperative therapy consisting of hospitalization, antibiotics, analgesia, nil by mouth, and nasogastric suction may be all that is necessary in patients who have mild illness. Patients with symptoms that do not improve with observation and medical therapy require prompt cholecystectomy. Many authors have demonstrated that a delay in surgery for biliary tract disease complications results in increased maternal and fetal morbidity and mortality. Cholecystectomy during pregnancy should be performed during the second trimester if possible. Several recommendations should be kept in mind when a patient requires cholecystectomy in the second half of pregnancy. Tocolytic therapy may be necessary and should be instituted if preterm labor occurs. There are no data to support or condemn the use of prophylactic tocolysis around the time of surgery. Surgery should be delayed until after delivery if possible when symptoms arise in the third trimester, although laparoscopic cholecystectomy has been performed safely even at that time.

Laparoscopic cholecystectomy is a safe procedure during pregnancy. The procedure has become the standard of care for treatment. Endoscopic management of biliary disease during pregnancy has been proposed. Endoscopic retrograde cholangiopancreatography (ERCP) has been shown to decrease morbidity, mortality, and costs as a definitive treatment alternative for pancreaticobiliary disease in pregnancy. However, further clinical evaluation of this aggressive endoscopic intervention during pregnancy is necessary.

Acute cholecystitis
The clinical manifestations of acute cholecystitis during pregnancy are the same as in the nonpregnant patient. Conservative medical management is the mainstay in the treatment of the pregnant patient with acute cholecystitis. This consists of nasogastric suction when necessary, analgesia, intravenous hydration, and antibiotics. Intravenous ampicillin or a cephalosporin are the drugs of choice. Most patients will respond to this medical management. Cholecystectomy should be reserved for those patients who have gallstone pancreatitis, jaundice, repeated attacks, or who fail medical management.

The Society of American Gastrointestinal Endoscopic Surgeons (SAGES) has adopted some guidelines to enhance operative safety in the pregnant patient including:
• When possible, operative intervention should be deferred until the second trimester, when fetal risk is low.
• Because pneumoperitoneum enhances lower extremity venous stasis already present in a gravid patient and because pregnancy is a hypercoagulable state, pneumatic compression devices must be used.
• Fetal and uterine status, as well as maternal endtidal carbon dioxide and arterial blood gases, should be monitored.
• The uterus should be protected with a lead shield if intraoperative cholangiography is a possibility. Fluroscopy should be used selectively.
• Given the enlarged gravid uterus, abdominal access should be attained using an open technique.
• Dependent positioning should be used to shift the uterus off the inferior vena cava.

- Pneumoperitoneum pressures should be minimized (8–12 mmHg) and not allowed to exceed 15 mmHg.
- Obstetric consultation should be obtained preoperatively.

Pancreatitis

The exact incidence of acute pancreatitis during pregnancy has been difficult to determine. It is not common. Pancreatitis can reoccur during the same or subsequent pregnancy or the puerperium. When pancreatitis develops in women of less than 30 years of age, half of them are pregnant.

The clinical picture of acute pancreatitis is characteristic. The symptoms and signs include a rapid onset of constant, central midepigastric pain that may radiate to the chest and back, and can be quite severe. In mild cases of pancreatitis, pain may be the only symptom that the patient experiences. Not infrequently, however, nausea and severe vomiting may occur alone or with pain. Low-grade fever and absent or decreased bowel sounds also aid in the diagnosis. The classic clinical presentation of a patient with pancreatitis is an individual rocking in the bed with her knees drawn up and trunk flexed in agony. The pain may also radiate to the flanks or shoulders due to the development of peritoneal irritation. Other symptoms include tachycardia in response to the pain, hypotension, ascites, pleural effusion, hypotonic bowel sounds or ileus, tenderness over the epigastrium, and generalized peritonitis. An adynamic ileus may be demonstrated on radiographic examination. The severity of the clinical features will depend on the severity of the pancreatitis and whether or not complications occur, such as pseudocyst or abscess formation.

Laboratory evaluation of the patient suspected to have pancreatitis may be helpful. Rarely is the white blood cell count above 30 000 cells/μL. It may even be within the range for normal pregnancy, 10 000–20 000 cells/μL. The serum amylase is the specific test used to diagnose pancreatitis and is usually elevated to more than 200 IU/mL. A serum amylase above 1000 IU/mL is almost always indicative of pancreatitis or an obstruction of the pancreatic duct. Serum amylase has been reported to be both increased and unchanged in the normal pregnancy.

Diagnostic ultrasound can be used to visualize the pancreas for the presence of pseudocyst or abscess. When inflamed, the pancreas can appear normal, swollen, or enlarged. At the same time, the gallbladder and biliary ducts can be visualized to rule out the presence of gallstones. The pancreas can also be evaluated during pregnancy by a CT scan. As both ultrasound and CT demonstrate pancreatitis, failure to demonstrate enlargement of the pancreas in a case of suspected acute pancreatitis should institute a search for other causes of hyperamylasemia.

Treatment for acute pancreatitis is primarily nonoperative. Management includes intravenous fluid hydration to correct hypovolemia and electrolyte imbalance, correction of hyperglycemia, enteric rest with nasogastric suction, broad-spectrum antibiotics, and adequate analgesia. Insulin may be necessary to reduce the blood sugar.

Maternal mortality is low when diagnosis is made promptly and appropriate management instituted. The prognosis for the fetus is also good unless severe peritonitis occurs, which predisposes the patient to spontaneous abortion or preterm birth.

Preterm labor occurs in 60% of patients when pancreatitis develops late in pregnancy. The mode of delivery is not affected by pancreatitis and, unless contraindicated for obstetric reasons, vaginal delivery is recommended.

Effects on the fetus of drugs used in treating gastrointestinal diseases

In 1979, the US Food and Drug Administration (FDA) established a system of five categories to indicate the potential of systemically absorbed drugs to be teratogenic. These risk categories were defined as A, B, C, D, and X and are used by manufacturers to rate their products for use during pregnancy. This classification is currently under revision by the FDA. A review of data on teratology by the American College of Obstetricians and Gynecologists found none of the commonly used drugs in the

Table 40.1 Gastrointestinal drugs frequently used in the treatment of gastrointestinal disorders during pregnancy.

Drugs	FDA risk category
Azathioprine	D
Cimetidine	B
Diazepam	D
Diphenoxylate	C
Doxylamine	B
Droperidol	C
Esomeprazole	B
Famotidine	B
Lansoprazole	B
Lidocaine	C
Loperamide	B
Meperidine	B
Mesalamine	B
Metoclyopramide	B
Misoprostol	X
Nizatidine	C
Olsalazine	C
Omeprazole	C
Pantoprazole	B
Prednisone	B
Prochlorperazine	C
Promethazine	C
Rabeprazole	B
Ranitidine	B
Sulcralfate	B
Tetracycline	D
Trimethobenzamide	C

treatment of gastrointestinal disease during pregnancy to be teratogenic. Table 40.1 lists drugs frequently used in the treatment of gastrointestinal diseases during pregnancy with their FDA risk category. The maternal condition, gestational age, treatment need, and benefit to the mother and risk to the fetus, especially of category C or X drugs, must be considered when these drugs are used during pregnancy.

Total parenteral nutrition in pregnancy

Pregnant patients unable to consume sufficient nutrients orally require an effective method of feeding. Alternative forms of nutrition are being used more frequently in obstetrics. Total parenteral nutrition (TPN), parenteral nutrition, hyperalimentation, intravenous hyperalimentation, and intravenous feedings are used synonymously and interchangeably to describe the various methods of providing all the required nutrients intravenously. Recently, numerous authors have reported long-term parenteral nutrition being provided with good results to a variety of hospitalized or outpatient pregnant patients at significant risk of malnutrition and poor fetal outcome. Patients at high risk of malnutrition during pregnancy may also benefit from TPN. TPN, whether in the pregnant or the nonpregnant patient, can be complicated by maternal death. Other complications include accidental pneumothorax or hemothorax, catheter infection, various metabolic disorders, glycosuria, hypoglycemia and, rarely, clinical sepsis. It has been demonstrated that enteral or parenteral nutrition can be safely and effectively administered during pregnancy. A team of qualified, knowledgeable individuals who are familiar with the techniques being used should explain it to the patient, obtain written consent, and manage the administration of the parenteral nutrition.

Further reading

Abell TL, Riely CA. Hyperemesis gravidarum. *Gastroenterol Clin North Am* 1992;21:835.

Baron TH, Richter JE. Gastresophageal reflux disease in pregnancy. *Gastroenterol Clin North Am* 1992;21:777.

Briggs GG, Freeman RK, Yaffee SJ, eds. *Drugs in pregnancy and lactation*, 7th edn. Philadelphia, PA: Lippincott, Williams and Wilkins, 2005.

Eliakim R, Abulafia O, Sherer DM. Hyperemesis gravidarum: a current review. *Am J Perinatol* 2000;17:207.

Cappell MS. Gastrointestinal disorders during pregnancy. Preface. *Gastroenterol Clin North Am* 2003;32:xi–xiii (Preface), 1–448.

Katz JA, Pore G. Inflammatory bowel disease and pregnancy. *Inflamm Bowel Dis* 2001;7:146.

Malangoni MA. Gastrointestinal surgery and pregnancy. *Gastroenterol Clin North Am* 2003;32:181.

Sharp HT. The acute abdomen during pregnancy. *Clin Obstet Gynecol* 2002;45:405.

Viktrup L, Hee P. Appendicitis during pregnancy. *Am J Obstet Gynecol* 2001;185:259.

Weiner CP, Buhimschi C, eds. *Drugs for pregnant and lactating women*. Philadelphia, PA: Churchill Livingstone, 2004.

41 Liver disease in pregnancy

Vivek Raj

Liver diseases in pregnancy (Table 41.1)

Pregnancy does not affect liver physiology in any significant manner. Hemodynamic and biochemical changes in normal pregnancy are outlined in Table 41.2. Aspartate aminotransferase (AST), alanine aminotransferase (ALT), bilirubin, gamma-glutamyltransferase (GGT), and serum bile acid concentration remain unchanged in pregnancy, while alkaline phosphatase (ALP) is mildly elevated (placental ALP). Elevation of any of these, or jaundice, warrants further investigation.

Liver diseases unique to pregnancy (Table 41.3)

Hyperemesis gravidarum

This condition is characterized by severe nausea and vomiting, frequently leading to dehydration and ketosis. It is seen in 1–1.5% of pregnancies, usually starts in the first trimester, and is more common in primiparous women. AST and ALT can be significantly elevated up to 500 IU/L, and bilirubin and ALP are mildly elevated. Liver biopsy is not necessary but, if performed, shows centrilobular vacuolation. Most patients respond to intravenous hydration, bowel rest, and symptomatic treatment of vomiting. There is no impact on the child. In severe cases, the birthweight may be low.

Intrahepatic cholestasis of pregnancy (ICP)

This is a benign cholestatic disorder that usually occurs during the second or third trimester and disappears shortly after delivery. It is characterized by pruritis, specifically involving the hands and feet, cholestatic liver test abnormalities, and occasionally jaundice (10–15% cases). Prevalence in the United States is 1–2 per 10 000 pregnancies. The exact cause is unknown. Liver biopsy shows cholestasis but no inflammation or necrosis. Total serum bile acids are increased, AST and ALT are elevated two- to 10-fold, and bilirubin up to sixfold. Prothrombin time may be elevated as a result of vitamin K malabsorption and should be corrected with vitamin K to avoid postpartum hemorrhage. ICP increases the risk of prematurity and stillbirth. Treatment is symptomatic with antihistaminics and phenobarbital. Ursodeoxycholic acid improves pruritis, liver test abnormalities, and may prevent prematurity. In severe cases, early delivery after 36 weeks should be considered.

Preeclampsia and liver disease

The commonest liver disease seen in preeclampsia is HELLP syndrome, which is characterized by hemolysis, elevated liver test values, and low platelets. It

Table 41.1 Liver diseases in pregnancy.

Liver diseases unique to pregnancy
  Hyperemesis gravidarum
  Intrahepatic cholestasis of pregnancy
  Preeclampsia and liver disease including HELLP syndrome, hepatic infarction, hepatic
    hematoma, and rupture
  Acute fatty liver of pregnancy

Common liver diseases occurring during pregnancy or exacerbated by pregnancy
  Acute viral hepatitis: A, B, C, E, Herpes simplex
  Drug hepatotoxicity
  Biliary and pancreatic diseases
  Budd–Chiari syndrome
  Other diseases

Pregnancy in the presence of chronic liver disease
  Cirrhosis and portal hypertension
  Chronic hepatitis B
  Chronic hepatitis C
  Autoimmune hepatitis
  Primary biliary cirrhosis
  Focal nodular hyperplasia and hepatic adenoma
  Liver transplantation

Table 41.2 Hemodynamic and biochemical changes in normal pregnancy.

Hemodynamic changes

Plasma volume	↑ Between weeks 6 and 36 by 50%. ↓ After delivery
Red cell volume	↑ By about 20%. ↓ After delivery
Cardiac output	↑ Until second trimester. Normalizes by term
Systemic vascular resistance	↓ Due to systemic vasodilation and placental circulation
Absolute hepatic blood flow	Unchanged

Biochemical changes

Serum albumin	↓ As pregnancy advances, due to hemodilution
ALP	↑ Mainly placental ALP
ALT	No change
AST	No change
Serum bilirubin	No change or mild ↓
Direct bilirubin	No change
Fasting total bile acid	No change
GGT	Mild ↓
Serum fibrinogen	↑
Prothrombin time/INR	No change

ALP, alkaline phosphatase; ALT, alanine aminotransferase; AST, aspartate aminotransferase; GGT, gamma-glutamyltransferase; INR international normalized ratio.

Table 41.3 Salient features of liver diseases in pregnancy by trimester.

Trimester of onset	Liver condition	Main symptoms	Laboratory test	Histology	Management
First	Hyperemesis gravidarum	Nausea, vomiting	↑ AST, ALT, ketosis	Central vacuolization	Intravenous hydration, bowel rest, antiemetics. TPN in severe cases
Second	Cholestasis of pregnancy	Pruritis, jaundice ±	↑ AST, ALT, total bile acids. Mild ↑ bilirubin	Cholestasis. No inflammation	Antihistaminics, phenobarbital, ursodeoxycholic acid. Early delivery ±
Third	HELLP syndrome	Abdominal pain, malaise, nausea, vomiting	Low platelets. ↑ AST, ALT, LDH. Hemolysis	Periportal hemorrhage, focal parenchymal necrosis	Supportive. Early delivery when possible
	Hepatic infarction	Severe abdominal or chest pain. Acute liver failure	↑ WBC, ↑↑ AST, ALT, ↑ bilirubin, coagulopathy. CT/MRI diagnostic	–	Supportive. May need ICU
	Hepatic rupture	Severe abdominal pain. Shock	Abdominal CT	–	Laparotomy. Prompt delivery
	Acute fatty liver of pregnancy	Nausea, vomiting, abdominal pain	↑ Prothrombin time, DIC. ↑ AST, ALT, bilirubin, ALP	Microvesicular fat in hepatocytes	Supportive care. Prompt delivery
Any	Viral hepatitis	Nausea, vomiting, jaundice	↑ AST, ALT, bilirubin. Hepatitis serology	Inflammation and hepatocyte necrosis	Supportive

ALP, alkaline phosphatase; ALT, alanine aminotransferase; AST, aspartate aminotransferase; CT, computed tomography; DIC, disseminate intravascular coagulation; ICU, intensive care unit; LDH, lactate dehydrogenase; MRI, magnetic resonance imaging; TPN, total parenteral nutrition; WBC, white blood cells.

Table 41.4 Diagnostic laboratory and pathological features of HELLP syndrome.

Hemolytic anemia
Decrease in Hb
Peripheral smear: schistocytes and burr cells
Total bilirubin > 1.2 mg/dL, mainly unconjugated
Lactate dehydrogenase > 600 U/L

Elevated liver enzymes
Serum AST > 70 U/L or > twice normal.
AST > ALT
AST and ALT up to 1000 IU/L

Thrombocytopenia
Platelet count < 100 000/mL

Liver biopsy
Periportal hemorrhage and periportal or focal parenchymal necrosis with hyaline deposits.
Fibrin microthrombi and fibrinogen deposits in sinusoids

ALT, alanine aminotransferase; AST, aspartate aminotransferase; Hb, hemoglobin.

complicates 0.1–0.6% of pregnancies and 4–12% of patients with severe preeclampsia. Some 70% of cases occur in the third trimester and the rest postpartum. Presentation varies from asymptomatic to severe life-threatening illness. Presenting symptoms are right upper quadrant or epigastric pain, malaise, nausea, and vomiting. Diagnostic laboratory abnormalities are listed in Table 41.4. It is associated with high perinatal mortality (35%), and significant maternal mortality (1–3%). Management is expectant and may require intensive care unit (ICU) care. Delivery is the definitive treatment and should be undertaken after 36 weeks, once fetal lungs have matured. Steroids may help the maternal platelet count and promote fetal lung maturity. Hepatic infarction, subcapsular hematoma, and hepatic rupture are rare complications of preeclampsia.

Acute fatty liver of pregnancy (AFLP)
AFLP is a rare disorder (1 in 7000–14 000 deliveries), occurring in the third trimester, and associated with a very high mortality rate (80% in old studies, 20% in recent). The etiology is unknown. It is more common in primiparous women or in women with more than one fetus. Patients present with acute onset of nausea, vomiting, abdominal pain, and flu-like symptoms. Fifty percent of patients have preeclampsia. Clinical, laboratory, and histological features are shown in Table 41.5. Ultrasound and computed tomography (CT) can show fatty liver but are not diagnostic. Most patients improve 1–4 weeks postpartum. If untreated, AFLP progresses rapidly to fulminant hepatic failure with encephalopathy, coagulopathy, disseminated intravascular coagulation (DIC), cerebral edema, renal failure,

Table 41.5 Diagnostic clinical, laboratory, and pathological features of acute fatty liver of pregnancy.

Clinical
Acute onset nausea, vomiting
Right upper quadrant or epigastric pain
Flu-like symptoms: malaise, anorexia, headache
Jaundice
Encephalopathy: somnolence, irritability, sleep alterations, asterexis, progressing to seizures and coma

Laboratory tests
Leukocytosis
Coagulation disorders: increased prothrombin time, decreased fibrinogen and clotting factors, thrombocytopenia, DIC
Elevated liver enzymes: AST, ALT (up to 1000 IU/L), bilirubin (up to 5–15 mg/dL), ALP
Hypoglycemia
Renal failure: elevated BUN and creatinine

Liver biopsy
Microvesicular steatosis with foamy appearance of cytoplasm. Mild inflammation and hepatocyte necrosis

---

ALP, alkaline phosphatase; ALT, alanine aminotransferase; AST, aspartate aminotransferase; BUN, blood urea nitrogen; DIC, disseminated intravascular coagulation.

gastrointestinal or uterine bleeding, seizures, coma, and death. Timely diagnosis, intensive monitoring, supportive management, and prompt delivery are key to a successful outcome. Liver transplantation is an option in postpartum patients who do not improve rapidly after delivery.

Further reading

Abell TL, Riely CA. Hyperemesis gravidarum. *Gastroenterol Clin North Am* 1992;21:835.
Bacq Y. Intrahepatic cholestasis of pregnancy. *Clin Liver Dis* 1999;3:1.
Bacq Y, Riely CA. The liver in pregnancy. In: *Schiffs textbook of liver disease*, Vol. 2, 9th edn. Lippincott Williams and Wilkins; 2003:1435.
Barron WM. The syndrome of preeclampsia. *Gastroenterol Clin North Am* 1992;21:851.
Davis A, Katz VL, Cox R. Gallbladder disease in pregnancy. *J Reprod Med* 1995;40:759.
Jaiswal SP, Jain AK, Naik G, et al. Viral hepatitis during pregnancy. *Int J Gynaecol Obstet* 2001;72:103.
Knox TA, Olans LB. Liver disease in pregnancy. *N Engl J Med* 1996;335:569.
Riely CA. Acute fatty liver of pregnancy. *Semin Liver Dis* 1987;7:47.
Riely CA. Liver diseases in pregnancy. In: Reece AE, Hobbins JC, eds. *Medicine of the fetus and mother*, 2nd edn. Philadelphia, PA: Lippincott-Raven Publishers; 1999:1153.
Sandhu BS, Sanyal AJ. Pregnancy and liver disease. *Gastroenterol Clin North Am* 2003; 32:407.

Schweitzer IL, Peters RL. Pregnancy in hepatitis B antigen positive cirrhosis. *Obstet Gynecol* 1976;48:53S.

Sherlock S, Dooley J. *Diseases of the liver and biliary system*. Blackwell Science, 2002.

Sibai BM, Ramadan MK, Usta I, et al. Maternal morbidity and mortality in 442 pregnancies with hemolysis, elevated liver enzymes, and low platelets (HELLP syndrome). *Am J Obstet Gynecol* 1993;169:1000.

42 Pregnancy complicated by renal disorders

Michelle W. Krause and Sudhir V. Shah

Recent epidemiological studies indicate that chronic kidney disease (CKD) is common and affects 20 million Americans.[1] This, coupled with the evidence that the incidence of pregnancy in women with CKD is rising, makes it important to understand how pregnancy affects the kidney as well as how kidney disease affects both the mother and the fetus. Advancement of medical technology in both obstetrics and neonatology has resulted in more favorable outcomes for pregnancy in women with renal disease.

Renal physiology and pregnancy

The marked decrease in the peripheral vascular resistance during pregnancy results in a reduction in blood pressure and significant changes in systemic and renal hemodynamics, including net retention of sodium and water, an increase in cardiac output, and an increase in the glomerular filtration rate (GFR) (Table 42.1).[2,3]

Acute renal failure in pregnancy

Pregnant women are at risk for the same causes of acute renal failure (ARF) as in the general population; however, etiologies specific for pregnancy-related ARF are depicted in Fig. 42.1. The evaluation of ARF in pregnancy consists of a detailed history and physical examination as well as evaluation of the urine, laboratory studies, and radiographic imaging of the kidneys and the collecting system to distinguish between prerenal ARF and intrinsic or postrenal ARF (Table 42.2). The treatment of ARF is based on correcting the underlying etiology. An intravenous fluid challenge to correct volume depletion and impaired renal perfusion is warranted in a hospitalized setting with careful monitoring for signs of volume overload to distinguish between prerenal ARF and intrinsic renal ARF.

Table 42.1 Systemic and renal physiologic changes in pregnancy.

	Normal	Pregnancy
Blood pressure	120/80 mmHg	110/60 mmHg
Cardiac output	4–5 L/min	6–7 L/min
Plasma volume	2.5–3.0 L	3.75–4.5 L
Renal plasma flow	650 mL/min	975–1000 mL/min
Glomerular filtration rate	100 mL/min/1.73 m²	140 mL/min/1.73 m²
Blood urea nitrogen	8–10 mg/dL	5–8 mg/dL
Creatinine	1.0–1.2 mg/dL	0.4–0.8 mg/dL
Sodium	135–145 mEq/L	130–135 mEq/L
Hematocrit	36–46%	30–36%
Serum bicarbonate	22–30 mEq/L	18–22 mEq/L

Table 42.2 Evaluation of acute renal failure in pregnancy.

	Prerenal ARF	Intrinsic renal ARF	Postrenal ARF
BUN:Cr ratio	20:1	10–15:1	10–15:1
Urinalysis			
Urine sodium	< 20 mEq/L	> 40 mEq/L	> 40 mEq/L
Hematuria	–	±	±
Proteinuria	–	±	±
Volume	Low	Low or normal	Low
Osmolality	High	Low	Low/normal
FeNa	< 1%	> 1%	> 1%
Volume status	Low	Normal/high	Normal/high
Renal ultrasonography	Normal	Normal	Abnormal

Cr, creatinine; FeNa, fractional excretion of sodium.

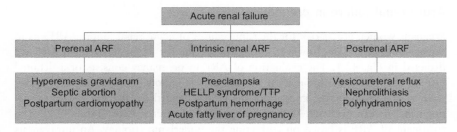

Figure 42.1 Etiologies of acute renal failure in pregnancy. TTP, thrombotic thrombocytopenic purpura.

Pregnancy and pre-existing renal disease

Renal disease in pregnancy can be classified into those with CKD diagnosed prior to conception, CKD unknown prior to conception but discovered during the pregnancy and, thirdly, renal disease that develops during pregnancy. Regardless of the etiology of CKD, with the exception of lupus nephritis, the degree of renal impairment at the time of conception largely defines the risk and outcome for both the mother and the fetus (Table 42.3).

The treatment of CKD in pregnant women is primarily directed at control of blood pressure with antihypertensive agents that are considered to be safe in pregnancy (Table 42.4) and monitoring and treatment of asymptomatic bacteriuria and urinary tract infections.

Pregnancy in endstage renal disease

Pregnancy is a relatively uncommon phenomenon in women with endstage renal disease (ESRD) on renal replacement therapy. The care of a pregnant dialysis patient is complex and begins with a dialysis prescription aimed at reducing the blood urea nitrogen (BUN) to less than 45–50 mg/dL.[4] This translates into > 20 hours/week on hemodialysis, often over five or six treatments. There needs to be judicious monitoring of calcium, phosphorous, and potassium, as levels may decrease with the increase in weekly dialysis.

Table 42.3 Pregnancy-related progressive renal failure in women with pre-existing renal disease.

	Creatinine < 1.5 mg/dL	1.5–3.0 mg/dL	> 3.0 mg/dL
Progressive renal failure during pregnancy	15%	30%	–
End stage renal disease (1 year)	6%	20%	45%

Table 42.4 Antihypertensive agents in pregnancy.

Central-acting adrenergic agents	*Calcium-channel blocking agents*
Methyldopa 0.25–3.0 g/day	Nifedipine 30–120 mg/day
Clonidine 0.1–1.2 mg/day	Diltiazem 60–360 mg/day
	Verapamil 80–480 mg/day
Beta-adrenergic blocking agents	
Atenolol 25–100 mg/day	*Vasodilators*
Metoprolol 25–400 mg/day	Hydralazine 50–300 mg/day
Labetalol 200–2400 mg/day	
Propranolol 40–240 mg/day	

Pregnancies in renal transplant recipients are more successful than those in women with ESRD on renal replacement therapy. Ideally, it is recommended that women wait until a year after their renal transplant to conceive when they are on a stable maintenance immunosuppressive regimen. Several immunosuppressive transplant medications have a long safety profile in pregnancy including prednisone, cyclosporine, and azathioprine.[5,6]

Conclusions

Although this unique group of women with renal disease and pregnancy is challenging to manage from a medical perspective, successful outcomes can be achieved with careful monitoring of both the fetus and the mother.

References

1 K/DOQI Advisory Board Members. Clinical Practice Guidelines for Chronic Kidney Disease. Part 4. Definition and Classification of Stages of Chronic Kidney Disease. *Am J Kidney Dis* 2002;39:S46.
2 Hytten FE, Leitch I. *The physiology of human pregnancy*, 2nd edn. Oxford, UK: Blackwell Scientific Publications, 1971.
3 Davison JM, Dunlop W. Renal hemodynamics in normal human pregnancy. *Kidney Int* 1980;18:152.
4 Jungers P, Chauveau D. Pregnancy in renal disease. *Kidney Int* 1997;52:871.
5 Bar Oz B, Hackman R, Einarson T, Koren G. Pregnancy outcome after cyclosporin therapy during pregnancy. *Transplantation* 2001;71:1051.
6 European Best Practice Guidelines (Part 2). *Nephrol Dial Transplant* 2002;17(Suppl. 4):50.

Neurological disorders in pregnancy

R. Lee Archer, Stacy A. Rudnicki, and
Bashir S. Shihabuddin

Headaches

Headaches can be a sign of many different neurological problems. A flow diagram to guide management is presented in Fig. 43.1. If headaches during pregnancy have been present for years, are unchanged in character, and the neurological examination is normal, then further attention is rarely warranted. Tension headaches should be managed without daily medication as a rule but, in severe cases, preventative treatment with low doses of tricyclic antidepressants (e.g., imipramine 10–50 mg at bedtime) may be justified. Migraine headaches constitute a large share of headaches

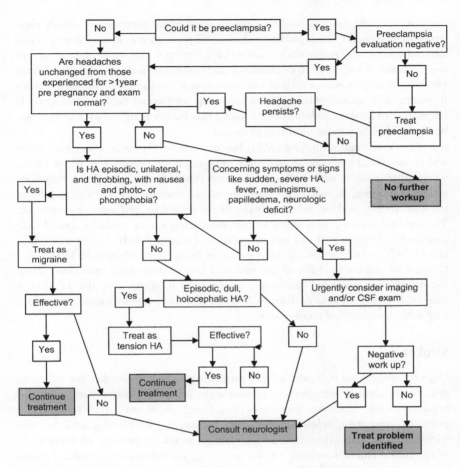

Figure 43.1 Flow diagram for headaches in pregnancy. CSF, cerebrospinal fluid; HA, headache.

in gravidas. They are often unilateral with a throbbing quality and may be accompanied by nausea, photophobia, and phonophobia. When necessary, migraine preventative medications may be used such as beta-blockers (e.g., atenolol 50–100 mg daily) or tricyclic antidepressants, but one should strive to manage migraineurs with limited doses (10–20 per month) of analgesics, particularly combinations of caffeine, butalbital, and acetaminophen (with codeine when necessary). The new onset of headaches or a significant change in the character or frequency of headaches during pregnancy should always cause concern. Preeclampsia is frequently accompanied by headache. Benign intracranial hypertension usually presents with a constant holocephalic headache and papilledema. Blindness may result without treatment. Treatments include serial lumbar punctures (the mainstay), cautious control of weight gain, occasionally acetazolamide (a class C drug) and, very rarely, surgical procedures such as lumboperitoneal shunting or optic nerve sheath fenestration. Regular ophthalmologic follow-up with visual field determination is imperative to confirm stability, as the visual loss occurs peripherally and may not be noticed by the patient until it is advanced.

Magnetic resonance imaging (MRI) has never been shown to cause fetal harm and is considered the imaging procedure of choice during pregnancy. When a cerebrovascular insult is suspected, consideration should be given to doing diffusion-weighted imaging, as well as magnetic resonance angiography and venography at the same sitting, as these will usually clarify the pathology and guide management. The very sudden onset of a severe or even moderately severe headache should raise concern for the possibility of a subarachnoid hemorrhage (SAH). A computed tomographic (CT) scan will discern the presence of blood more often than MRI, but a CT scan will miss a SAH 5% of the time, so a lumbar puncture is mandatory when the diagnosis is suspected (preferably after urgent imaging). The risk of SAH is increased around the time of delivery. Immediate workup and treatment are mandatory with neurosurgical consultation.

Strokes

Urgent evaluation is indicated for the pregnant patient with stroke, just as in the general population. Intracerebral hemorrhages generally present with profound hemiparesis and headache, sometimes progressing quickly to coma. Treatment is primarily supportive, unless the size of the hemorrhage or bleeding into the ventricular system necessitates surgical intervention to relieve pressure on other parts of the brain. Nonhemorrhagic strokes are either thrombotic or embolic. Thrombotic strokes may be arterial or venous. Venous sinus thrombosis is more common in the puerperium, and the new onset of headaches with any neurological symptoms or signs (such as papilledema) during this period should prompt concern for this diagnosis. Other cerebrovascular disorders associated with or more common during pregnancy include air or amniotic fluid embolism, embolic strokes caused by right to left shunts through a patent foramen ovale, hypercoagulable states (such as antiphospholipid syndrome), and metastatic choriocarcinoma. Appropriate testing and treatment are evolving rapidly in this field, with clot retrieval devices recently becoming available and intra-arterial thrombolysis an option at many institutions, so that management should involve neurological consultation. Anticoagulation has been proven to be of benefit only with atrial fibrillation, but one should consider using it with venous sinus thrombosis, arterial dissections, hypercoagulable states, and with embolic strokes associated with cardiac problems. Heparin (particularly low-molecular-weight heparin) is considered by many the anticoagulant of choice in pregnancy as warfarin crosses the placenta and is teratogenic in the first trimester.

Multiple sclerosis

A diagnosis of multiple sclerosis does not contraindicate pregnancy, but the post-partum period is associated with an increased incidence of exacerbations, and any neurological disability present (such as paraplegia) can certainly complicate management. None of the available treatments is approved during pregnancy, but anecdotal reports suggest that glatiramer acetate may be safe. There are no known anesthetic contraindications.

Focal neuropathies during pregnancy

Up to 62% of pregnant women have symptoms of carpal tunnel syndrome. Wrist splints at night are beneficial, and steroid injections may be used when symptoms are severe. Spontaneous resolution following delivery is common. Bell's palsy is associated with an increased risk of preeclampsia and hypertension. Prognosis for an incomplete Bell's palsy is excellent but, for a complete Bell's palsy, pregnancy is associated with a worse prognosis. Meralgia paresthetica causes numbness or burning pain in the lateral thigh. Symptoms generally resolve within a few months of delivery as weight is lost. For patients who have significant pain, topical capsaicin may be beneficial. Approximately 1% of postpartum women have leg numbness or weakness confirmed by neurological examination. Common nerves involved are the femoral and lateral femoral cutaneous nerves. Recovery may take anywhere from a week to 18 months, with some patients having persistent problems.

Peripheral neuropathy

Thiamine deficiency may occur with hyperemesis gravidarum, resulting in either a peripheral neuropathy or Wernicke's encephalopathy. Intravenous thiamine may reverse the encephalopathy, but the neuropathy, which may be severe, improves slowly, and recovery may be incomplete. Guillain–Barré syndrome may occur during pregnancy, although pregnant women do not appear to be at increased risk, and plasmapheresis for it appears to be safe.

Neuromuscular junction and muscle disorders

Myasthenia gravis (MG) exacerbations occur during pregnancy in 15–41% of myasthenics, and in an additional 16–30% during the puerperium. The latter is not influenced by mode of delivery.

Magnesium should be used very cautiously in treating preeclampsia and eclampsia in myasthenics. Neuromuscular blocking agents should be avoided. Both increased incidences of preterm labor and a higher rate of Cesarean sections occur in women with myotonic dystrophy (the most common muscular dystrophy of adulthood). Treatment of any of the autoimmune neurological diseases should be done in conjunction with a neurologist, as the risks of immunosuppression in a pregnant patient must be carefully weighed against the risks of untreated disease. Prednisone is generally considered to be safe during pregnancy, and azathiaprine, a class D drug, may be safest of the other immune suppressants.

Epilepsy

Although women with epilepsy have an increased risk of obstetric complications, worsening seizure control, and adverse neonatal outcomes, most of them have an uncomplicated pregnancy course and give birth to normal offspring. Factors leading to increased seizure frequency during pregnancy include declining antiepileptic drug (AED) concentrations, noncompliance, stress, and sleep deprivation. Serum AED concentrations start declining in the first trimester, reach a nadir near term, then return to preconception levels within 4–12 weeks postpartum. Anticonvulsant levels should be checked every 1–3 months, and the dosage of medication adjusted to maintain prepregnancy levels. Changing anticonvulsants for fetal safety should be entertained before pregnancy and rarely during pregnancy. Infants born to women with epilepsy are at increased risk of congenital malformations, cognitive impairment, and developmental delays. Contributing factors to these adverse outcomes are intrauterine AED exposure, folic acid deficiency, seizure control, seizure type, genetics, maternal health, smoking, and lower socioeconomic class. The incidence of major congenital malformations in infants born to women with epilepsy is 4–8%, a twofold increase over the incidence in the general population. Folic acid deficiency is associated with the development of congenital malformations, mainly neural tube defects (NTDs). Folic acid levels decline during pregnancy, and the antifolate effect of some AEDs predisposes women with epilepsy to folic acid deficiency. Folic acid supplements of 0.4–4 mg daily, beginning 1 month before conception and continuing through pregnancy, reduce the incidence of NTDs by 50–70%. The higher dose of 4 mg daily is used in women who have a prior history of offspring with NTDs. Infants born to women taking enzyme-inducing AEDs are also at greater risk of hemorrhagic complications because of the reduced activity of vitamin K-dependent clotting factors and should be treated with oral vitamin K 10–20 mg daily during the last month of pregnancy. Infants should receive vitamin K 1 mg intramuscularly at birth and, if needed, fresh frozen plasma.

Further reading

Devinsky O, Yerby MS. Women with epilepsy: reproduction and effects of pregnancy on epilepsy. *Neurol Clin* 1994;12:479.

Djelmis J, Sastarko M, Mayer D, et al. Myasthenia gravis in pregnancy: report on 69 cases. *Eur J Obstet Gynecol Reprod Biol* 2002;104:21.

Ferrero S, Pretta S, Ragni N. Multiple sclerosis: management issues during pregnancy. *Eur J Obstet Gynecol Reprod Biol* 2004;115:3.

Martin SR, Foley RF. Approach to the pregnant patient with headache. *Clin Obstet Gynecol* 2005;48:2.

Sawhney H, Vasishta K, Suri V, et al. Pregnancy with epilepsy – a retrospective analysis. *Int J Gynaecol Obstet* 1996;54:17.

Shehata HA, Okosun H. Neurological disorders in pregnancy. *Curr Opin Obstet Gynecol* 2004;16:117.

Shmorgun D, Chan WS, Ray JG. Association between Bell's palsy in pregnancy and pre-eclampsia. *Q J Med* 2002;95:359.

Steeger-Theunissen RPM, Renier WO, Borm GF, et al. Factors influencing the risk of abnormal pregnancy outcome in epileptic women: a multi-centre prospective study. *Epilepsy Res* 1994;18:261.

Turan TN, Stern GJ. Stroke in pregnancy. *Neurol Clin* 2004;22:821.

Wong CA, Scavone BM, Dugan S, et al. Incidence of postpartum lumbosacral spine and lower extremity nerve injuries. *Obstet Gynecol* 2003;101:279.

44 Thromboembolic disorders of pregnancy

Michael J. Paidas, Christian M. Pettker, and Charles J. Lockwood

Venous thromboembolism (VTE) complicates 1 in 1000 pregnancies, but the precise frequency of thromboembolism is probably underestimated. Pregnancy has been associated with a sixfold higher incidence of VTE compared with age-matched nonpregnant women, and pulmonary embolism (PE) remains a leading cause of maternal mortality. In the United States, death from PE occurs in 2 in 100 000 deliveries and represents 11% of maternal deaths. Postpartum deep venous thrombosis (DVT) is more common than antepartum DVT, with reported rates of 0.61 in 1000 and 0.13 in 1000 pregnancies respectively.

Hematologic changes in pregnancy

Substantial changes must occur in local decidual and systemic coagulation, anticoagulant and fibrinolytic systems to meet the hemostatic challenges of pregnancy, including avoidance of hemorrhage at implantation, placentation, and the third stage of labor. Pregnancy is associated with significant elevations in a number of clotting factors. Fibrinogen concentration is doubled, and 20–1000% increases in factors VII, VIII, IX, X, XII, and von Willebrand factor are observed, with maximum levels reached at term (Table 44.1). Prothrombin and factor V levels remain unchanged, while levels of factors XIII and XI decline modestly. Protein S levels decrease significantly in normal pregnancy. Mean protein S free antigen levels have been reported to be 38.9 ± 10.3% and 31.2 ± 7.4% in the second and third trimesters respectively.

Table 44.1 Coagulation parameters in pregnancy.

Variables (mean ± SD)	First trimester*	Second trimester*	Third trimester*	Normal range
Platelet (× 10⁹/L)	275 ± 64	256 ± 49	244 ± 52	150–400
Fibrinogen (g/L)	3.7 ± 0.6	4.4 ± 1.2	5.4 ± 0.8	2.1–4.2
Prothrombin complex (%)	120 ± 27	140 ± 27	130 ± 27	70–30
Antithrombin (U/mL)	1.02 ± 0.10	1.07 ± 0.14	1.07 ± 0.11	0.85–1.25
Protein C (U/mL)	0.92 ± 0.13	1.06 ± 0.17	0.94 ± 0.2	0.68–1.25
Protein S, total (U/mL)	0.83 ± 0.11	0.73 ± 0.11	0.77 ± 0.10	0.70–1.70
Protein S, free (U/mL)	0.26 ± 0.07	0.17 ± 0.04	0.14 ± 0.04	0.20–0.50
Soluble fibrin (nmol/l)	9.2 ± 8.6	11.8 ± 7.7	13.4 ± 5.2	< 15
Thrombin–antithrombin (µg/L)	3.1 ± 1.4	5.9 ± 2.6	7.1 ± 2.4	< 2.7
D-Dimers (µg/L)	91 ± 24	128 ± 49	198 ± 59	< 80
Plasminogen activator inhibitor-1 (AU/mL)	7.4 ± 4.9	14.9 ± 5.2	37.8 ± 19.4	< 15
Plasminogen activator inhibitor-2 (µg/l)	31 ± 14	84 ± 16	160 ± 31	< 5
Cardiolipin antibodies positive	2/25	2/25	3/23	0
Protein Z (µg/mL)†	2.01 ± 0.76	1.47 ± 0.45	1.55 ± 0.48	–
Protein S, free antigen (%)†	–	38.9 ± 10.3	31.2 ± 7.4	–

Table modified from Bremme K. Haemostatic changes in pregnancy. *Best Pract Res Clin Haematol* 2003;16:153–168, and †Paidas MJ, Ku DW, Lee MJ, et al. Protein Z, protein S levels are lower in patients with thrombophilia and subsequent pregnancy complications. *J Thromb Haemost* 2005;3:497–501.

*First trimester, weeks 12–15; second trimester, week 24; third trimester, week 35.

†First trimester, 0–14 weeks; second trimester, 14–27 weeks; third trimester, ≥ 27 weeks.

Acquired and inherited thrombophilias

Inherited thrombophilias are a heterogeneous group of disorders associated with varying degrees of increased thrombotic risk (Table 44.2). Specific concerns include increased risks of DVT, PE, and a variety of adverse pregnancy outcomes, consisting of preeclampsia, intrauterine growth restriction (IUGR), abruptio placentae, and fetal loss. The high-risk thrombophilias include antithrombin III (ATIII) deficiency, factor V Leiden homozygosity, and prothrombin gene (G20210A) mutation. Heterozygous factor V Leiden is associated with a 0.2% risk of thromboembolism during pregnancy, while heterozygous prothrombin gene mutation is associated with a 0.5% risk. Compound heterozygous factor V Leiden and prothrombin gene mutation is associated with a 4.6% risk of thromboembolism. Other inherited thrombophilic mutations, including methylene tetrahydrafolate reductase (MTHFR) C667T and A1298C (often associated with hyperhomocysteinemia) and plasminogen activator inhibitor (PAI) gene mutations 4G/4G, 4G/5G, and 5G/5G, have been weakly associated, if at all, with thrombotic risk and pregnancy complications. The well-characterized antiphospholipid antibody syndrome is defined by the combination of VTE, obstetric complications, and antiphospholipid antibodies (APA). By definition, APA-related thrombosis can occur in any tissue or organ except superficial veins, whereas accepted associated obstetric complications include at least one fetal death at or beyond the 10th week of gestation, or at least one premature birth at or before the 34th week, or at least three consecutive spontaneous abortions before the 10th week. All other causes of pregnancy morbidity must be excluded. Antiphospholipid antibodies must be present on two or more occasions at least 6 weeks apart, and are immunoglobulins directed against proteins bound to negatively charged surfaces, usually anionic phospholipids.

Prevention and treatment strategies

The selection of suitable patients for thrombophilia screening and the thrombophilia workup continues to evolve. At this time, suitable candidates for thrombophilia screening include those with a history of unexplained fetal loss at ≥ 10 weeks; a history of severe preeclampsia/HELLP at < 36 weeks; a history of abruptio placentae; a history of IUGR $\leq$ 5th percentile; a personal history of thrombosis; and a family history of thrombosis. Initial thrombophilia evaluation should include: Protein C (functional level); protein S (functional/free antigen level); ATIII (functional level); factor V Leiden (PCR); prothrombin gene mutation 20210A (PCR); lupus anticoagulant; anticardiolipin antibody IgG, M, A; and platelet count. Heparins are the mainstay in the treatment and prevention of thromboembolism in pregnancy. Unfractionated heparin enhances antithrombin activity, increases factor Xa inhibitor activity, and inhibits platelet aggregation. Low-molecular-weight heparin (LMWH) is generated by chemical or enzymatic manipulation of unfractionated heparin from a molecular weight of 15 000 Da to 4000–6500 Da. The smaller size impedes its antithrombin but not antifactor Xa effects. Both LMWH

Table 44.2 Inherited thrombophilias and their association with VTE.

Thrombophilia	Inheritance	Prevalence in European populations (from large cohort studies)	Prevalence in patients with VTE (range)	Relative risk or odds ratio (OR) of VTE [95% CI] (lifetime)	Reference
Factor V Leiden (FVL) (homozygous)	AD	0.07%*	< 1%*	80 [22–289]	54–56
FVL (heterozygous)	AD	5.3%	6.6–50%	2.7 [1.3–5.6]	54, 55
Prothrombin G20201A (PGM) (homozygous)	AD	0.02%*	< 1%	> 80-fold*	57
PGM (heterozygous)	AD	2.9%	7.5%	3.8 [3.0–4.9]	58
FVL/PGM (compound heterozygous)	AD	0.17%*	2.0%	20.0 [11.1–36.1]	58
Hyperhomocysteinemia	AR	5%	< 5%	3.3 [1.1–10.0]†	56, 59
Antithrombin deficiency (< 60% activity)	AD	0.2%	1–8%	17.5 [9.1–33.8]	56, 60
Protein S deficiency Heerlen S460P mutation or free S antigen < 55%	AD	0.2%	3.1%	2.4 [0.8–7.9]	61
Protein C (< 60% activity)	AD	0.2%	3–5%	11.3 [5.7–22.3]	56, 60

AD, autosomal dominant; AR, autosomal recessive; CI, confidence interval.
*Calculated based on a Hardy–Weinberg equilibrium.
†OR adjusted for renal disease, folate, and B12 deficiency, while odds ratios are adjusted for these confounders.

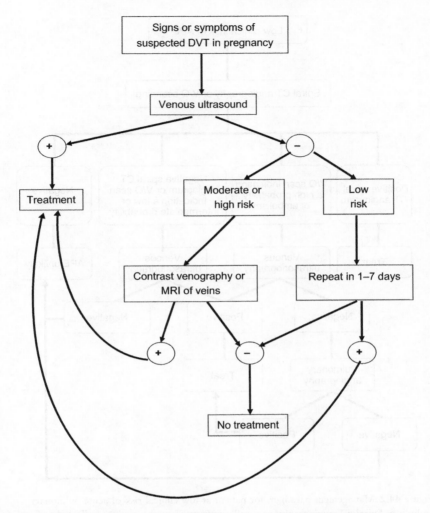

Figure 44.1 Management of suspected DVT in pregnancy. Once a DVT (deep venous thrombosis) is suspected, a venous ultrasound should be performed to establish the diagnosis of DVT. If positive, anticoagulation should be instituted. If negative, additional testing or repeat venous ultrasound may be indicated, depending upon the level of suspicion for the presence of DVT.

and unfractionated heparin cross the placenta, are considered safe for pregnancy, and are compatible with breastfeeding. Complications associated with heparins include hemorrhage, osteoporosis, and thrombocytopenia.

In pregnancy, the diagnosis of VTE is based on history, physical examination, and diagnostic studies. The typically cited signs and symptoms of DVT include erythema, warmth, pain, edema, tenderness, and a positive Homan's sign. Venous ultrasound

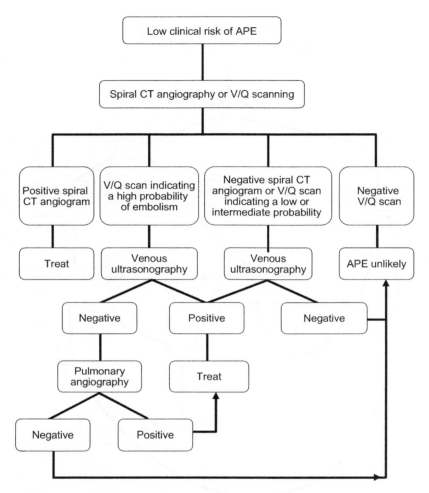

Figure 44.2 Management paradigm for patient at low clinical risk of acute pulmonary embolism. Spiral CT angiography or ventilation/perfusion scanning are indicated as first line imaging modalities. Anticoagulation is indicated in the setting of: a positive spiral CT angiography; a high probability V/Q scan along with a positive venous ultrasound; a positive pulmonary angiogram; negative spiral CT and positive venous ultrasound; low or intermediate V/Q scan and a positive venous ultrasound.

with or without color Doppler has become the primary diagnostic modality for evaluating patients at risk of DVT (Fig. 44.1). Clinical features of acute pulmonary embolism can include tachypnea, tachycardia, dyspnea, pleuritic chest pain, and presyncope and syncope in severe cases. Electrocardiographic changes may be present in 87% of patients with proven acute PE (APE). The alveolar–arterial oxygen tension difference appears to be a more useful indicator of disease, with

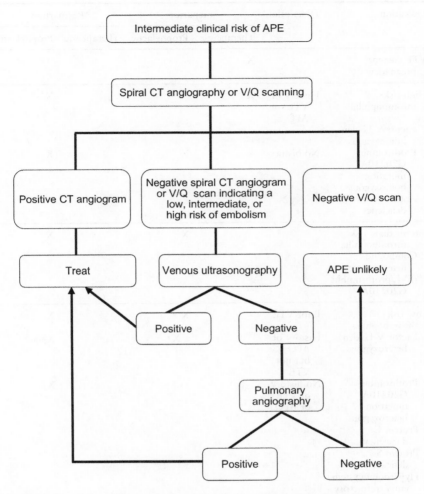

Figure 44.3 Management paradigm for patient at intermediate clinical risk of acute pulmonary embolism. Spiral CT angiography or ventilation/perfusion scanning are indicated as first line imaging modalities. Pulmonary angiography remains the gold standard for the diagnosis of APE. If there is a high clinical risk of acute pulmonary embolism, pulmonary angiography should be performed even if initial tests (spiral CT angiography or V/Q scanning) do not suggest APE (acute pulmonary embolism).

alveolar–arterial differences of > 20 mmHg present in 86% patients with APE. To confidently diagnose PE, one or more specific diagnostic studies must be performed (Figs 44.2 and 44.3). Active thromboembolism in pregnancy and other high-risk settings requires therapeutic anticoagulation (Table 44.3). Prophylactic anticoagulation is appropriate in the setting of thrombophilia and a history of adverse pregnancy outcome.

Table 44.3 Anticoagulation in pregnancy: indications and dosing.

Indication	Description	Antepartum		Postpartum	
		Therapeutic	Prophylactic	Therapeutic	Prophylactic
VTE current pregnancy		X		*	
High-risk thrombophilia	History of VTE or APO*	X			X
Factor V Leiden homozygous					
Prothrombin G20210A mutation homozygous Antithrombin III deficiency	No history		X		X
Intermediate-risk thrombophilia Compound heterozygote (FVL/prothrombin G20210A)			X		X
Low-risk thrombophilia Factor V Leiden heterozygous	Prior VTE		X		X
	History of APO† but not VTE		± X‡		X§
Prothrombin G20210A mutation heterozygous Protein C deficiency Protein S deficiency Hyperhomocystein emia (refractory to folate therapy)	No history of VTE or APO†				X§
No thrombophilia	Prior VTE				X
Hyperhomo-cysteinemia	Prior VTE or		X		X§§

*VTE during current pregnancy should receive therapeutic anticoagulation for 20+ weeks during pregnancy, followed by prophylactic therapy for up to 6 weeks postpartum.

†Adverse pregnancy outcome (APO) includes early-onset severe preeclampsia, unexplained recurrent abruptio placentae, severe IUGR, intrauterine fetal demise (>10 weeks) with placental thrombosis or infarction.

‡Patients with less thrombogenic thrombophilias and histories of APO should be treated prophylactically in the antepartum period if the clinical scenario suggests a high risk of recurrence or there are other thrombotic risk factors (obesity, immobilization, etc.).

(Continued)

Table 44.3 *Continued.*

§If Cesarean delivery or first-degree relative with history of VTE.

§§Cases of hyperhomocysteinemia unresponsive to folate, vitamin B6, and vitamin B12 therapy.

Notes:
Unfractionated heparin (UFH)
  • Initial dose of UFH for acute VTE to keep activated partial thromboplastin time (aPTT) 1.5–2.5 times control. Thereafter, UFH may be given subcutaneously q 8–12 h to keep aPTT 1.5–2 times control (when tested 6 h after injection) for therapeutic levels.
  • Prophylactic doses may range from 5000 to 10 000 units subcutaneously q 12 h and can be titrated to achieve heparin levels (by protamine titration assay) of 0.1–0.2 U/mL.

Low-molecular-weight heparin (LMWH)
  • Therapeutic doses of Lovenox (enoxaparin) may start at 1 mg/kg subcutaneously q 12 h. Therapeutic doses should be titrated to achieve antifactor Xa levels of 0.6–1.0 U/mL (when tested 4-6 h after injection).
  • Prophylactic doses of Lovenox (enoxaparin) may start at 40 mg subcutaneously q 12 h. Prophylactic doses should be titrated to achieve antifactor Xa levels of 0.1–0.2 U/mL 4 h after injection.
  • Regional anesthesia is contraindicated within 18–24 h of LMWH and thus LMWH should be converted to UFH at 36 weeks or earlier if clinically indicated.

Postpartum
  • Heparin anticoagulation (LMWH or UFH) may be restarted 3–6 h after vaginal delivery and 6–8 h after Cesarean.
  • Warfarin anticoagulation may be started on postpartum day 1.
  • Therapeutic doses of LMWH or UFH must be continued for 5 days and until the international normalized ratio (INR) reaches the therapeutic range (2.0–3.0) for 2 successive days.

Maternal and fetal surveillance
  • Fetal growth should be monitored every 4–6 weeks beginning at 20 weeks in all patients on anticoagulation.
  • Nonstress tests (NSTs) and biophysical profiles (BPPs) may be appropriate at 36 weeks or earlier as clinically indicated.

Further reading

Brill-Edwards P, Ginsberg JS, Gent M, et al. Safety of withholding heparin in pregnant women with a history of venous thromboembolism. Recurrence of clot in this pregnancy study group. *N Engl J Med* 2000;343:1439–1444.

Clinical Updates in Women's Health. *Thrombosis, thrombophilia and thromboembolism in women.* American College of Obstetricians and Gynecologists, in press.

Cochrane E. Antiphospholipid antibody and recurrent pregnancy loss. *Obstet Gynecol* 2002;99:135–144.

Greer IA, Nelson-Percy C. Safety and efficacy of LMWH: thromboprophylaxis and treatment of venous thromboembolism (64 reports, 2777 pregnancies). *Blood* 2005;106:401–407.

Gris JC, Mercier E, Quere II, et al. Low-molecular-weight heparin versus low-dose aspirin in women with one fetal loss and a constitutional thrombophilic disorder. *Blood* 2004; 103:3695–3699.

Paidas MJ, Ku DH, Langhoff-Roos J, Arkel YS. Inherited thrombophilias and adverse pregnancy outcome: screening and management. *Semin Perinatol* 2005;29:150–163.

Preston FE, Rosendaal FR, Walker ID, et al. Increased fetal loss in women with heritable thrombophilia. *Lancet* 1996;348:913–916.

Rand JH, Wu XX, Andree HA, et al. Pregnancy loss in the antiphospholipid-antibody syndrome – a possible thrombogenic mechanism. *N Engl J Med* 1997;337:154–160.

Rey E, Kahn SR, David M, Shrier I. Thrombophilic disorders and fetal loss: a meta-analysis. *Lancet* 2003;361:901–908.

Tapson VF, Carroll BA, Davidson BL, et al. The diagnostic approach to acute venous thromboembolism. Clinical practice guideline. American Thoracic Society. *Am J Respir Crit Care Med* 1999;160:1043–1066.

45 Coagulation and hematological disorders of pregnancy

Carl P. Weiner and Chien Oh

Red blood cell disorders/anemia

Normal physiological changes
Dilution of pregnancy causes a physiological anemia in pregnancy. Per the Centers for Disease Control (CDC), anemia is defined as a hemoglobin level < 11 g/dL in the first and third trimesters or < 10.5 g/dL in the second trimester. For a laboratory workup of anemia, see Fig. 45.1.

Nutritional anemias

Iron deficiency
This is the most common cause of anemia. It is confirmed by low ferritin levels and elevated total iron-binding capacity (TIBC). Treat this deficiency with oral iron 2–3 times a day. Parenteral treatment of anemia if severe or if oral therapy is not tolerated. The effect on pregnancy is controversial.

Megaloblastic anemia
This is usually caused by a deficiency in folic acid or vitamin B12. Check serum levels and treat accordingly.

Normocytic anemia
It is sometimes difficult to find the etiology. Check thyroid, renal, and hepatic function as well as iron studies.

Hemoglobinopathies

Thalassemias
Classification based on the poorly produced hemoglobin (Hgb) chain, α or β. Severity depends on the number of gene deletions of the α-globulin chain for α-

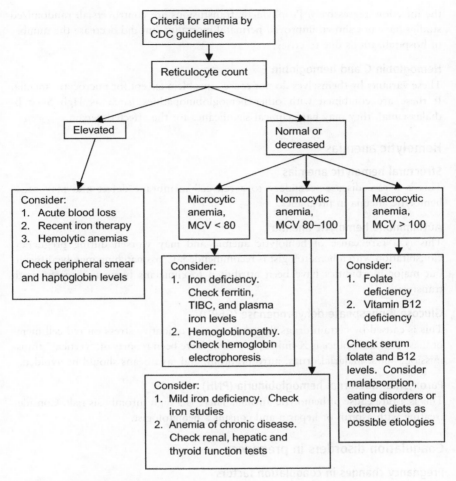

Figure 45.1 Workup algorithm for anemia.

thalassemia, or the amount of β-globulin chain produced. If this is diagnosed, there are genetic implications.

Sickle cell anemia, disease, and crisis

The major form is caused by Hgb SS. "Milder" forms are Hgb SC (this does not mean "hemoglobin sickle cell") or Hgb S/β-thalassemia. The "milder" forms may have a worse prognosis during pregnancy because of a healthier spleen. Antenatal surveillance is strongly recommended. Neurologic and pulmonary diseases may manifest because of sickle cell disease (SCD). Be aware of acute chest syndrome. Consult a hematologist or pulmonologist for lung findings with leukocytosis. Treatment for crises are pain relief, rule out infection, hydration, and oxygenation. Treat the infection aggressively. Prophylactic transfusions are controversial: randomized studies have not shown improved perinatal mortality, but did decrease the number of hospitalizations due to crises.

Hemoglobin C and hemoglobin E

These variants by themselves do not cause a problem except for microcytic anemia. If these are combined with other hemoglobinopathies (such as Hgb S or β-thalassemia), they may have clinical significance for the affected person.

Hemolytic anemias

Structural hemolytic anemias

This is a rare disease secondary to a red cell membrane defect and may cause hemolytic anemia in pregnancy.

Autoimmune hemolytic anemia

This is a rare cause of hemolytic anemia and may worsen during pregnancy. Consultation with a hematologist is recommended. Crossmatching may be difficult, but major morbidities have been attributed to clinicians being too careful with transfusion.

Glucose 6-phosphate dehydrogenase (G6PD)

This is caused by certain drugs that may worsen oxidative stress on red cell membranes. The inheritance is X-linked, and there have been reports of "vertical" transmission. Sulfa, malarial drugs, nitrofurantoin, and fava beans should be avoided.

Paroxysmal nocturnal hemoglobinuria (PNH)

This is a rare cause of hemolytic anemia. There is a high thrombosis risk. Consider treating with aspirin or heparin and consult a hematologist.

Coagulation disorders in pregnancy

Pregnancy changes in coagulation factors

Delicate balance in nonpregnant state now favors thrombosis. Entire coagulation (and anticoagulation) system upregulated.

Laboratory workup of coagulation

Complete blood count (CBC), prothrombin time (PT), activated partial thromboplastin time (PTT), and fibrinogen. Bleeding time is not a standard laboratory test for coagulation panel.

Thrombocytopenia

Gestational thrombocytopenia (GT)

This affects 8% of pregnancies and has no clear etiology. However, it is of little clinical significance, especially if the platelet count is > 100 000/μL. If the platelet count is < 100 000/μL, then discuss with anesthesiologist about regional anesthesia.

Immune thrombocytopenia purpura (ITP)

This is thrombocytopenia due to antiplatelet antibodies. Consider treatment to raise the platelet count to over 50 000/μL by the time of delivery or 20 000/μL during pregnancy. First-line treatment is corticosteroids (1 mg/kg/day of prednisone in divided doses, then taper to minimally effective doses). Second-line treatment is intravenous immunoglobulin (IVIG). If both fail, then get a hematology consultation, and splenectomy should possibly be considered. The fetal platelet count is often in the thrombocytopenic range, but is not an indication for Cesarean section.

Differentiating between GT and ITP

No clear method for differentiating the two processes exists. Differentiation is mainly based on platelet count but, even with significant overlap, no change in clinical management is necessary. If the platelet count is < 50 000/μL, the diagnosis is probably ITP.

Alloimmune thrombocytopenia purpura

This is the platelet form of rhesus (Rh) disease, but it can occur in a first pregnancy. Prognosis is poorer for the fetus even with similar platelet counts compared with ITP. Consultation with a maternal–fetal specialist is strongly recommended.

Other causes of thrombocytopenia

1 Preeclampsia;
2 HELLP: consider treatment with higher doses of dexamethasone (12 mg × 2 q12 h, 6 mg × 2 q12 h) either antepartum or postpartum. May use betamethasone for initial treatment (12 mg intramuscularly q12 h);
3 Thrombotic thrombocytopenic purpura (TTP): treatment with plasmapheresis;
4 Hemolytic uremic syndrome (HUS): treatment with plasmapheresis.

Other platelet disorders

Thrombocytosis

Consider other primary etiologies (Table 45.1). If the platelet count is consistently above 450 000/μL, consider aspirin therapy.

Platelet qualitative disorders

The most common cause of these disorders is drug inhibition of platelet function, most commonly aspirin. Platelet function is irreversibly damaged for the lifespan (approximately 10 days), but 60 mg/day has been shown to have no effect on maternal or fetal outcome, even with regional anesthesia.

Inherited bleeding disorders

von Willebrand's disease (vWD)

This is the most common inherited bleeding disorder in the general population.

Table 45.1 Differential diagnosis for thrombocytosis.

Primary causes
  Myeloproiferative syndromes
  Essential thrombocytosis
  Polycythemia vera
  Chronic myelogenous leukemia
  Myelofibrosis
Secondary causes
  Infectious diseases
  Inflammatory diseases
  Rebound after recovery from thrombocytopenia
  Asplenia
  Iron deficiency
  Parturition
  Exercise

Treatment depends on the type of vWD: type 1 and type 2A can initially be treated with vasopressin (one spray/nostril in active labor, good for 12 h). In type 3 vWD, vasopressin is ineffective and, in type 2b, vasopressin is contraindicated. For these types, blood products may be necessary for treatment.

Hemophilia

This is an X-linked disease, but may affect females occasionally. Treatment with blood products is necessary. Genetic counseling for carriers is a must, but one should first confirm the disease by checking factor VIII or factor IX levels.

Disseminated intravascular coagulation (DIC)

Management is first to identify the underlying pathological process and, second, to prevent hypovolemia and hypoxemia.

1 Abruptio placentae: this is the most common cause of DIC in the obstetric patient. Delivery is the usual treatment, especially in association with clinical laboratory abnormalities. Heparin is not recommended.

2 Intrauterine fetal demise (IUFD): treatment is delivery soon after diagnosis. DIC is not usually seen until weeks after demise. Heparin may be useful in these circumstances.

3 Amniotic fluid embolism (AFE): there is no standard protocol for the treatment of this rare, but severe, occurrence. Basic and advanced life support is necessary initially. If the patient survives, DIC may develop soon after. Treat coagulopathy with blood products. Pulmonary artery catheter placement is recommended.

4 Septic abortion: treatment consists of the aggressive use of antibiotics and evacuation of the uterus. Heparin use can be considered after evacuation of the pregnancy.

Thrombophilias in pregnancy

Acquired thrombophilias

Obstetric antiphospholipid syndrome (APS) is a diagnosis of antiphospholipid antibodies (either lupus anticoagulant or anticardiolipin antibodies) along with adverse pregnancy outcomes. Current recommendations for treatment include the use of prophylactic heparin (5000–10 000 U b.i.d. depending on trimester) and aspirin (81 mg q.d.).

Inherited thrombophilias

Interest has been growing in these thrombophilias. Is there truly an association? Who should be tested? How should patients then be managed?

1 Factor V Leiden (activated protein C resistance): this is the most common mutation causing activated protein C resistance. It is present in approximately 5–9% of the northern European population. This mutation causes factor V to be resistant to neutralization by the protein C/S complex. The role of heterozygosity in adverse pregnancy outcome is still being elucidated. Some experts recommend treatment with prophylactic heparin.

2 Protein C: this impedes the coagulation process. It is an autosomal-dominant trait. Activity level is lowered by warfarin or acute thrombosis. Testing should occur 10 days off warfarin and with no acute thrombosis. Activities of less than 55–65% are considered to be suspicious of genetic abnormality.

3 Protein S: cofactor to protein C to stop the coagulation process. Lowered in both pregnancy and oral contraceptive use. Levels also lowered by warfarin and acute thrombosis. Testing should occur 10 days off warfarin and with no acute thrombosis. Levels of less than 20–25% in pregnancy without other factors (warfarin use or thrombosis) are suspicious of genetic abnormality.

4 Antithrombin (III) activity: autosomal dominant. Many experts consider this to be the most thrombogenic of the inherited thrombophilias. Activity levels of < 70% are suspicious of deficiency. Consider at least prophylactic anticoagulation; some experts even suggest therapeutic anticoagulation.

5 Prothrombin gene mutation (G20210A): this is perhaps the second most common thrombophilia. This mutation causes thrombin to be expressed at a higher rate. Heterozygosity can confer increased risk of thrombosis. There is very little information available with regard to pregnancy risk. Consider prophylactic anticoagulation with heterozygotes; therapeutic anticoagulation with homozygotes.

6 Hyperhomocysteinemia: homocysteine causes endothelial damage. Levels of 10–15 µmol/L are associated with a twofold increase in the rate of stillbirth, and levels above 15 µmol/L with a sevenfold increase. There are two general causes:

either enzyme deficiency [can check for methylenetetrahydrofolate (MTHFR) homozygous mutation] or nutritional deficiency (start folic acid, vitamin B6).

Further reading

ACOG Technical Bulletin no. 6, September 1999.

British Committee for Standards in Haematology General Haematology Task Force. Guidelines for the investigation and management of idiopathic thrombocytopenic purpura in adults, children and in pregnancy. *Br J Haematol* 2003;120:574.

Centers for Disease Control. Anemia during pregnancy in low-income women – United States, 1987. *Morbid Mortal Weekly Rep* 1990;39:73.

Koshy M, Burd L, Wallace D, et al. Prophylactic red cell transfusion in pregnant patients with sickle cell disease. A randomized cooperative study. *N Engl J Med* 1988;319:1447.

Kujovich JL. Thrombophilia and pregnancy complications. *Am J Obstet Gynecol* 2004:191:412.

Lassere M, Empson M. Treatment of antiphospholipid syndrome in pregnancy – a systematic review of randomized therapeutic trials. *Thromb Res* 2004;114:419.

National Institutes of Health Consensus Development Conference. Prevention of venous thrombosis and pulmonary embolism. *JAMA* 1986;256:744.

O'Brien JM, Milligan DA, Barton JR. Impact of high-dose corticosteroid therapy for patients with HELLP (hemolysis, elevated liver enzymes, and low platelet count) syndrome. *Am J Obstet Gynecol* 2000;183:921.

Stasi R, Provan D. Management of immune thrombocytopenic purpura in adults. *Mayo Clin Proc* 2004;79:504.

Thomas R. Hypercoagulabililty syndromes. *Ann Intern Med* 2001;161:2433

Tuffnell DJ. Amniotic fluid embolism. *Curr Opin Obstet Gynecol* 2003;15:119.

Vichinsky EP, Neumayr LD, Earles AN, et al. Causes and outcomes of the acute chest syndrome in sickle cell disease: National Acute Chest Syndrome Study Group. *N Engl J Med* 2000;342:1855.

 # Maternal alloimmunization and fetal hemolytic disease

Carl P. Weiner and Anita C. Manogura

Rhesus (Rh) functionality

The function of the Rh antigen is unclear. It may have a role in maintaining erythrocyte integrity, as well as contributing to electrolyte and volume flux across the erythrocyte membrane. Rh_{null} (lacking all Rh antigens) individuals suffer multiple membrane defects, osmotic fragility, and abnormal shapes.

Pathogenesis of maternal alloimmunization

For Rh alloimmunization to occur:
• The woman must be Rh negative and the fetus Rh positive.
• Fetal erythrocytes must enter the maternal circulation in sufficient quantity.
• The mother must be immune competent.

Transplacental hemorrhage

In 1954, Chown proved that fetal-to-maternal transplacental hemorrhage (TPH) caused Rh immunization. Seventy-five percent of women have a fetal TPH some time during pregnancy or at delivery. The volume of the hemorrhage is usually small, but exceeds 5 mL in 1% and 30 mL in 0.25% of women.

Rh immune response

The primary Rh immune response develops slowly, typically over 6–12 weeks. It is usually weak and predominantly IgM, which does not cross the placenta. Most immunized women convert quickly to IgG anti-D production, which can readily cross the placenta. The anti-D coats Rh-positive fetal erythrocytes and triggers hemolysis. With a second TPH, the response is rapid (days) and is usually IgG.

ABO incompatibility

ABO incompatibility between the Rh-positive fetus and the Rh-negative mother reduces the risk of immunization to 1.5–2%. The partial protection reflects at least in part rapid intravascular hemolysis of the fetal ABO-incompatible cells and their sequestration in the liver. ABO incompatibility confers no protection once Rh immunization has developed.

Pathogenesis of fetal hemolytic disease

Maternal IgG anti-D crosses the placenta and coats the D-positive fetal red cells. The fetal red cells are destroyed extravascularly, primarily in the spleen, as anti-D does not fix complement. The resulting anemia stimulates fetal erythropoietin synthesis and release. Should marrow red cell production fail to compensate, extramedullary erythropoiesis occurs. Nucleated red cell precursors from normoblasts to primitive erythroblasts are released into the circulation.

Degrees of Rh hemolytic disease

Mild disease
Approximately 50% of affected fetuses do not require treatment postnatally. Their

umbilical cord blood hemoglobin is above 12 g/dL, and their umbilical cord serum bilirubin is less than 68 μmol/L.

Intermediate disease

Some 25–30% of affected fetuses have intermediate disease. They are born at or near term in good condition, with an umbilical cord blood hemoglobin between 9 g/dL and 12 g/dL. Extramedullary erythropoiesis is modest and liver function normal. Some of these infants develop severe hyperbilirubinemia. The mortality rate is up to 90%. In the remaining 10%, the jaundice fades and spasticity lessens. However, they show severe central nervous system dysfunction over time with profound neurosensory deafness and choreoathetoid spastic cerebral palsy. Intellectual retardation may be relatively mild, but learning and functioning are hindered by deafness and spastic choreoathetosis.

Severe disease

The 20–25% of most severely affected fetuses, despite maximal red cell production, become progressively more anemic. Ascites with anasarca (generalized edema) occurs. Half of these fetuses become hydropic between 18 and 34 weeks' gestation; the other half between 34 weeks and term. Cardiac dysfunction secondary to severe fetal anemia and the resultant inadequate oxygen-carrying capacity is evident in at least 90% of hydropic fetuses.

Monitoring the mother and fetus at risk

A blood sample is obtained from every woman during her first prenatal visit for blood type and antibody screening, and the Rh status of her husband should be determined as needed. Cesarean section and manual removal of the placenta increase the frequency and size of fetal–maternal TPH, increasing the risk of immunization if the fetus is Rh positive. Amniocentesis for genetic purposes or for the determination of pulmonary maturity carries a 2% risk of immunization if performed under constant ultrasound guidance. At delivery, umbilical cord and maternal blood are tested: umbilical cord blood for ABO, Rh type, and the direct Coombs' status, and maternal blood for the presence of Rh antibody and fetal red cells. Rhogam should be administered in sufficient quantities.

Predicting the severity of Rh hemolytic disease

History

The risk of hydrops is 8–10% in a first sensitized pregnancy. If a woman has had a hydropic fetus, there is a 90% chance that the next affected fetus will also develop hydrops without intervention, typically at the same or an earlier time in gestation.

Generally speaking, an albumin titer of 16 or an indirect antiglobulin titer of 32–64 carries a 10% risk that the fetus will become hydropic without intervention. Titers of at-risk women should be repeated monthly after the first prenatal visit.

Amniotic fluid analysis

Optical density readings of centrifuged amniotic fluid (protected from light which can destroy the bilirubin) are made over the visual wavelength spectrum from 700 to 350 nm. The readings are plotted on semilogarithmic graph paper (with wavelength as the horizontal linear coordinate and optical density as the vertical logarithmic coordinate). The deviation from linearity at 450 nm (the ΔOD 450 reading) correlates directly with disease severity. Liley divided a plot of single amniotic fluid sample ΔOD 450 readings from 101 pregnancies after 28 weeks' gestation into three zones and related them to neonatal outcome. Readings in zone 1 indicated mild or no disease, but did not exclude the possibility that treatment would be required after birth. Readings in zone 2 were felt to indicate intermediate disease, increasing in severity as the zone 3 boundary was approached. It is necessary to repeat the amniotic fluid analyses to establish the ΔOD 450 trend. Thus, a decision to rely on amniotic fluid ΔOD 450 measurements is a decision to do at least two invasive procedures (Figs 46.1 and 46.2).

Hazards of amniocentesis

The risks of amniocentesis include placental trauma causing TPH, rising titers, and increasing severity of fetal hemolytic disease, amnionitis, and premature rupture of membranes. Any invasive procedure should be performed under continuous ultrasound visualization.

Fetal blood sampling

This procedure, which usually precedes fetal intravascular transfusion (IVT), allows the measurement of all blood parameters that can be measured after birth (i.e.,

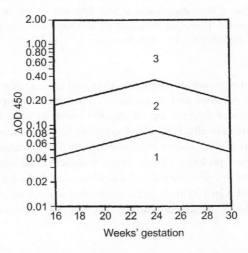

Figure 46.1 Modification of Liley's ΔOD 450 reading zone boundaries before 24 weeks' gestation. From Bowman et al. 1992.

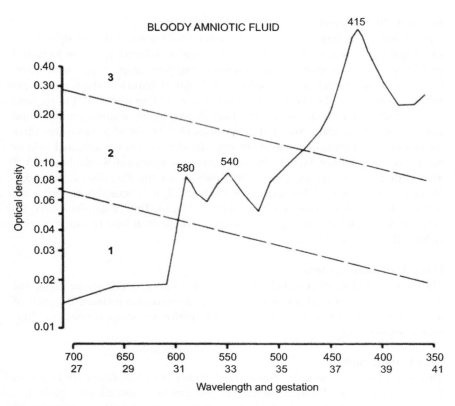

Figure 46.2 Spectrophotometric curve (Liley method) of amniotic fluid grossly contaminated with blood. Note sharp peaks at 580, 540, and 415 nm that obscure the 450-nm rise (Bowman JM. Hemolytic disease of the newborn. In: Conn HF, Conn RB, eds. *Current diagnosis 5.* Philadelphia, PA: W.B. Saunders; 1977:1107).

hemoglobin, hematocrit, serum bilirubin, direct and indirect platelet count, leukocyte count, serum proteins, and blood gases). Fetal blood sampling is by far the most accurate means of determining the degree of severity of hemolytic disease, in the absence of hydrops fetalis. Fetal blood sampling has an associated mortality rate of less than 1%. Morbidity occurs in approximately 5% of patients sampled using a freehand technique; prolonged bradycardia, umbilical cord hematoma, amnionitis with maternal adult respiratory distress syndrome, and placental abruption have each been described. Cordocentesis is recommended when a screening tool such as measurement of the middle cerebral artery (MCA) peak velocity is abnormal.

Ultrasound

Ultrasound has a central role in the management of the alloimmunized pregnancy.

First, it is used early to accurately establish gestational age. Second, many investigators have searched for alternative ultrasound parameters that could predict mild to moderate anemia. Lastly, hydrops fetalis can easily be detected with ultrasound.

Doppler ultrasonography

The peak systolic velocity in the fetal MCA has proved more accurate. Mari et al. (1995) established normative data for gestational age. Using a threshold value of 1.5 multiples of the mean (MoM) to predict moderate to severe anemia, more than 70% of invasive tests were avoided. Since 2000, multiple reports have confirmed the high sensitivity of the peak MCA velocity in detecting moderate to severe fetal anemia.

Management of the Rh-immunized woman (nonsensitized) and her fetus

When the maternal indirect Coombs' antibody titers are below the threshold (below which severe fetal hemolytic disease does not occur), they should be repeated monthly. Once the critical titer is exceeded, the fetus is followed with serial measurements of the peak MCA velocity. Invasive fetal evaluation following a positive Doppler finding consists of cordocentesis. The principal concern with cordocentesis is safety—vascular accidents and maternal sensitization are known to occur. Approximately 50% of isoimmunized women will require only one cordocentesis and, with the use of Doppler ultrasound, delivery may be safely deferred until term.

Management of the Rh-immunized woman with a previously affected fetus

Patients should be referred to a tertiary care center if they have documented isoimmunization. Maternal titers are not predictive of the degree of fetal anemia. If the paternal phenotype is heterozygous, an amniocentesis is performed at 15 weeks to determine fetal Rh D status. If the fetus is antigen positive, initiate serial MCA Doppler measurements by 18 weeks to monitor these pregnancies. Testing should be repeated every 1–2 weeks as long as they are normal. If a rising value for peak MCA Doppler velocity greater than 1.5 MoM is found, a cordocentesis is performed, and the fetus is transfused if the hematocrit is < 30%.

Intraperitoneal fetal transfusion

This is the original, but least preferred, method of fetal transfusion. Red cells placed in the peritoneal cavity of any animal with a diaphragm are absorbed intact into the circulation via the subdiaphragmatic lymphatics and the right thoracic duct. Diaphragmatic contractions are necessary for the absorption. In the absence of hydrops, 10–12% of transfused red cells are absorbed each day after transfusion. Absorption is greatly diminished and unpredictable in the presence of hydrops. The volume of blood injected is limited by the capacity of the peritoneal space. If the volume transfused is such that intraperitoneal pressure exceeds umbilical venous pressure, blood flow from the placenta to the fetus stops and the fetus dies. The intraperitoneal transfusion (IPT) volume can be calculated by the following formula: IPT volume = (weeks' gestation−20) × 10 mL (i.e., 50 mL at 25 weeks, 90 mL at 29 weeks). Calculation of residual donor hemoglobin concentration is necessary to space IPTs optimally so that the fetus undergoes the minimal number of procedures. IPT has several disadvantages. There is slow correction of the fetal anemia and a higher risk of trauma. There is the added risk of obstructing cardiac return if the intra-abdominal pressure becomes too high.

Direct intravascular fetal transfusion

Transfusion therapy is initiated when the fetal hematocrit is < 30%, a value less than the 2.5 per centile at all gestational ages above 20 weeks. The blood should be from a fresh donor, group O, and negative for the antigen (or antigens) to which the mother is sensitized (D negative if the mother is Rh negative with anti-D). It should also be negative for hepatitis B surface antigen (HBsAg), anti-human immunodeficiency virus (HIV), anti-hepatitis C (HCV), and anti-cytomegalovirus (CMV). Excluding the first transfusion of a hydropic fetus, the target for the post-transfusion fetal hematocrit is 48–55%. Consequently, the volume infused depends on the gestational age and the initial hematocrit. Except for the hydropic fetus, the second transfusion is generally performed 2 weeks after the first transfusion. The decline in fetal hematocrit thereafter is more predictable and generally, by 34–35 weeks, delivery may be delayed 4–5 weeks without another transfusion. The complications of hyperbilirubinemia are less if at least two transfusions are performed 3 weeks apart. The last transfusion is done between 34 and 35 weeks' gestation, and delivery is planned at 38–39 weeks. Transfusion therapy is not an indication for Cesarean delivery.

Intrauterine transfusion (IUT) in the presence of hydrops fetalis

Most hydropic fetuses have myocardial dysfunction. As a result, they frequently fail to tolerate the typical volume load. Thus, their target hematocrit after the first transfusion should be no more than 25%. A day later, the hematocrit can safely be brought up to the target 48–55% with a second transfusion. Umbilical vein pH (UVpH) maintenance is especially important in the hydropic fetus. During a transfusion, the UVpH normally declines because the pH of the transfused blood is 6.98–7.01. The red blood cell is the principal buffer in the human fetus. In the authors' experience, all losses of hydropic fetuses after the era of umbilical venous pressure measurement began were associated with profound acidemia and occurred hours after the transfusion. Consequently, the authors now infuse bicarbonate in

1-mEq increments to maintain UVpH above 7.30. The overall survival rate for hydrops (since beginning IVT) now exceeds 94%.

Survival after fetal transfusion

Survival after IUT varies with center experience and with the presence or absence of hydrops. Overall survival in one review was 84%. However, fewer hydropic fetuses survived after (IUT 70%) compared with fetuses who were not hydropic (92%). Mild hydrops reversed in 88% of cases, whereas severe hydrops only reversed in 39%, a finding clearly linked to overall perinatal survival: 98% of fetuses survived after reversal of hydrops. With persistent hydrops, only 39% of fetuses survived; if the hydrops was severe and persisted, only a quarter survived.

Delivery of the fetus after intrauterine transfusion

Generally, the last transfusion is administered around 34–35 weeks' gestation. If the fetal hematocrit at the end of the last transfusion was approximately 50%, then it will still be above 35% at delivery 4 weeks later. Consequently, there is no justification for preterm induction of labor if a transfusion can be performed.

Prevention of Rh immunization

Clinical trials were performed in which Rh-negative unimmunized women were given rhesus immune globulin (RhIG) after the delivery of a Rh-positive infant. All such trials were successful. As a result of these trials, RhIG was licensed in 1968 for use in North America. The standard dose in the United States is 300 μg given intramuscularly (i.m.). Smaller doses of 100–125 μg i.m. are used in Canada, Europe, and Australia. All these doses appear to be effective. RhIG prevents Rh immunization with two provisos: it must be given in an adequate amount, and it must be given before Rh immunization has begun. RhIG administration does not suppress Rh immunization once it has begun, no matter how weak the immunization. The precise mechanism of action of RhIG is unknown. There are three theories: antigen deviation, antigen blocking–competitive inhibition, and central inhibition (most likely). It is recommended in the United States that 300 μg of RhIG be administered within 72 h of delivery of a Rh-positive infant. This dose will protect against sensitization from a fetal–maternal hemorrhage (FMH) of 30 mL of fetal whole blood. Approximately 1 in 1000 deliveries will exceed this volume, and risk factors identify only 50%. Therefore, routine screening at delivery for excessive FMH is indicated. Universal antenatal prophylaxis combined with universal postpartum, postabortion, and postamniocentesis prophylaxis will reduce the prevalence of Rh immunization by 97% from the preprophylaxis incidence of approximately 13% to 0.27%.

Current recommendations for Rh prophylaxis

Every Rh-negative unimmunized woman who delivers a Rh-positive baby must be given one prophylactic dose of RhIG as soon as possible after delivery. Every Rh-negative unimmunized woman who aborts or threatens to abort must be given RhIG, unless her husband (or father of the baby) is known to be Rh negative. Every Rh-negative unimmunized woman who undergoes amniocentesis or chorionic villus sampling, unless her husband (or father of the baby) is known to be Rh negative, must be given 300 μg of RhIG at the time of the procedure, with subsequent doses at 12-week intervals until delivery. Every Rh-negative unimmunized woman whose husband (or father of the baby) is either Rh positive or Rh unknown should be given 300 μg of RhIG at 28 weeks' gestation. A second dose should be given 12.5 weeks later if delivery has not taken place, but then need not be repeated postpartum if delivery occurs within 3 weeks. If massive TPH is diagnosed, 300 μg of RhIG should be given i.m. for every 25 mL of fetal blood or fraction thereof in the maternal circulation. The dose may be reduced by one-third if RhIG is given intravenously. One prophylactic dose of RhIG should be given antepartum to the mother who has an Rh antibody detectable only by AutoAnalyzer (AA; Technicon Instruments Corp., Tarrytown, NY, USA) and again after delivery, if she delivers a Rh-positive baby. If the antibody is detectable by a manual enzyme method, administration of RhIG will not prevent progressive immunization. However, it should be given if there is any question about the specificity of the enzyme reactions.

ABO hemolytic disease

Although ABO-incompatible hemolytic transfusion reactions are intravascular and much more serious than extravascular Rh-incompatible hemolytic transfusion reactions, ABO hemolytic disease is much milder than Rh hemolytic disease. ABO hemolytic disease is mild because A and B antigens are not well developed on the fetal red cell membrane, because most anti-A and anti-B is IgM and does not cross the placenta, and because most of the small amounts of IgG anti-A and anti-B that do cross become attached to numerous other tissue and fluid A or B antigens. Thus, only a small amount of A or B antibody traversing the placenta binds to red cell antigenic sites. The management of ABO erythroblastosis is entirely a pediatric concern. Amniocentesis and other fetal investigative measures are not required in the ABO-incompatible pregnancy.

Hemolytic disease caused by atypical blood group antibodies

NonD alloimmunization has increased partly because of increased screening of pregnant D-positive women. It may also be because of a real increase in the occurrence of nonD alloimmunization because of the increased frequency of blood transfusion (transfused blood being only ABO and D compatible). The alloantibodies causing hemolytic disease of the newborn are numerous (Table 46.1).

Table 46.1 Association of hemolytic disease with maternal blood group antibodies.

Common	c(cE)—incidence high, disease common, may be severe
	Kell—incidence high, disease uncommon but, if present, may be severe
	E—incidence high, disease uncommon, usually mild, rarely severe
	C(Ce, C^w)—incidence moderate, disease common, usually mild
Uncommon	k—rarely present but, when present, may be very severe
	Kp^a(Kp^b)—rare, disease may require treatment, very rarely severe
	Jk^a—uncommon, may require treatment, rarely severe
	Fy^a—uncommon, usually mild, may require treatment, rarely severe
	S—uncommon, usually mild, may require treatment, rarely severe
Rare	s, U, M, Fy^b, N, Do^a, Di^a, Di^b, Lu^a, Yt^a, Jk^b—rarely cause hemolytic disease
Never	Le^a, Le^b, P—never cause hemolytic disease

However, the only antibodies implicated in moderate to severe disease are all those in the Rh blood group system plus anti-K, -Jk^a, -Js^a, -Js^b, -Ku, -Fy^a, -M, -N, -s, -U, -PP$_1$p^k, -Di^b, -Lan, -LW, -Far, -Good, -Wr^a, and -Zd. Although this list seems overwhelming, it must be considered in conjunction with the frequency with which such antibodies occur and the frequency with which they cause significant hemolytic disease of the newborn. Pregnant women with atypical antibodies [i.e., c(cE), Kell, E, C(Ce, C^w), k, Kp^a(Kp^b), Jk^a, Fy^a, S] should be managed in exactly the same manner as if they were Rh negative and Rh D immunized. The management of Kell isoimmunization is the same as for Rh disease, and based on serial MCA peak velocity measurements and cordocentesis when abnormal.

Further reading

Bowman JM, Pollock JM, Manning FA, et al. Maternal Kell blood group alloimmunization. *Obstet Gynecol* 1992;79:239.

Giancarlo M. Noninvasive diagnosis by Doppler ultrasonography of fetal anemia due to maternal red-cell alloimmunization. *N Engl J Med* 2000;342:9.

Mari G, Adrignolo A, Abuhamad AZ, et al. Diagnosis of fetal anemia with Doppler ultrasound in pregnancy complicated by maternal blood group immunization. *Ultrasound Obstet Gynecol* 1995;5:400.

Nicolaides KH, Warenski JC, Rodeck CH. The relationship of fetal protein concentration and haemoglobin level to the development of hydrops in rhesus isoimmunization. *Am J Obstet Gynecol* 1985;152:341.

Vyas S, Nicolaides KH, Campbell S. Doppler examination of the middle cerebral artery in anemic fetuses. *Am J Obstet Gynecol* 1990;162:1066.

Weiner CP Human fetal bilirubin and fetal hemolytic disease. *Am J Obstet Gynecol* 1992;116:1449.

Weiner CP, Pelzer GD, Heilskov J, et al. The effect of intravascular transfusion on umbilical venous pressure in anemic fetuses with and without hydrops. *Am J Obstet Gynecol* 1989; 161:149E.

Wiener CP, Heilskov J, Pelzer G, et al. Normal values for human umbilical venous and amniotic fluid pressures and their alteration by fetal disease. *Am J Obstet Gynecol* 1989;161:714.

Weiner CP, Wenstrom KD, Sipes SL, Williamson RA. Risk factors for cordocentesis and fetal intravascular transfusions. *Am J Obstet Gynecol* 1991;165:1020.

Weiner CP, Williamson RA, Wenstron KD, et al. Management of fetal hemolytic disease by cordocentesis: I. Prediction of fetal anemia. *Am J Obstet Gynecol* 1991;165:546.

Weiner CP, Williamson RA, Wenstrom KD, et al. Management of fetal hemolytic disease by cordocentesis: II. Outcome of treatment. *Am J Obstet Gynecol* 1991;165:1302.

 # Maternal infections, human immunodeficiency virus infection, and sexually transmitted diseases in pregnancy

Richard L. Sweet and Howard Minkoff

Maternal infections during pregnancy

The altered immune state of pregnancy increases the risk of infection for the adult host. Both the frequency and the severity of infection can be increased. Most of the studies of humoral immune response in pregnancy show reactions similar to those found in nonpregnant women. In contrast, the cellular immune response has generally been diminished.

Immunization of adult women

Immunization programs are a major part of our infectious disease prevention strategy. Of critical importance is the recognition that adult immunization programs are an integral part of this strategy. It has been estimated that over 60 000 adults die annually in the United States from vaccine-preventable diseases. Obstetrician–gynecologists should play an important role in adult immunization.

Tetanus–diphtheria

The Centers for Disease Control (CDC) recommends that adults, including pregnant women with an uncertain history of a complete primary vaccination series, should receive a primary series of tetanus and diphtheria (Td). For those women who have received the primary series, one booster dose should be administered every 10 years.

Measles, mumps, and rubella
Antibody testing should be done to confirm susceptibility. If the patient has no antibodies, she should be offered immunization. Because this is an attenuated live virus, the patient should be counseled to avoid getting pregnant for 3 months after the immunization.

Hepatitis B
Hepatitis B is an important disease for American women. It causes short-term illness and, for those chronic carriers of the virus, there is the possibility of serious long-term morbidity with cirrhosis or a hepatic carcinoma. Pre-exposure vaccination to prevent hepatitis B virus (HBV) infection addresses three groups of patients: (1) routine vaccination of all newborns/infants; (2) catch-up vaccination of susceptible children and adolescents; and (3) vaccination of high-risk adults (Table 47.1).

Hepatitis B vaccine is recommended for all newborns/infants; those born to mothers who are hepatitis surface antigen positive should receive the first dose of vaccine within 12 h of birth and a concomitant injection of hepatitis B immune globulin (HBIG).

Varicella
Varicella is a potentially serious illness for adults, resulting in pneumonia in some cases, and progressing to death in a few, especially in pregnant women. In addition, acquisition during pregnancy can be damaging to the fetus. Susceptibility should be determined by antibody testing and, if susceptible, immunization should be offered. Varicella vaccine is a live attenuated virus vaccine and thus, because of a theoreti-

Table 47.1 Groups at high risk of hepatitis B infection.

Sexually active heterosexual persons with recent STD, identified as prostitutes, having more than one sexual partner in the past 6 months, or seen in an STD clinic

Homosexual or bisexual men

Household contacts and sexual partners of HbsAg-positive persons

Intravenous drug abusers

Persons at occupational risk through exposure to blood or infected body fluids (i.e., healthcare workers, public safety workers)

Clients and staff of institutions for the developmentally disabled

Patients on hemodialysis

Patients receiving clotting factor concentrate

Adoptees from countries where HBV infection is endemic

International travelers to areas where HBV is endemic who will have close contact with the local population

Inmates of long-term correctional facilities

STD, sexually transmitted disease; HBsAg, hepatitis B surface antigen; HBV, hepatitis B virus.

cal risk, should not be given to pregnant women or those planning on becoming pregnant in the next 1 (Advisory Committee on Immunization Practices; ACIP) to 3 (Merck) months. Breastfeeding is not a contraindication to varicella vaccine.

Influenza

Influenza vaccines are inactivated viral vaccines and, as a result, are safe to use during any trimester of pregnancy. Pregnant women suffered excess deaths due to influenza during the pandemics of 1918–1919 and 1957–1958. Thus, the benefits of influenza vaccination in pregnant women clearly outweigh the potential risks. Women who will be pregnant during the influenza season should be inoculated with the influenza vaccine prior to the influenza season, regardless of the stage of pregnancy.

Pneumococcal pneumonia

Pneumococcal infections caused by *Streptococcus pneumoniae* are a major source of morbidity and mortality. The ACIP recommends pneumococcal vaccine for all persons aged $\geq$ 65 years and for those individuals between 2 and 65 years of age who are at increased risk of serious pneumococcal infection. While the safety of pneumococcal vaccine use in pregnancy has not been determined, there is no reason to suspect that the vaccine would have an adverse effect on the fetus or mother and, thus, pneumococcal vaccine is not contraindicated during any stage of pregnancy.

Hepatitis A

Hepatitis A vaccine is recommended for those aged $\geq$ 2 years who are at increased risk of hepatitis A virus (HAV) infection (Table 47.2).

Hepatitis A vaccine is an inactivated virus and thus is not specifically contraindicated during pregnancy, and is safe in breastfeeding mothers. However, it is recommended by the CDC that hepatitis A vaccine should be given in pregnancy only if clearly indicated (e.g., exposure to an infected contact or travel to an endemic region).

Table 47.2 Groups at high risk of hepatitis A infection.

International travelers to countries where HAV is endemic
Military personnel
High-risk ethnic or geographic populations (e.g., Native Americans, Alaskan natives)
Men who have sex with men
Intravenous drug abusers
Regular recipients of blood or plasma-derived products
Persons engaged in high-risk employment (primate handlers, employees of institutions for the developmentally challenged, day-care staff
Persons chronically infected with hepatitis C

Urinary tract infections

Approximately 2–10% of pregnant women have asymptomatic bacteriuria (ASB). The physiologic changes associated with pregnancy predispose the pregnant women to develop upper urinary tract infection.

Prevention of pyelonephritis

An estimated 25–30% of women with asymptomatic bacteriuria at the time of their first antepartum visit who are not treated will subsequently develop pyelonephritis. In addition, ASB has been associated with an increased risk of preterm delivery and low birthweight.

Although other screening tests are available, they lack sensitivity, and the standard remains the screening culture. When voided urine culture tests are employed, a significant test result has > 100 000 colonies/mL of one bacterial species. The treatment of women who are culture positive is based on the recognition that, as in nonpregnant women, *Escherichia coli* is the predominant pathogen isolated (80–90% of cases). Other important pathogens include *Staphylococcus saprophytieus* and group B streptococci.

When the presence of ASB is identified, empiric treatment is instituted based on the above described causative microorganisms. Treatment is instituted with a 3-day course of trimethoprim-sulfamethoxazole (1 double-strength tablet b.i.d.) or nitrofurantoin 100 mg b.i.d. In geographic areas where *E. coli* remains sensitive to ampicillin, amoxicillin 500 mg t.i.d. is an alternative. Continuous monitoring of patients for recurrent or persistent ASB is critical. If infection recurs, treatment should be based on antimicrobial susceptibility studies, and the patient should be maintained on suppressive antimicrobials (nitrofurantoin 100 mg h.s.) for the remainder of the pregnancy.

Pyelonephritis

Acute pyelonephritis is one of the most frequent medical complications of pregnancy, occurring in 1–2.5% of obstetric patients.

Premature labor can occur in these women. Occasionally, some of these women become critically ill. Although uncommon, septic shock and adult respiratory distress syndrome may occur. Thus, these women require close medical supervision.

Initially, treatment for acute pyelonephritis is empiric, with antimicrobial therapy dictated by knowledge of the most common etiologic organisms and the need for bactericidal drugs. The organisms most commonly recovered from pregnant women with acute pyelonephritis include *E. coli* (80–85%) and, less commonly, the *Klebsiella–Enterobacter* group. Gram-positive bacteria, such as group B streptococci and enterococci, have increasingly been recognized as pathogens in acute pyelonephritis in pregnant women. The authors recommend that empiric therapy for acute pyelonephritis during pregnancy be instituted with ceftriaxone 1–2 g intravenously as a single daily dose; it provides coverage against most major uropathogens other than *Enterococcus* and, because of once-daily administration, facilitates home parenteral therapy after initial in-hospital treatment and

369

stabilization. Trimethoprim-sulfamethoxazole 160/800 mg intravenously b.i.d. is also appropriate in geographic areas where *E. coli* resistance to this agent has not occurred. A combination of either ampicillin (1–2 g intravenous q6h) or cefazolin 1–2 g intravenous q8h) in combination with gentamicin (1 mg/kg q8h) is an alternative approach. When patients have been afebrile for 24–48 h, they can be switched to an oral agent or home parenteral therapy to complete 10 days of therapy.

Economic pressures have altered this inpatient treatment emphasis, and there is evidence suggesting that selected patients might be treated as outpatients.

HIV in pregnancy

According to United Nation statistics, close to thirty million people were alive with HIV infection in 2003. During that year, nearly five million new infections were recorded, and almost three million people died. Women now comprise about half of all HIV-infected individuals, and there are approximately 2000 new infections of children under the age of 15 years (the vast majority secondary to mother-to-child transmission) every day. Over 95% of infections occur in sub-Saharan Africa. However, if recent projections prove correct, the bulk of new infections will be occurring in other parts of the world by the end of this decade. It is now predicted that India, Nigeria, China, Ethiopia, and Russia (in decreasing order of new infections) will have as many as 70 million infected individuals within 5 years.

In the United States, the CDC estimates that 40 000 new HIV infections occur every year. From the beginning of the epidemic in 1981 to 2000, an estimated 1.3–1.4 million Americans have been infected with HIV, and approximately one-third (450 000) of those have died. It is further estimated that, as of 2000, between 850 000 and 950 000 people are alive with HIV.

Virology and pathophysiology

HIV-1 and HIV-2 are members of the lentivirus subfamily of Retroviridae and are single-stranded ribonucleic acid (RNA) enveloped viruses that have the ability to become incorporated into cellular deoxyribonucleic acid (DNA). HIV preferentially infects cells with the CD4 antigen, particularly helper lymphocytes, but also macrophages, cells of the central nervous system and, according to some evidence, cells of the placenta. At least two other cell-surface molecules help HIV to enter the cells. These co-receptors for HIV, called CXCR4 and CCR5, are receptors for chemokines. Once the virus is internalized, its RNA is released from the nucleo-capsid and is reverse transcribed into proviral DNA. The provirus is inserted into the genome and then transcribed into RNA; the RNA is translated, and virions assemble and are extruded from the cell membrane by budding. The virus is composed of core (p18, p24, and p27) and surface (gp120 and gp41) proteins, genomic RNA, and the reverse transcriptase enzyme surrounded by a lipid bilayer envelope.

Untreated, HIV infection leads to progressive debilitation of the immune system, rendering infected individuals susceptible to opportunistic infections (e.g., *Pneu-*

mocystis carinii pneumonia and central nervous system toxoplasmosis) and neoplasias (e.g., Kaposi's sarcoma) that rarely afflict patients with intact immune systems. For an HIV-infected patient with one of several specific opportunistic infections, neoplasia, dementia encephalopathy, or wasting syndrome, the diagnosis of acquired immunodeficiency syndrome (AIDS) is assigned. In 1993, the CDC changed the case definition to include all individuals with HIV infection whose CD4 counts drop below 200 CD4 lymphocytes/μL as well as HIV-infected individuals with advanced cervical cancer, pulmonary tuberculosis, and recurrent pneumonia.

At the time of initial infection, there is an immediate viremia of substantive proportions (up to a billion viral particles turned over per day) and an equally impressive immune response with similar levels of T-cell turnover. After the initial viremia, the level of virus returns to a "set point" The level of virus in the plasma at that time can provide an estimate of the probability that an individual, if left untreated, will develop AIDS within 5 years. Antibodies are usually detectable 1 month after infection and are almost always detectable within 3 months.

Management of the HIV-infected pregnant women

Appropriate management of HIV-infected pregnant women requires an understanding of testing, monitoring and medical therapy. The latter issue is the most complex and the most rapidly changing. In order to stay abreast of those changes, the International AIDS Society and the Public Health Service provide continuing updates, the latter on a web site, to which the reader should refer as new drugs and protocols emerge. The Public Health Service ("AIDSinfo") website also provides guidelines specifically for the care of pregnant women.

Testing

A great deal can now be offered to HIV-infected individuals. As will be detailed below, therapy is now available that can reliably reduce both disease progression and mother-to-child transmission (MTCT). All the available treatments work best when they are initiated before clinical disease or advanced immune compromise occurs. Thus, it is essential that obstetricians ascertain the serostatus of all their patients as early in pregnancy as possible. Opt-in testing is the most common testing strategy employed in the United States. It requires counseling and written consent. However, it is neither the most successful nor the currently recommended strategy for testing. In the antepartum setting, identification of infected women is best accomplished using a "routine" right-of-refusal approach and employing standard enzyme-linked immunosorbent assay (ELISA) and Western blot technologies.

Despite the implementation of routine testing protocols in prenatal settings, there will still be circumstances in which rapid testing will play an important role. It is estimated that 40–85% of infants infected with HIV are born to women whose HIV infection is unknown prior to delivery. A number of studies have been published that demonstrate the ability of antiretroviral therapy, even when first introduced in the intrapartum or immediate neonatal period, to prevent some cases of pediatric HIV infection. When selecting a rapid HIV test for use during labor and delivery,

371

it is important to consider the accuracy of the test and the site (i.e., hospital laboratory versus point-of-care testing in labor and delivery) at which testing will be performed. Performance evaluations on three United States Food and Drug Administration (FDA)-approved rapid HIV tests (OraQuick, Reveal, and Uni-Gold) indicate a sensitivity of 100%, 99.8%, and 100% (95% confidence interval), respectively, and a specificity of 99.9%, 99.1% (serum), and 99.7% (95% confidence interval) respectively.

Monitoring

The advent of highly active antiretroviral therapy (HAART) has made HIV, in many ways, a chronic illness similar to diabetes. Just as no clinician would think about managing a diabetic without ongoing assessments of their disease state and the impact of their therapy (e.g., monitoring of blood glucose levels), so no HIV-specialist would be able to manage his/her patient without tracking their immune status, viral status, and viral resistance as appropriate.

During pregnancy, viral load status should be determined every month until the virus is no longer detectable. Viral load should drop by approximately 1–2 logs per month if effective therapy is being used. Once the virus is no longer detectable, testing can be performed every 3 months. The CD4 count can be used to decide when it is necessary to institute prophylaxis for opportunistic infections. No such medications are required if the CD4 count is higher than 200/µL. If such therapy is begun at a lower count, but the CD4 count rises back above 200/µL consequent to HAART, the prophylaxis can be discontinued once the count has remained over that threshold for 6 months.

Failure to achieve the "undetectable" benchmark often reflects the development of a resistant organism. The life cycle of HIV predisposes to mutations and, hence, resistance because of the combination of the rapid turnover of HIV (10^7–10^8 rounds of replication/day) and the high error rate of reverse transcriptase when replicating the nearly 10 000 nucleotides present in the HIV genome. When incompletely suppressive drug regimens are used, they provide the evolutionary pressure that selects those mutations that cause resistance to antiretroviral agents.

Medical therapy: when to start

Once a diagnosis of HIV infection has been made and the individual's clinical, virologic, and immune status has been assessed, the clinician must determine whether antiretroviral therapy is appropriate.

If the patient has severe immune compromise or a clinical diagnosis of AIDS, then the decision is clear. Randomized clinical trials have demonstrated a survival benefit with the use of antiretroviral therapy in those circumstances. For less severely compromised individuals (i.e., asymptomatic individuals with CD4 cell counts ≥ 200/µL), the data are not as clear cut. The largest study, which analyzed data from more than 10 000 patients, concluded that prognosis could be best predicted by CD4 cell count and HIV RNA response after 6 months of treatment, independent of pretreatment values. Another study analyzed data from 1464 patients from several clinics in the United States and found that, after 4 years of follow-up, patients with baseline CD4 cell counts between 200/μL and 350/μL who started antiretroviral therapy had lower mortality rates than those who waited until their CD4 cell count was below 200/μL.

Thus, delay in initiation of therapy carries with it some risk of poorer prognosis. However, there are countervailing considerations. These include concerns over the long-term safety of therapy, toxic effects, potential cardiovascular consequences, and the negative impact of fat maldistribution on quality of life.

In sum, these data from observational cohorts strongly suggest that antiretroviral therapy may decrease the incidence of potentially life-threatening conditions. That finding, in conjunction with long-term safety data on some regimens, and the availability of newer drugs that are safer and easier to take, would support the initiation of therapy before HIV-related disease becomes clinically manifest.

In reviewing all the aforementioned data, the International AIDS Society drew several conclusions. They felt that therapy should be recommended for all patients with symptomatic HIV disease. They also recommend antiretroviral treatment initiation before CD4 cell counts reach 200/μL. However, initiation of therapy in patients with CD4 cell counts below 350/μL but above 200/μL should be individualized. Finally, initiation of therapy is generally not recommended for patients with CD4 cell counts between 350/μL and 500/μL, but it may be considered in cases with high plasma viral load or a rapid decline in CD4 cell count.

More recently, the Panel on Clinical Practices for Treatment of HIV Infection convened by the Department of Health and Human Services modified their recommendations for when to initiate therapy for asymptomatic treatment-naïve patients with CD4 cell counts > 350 cells/μL. The viral load recommendation to defer or to consider therapy was increased from 55 000 to 100 000 copies/mL. They based this change on the belief that, even at those CD4 and viral load levels, the chance of disease progression is relatively low.

Medical therapy: what to start

Over the last several years, arrays of antiretroviral therapies have come on the market. They vary in price, efficacy, and toxicity. Some are inappropriate for use in pregnancy. The obstetrician should be comfortable with a few regimens that are most appropriate for use in pregnancy and be liberal in consulting with experts in HIV infection in those circumstances (e.g., resistance) in which their usual choices are no longer appropriate.

A HAART regimen using a non-nucleoside reverse transcriptase inhibitor (NNRTI) is often the initial regimen of choice because of convenience, superior virological suppression, lower rates of toxic effects, and fewer interactions between drugs than seen with regimens that utilize a boosted protease inhibitor. However, during pregnancy, that approach may require modification because the preferred NNRTI, efavirenz, is contraindicated in women who are or wish to become pregnant because of potential teratogenicity. Nevirapine (NVP), which is a reasonable option under other circumstances, has the disadvantage of potential toxic effects that are particularly common among pregnant women with relatively high CD4 counts (> 250/µL).

The alternative to an NNRTI backbone in a HAART regimen is a protease inhibitor (PI) backbone. Some of these regimens involve two PIs with one drug acting to "boost" the availability of the other. Regimens that are ritonavir boosted are often recommended because of the improvement in PI pharmacokinetics and potency.

A large number of nucleoside reverse transcriptase inhibitor (NRTI) combinations are available for use as the backbone of HAART regimens in nonpregnant women. These include zidovudine (ZDV) plus lamivudine or emtricitabine; tenofovir plus lamivudine or emtricitabine; or emtricitabine plus didanosine. In pregnancy, the first choice is ZDV plus lamivudine. There are a few combinations that should be avoided. Combining stavudine and ZDV is contraindicated; combinations of stavudine and didanosine or combinations with zalcitabine are not recommended because of increased toxic effects.

Prevention of transmission
Drugs
Since the results of ACTG 076 were first reported in 1994 (monotherapy with ZDV reduced MTCT from 25.5% to 8.3%), it has been apparent that antiretroviral therapy can substantially reduce the rate of MTCT. Since that time, research has advanced in two directions. In the developing world, there have been a large number of studies designed to see whether cheaper, shorter regimens could have benefits similar to those seen with more expensive, cumbersome approaches. In the developed world, the focus has been on improved efficacy, as opposed to reduced cost. Both avenues of research have borne fruit.

The most dramatic result, from the perspective of simplicity and cost, came from the HIVNET 012 trial, which documented the efficacy of oral NVP when given just twice, once in the intrapartum period and once to the neonate. Subsequent studies have highlighted the public health risks attendant on this approach. Fairly high frequencies of resistant virus in the postpartum period have been reported among mothers who have used NVP in the intrapartum period and, more alarmingly, there is some evidence that women who took NVP to prevent MTCT were more likely to fail NVP-based HAART when they became eligible for treatment later in life.

In the United States, data have accumulated fairly quickly demonstrating that the results obtained with monotherapy could be exceeded with more aggressive antiretroviral therapy. As HAART became the standard of care for HIV infection, several authors noted that those pregnant women who were on HAART for their own care had remarkably low rates of MTCT, independent of the mode of delivery. In fact, there are now preliminary data, summarized in the next section, that HAART therapy *per se* may be as efficacious as Cesarean section in preventing MTCT.

In determining which regimen should be used for the prevention of MTCT, the first question to be asked is what regimen does the mother need for her own health and is there any need to modify that regimen in order to minimize rates of MTCT? If the patient meets the criteria for antiretroviral therapy (as detailed above), then she should be on a HAART regimen. The obstetrician should review the regimen that the patient is taking. If it is effective (viral load is undetectable), then it should only be changed if some component of the regimen is contraindicated in pregnancy (e.g., efavirnez). If it is failing, then it should be changed, taking into consideration both the results of resistance testing and the safety of individual agents for use during pregnancy.

Mode of delivery

Evidence of the potential benefit of Cesarean section for reducing MTCT antedates the use of antiretroviral therapy. Studies from that era showed substantive reductions in transmission (55–80%) when surgery was performed before labor or rupture of membranes occurred.

The most compelling data from that time were observational data from a meta-analysis and from an international randomized study. The former included observations from 15 prospective cohort studies, including more than 7800 mother–child pairs, and found that the rate of perinatal HIV-1 transmission among women undergoing elective Cesarean delivery was significantly lower than that among similar women having either nonelective Cesarean or vaginal delivery, regardless of whether they received ZDV, the only antiretroviral in use at the time. In the latter, transmission was 1.8% among women randomized to elective Cesarean delivery, many of whom received ZDV. The American College of Obstetricians and Gynecologists' (ACOG) Committee on Obstetric Practice, after reviewing these data, issued a Committee Opinion concerning the route of delivery, recommending consideration of scheduled Cesarean delivery for HIV-1-infected pregnant women. However, as data were also available demonstrating low rates of transmission, independent of mode of delivery, when the viral load was < 1000 copies/mL, the committee limited their recommendation to those women with HIV-1 RNA levels of > 1000 copies/mL near the time of delivery.

Transmission, viral load, and combination antiretroviral therapy

As noted, the studies mentioned above were performed on the cusp of the era of HAART. Given the dramatic reductions in MTCT that have followed in the wake of these therapies, it is becoming increasingly difficult to document an effect of operative delivery above and beyond that which can be obtained with medical therapy alone.

Even the most recent data fail to clarify the proper role for Cesarean section in the era of HAART, with some suggesting a role for Cesarean section even in the presence of HART and others seeming to demonstrate that HAART alone will have maximal benefits. Thus, data from PACTG 367, including 2756 women, do not demonstrate any benefit from elective Cesarean delivery among either women with HIV RNA levels below 1000 copies/mL or those on multiagent antiretroviral therapy. Specifically, women with HIV RNA levels below 1000 copies/mL on multiagent therapy had transmission rates of 0.8% with elective Cesarean delivery and 0.5% with all other delivery modes [odds ratio (OR) 1.4, 95% CI 0.2–6.4], and those on single-agent therapy, usually ZDV, had a transmission rate of 4.3% after elective Cesarean delivery and 1.8% with all other delivery modes (OR 2.5, 95% CI 0.04–50.0). Women on multiagent therapy with HIV RNA levels over 1000 copies/mL near delivery had a transmission rate of 3.6% with elective Cesarean and 2.3% with other delivery modes (OR 1.6, 95% CI 0.6–4.3). Data from the 4377 women who participated in the European Collaborative Study yielded strikingly divergent results, suggesting a reduction in perinatal transmission of HIV with scheduled Cesarean delivery even among women on HAART or with undetectable HIV RNA levels. While the overall transmission rate among women on HAART was a reassuringly low 10 out of 678 (1.5%), a logistic regression, adjusting for antenatal antiretroviral therapy, CD4+ lymphocyte count, gender, and time period, revealed that scheduled Cesarean delivery was still associated with a reduced risk of transmission (AOR 0.51, 95% CI 0.31–0.82).

Intrapartum management

If a decision has been made to effect delivery via scheduled Cesarean delivery, then antiretroviral therapy should be part of the preoperative protocol. Intravenous ZDV should begin 3 h before surgery, according to standard dosing recommendations, and the infant should receive ZDV for 6 weeks after birth. Other maternal drugs should be continued on schedule as much as possible to provide maximal effect and minimize the chance of development of viral resistance.

As noted above, infectious morbidity is an important consideration, and consideration should be given to the initiation of prophylactic antibiotics. If vaginal delivery is planned and if labor is progressing and membranes are intact, artificial rupture of membranes or invasive monitoring should be avoided.

The most problematic clinical dilemmas involve circumstances in which the fetus may be exposed to prolonged periods of membrane rupture. If a vaginal delivery had been planned, i.e., the viral load is low, then continuing antiviral therapy and aggressively moving toward vaginal delivery seems the most appropriate management plan. However, if a Cesarean section was planned, it is unclear how long after membranes rupture that Cesarean section will continue to offer a benefit with regard to a lowered MTCT rate. Much of the data linking duration of rupture to increased risk of transmission antedate the use of antiretroviral therapy, and their utility for predicting events in the HAART era is thereby limited. The data from more recent studies are less uniform in their conclusions.

Postpartum management

The first management decision that the obstetrician and parturient confront in the immediate postpartum period is whether to continue the medications that the woman had been on during pregnancy. If the woman had been on HAART prior to pregnancy and her viral load had continued to be suppressed throughout gestation, then she should be maintained on the same regimen at least until she re-establishes contact with her primary HIV care provider. Alternatively, if the patient had not met the criteria for HAART during the prepregnancy period, but had been started merely as part of a strategy to reduce the risk of MTCT, the discontinuation of therapy would be appropriate. In that circumstance, all medications should be discontinued simultaneously to avoid prolonged exposure to monotherapy and the consequent risk of development of resistant virus.

Sexually transmitted diseases in pregnancy

The epidemic of STDs remains unabated in America. In 1993, the Institute of Medicine (IOM) estimated that 12 million new cases of STDs occurred annually in the United States at an estimated annual cost of US$17 billion. Subsequently, the estimate of new STD cases is nearly 19 million annually.

Gonorrhea

Gonorrhea, caused by the Gram-negative diplococcus, *Neisseria gonorrhoeae*, is the second most commonly reported communicable disease in the United States with over 335 000 cases reported in 2003. As a result of underreporting, it is estimated that approximately 750 000 cases actually occur annually in the United States.

Clinical manifestations

Acute symptomatic anogenital infections in women are characterized by dysuria, increased urinary frequency, increased vaginal discharge secondary to an exudative endocervicitis, abnormal menstrual bleeding, or anorectal discomfort.

Maternal and fetal risks

The association between maternal gonorrheal infection and ophthalmia neonatorum has been appreciated for over a century. Before routine administration of silver nitrate, this disease occurred in 10% of newborns. The institution of routine neonatal prophylaxis reduced this rate dramatically.

Subsequently, gonococcal infection during gestation has been linked to a wide variety of perinatal complications. Postabortal and postpartum endometritis occur more frequently in women with untreated gonococcal cervicitis at the time of delivery. Intra-amniotic infection has also been described. A chronic, low-grade infection may ensue, with resultant intrauterine growth retardation. The incidence of preterm delivery in women with untreated cervical gonorrhea has been recorded to be as high as 67%.

Laboratory diagnosis

The diagnosis of gonococcal infection in women requires identification of N. *gonorrhoeae* at infected sites. Available methods include culture, immunochemical detection, or molecular diagnostic techniques.

Selective plates, such as Thayer–Martin, provide optimal conditions for isolation of the organism. *N. gonorrhoeae* forms oxidase-positive colonies that can be differentiated from other *Neisseria* species.

The traditional method of gonorrhea detection in women was culture of the cervix. With the introduction of nonculture assays for detection of *N. gonorrhoeae*, these newer methodologies have replaced culture. Nonamplified DNA probe tests were the first widely accepted alternative to culture and became the most common nonculture method for the detection of *N. gonorrhoeae* in the United States. Nucleic acid amplification tests have become available more recently and include polymerase chain reaction (PCR), ligase chain reaction (LCR), and transcription-mediated amplification (TMA). These amplification methods have excellent sensitivity and specificity.

Treatment

Chlamydial infection coexists with gonorrhea in up to 30% of patients. Patients with gonococcal infections should be treated with regimens effective against both pathogens. The CDC recommendations are given in Table 47.3. For pregnant women, the recommended regimens include ceftriaxone or cefixime plus erythromycin. Alternative cephalosporins for the pregnant patient include cefotaxime, ceftizoxime, cefotetan, and cefoxitin. For patients who cannot tolerate cephalosporins, spectinomycin is the preferred alternative. The incidence of treatment failure among those treated with ceftriaxone or cefixime is extremely rare, obviating the need for test-of-cure for *N. gonorrhoeae*. These women should be screened for reinfection after 2–3 months.

Table 47.3 Centers for Disease Control 2002 recommended treatment guidelines for uncomplicated anogenital gonorrhea during pregnancy.

Recommended regimens
  Ceftriaxone, 125 mg i.m. once
  or
  Cefixime, 400 mg p.o. in a single dose
  plus
  Erythromycin, 500 mg p.o. q.i.d. for 7 days
  or
  Amoxicillin 500 mg p.o. q.i.d. for 7 days

Alternative regimens
  Spectinomycin, 2 g i.m. in a single dose
  Cefotaxime, 500 mg i.m. once
  Ceftizoxime, 500 mg i.m. once
  Cefotetan, 1 g i.m. once
  Cefoxitin, 2 g i.m. once

Syphilis

Syphilis is a chronic, debilitating systemic infection caused by the spirochete *Treponema pallidum*.

Clinical manifestations

Primary The first sign of primary infection is the development of a single, nontender lesion (chancre) at the site of entry. The most customary sites of infection in women include the vulva, introitus, or cervix. The syphilitic chancre is a painless, dull red macule, which becomes a papule and then ulcerates.

Secondary The symptoms of secondary syphilis typically emerge 3–6 weeks later. By this time, the infection is widely disseminated, and most symptoms are due to immune complex deposition. A classic faint macular rash develops over the trunk and flexor surfaces in the vast majority of infected individuals. The rash spreads over the whole body, including the palms and soles, and becomes first dull red and papular, then squamous. Superficial ulcerations called mucous patches appear in the mucous membranes in 30% of patients.

Latent By definition, this stage lacks clinical manifestations. The early latent phase (less than 1 year) has been associated with recurrence of secondary mucocutaneous lesions. Although late latent syphilis (more than 1 year) cannot be transmitted sexually, vertical transmission to the fetus persists.

Tertiary One-third of untreated patients develop tertiary syphilis. This is characterized by involvement of the cardiovascular, central nervous, or musculoskeletal systems. The presence of gummas in various tissues designates late benign tertiary syphilis. Aortic aneurysms and aortic insufficiency are characteristic cardiovascular lesions, whereas generalized paresis, tabes dorsalis, and optic atrophy with the Argyll Robertson pupil that accommodates, but does not react to, light are all features of neurosyphilis.

Laboratory diagnosis

The gold standard for diagnosis of early syphilis is the detection of treponemes on darkfield examination of ulcer scrapings or tissue samples. Indirect diagnosis of syphilis can be made using two types of serologic tests. Nontreponemal tests such as the Venereal Disease Research Laboratory (VDRL) test and rapid plasma regain (RPR) show reactive results approximately 2 weeks after development of the initial lesion. Treponemal-specific tests, which confirm the diagnosis, include the fluorescent treponemal antibody absorbed (FTA-ABS) assay and microhemagglutination assay for antibody to *T. pallidum* (MHATP).

The CDC recommends that all pregnant women should be screened for syphilis at their first prenatal visit. Where prenatal care is problematic, the RPR card test screening (a rapid screen for syphilis) is recommended when pregnancy is diagnosed and treatment given if positive. For women at high risk of syphilis and in

379

Table 47.4 Centers for Disease Control 2002 recommended treatment guidelines for syphilis in pregnancy.

Early syphilis recommended regimen (primary, secondary, and early latent syphilis)
 Benzathine penicillin G, 2.4 million units (U) i.m. once (1.2 million U in each buttock)

Late latent and tertiary syphilis recommended regimen
 Benzathine penicillin G, 7.2 million U total administered as three doses of 2.4 million
  U i.m. given 1 week apart for 3 consecutive weeks

Neurosyphilis recommended regimen
 Aqueous crystalline penicillin G, 12–24 million U administered 2–4 million U i.v. q4h
  for 10–14 days

Neurosyphilis alternative regimen
 Procaine penicillin, 2.4 million U i.m. daily with
 Probenecid, 500 mg p.o. q.i.d., both for 10–14 days

---

populations with a high prevalence of syphilis, additional serologic testing at 28 weeks' gestation and at delivery are recommended.

Patients with neurologic or ophthalmic signs or symptoms, evidence of tertiary syphilis, treatment failure, or HIV infection with late latent syphilis of unknown duration should have cerebrospinal fluid obtained to test for neurosyphilis.

The diagnosis of neurosyphilis is challenging, because no one test is reliable. The cerebrospinal fluid should be tested for cell count, protein, and with the VDRL test. An elevated count of more than five white blood cells/µL is a relatively sensitive indicator of active infection. A positive cerebrospinal fluid VDRL result is diagnostic for neurosyphilis.

Treatment

Treatment regimens in pregnancy are listed in Table 47.4. Pregnant patients who are allergic to penicillin should be treated with penicillin after desensitization.

Maternal and fetal risks

Pregnancy does not appear to alter the course of syphilis; however, *T. pallidum* adversely affects pregnancy. It crosses the placenta and has been associated with preterm delivery, stillbirth, congenital infection, and neonatal death, depending on the timing of infection. The majority of infants with congenital syphilis are born to mothers with early syphilis or secondary infection. Fetal infection during the first and second trimesters carries significant morbidity, whereas third-trimester exposure results in asymptomatic infection. Fiumara et al. reported that, with untreated primary or secondary syphilis, 50% of the infants were premature, stillborn, or died as neonates, and the remaining 50% developed congenital syphilis. With early latent syphilis, 20–60% of infants were normal, 20% premature, and 16% stillborn; 40%

had congenital syphilis. For late untreated syphilis, the congenital syphilis rate was 10%, stillbirth rate was 10%, premature rate was 9%, and healthy infants made up 70%. More recently, studies have confirmed the significant adverse effect of untreated syphilis on pregnancy outcome.

Chlamydial infections
Chlamydia trachomatis is the most frequently diagnosed bacterial STD in the United States with an estimated prevalence of more than 4 million cases and an annual cost of more than US$1 billion. It has been estimated that between 20% and 40% of sexually active women in the United States have been exposed to *C. trachomatis*. The prevalence among pregnant women depends on the population sampled, varying from 2% to 37%.

Clinical manifestations
Endocervicitis The most commonly infected site in the female genital tract is the endocervix. The majority of infected women are asymptomatic. Findings on physical examination extend from normal to cervical erosion and mucopurulent cervicitis.

Acute urethral syndrome Chlamydial infection has also been implicated in the etiology of 25% of patients with acute urethral syndrome. Such women present with dysuria and increased urinary frequency in the face of sterile urine.

Maternal and fetal risks
Vertical transmission rates secondary to passage through an infected cervix are as high as 60–70%. Inclusion conjunctivitis develops during the first 2 weeks of life in 25–50% of these neonates, whereas another 10–20% develop chlamydial pneumonia within 4 months of birth.

The role of endocervical *C. trachomatis* infection in the development of spontaneous abortion, fetal death, premature rupture of membranes (PROM), preterm delivery, and intrauterine growth retardation is debated.

Laboratory diagnosis
In the past, culture was considered the optimal means of making the diagnosis of chlamydial infection. However, isolation of *C. trachomatis* was challenging, because the organism requires a susceptible tissue culture cell line, using a technically arduous procedure whereby these cells are inoculated with specimen and then examined 24–72h later for the development of inclusions.

The first major advancement in making *Chlamydia* testing more available was the introduction of chlamydial antigen detection products in the late 1980s. One is fluorescent monoclonal antibody staining of chlamydial elementary bodies (Microtrac-Syva Co., Palo Alto, CA, USA), and the other is an enzyme-linked immunosorbent assay (ELISA; Chlamydiazyme, Abbott Laboratories, Chicago, IL, USA). These antigen detection tests were largely replaced in the 1990s by methods using DNA

Table 47.5 Centers for Disease Control 2002 recommended treatment guidelines for chlamydial infections in pregnancy.

Recommended regimen
  Erythromycin base, 500 mg p.o. q.i.d. for 7 days
  or
  Amoxicillin 500 mg p.o. q.i.d. for 7 days

Alternative regimens
  Erythromycin base, 250 mg p.o. q.i.d. for 14 days
  or
  Erythromycin ethylsuccinate, 800 mg p.o. q.i.d. for 7 days
  or
  Azithromycin 1 g p.o. as a single dose

---

probe hybridization (PACE 2 test; Gen. Probe, San Diego, CA, USA). An important advantage of the DNA probe is that it can be used in conjunction with a probe for the detection of *N. gonorrhoeae* in a single swab. Most recently, DNA amplification methodology has been introduced into clinical practice. Both the PCR and LCR tests for *C. trachomatis* have excellent sensitivity, specificity, and positive predictive value.

Treatment

The CDC recommendations for the treatment of chlamydial genital tract infection during pregnancy are provided in Table 47.5. As doxycycline and fluoroquinolones are contraindicated for pregnant women, erythromycin base and amoxicillin are the CDC-recommended regimens for the treatment of chlamydial infection during pregnancy.

Human papillomavirus

Human papillomavirus (HPV) is a member of the papovavirus family and is composed of double-stranded DNA. More than 100 types have been identified, of which 35 primarily infect the genital tract. Genital HPV types are generally divided into two major groups based upon their oncogenic potential. The high-risk or oncogenic group includes HPV types 16, 18, 31, 33, 35, and 39. The low-risk group includes HPV types 6, 11, 42, 43, and 44. These low-risk HPV types are associated with genital warts (condyloma acuminata), cervical condyloma, and some cases of low-grade squamous intraepithelial lesions (LGSIL).

Epidemiology

Sexual transmission of HPV is the primary route of transmission and results in urogenital and anorectal lesions. The highest risk groups are sexually active teenagers and young adults. Transmission rates are high, with 65% of sexual contacts becoming infected.

According to the CDC an estimated 24 million Americans are infected with HPV, and between 500 000 and 1 million new cases of HPV-induced genital warts occur each year in the United States. The use of PCR technology has shown that the prevalence of subclinical HPV is higher, and recent serologic studies have suggested that at least 50% of sexually active women have been infected with one or more HPV types.

Treatment

Treatment for warts of the genital tract depends upon the anatomic location of disease (external genitalia/perianal, cervical, vaginal, or urethral), the clinical presentation of disease (clinical versus subclinical), and the extent of disease.

For external genital/perianal warts (condyloma acuminata), the recommended therapeutic measures are listed in Table 47.6. According to the CDC, none of the currently available treatments is superior to other treatments, and no single treatment is ideal for all patients or all warts.

The use of podophyllin, podofilox, and imiquimod is contraindicated in pregnancy. During pregnancy, the best approach to treatment is removal of lesions by excision, electrocautery, or cryosurgery. Trichloroacetic acid (TCA) application has been used in pregnancy without adverse effects.

Table 47.6 Centers for Disease Control 2002 recommendations for treatment of external genital warts.

Recommended treatments
Patient applied
Podofilox 0.5% solution or gel. Apply podofilox solution with a cotton swab, or podofilox gel with a finger, to visible genital warts b.i.d. for 3 days, followed by 4 days of no therapy. Cycle may be repeated as necessary for a total of four cycles
   or
Imiquimod 5% cream. Apply with finger at bedtime, three times a week for up to 16 weeks

Provider administered
Cryotherapy with liquid nitrogen or cryoprobe. Repeat every 1–2 weeks
   or
Podophyllin resin 10–25% in compound tincture of benzoin. Repeat weekly if necessary
   or
TCA or BCA 80–90%. Repeat weekly if necessary
   or
Surgical removal by tangential scissors excision, tangential shave excision, curettage, or electrosurgery

Alternative treatments
Intralesional interferon
   or
Laser surgery

BCA, bichloroacetic acid; TCA, trichloroacetic acid.

Maternal and fetal risks

Warty lesions have a tendency to grow and become more vascularized during pregnancy. The only contraindications to a vaginal delivery are extensive lesions that might result in dystocia and lesions that might bleed heavily with birth trauma. Vertical transmission of HPV is rare, but can result in respiratory papillomatosis in the exposed infant. The exact mode of spread is unknown. Thus, Cesarean section is not recommended in the presence of genital warts in order to prevent vertical transmission of HPV.

Herpes simplex virus

Herpes simplex virus (HSV) is a double-stranded DNA virus. Two major serotypes are recognized: HSV-1 and HSV-2.

Epidemiology

There are an estimated 1 million new cases of genital HSV in the United States each year. While approximately 5 million American adults have a history of genital herpes, serologic surveys utilizing type-specific HSV-2 antibodies to glycoprotein G have demonstrated a seroprevalence for HSV-2 in 30% of adults; thus, an estimated 45 million Americans have been infected with HSV-2.

Three types of genital herpes infections are recognized on the basis of clinical history, serologic testing, and HSV typing. Primary infection is an initial infection with either HSV-1 or HSV-2 in an individual without serologic evidence of prior exposure to either HSV-1 or HSV-2. Nonprimary first clinical episode is an initial episode (clinical or subclinical) with HSV-1 or HSV-2 in an individual with serologic evidence of prior exposure to the other serotype. Recurrent genital herpes is reactivation of latent virus.

Clinical manifestations

As noted above, there are three types of herpetic episodes. Primary infections occur in previously unexposed hosts and are characterized by multiple painful vesicular lesions that ulcerate, with inguinal lymphadenopathy and flu-like symptoms, including fever, malaise, nausea, headaches, and myalgias.

First-episode nonprimary genital herpes occurs in an individual with previous nongenital exposure to HSV-1 or HSV-2. Its presentation is generally much milder than primary infections.

Recurrent HSV is more frequent after HSV-2 infection. Approximately half of infected individuals experience a recurrence within 6 months. Most of these episodes are prefaced by a 1- or 2-day prodrome consisting of localized pruritus, pain, and paresthesias. Systemic manifestations are absent. The episode usually lasts approximately half as long as the primary outbreak, with only 4–5 days of viral shedding.

Laboratory diagnosis

Until recently, viral culture was the gold standard for diagnosis of HSV infection. Cultures are more likely to be positive among patients with first episodes of HSV infection and those with vesicles or pustules rather than ulcerative or crusted lesions. Detection of HSV in culture has been facilitated by the use of monoclonal antibodies in immunofluorescence or immunoassay tests.

The introduction of nucleic acid amplification tests such as PCR has revolutionized the laboratory diagnosis of HSV. Compared with culture, PCR has excellent sensitivity and specificity for the detection of HSV. The clinical implications of PCR detection of low viral load, especially among pregnant women at term, remain to be determined.

Diagnosis of HSV infection has been further enhanced by the introduction of type-specific serology. Identifiable proteins for each HSV type are present in a characteristic protein coat; glycoprotein G-1 is associated with HSV-1 and glycoprotein G-2 with HSV-2. Type-specific serologic assays are now commercially available.

While serologic screening for HSV-1 and HSV-2 infection in the general population is not currently recommended, screening may be useful in counseling couples in which one partner has a history of genital herpes and the other does not, especially preconception or in pregnant couples.

Maternal and fetal risks

The major adverse impact of genital herpes in pregnancy is the development of neonatal herpes infection. An estimated 700–1000 cases of neonatal herpes infection occur each year in the United States, resulting in an incidence ranging from 1 in 3500 to 1 in 5000 births. Infection may be vertically transmitted either transplacentally or perinatally. Fortunately, transplacental transmission is rare.

During the past two decades, risk factors associated with transmission of HSV from mother to neonate have been elucidated. These include: (1) HSV type (HSV-2 > HSV-1); (2) maternal clinical stage of infection (primary > recurrent); (3) anatomic site of viral shedding (cervix > labia); (4) use of fetal scalp electrode; and (5) presence and specificity of transplacental passively transferred HSV antibodies from mother to infant. With recently acquired first-episode genital HSV infection, neonates have a 10-fold greater risk of acquiring HSV infection than infants born to mothers with recurrent infection. First-episode genital herpes infection, whether primary or nonprimary, is associated with neonatal infection rates of 40% and 31% respectively. Passive transplacental passage of maternal antibodies to HSV-2 (but not HSV-1) is protective. With recurrent genital herpes, the estimated risk of neonatal infection is < 1–4%. The estimated risk of neonatal herpes occurring from an asymptomatic mother with a history of recurrent genital HSV is less than 1 in 1000.

Until the mid-1980s, the approach for the prevention of neonatal herpes focused on the use of weekly cultures for HSV starting at 34–36 weeks' gestation in women with a history of recurrent genital herpes.

Because weekly maternal vaginal cultures in the third trimester do not predict viral shedding at the time of delivery, this approach was abandoned. The Infectious

Disease Society for Obstetrics and Gynecology developed a position paper on the peripartum management of women with a history of HSV. They made the following suggestions:
- Weekly antenatal cultures should be abandoned.
- In the absence of genital lesions, Cesarean sections should be performed for obstetric considerations only.
- A culture should be obtained from the mother or neonate at delivery in order to identify exposed infants.
- Women with genital lesions should undergo Cesarean section, preferably within 6 h of membrane rupture, to prevent HSV exposure in the neonate.
- The mother should not be isolated from her infant.

Shortly thereafter, the ACOG issued a Technical Bulletin, which basically agreed with these recommendations. Until recently, limited experience with active herpetic lesions in the face of preterm premature ruptured membranes (PPROM) suggested that expectant management may be successful. More recently, Major et al. reported a series of 29 patients with PPROM complicated by active recurrent genital HSV infection. The mean gestational age of the women was 28.7 weeks (range 24.6–31 weeks), and the mean latency from development of herpes lesions to delivery was 13.2 days (range 1–35 days). There were no cases of neonatal herpes infection among the delivered newborns, and all neonatal cultures for HSV were negative (95% CI 0–10.4%).

Treatment

The current CDC-recommended treatment guidelines for HSV infections are listed in Table 47.7.

Interest has focused on the use of acyclovir prophylaxis during late pregnancy to prevent recurrent HSV infection at delivery. While the CDC suggested that insufficient data exist to recommend prophylaxis in pregnancy, the ACOG suggest that the use of acyclovir to suppress recurrent HSV infection in late pregnancy is acceptable. ACOG notes that, for women at or beyond 36 weeks of gestation who are at risk of recurrent HSV, antiviral therapy may be considered. However, they caution that such therapy may not reduce the likelihood of Cesarean delivery.

The following recommendations have been suggested for the management of genital herpes infection in pregnancy:
- Women with primary HSV infection during pregnancy should be treated with antiviral therapy.
- Cesarean delivery should be performed on women with first-episode HSV infection who have active lesions at the time of delivery.
- For women of ≥ 36 weeks' gestation with a first episode of HSV infection during the current pregnancy, antiviral therapy should be considered.
- Cesarean delivery should be performed on women with recurrent herpes who have active lesions or prodrome at labor and delivery.
- Expectant management of patients with preterm labor or PPROM and active HSV lesion(s) may be warranted.

• For women of ≥ 36 weeks' gestation who are at risk of recurrent HSV infection, antiviral therapy may also be considered.
• In women with no active lesions or prodrome during labor, Cesarean delivery should not be performed on the basis of a history of recurrent herpes.

Trichomonas vaginalis

It has been estimated that 2–3 million women in the United States contract the infection annually. More recently, Cates (1999) estimated that 5 million new cases of trichomoniasis occur each year in the United States.

Clinical manifestations

It appears that this pathogen confines itself to the genitourinary system. Although most men are asymptomatic, anywhere from 50–90% of infected women become symptomatic at some time.

An abnormal vaginal discharge is noted by 50–75% of symptomatic women. In only 10% of these women is the exudate malodorous. Pruritus, dysuria, and dyspareunia are experienced in up to half of them.

Physical examination findings are normal in 15% of infected patients. Vaginal erythema and an excessive vaginal discharge are present in up to 75%, whereas vulvar inflammation is much less common. The so-called classic findings of a yellowish-green frothy discharge and strawberry cervix are relatively uncommon, seen in 25% and 2% respectively.

Table 47.7 Centers for Disease Control 2002 recommendations for the treatment of genital herpes.

Recommended regimens: first clinical episode
  Acyclovir 400 mg orally, three times a day for 7–10 days
  Acyclovir 200 mg orally, five times a day for 7–10 days
  Famciclovir 250 mg orally, three times a day for 7–10 days
  Valacyclovir 1 g orally, twice a day for 7–10 days

Recommended regimens: episodic recurrent regimens
  Acyclovir 400 mg orally, three times a day for 5 days
  Acyclovir 200 mg orally, five times a day for 5 days
  Acyclovir 800 mg orally, twice a day for 5 days
  Famciclovir 125 mg orally, twice a day for 5 days
  Valacyclovir 500 mg orally, twice a day for 3–5 days
  Valacyclovir 1 g orally, once a day for 5 days

Recommended regimens: suppression recurrent episodes
  Acyclovir 400 mg orally, twice a day
  Famciclovir 250 mg orally, twice a day
  Valacyclovir 500 mg orally, once a day*
  Valacyclovir 1 g orally, once a day

---

*Valacyclovir 500 mg once a day might be less effective than other dosing regimens in patients who have frequent (≥ 10 episodes per year) recurrences.

Laboratory diagnosis

Because clinical manifestations are so nonspecific, the clinician must rely on laboratory parameters to make the diagnosis. Most commonly, the diagnosis is made by light microscopic examination of a saline wet mount. The vaginal pH is ≥ 4.5 in the majority of patients. Performance of a Pap smear makes the diagnosis nearly 70% of the time.

Collection of a sample of vaginal discharge for wet mount or culture is the diagnostic procedure of choice. Large numbers of polymorphonuclear leukocytes (PMNs) are generally present. *T. vaginalis* can be seen as motile ovoids that appear slightly larger than PMNs. The sensitivity of the wet mount ranges between 40% and 80%, matching that of the Pap smear. Culture is the optimum method currently available for detecting the presence of *T. vaginalis*. While easily performed, culture for *T. vaginalis* requires the use of special medium such as Diamond or Kupferberg.

Treatment

In the 1960s, the 5-nitroimidazoles, including metronidazole, were developed and found to be effective in the treatment of this infection. Recent years have seen the development of isolated clusters of resistant organisms.

The original regimen of metronidazole therapy lasted 7 days. This has been shortened to a single oral dose in order to improve compliance, decrease the total dose, and deal with the problems of alcohol use during treatment.

Relative resistance of *T. vaginalis* to metronidazole is documented. For treatment failures, the CDC recommends retreatment with metronidazole 500 mg twice daily for 7 days. If failure occurs again, a single 2-g dose once daily for 3–5 days is recommended. For patients still having persistent trichomoniasis, the CDC suggests excluding reinfection, evaluating the *in vitro* susceptibility of the isolate, and managing in consultation with an expert. In May 2004 tinidazole (Tindamax) was approved by the FDA for the treatment of trichomoniasis with a suggested treatment regimen of a single 2-g oral dose.

Maternal and fetal risks

Studies with conflicting results have been published on the potential association of *T. vaginalis* with adverse pregnancy outcomes. The Vaginal Infection and Prematurity Study demonstrated that *T. vaginalis* in midpregnancy was significantly associated with preterm low birthweight (OR 1.6, 95% CI.1.3–1.9). However, a recent prospective randomized trial of metronidazole versus placebo sponsored by the National Institutes of Health (NIH) demonstrated that metronidazole treatment of asymptomatic pregnant women with trichomoniasis (identified by culture) during the midtrimester resulted in an increased risk of preterm birth.

Prevention

Because this infection is sexually transmitted, its diagnosis should serve as a reminder to test carefully for the coexistence of other, more dangerous STDs.

Further reading

American College of Obstetricians and Gynecologists. Prenatal and perinatal human immuno-deficiency virus testing: expanded recommendations. ACOG Committee Opinion No. 304. *Obstet Gynecol* 2004;104:1119–1124.

Cates W and The American Social Health Panel. Estimates of the incidence and prevalence of sexually transmitted diseases in the United States. *Sex Transm Dis* 1999;26(Suppl.):S2–S7.

Centers for Disease Control and Prevention. 2002 Sexually transmitted diseases treatment guidelines. *Morbid Mortal Wkly Rep* 2002;51:1–77.

Centers for Disease Control and Prevention. Recommended adult immunization schedule – United States, October 2004–September 2004. *Morbid Mortal Wkly Rep* 2004;53:Q1–4.

Eng TR, Butler WT, eds. *The hidden epidemic: confronting sexually transmitted diseases.* Committee on Prevention and Control of Sexually Transmitted Diseases. Washington, DC: Institute of Medicine National Academy Press, 1997.

Fiumara NJ, Fleming WI, Downing JG, et al. The incidence of prenatal syphilis at the Boston City Hospital. *N Engl J Med* 1952;247:48–52.

Gayle HD. Curbing the global AIDS epidemic. *N Engl J Med* 2003;348:1802–1805.

HIV/AIDS update: a glance at the HIV epidemic. Atlanta, GA: Centers for Disease Control and Prevention. Available at http//www.cdc.gov/nchstp/od/news/At-a-Glance.pdf. Retrieved November 22, 2004.

Major CA, Towers CV, Lewis DF, Garite TJ. Expectant management of preterm premature rupture of membranes complicated by active recurrent genital herpes. *Am J Obstet Gynecol* 2003;188:1551–1555.

Minkoff H. HIV infections in pregnancy. *Obstet Gynecol* 2003;101:797–810.

Sweet RL, Gibbs RS. Sexually transmitted diseases. In: Sweet RL, Gibbs RS, eds. *Infectious diseases of the female genital tract.* Philadelphia, PA: Lippincott-Williams & Wilkins; 2002:118–175.

Sweet RL, Gibbs RS. Urinary tract infection. In: Sweet RL, Gibbs RS, eds. *Infectious diseases of the female genital tract.* Philadelphia, PA: Lippincott Williams and Wilkins; 2002:413–448.

Yenni PG, Hammer SM, Hirsch MS, et al. Treatment for adult HIV infection 2004. Recommendations of the International AIDS Society–USA Panel. *JAMA* 2004;292:251–265.

48 Rheumatologic and connective tissue disorders in pregnancy

Gustavo F. Leguizamón and E. Albert Reece

Systemic lupus erythematosus

Systemic lupus erythematosus (SLE) is a chronic autoimmune condition of unknown etiology with an overall incidence of approximately 7 per 100 000. A strong predilection for women is observed with a female to male ratio of 7:1. African–Americans and Hispanics have an excess risk of two- to fourfold. The onset is often subtle and can compromise one or multiple organ systems characterized by periods of disease activity alternating with quiescence. Systemic signs and symptoms are common and usually involve fatigue, fever, malaise, and weight loss. Diagnosis is based on the revised American College of Rheumatology (ACR) criteria (Table 48.1).

Table 48.1 The 1982 revised criteria for the classification of systemic lupus erythematosus.

Criterion	Definition
1. Malar rash	Fixed erythema, flat or raised, over the malar eminences, tending to spare the nasolabial folds
2. Discoid rash	Erythematous raised patches with adherent keratotic scaling and follicular plugging; atrophic scarring may occur in older lesions
3. Photosensitivity	Skin rash as a result of unusual reaction to sunlight, by patient history or physician observation
4. Oral ulcers	Oral or nasopharyngeal ulceration, usually painless, observed by physician
5. Arthritis	Nonerosive arthritis involving two or more peripheral joints, characterized by tenderness, swelling, or effusion
6. Serositis	a) Pleuritis – convincing history of pleuritic pain or rubbing heard by a physician or evidence of pleural effusion or b) Pericarditis – documented by ECG or rub or evidence of pericardial effusion
7. Renal disorder	a) Persistent proteinuria >0.5 g/day or > 3+ if quantitation not performed or b) Cellular casts – may be red cell, hemoglobin, granular, tubular, or mixed
8. Neurologic disorder	a) Seizures – in the absence of offending drugs or known metabolic derangements, e.g., uremia, ketoacidosis, or electrolyte imbalance or b) Psychosis – in the absence of offending drugs or known metabolic derangements, e.g., uremia, ketoacidosis, or electrolyte imbalance
9. Hematologic disorder	a) Hemolytic anemia – with reticulocytosis or b) Leukopenia – < 4000/μL total on two or more occasions or c) Lymphopenia – < 1500/μL on two or more occasions or d) Thrombocytopenia – less than 100000/μL in the absence of offending drugs
10. Immunologic disorder	a) Anti-DNA: antibody to native DNA in abnormal titer or b) Anti-Sm: presence of antibody to Sm nuclear antigen or c) Positive finding of antiphospholipid antibodies based on: an abnormal serum level of IgG or IgM anticardiolipin antibodies or a positive test result for lupus anticoagulant using a standard method or a false-positive serologic test for syphilis known to be positive for at least 6 months and confirmed by *Treponema pallidum* immobilization or fluorescent treponemal antibody absorption test
11. Antinuclear antibody	An abnormal titer of antinuclear antibody by immunofluorescence or an equivalent assay at any point in time and in the absence of drugs known to be associated with "drug-induced lupus" syndrome

From ref 3.
ECG, electrocardiogram.

Table 48.2 Antibodies of clinical significance in SLE.

Antibody	Frequency (%)	Feature
Anti-ds DNA	60–90	Specific for SLE
		Associated with activity and nephritis
Anti-Sm	10–30	Specific for SLE
		Lupus nephritis?
Anti-La	20–40	Neonatal lupus
Anti-Ro	20–40	Neonatal lupus
Anti-RNP	10	Mixed connective tissue disorder

Laboratory evaluation

Antinuclear antibodies (ANA) are the most sensitive screening laboratory tool for evaluating patients with clinical suspicion of SLE, and approximately 90% of patients with SLE will present a positive test for ANA. Although false positives are common, a negative ANA result makes the diagnosis of lupus very unlikely, whereas a positive result (> 1/80) favors the diagnosis. The presence of anti-Ro (SS-A) and anti-LA (SS-B) antibodies is of clinical significance as they are associated with neonatal lupus. These antibodies are present in 20–60% of patients with SLE. Table 48.2 depicts relevant clinical information about different lupus-related antibodies.

Effects of pregnancy on systemic lupus erythematosus

The impact of pregnancy on SLE is not fully elucidated. Overall, the incidence of lupus flare during pregnancy ranges from 15% to 63%. Early uncontrolled studies suggested that exacerbations were common during pregnancy or the puerperium. More recent reports have shown contradictory results. While some authors report no increases in lupus flares during pregnancy, others have observed increased exacerbations.

Patients with lupus nephritis have a small but crucial risk of permanent renal function deterioration during pregnancy. In one study, 7% of the patients had permanent renal failure, 26% experienced a transient deterioration in renal function, and 60% demonstrated no significant change in renal function. Conditions associated with improved outcomes include prepregnancy remission of at least 6 months, serum creatinine < 1.5 mg/dL, creatinine clearance of 60 mL/min or more, and proteinuria of 3 g/24 h or less.

Effects of systemic lupus erythematosus on pregnancy

SLE can increase the risk of early and late pregnancy losses because of hypertension, renal dysfunction, placental insufficiency, and its association with antiphospholipid antibody syndrome (APAS). It is also an important cause of fetal and neonatal heart block. Finally, it increases the risk of spontaneous as well as medically indicated preterm labor.

Preeclampsia

Women with SLE have an increased risk of developing preeclampsia with an incidence of 15–32%. Risks factors have been identified such as lupus nephritis, APAS, and chronic hypertension. Making the differential diagnosis between the onset of preeclampsia and lupus flare can be a difficult challenge for the obstetrician. Both can present with hypertension, deteriorating renal function, proteinuria, and edema. Decreased complement levels (C3-C4-CH50), increased anti-double-stranded (ds) DNA, leukopenia, hematuria, and the presence of casts in urine should raise the suspicion of an SLE flare, while the presence of microangiopathic hemolytic anemia, abnormal liver function tests, and hyperuricemia most likely indicates preeclampsia.

Fetal outcome

Women with SLE present an excess risk of pregnancy loss. Prospective studies addressing this issue are in agreement and report a median incidence of pregnancy loss of approximately 20%. The incidence of preterm labor in this population has been reported to be from 20% to 50%. The incidence of intrauterine growth restriction (IUGR) is also increased, and it has been reported in the range of 12–32%. Several risk factors for poor fetal outcome have been described and include anti-β2 glycoprotein I, hypertension at conception, and hypocomplementemia. The presence of anticardiolipin antibodies and hypertension during pregnancy as well as lupus nephritis is associated with IUGR and prematurity. Renal disease is a predictor of poor fetal outcomes. Although most pregnancies of women with SLE do well, women with these risk factors need to be monitored aggressively throughout pregnancy.

Neonatal lupus syndrome (NLS)

One or more of the following findings are characteristic of NLS and include congenital heart block (CHB), cardiomyopathy, cutaneous lesions, thrombocytopenia, and hepatobiliary disease. The most frequent and severe finding in NLS is CHB, which is associated with the presence of anti-SS-A/Ro and anti-SS-B/La antibodies. In pregnancies with CHB and positive anti-SS-A/Ro and anti-SS-B/La antibodies, no major structural abnormalities were observed. The majority (82%) were diagnosed by ultrasound before 30 weeks of gestation. A significant mortality was found (19%), most frequently occurring in the first 3 months of life. Although the cumulative 3-year survival was 79%, significant morbidity was present as 63% of neonates required pacemaker placement. Finally, for women with a previous child with CHB, the recurrence rate was 16%.

Drug therapy

Cyclophosphamide

This drug has been associated with decreased fertility as well as teratogenicity. Certain risk factors are associated with a higher risk of toxicity: age ($\geq$ 32 years) and the cumulative dose. For those patients under treatment, an adequate method of contraception is mandatory as this drug has been associated with spontaneous abortion and teratogenicity when used during the first trimester.

Aspirin

When used during the first trimester, aspirin has no teratogenic effect; however, it has been associated with an increased incidence of miscarriages. During the last weeks of gestation, nonsteroidal anti-inflammatory drugs (NSAIDs) and aspirin have been associated with a reduction in amniotic fluid volume and constriction of the fetal ductus arteriosus.

Corticosteroids

Potential maternal side-effects secondary to corticosteroids include gastro-intestinal discomfort, fluid retention and hypertension secondary to the mineralo-corticoid activity, bone demineralization, avascular necrosis, acne, and gestational diabetes. No teratogenic effect in humans has been described with these drugs. Prednisone, prednisolone, and methylprednisone cross the placenta minimally (~ 10%). Fluorinated steroids (β-methasone and dexamethasone) should be avoided when steroids are administered for maternal indications as they readily cross the placenta.

Hydroxychloroquine

Recent reports have shown a lack of teratogenicity or other significant fetal effects. Furthermore, discontinuing hydroxychloroquine in high-risk patients could be associated with a poor prognosis. No congenital anomalies as well as normal neuro-ophthalmological and auditory evaluations were observed at 1.5–3 years of age. Based on these data, it would be prudent to continue hydroxychloroquine therapy in pregnant patients with SLE.

Azathioprine

This has been widely used throughout gestation in patients with renal transplants and is the only cytotoxic agent that can be considered safe during pregnancy. Aza-thioprine is well tolerated during pregnancy with no significant increase in congen-ital malformations.

Rheumatoid arthritis

Rheumatoid arthritis (RA) is a systemic, autoimmune, and inflammatory disorder that primarily affects synovial tissue and is characterized by involvement of the peripheral joints such as metacarpophalangeal, proximal interphalangeal, wrist, and metatarsophalangeal, with characteristic cartilage destruction and eventually joint distortion. The diagnosis is not made by a single finding but rather by a combina-tion of clinical and laboratory findings together with the clinical course. The ACR published the revised criteria depicted in Table 48.3. These guidelines are based on the presence of the following: morning stiffness, arthritis of three or more joint

Table 48.3 1987 criteria for the classification of acute arthritis of rheumatoid arthritis (ACR).

Criterion	Definition
1. Morning stiffness	Morning stiffness in and around the joints, lasting at least 1 h before maximal improvement
2. Arthritis of three or more joint areas	At least three joint areas simultaneously have had soft tissue swelling or fluid (not bony overgrowth alone) observed by a physician. The 14 possible areas are right or left PIP, MCP, wrist, elbow, knee, ankle, and MTP joints
3. Arthritis of hand joints	At least one area swollen (as defined above) in a wrist, MCP, or PIP joint
4. Symmetric arthritis	Simultaneous involvement of the same joint areas (as defined in 2) on both sides of the body (bilateral involvement of PIPs, MCPs, or MTPs is acceptable without absolute symmetry)
5. Rheumatoid nodules	Subcutaneous nodules, over bony prominences, or extensor surfaces, or in juxta-articular regions, observed by a physician
6. Serum rheumatoid factor	Demonstration of abnormal amounts of serum rheumatoid factor by any method for which the result has been positive in < 5% of normal control subjects
7. Radiographic changes	Radiographic changes typical of rheumatoid arthritis on posteroanterior hand and wrist radiographs, which must include erosions or unequivocal bony decalcification localized in or most marked adjacent to the involved joints (osteoarthritis changes alone do not qualify)

MCP, metacarpophalangeal; MTP, metatarsophalangeal; PIP, proximal interphalangeal. For classification purposes, a patient shall be said to have rheumatoid arthritis if he/she has satisfied at least four or these seven criteria. Criteria 1 through 4 must have been present for at least 6 weeks. Patients with two clinical diagnoses are not excluded. Designation as classic, definite, or probable rheumatoid arthritis is *not* to be made.

From Arnett FC, Edworthy SM, Bloch DA, et al. The American Rheumatism Association 1987 revised criteria for the classification of rheumatoid arthritis. *Arthritis Rheum* 1988;31:315–324.

areas, arthritis of hand joints, symmetric arthritis, rheumatoid nodules, serum rheumatoid factor, and radiographic changes. Serum rheumatoid factor is present in approximately 80% of affected patients, but it is not specific.

It has been reported that pregnancy induces improvement in RA symptoms in approximately 75% of women. During the puerperium, however, the relapse rate is approximately 90%. The considerable increase in prolactin secretion during breastfeeding is thought to be involved in the increase in disease activity. Finally, the risk of adverse perinatal outcome or infertility does not seem to be increased in women with RA. The goals of treatment are initially to attain remission of symptoms, maintain the remission over time, and insure adequate joint function. NSAIDs are useful in decreasing symptoms. During pregnancy and the preconception period, patient education and guidance regarding drug side-effects is of utmost importance in achieving a good perinatal outcome. Frequently, the decreased disease activity during gestation and subsequent reduction in symptom severity allows analgesics such as acetaminophen, which have been shown to be safe for the fetus, to be utilized. If NSAIDs are needed, they can be used with caution after the first trimester and up to 32 weeks' gestation. As the potential risk of decreased amniotic fluid is well proven, it is recommended that serial amniotic fluid volumes should be performed with ultrasonography during treatment. When steroids are required to control the symptoms of arthritis, they are generally considered safe to use in pregnancy and lactation. Most disease-modifying antirheumatic drugs (DMARDs) are contraindicated during pregnancy, lactation, and the preconception period.

Ankylosing spondylitis

Ankylosing spondylitis is an inflammatory condition with unknown etiology and a strong genetic predisposition. It most frequently affects the axial skeleton with insidious lumbar pain and morning stiffness. Diagnosis of ankylosing spondylitis is based on the modified New York criteria of 1984 which include: (1) a history of inflammatory back pain; (2) limitation of motion of the lumbar spine in the sagittal and frontal planes; (3) limited chest expansion; and (4) evidence of radiographic sacroiliitis.

Unlike rheumatoid arthritis, ankylosing spondylitis does not usually undergo remission during pregnancy; however, women with ankylosing spondylitis can be reassured that the perinatal outcome is not significantly affected by the disease. Children of women with ankylosing spondylitis seem to have an increased incidence of the disease over the general population. Treatment during pregnancy is oriented to maintaining functional capacity as well as ameliorating pain. NSAIDs can be used with caution.

Scleroderma

This multisystem disorder is characterized by fibrosis of the skin, blood vessels, gastrointestinal tract, lungs, kidneys, and heart. Two subsets can be described: the diffuse cutaneous scleroderma and the limited cutaneous scleroderma. In general, the prognosis of the limited form is more positive. Recent studies suggest that, with careful planning and intensive monitoring, maternal and fetal prognosis are in general favorable. Generally, scleroderma symptoms remain unchanged or can even improve during pregnancy. Renal crisis is probably the most problematic complication, and its diagnosis represents a difficult challenge. Differential diagnosis with preeclampsia–HELLP syndrome is difficult and is based on normal liver function tests, the rapid progression of renal deterioration with daily increases in serum creatinine, lack of proteinuria, as well as a history of diffuse scleroderma diagnosed less than 5 years ago. Most authorities suggest that, if renal crisis is diagnosed in pregnancy, the parents should be counseled and angiotensin-converting enzyme (ACE) inhibitors offered as this therapy could be life-saving. Overall, perinatal outcomes are good for women who showed stable disease before conception, especially for patients with localized forms. Preterm labor is the most frequent complication, and recent studies show an incidence of approximately 30%.

Further reading

Boumpas DT, Austin HA, 3rd, Vaughan EM, Yarboro CH. Risk for sustained amenorrhea in patients with systemic lupus erythematosus receiving intermittent pulse cyclophosphamide therapy. *Ann Intern Med* 1993;119:366–369.

Cervera R, Khamashta MA, Font J, et al. Systemic lupus erythematosus: clinical and immunologic patterns of disease expression in a cohort of 1,000 patients. The European Working Party on Systemic Lupus Erythematosus. *Medicine (Baltimore)* 1993;72:113–124.

Hahn BH. Mechanism of disease: antibodies to DNA. *N Engl J Med* 1998;338:1359–1368.

Hochberg MC. Updating the American Collage of Rheumatology revised criteria for the classification of systemic lupus erythematosus. *Arthritis Rheum* 1997;40:1725.

Khamashta MA, Buchanan NM, Hughes GR. The use of hydroxychloroquine in lupus pregnancy: the British experience. *Lupus* 1996;5(Suppl. 1):S65.

O'Dell JR. Therapeutic strategies for rheumatoid arthritis. *N Engl J Med* 2004;350:2591–2602.

Ostensen M, Ostensen H. Ankylosing spondylitis – the female aspect. *J Rheumatol* 1998;25:120–124.

Piper JM, Ray WA, Rosa FW. Pregnancy outcome following exposure to angiotensin converting enzyme inhibitors. *Obstet Gynecol* 1992;80:429–432.

Steen VD. Pregnancy in women with systemic sclerosis. *Obstet Gynecol* 1999;94:15–20.

Yasmeen S, Wilkins EE, Field NT, et al. Pregnancy outcomes in women with systemic lupus erythematosus. *J Matern Fetal Med* 2001;10:91–96.

49 Dermatologic disorders during pregnancy

Thomas D. Horn and Jerri Hoskyn

Pigmentary alterations

Hyperpigmentation is the most common skin change during pregnancy, and is most pronounced in scars, melanocytic nevi and ephelides, areolae, and genital, perineal, and axillary skin. Any melanocytic nevus undergoing significant change, however, should be sampled to explore the rare possibility of melanoma. Prognosis of

Table 49.1 Melanoma TNM classification.

T classification	Thickness	Ulceration status
T1	≤ 1.0 mm	a: Without ulceration and level II/III b: With ulceration or level IV/V
T2	1.01–2.0 mm	a: Without ulceration b: With ulceration
T3	2.01–4.0 mm	a: Without ulceration b: With ulceration
T4	> 4.0 mm	a: Without ulceration b: With ulceration

N classification	No. of metastatic nodes	Nodal metastatic mass
N1	1 node	a: Micrometastasis* b: Macrometastasis†
N2	2–3 nodes	a: Micrometastasis* b: Macrometastasis† c: In transit met(s)/satellite(s) without metastatic node(s)
N3	4 or more metastatic nodes, or matted nodes, or in transit met(s)/satellite(s) with metastatic node(s)	

M classification	Site	Serum lactate dehydrogenase
M1a	Distant skin, subcutaneous, or nodal metastases	Normal
M1b	Lung metastases	Normal
M1c	All other visceral metastases Any distant metastasis	Normal Elevated

Reprinted with permission from Bolognia JL, Jorizzo JL, Rapini RP, et al. *Dermatology*. London: Mosby, 2003.

*Micrometastases are diagnosed after sentinel or elective lymphadenectomy.

†Macrometastases are defined as clinically detectable nodal metastases confirmed by therapeutic lymphadenectomy or when nodal metastasis exhibits gross extracapsular extension.

melanoma appears to be the same, based upon the characteristics of the tumor, as in nonpregnant women (Tables 49.1 and 49.2). The linea alba may darken, becoming the linea nigra. Melasma is common in pregnancy or in patients taking oral contraceptives and generally resolves postpartum without treatment.

Table 49.2 Proposed stage groupings for cutaneous melanoma.

	Survival (%)*	Clinical staging†			Pathologic staging‡		
		T	N	M	T	N	M
0		Tis	N0	M0	Tis	N0	M0
IA	95	T1a	N0	M0	T1a	N0	M0
IB	90	T1b	N0	M0	T1b	N0	M0
		T2a			T2a		
IIA	78	T2b	N0	M0	T2b	N0	M0
		T3a			T3a		
IIB	65	T3b	N0	M0	T3b	N0	M0
		T4a			T4a		
IIC	45	T4b	N0	M0	T4b	N0	M0
III§		Any T	N1	M0			M0
			N2				
			N3				
IIIA	66				T1-4a	N1a	M0
					T1-4a	N2a	
IIIB	52				T1-4b	N1a	M0
					T1-4b	N2a	
					T1-4a	N1b	
					T1-4a	N2b	
					T1-4a/b	N2c	
IIIC	26				T1-4b	N1b	M0
					T1-4b	N2b	
					Any T	N3	
IV	7.5–11	Any T	Any N	Any M1	Any T	Any N	Any M1

Reprinted with permission from Bolognia JL, Jorizzo JL, Rapini RP, et al. *Dermatology*. London: Mosby, 2003.

*Approximate 5-year survival as a percentage.

†Clinical staging includes microstaging of the primary melanoma and clinical/radiologic evaluation for metastases. By convention, it should be used after complete excision of the primary melanoma with clinical assessment for regional and distant metastases.

‡Pathologic staging includes microstaging of the primary melanoma and pathologic information about the regional lymph nodes after partial or complete lymphadenectomy. Pathologic stage 0 or stage IA patients are the exception.

§There are no stage III subgroups for clinical staging.

Vascular alterations

Spider angioma, capillary hemangioma, pyogenic granuloma, palmar erythema, varicosities and hemorrhoids, livedo reticularis, gingival hyperemia and hyperplasia, and dependent edema arise in pregnancy. Treatment of pyogenic granuloma is usually indicated to stop the nearly constant erosion and bleeding.

Connective tissue alterations

Striae, also known as striae distensae, are common in pregnancy, usually arising in the third trimester on the abdomen, breasts, thighs, hips, and buttocks. Vaginal lacerations during delivery have been associated with the development of striae. Skin tags, or acrochordons, may proliferate during pregnancy, typically on the neck, axillae, and groin.

Hair and nail alterations

Both hirsutism (development of a male pattern of hair growth in a woman) and hypertrichosis (increased amount of hair) may arise during pregnancy, but neither condition warrants concern or treatment. Telogen effluvium is a shedding of hair that begins 2–4 months after delivery, lasts for 2–4 months, and resolves over many months without intervention. Nail changes are common and may include brittleness, an increased rate of growth, or Beau's lines.

Dermatoses of pregnancy

The dermatoses of pregnancy are a group of skin conditions unique to pregnancy or directly related to the products of conception (Table 49.3).

Polymorphic eruption of pregnancy

Polymorphic eruption of pregnancy (PEP) is the most common of the pregnancy dermatoses. Pruritic urticarial papules first appear on the abdomen, often in the striae, then progress to involve the thighs, buttocks, arms, and trunk (Fig. 49.1). The periumbilical skin is characteristically spared. Typically, PEP presents in primigravidas late in the third trimester, but earlier in multiple gestation. PEP is self-limited and seldom recurs in subsequent pregnancies. Diagnosis of PEP is clinical but, if there is uncertainty, it is essential to rule out pemphigoid gestationis (PG) with a skin biopsy and direct immunofluorescence (DIF). DIF is negative in PEP. The prognosis for mother and baby is excellent, and treatment is symptomatic, usually consisting of moderate- to high-potency topical steroids in the majority of cases.

Pemphigoid gestationis

PG is an uncommon autoimmune blistering disorder unique to pregnancy that is caused by autoantibodies to the basement membrane zone. In classic PG, pruritic urticarial papules and plaques appear on the periumbilical skin during the second or third trimester and evolve into vesicles and tense bullae within days to weeks (Figs 49.2–49.5). Palmoplantar involvement is common, but the face and mucous membranes are usually spared. During the third trimester, PG may remit or clear, but a postpartum flare is the rule, with clearance within 2–6 months. PG recurs in subsequent pregnancies, and oral contraceptives and menses may precipitate flares.

399

Table 49.3 Key features of the dermatoses of pregnancy.

	Incidence	Key signs/symptoms	Presentation	Diagnosis	Course	Risks to mother or fetus	Recurrence	Treatment
PEP	1:150–160	Abdominal urticarial papules favoring striae, periumbilical sparing	36–39 weeks, rarely postpartum	Clinical Negative DIF	Self-limited, with resolution in 6 weeks	No	No	Symptomatic Systemic steroids in severe cases
CP	1:100–200	Pruritus ± jaundice	> 30 weeks in 80%	Clinical Elevated serum bile salts	Resolution with delivery. Pruritus remits before laboratory values normalize	Yes, fetal distress	Yes	Symptomatic UDCA Delivery
PG	1:40000–60000	Periumbilical urticarial papules, vesicles, bullae	Second and third trimesters	Clinical Skin biopsy Positive DIF	Remission in third trimester with postpartum flare. Resolution in 2–6 months	Yes, low birthweight, small for dates, prematurity	Yes Flare with OCP or menses	Systemic steroids

IH	Rare (case reports)	Grouped sterile pustules, favor flexural areas, constitutional symptoms	Second and third trimesters	Clinical Skin biopsy Negative DIF	Resolution with delivery	Yes, placental insufficiency	Yes Flare with OCP or menses	Systemic steroids Delivery or termination
PP	1:300	Red papules, most excoriated, on trunk and extremities	Third trimester	Clinical	Resolution by 3 months postpartum	No	Rare	Symptomatic
PFP	Case reports	Small follicular papules and pustules on the trunk	Third trimester	Clinical	Resolution with delivery	No	Unknown	Symptomatic

PEP, polymorphic eruption of pregnancy; CP, cholestasis of pregnancy; PG, pemphigoid gestationis; IH, impetigo herpetiformis; PP, prurigo of pregnancy; PFP, pruritic folliculitis of pregnancy; DIF, direct immunofluorescence; OCP, oral contraceptive pills; UDCA, ursodeoxycholic acid.

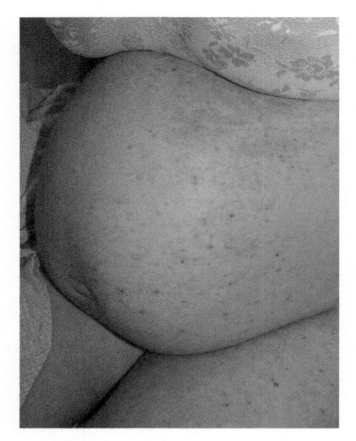

Figure 49.1 Polymorphic eruption of pregnancy. Erythematous papules on the abdomen, sparing the umbilicus. Excoriations are present here, but are not typical. Image courtesy of Susan Mallory, MD.

The diagnosis can be confirmed with a skin biopsy and positive DIF. Fetal risks include prematurity, low birthweight, and small size for gestational age. Systemic steroids are usually required to control symptoms. Some newborns may have a transient eruption, which can be treated with topical steroids alone.

Impetigo herpetiformis

Impetigo herpetiformis (IH) is a very rare dermatosis similar to pustular psoriasis that occurs exclusively in pregnancy. IH presents in the third trimester with fever and erythematous patches with tiny sterile pustules appearing first in the groin, axillae, and neck. Resolution follows delivery, and recurrence in subsequent pregnancies and with oral contraceptives is typical. Skin biopsy is consistent with pustular psoriasis, with negative DIF. IH is associated with placental insufficiency, placing the fetus at risk of stillbirth, neonatal death, and fetal abnormalities. Sys-

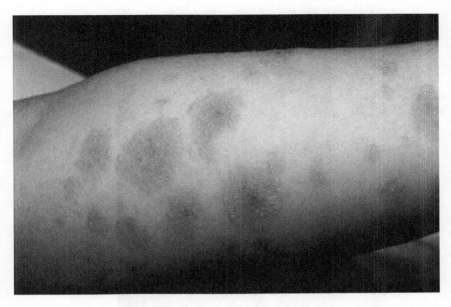

Figure 49.2 Pemphigoid gestationis. Urticarial plaques with small vesicles. Image courtesy of Susan Mallory, MD.

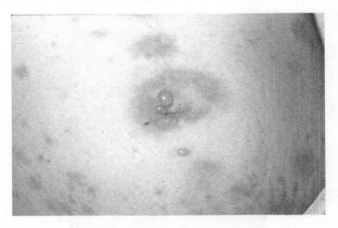

Figure 49.3 Pemphigoid gestationis. Typical periumbilical involvement. Image courtesy of Jeffrey Callen, MD.

temic steroids are the treatment of choice, but severe or refractory cases may necessitate early delivery or termination.

Cholestasis of pregnancy
Cholestasis of pregnancy (CP) is characterized by pruritus and intrahepatic

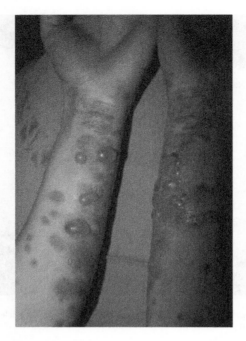

Figure 49.4 Pemphigoid gestationis. Urticarial plaques surmounted by tense bullae. Image courtesy of Jeffrey Callen, MD.

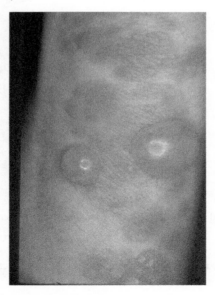

Figure 49.5 Pemphigoid gestationis. The characteristic tense bullae seen in PG. Image courtesy of Jeffrey Callen, MD.

cholestasis, with or without jaundice, occurring late in pregnancy. There are no primary skin lesions, but excoriations may be seen. In the third trimester, pruritus begins on the palms and soles and later spreads to include the trunk, extremities, and face. In a minority of patients, jaundice may follow pruritus by 2–4 weeks. The pruritus remits within 1–2 weeks of delivery, with the biochemical abnormalities normalizing over 4–6 weeks. CP usually recurs in subsequent pregnancies. The diagnosis of CP is largely clinical. Laboratory abnormalities are variable. Fetal complications can include fetal distress, meconium staining, preterm labor, and increased perinatal mortality. In mild cases, symptomatic treatment may suffice but, in more severe cases, systemic therapy or early delivery may be required.

Miscellaneous eruptions during pregnancy

Pruritic folliculitis of pregnancy is characterized by sterile follicular pustules appear-

Table 49.4 Common skin disorders that may cause pruritus in pregnancy.

Category	Skin disorder	Clinical features
Allergic/atopic	Urticaria (hives)	Transient wheals
	Atopic dermatitis	Scaly plaques with lichenification. Often coexists with allergic rhinitis and asthma
	Contact dermatitis	Pattern of rash often suggestive
	Drug reactions	History of drug ingestion or change in medication. Morphology varies
Infection/infestation	Scabies	Excoriated papules favor fingerwebs, areola. Burrow is diagnostic
	Infectious folliculitis	Follicle-based pustules. May follow hot-tub exposure
	Tinea (ringworm)	Annular or round scaly plaques. May have affected child or pet
	Other arthropod bites	Scattered excoriated or urticarial papules. Flea bites usually on legs. Chigger bites favor areas where clothing fits tightly. Head or pubic lice in characteristic location
Others	Psoriasis	Scaly red plaques on extensor limbs, scalp. May be generalized
	Pityriasis rosea	Oval plaques with fine scale on trunk. May be preceded by a larger "herald patch"
	Miliaria (prickly heat)	Tiny vesicles appear in hot weather
	Polymorphous light eruption	Pink papules, papulovesicles on sun-exposed areas of arms, chest. Appears in spring or after sunny vacation in winter. Improves over summer
	Xerosis	Dry skin

Table 49.5 Some causes of pruritus without rash.

Medications (e.g., opiates)	Malignancy (especially lymphoma)
Drug reactions	Hyperthyroidism
Hepatitis	Iron deficiency
Cholestatic or obstructive biliary disease	Acquired immunodeficiency syndrome
Chronic renal failure	

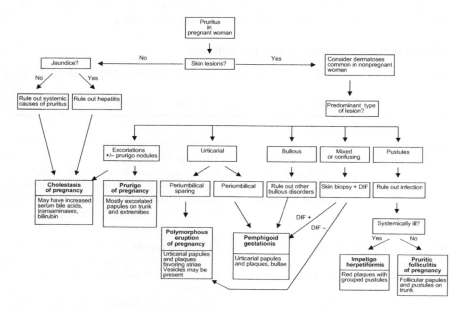

Figure 49.6 Approach to the pregnant patient with pruritus.

ing on the trunk in the latter half of pregnancy and clearing spontaneously after delivery. Prurigo of pregnancy presents in the second or third trimester with excoriated papules on the trunk and extremities. These entities are less well characterized, and it is unclear whether they represent truly separate diseases or are part of a poorly understood spectrum of overlapping disorders.

Approach to the patient

Pruritus is common in pregnancy, and the differential diagnosis is broad, encompassing not only the specific dermatoses of pregnancy but many conditions that cause pruritus with or without rash in the nonpregnant population (Tables 49.4 and 49.5). It is especially important to exclude the dermatoses of pregnancy that are associated with fetal complications, chiefly PG and CP (Fig. 49.6).

Further reading

Dacus JV. Pruritus in pregnancy. *Clin Obstet Gynecol* 1990;33(4):738–745.

Jenkins RE, Hern S, Black MM. Clinical features and management of 87 patients with pemphigoid gestationis. *Clin Exp Dermatol* 1999;24(4):255–259.

Kroumpouzos G. Intrahepatic cholestasis of pregnancy: what's new. *J Eur Acad Dermatol Venereol* 2002;16(4):316–318.

Kroumpouzos G, Cohen LM. Dermatoses of pregnancy. *J Am Acad Dermatol* 2001;45(1):1–19.

Muzaffar F, Hussain I, Haroon TS. Physiologic skin changes during pregnancy: a study of 140 cases. *Int J Dermatol* 1998;37:429–431.

Pennoyer JW, Grin CM, Driscoll MS, et al. Changes in size of melanocytic nevi during pregnancy. *J Am Acad Dermatol* 1997;36(3 Pt 1):378–382.

Roger D, Vaillant L, Fignon A, et al. Specific pruritic diseases of pregnancy. A prospective study of 3192 pregnant women. *Arch Dermatol* 1994;130(6):734–739.

Shornick JK, Black MM. Fetal risks in herpes gestationis. *J Am Acad Dermatol* 1992;26(1):63–68.

Wahman AJ, Finan MA, Emerson SC. Striae gravidarum as a predictor of vaginal lacerations at delivery. *South Med J* 2000;93:873–876.

Yancey KB, Hall RP, Lawley TJ. Pruritic urticarial papules and plaques of pregnancy. Clinical experience in twenty-five patients. *J Am Acad Dermatol* 1984;10(3):473–480.

50 Cancer and other neoplasms in pregnancy

Peter E. Schwartz and Masoud Azodi

In the United States, benign gynecologic masses account for more than 1 million hospital admissions per year. Benign masses may occur in pregnancy, and their management is complicated by the risk to the fetus. Knowledge of the natural history of these masses during pregnancy is essential to their proper management. Cancer during pregnancy is unusual. As a result of physiologic changes that normally occur in pregnancy, cancer during pregnancy may be more advanced because the diagnosis is not recognized as early as it otherwise might have been. However, stage for stage, cancer during pregnancy is no more virulent than cancer occurring in the nonpregnant state. The routine interruption of pregnancy to influence cancer progression has not been established.

Benign masses in pregnancy

Uterine myomas

Myomas are very common in the general population, especially in nonwhite women. Complications occur in about 10% of pregnancies with uterine myomas. Non-growing myomas can cause symptoms during pregnancy as a result of the enlarging uterus displacing them out of the pelvis. Symptoms may develop as asymptomatic myomas compress abdominal organs. Uterine myomas can undergo central necrosis and degeneration, causing localized pain. Placental abruption, postpartum hemorrhage, and retained placenta are thought to be complications of uterine myomas during pregnancy. Medical management is the primary means of treatment in pregnancy. Surgical management is usually avoided during pregnancy.

Adnexal masses in pregnancy

Benign adnexal tumors are sometimes associated with normal pregnancies. Clinical features suspicious of malignancy, particularly ovarian cancer, include the presence of a fixed mass, lymphadenopathy, ascites, and constitutional symptoms such as pain, abdominal distention, dyspareunia, frequency, or constipation. Sonographic features of adnexal masses suspicious of malignancy include a size greater than 6 cm, thick septations, papillary projections, mixed or high echogenicity, and the presence of ascites.

When a pelvic mass is symptomatic but not suspicious for malignancy, there are two management options: (1) prophylactic excision during pregnancy for protection against torsion, rupture, or intra-abdominal hemorrhage; or (2) expectant management with re-evaluation postpartum (or at the time of Cesarean section).

The most common benign pelvic masses in pregnancy are persistent corpus luteum cysts, benign cystic teratomas, paratubal cysts, cystadenomas, and pedunculated myomas. Although the vast majority of benign pelvic neoplasms discovered during pregnancy are present before the beginning of the pregnancy, the hormonal changes of pregnancy, particularly the production of human chorionic gonadotropin (hCG), are associated with luteomas, theca-lutein cysts, hyperreactio luteinalis, and large solitary luteinized follicular cyst of pregnancy.

Cancers in pregnancy

Incidence

Estimates of cancer during pregnancy vary considerably (Table 50.1). The uterine cervix remains the most common site for neoplasia to develop in pregnancy. The breast is the second most common site. A fear expressed by pregnant patients is that the cancer might spread to the fetus. Information collected during the past two decades suggests that transplacental metastasis is extremely unusual, and metastases to the fetus are so rare as to preclude this as an indication for termination of a pregnancy complicated by cancer. The most common malignancy to be associated with fetal metastases is malignant melanoma.

Surgery in pregnancy

Patients may undergo successful surgical procedures when they are pregnant without

Table 50.1 Estimate of cancer occurring in pregnancy.

Site	Estimated incidence	Authors
Skin, melanoma	2.8/1000	Smith and Randal[237]
Cervix		
Carcinoma *in situ*	1/767	Sokol and Lessmann[34]
Invasive	1/2205	Sokol and Lessmann[34]
Breast	1/3000	Benedet et al.[35]
	10–39/100 000	Wallack et al.[47]
Vulva	1/8000	Nugent and O'Connell[229]
Ovary	1/9000	Nugent and O'Connell[229]
	1/25 000	Ribeiro and Palmer[230]
Leukemia	Less than 1/75 000	Applewhite et al.[231]
	1/100 000	Haas[37]
Hodgkin's disease	1/1000	Riva et al.[234]
	1/6000	Morgan et al.;[235] Stewart and Monto[236]
Colorectal	1/100 000	Fisher et al.;[232] Clark et al.[233]

jeopardizing the fetus. In general, surgery should be delayed until the second trimester, which seems to be the safest time in terms of avoiding patients going into labor. Corpus luteum function is replaced by the placenta after the 12th week of gestation. Pathologic ovaries may be removed safely once the patient has entered the second trimester.

Radiation in pregnancy

Radiation is commonly employed in the routine management of cancers that may occur in pregnancy. Deleterious effects that the fetus may experience from being exposed to radiation therapy have been recognized for many years. Three phases of pregnancy must be considered with regard to radiation damage. The preimplantation phase lasts for approximately 7–10 days and represents the time from fertilization to the implantation of the blastocyst into the uterine wall. Spontaneous abortion is the most likely consequence of an embryo being exposed to radiation in the preimplantation phase. Organogenesis, the period from the first to the 10th week of gestation, represents the most sensitive time for the fetus with regard to radiation injury. This is the time of major organ formation and the time at which the fetus is most susceptible to teratogenic agents. However, the central nervous system, the eyes, and the hematopoietic system remain highly sensitive to the effects of radiation throughout the entire pregnancy.

Chemotherapy and pregnancy

Although certain drugs must be avoided during early pregnancy, others might

409

be life-saving and might not cause congenital anomalies in the fetus. Prematurity and low birthweight are frequent complications of chemotherapy exposure in any trimester of pregnancy. Children who have been born after *in utero* exposure to chemotherapeutic agents during the second and third trimesters have not been noted to have significant congenital abnormalities (see Table 50.2).

Cervical cancer

The cervix remains the most common site for precancerous and cancerous changes in pregnancy. The most common histologic types of cancer occurring in the cervix are squamous cell (93.1%).

Cervical intraepithelial neoplasia

The presence of cervical intraepithelial neoplasia (CIN) in pregnancy is usually identified by Pap smear and confirmed by colposcopically directed biopsies. In general, colposcopy will show the entire transformation zone, as the squamocolumnar junction tends to be present well out on the exocervix during pregnancy. It has been a successful policy to biopsy the worst colposcopically identified site and, if the cervical biopsy and Pap smear are consistent, simply to follow the patient throughout the pregnancy with Pap smears every 3 months. If the assessment at 36 weeks remains consistent with CIN, the patient and her physician are advised that the patient may deliver vaginally, if obstetrical indications are appropriate. No attempt is routinely made to perform Cesarean hysterectomies in the management of CIN. Assessment of precancerous changes can readily be done 8–12 weeks following delivery.

Microinvasive cancer of the cervix

Microinvasive cancer of the cervix is defined as a lesion that has only microscopically penetrated through the basement membrane. The current International Federation of Gynecology and Obstetrics (FIGO) staging system is given in Table 50.3. In general, patients with microinvasive cancer are found to have abnormal Pap smears and undergo routine colposcopic assessment. Confirmation of the extent of disease is extremely important in pregnancy. It may require a more extensive biopsy in the form of a hemicone biopsy or a cone biopsy of the cervix. If surgical margins are histologically free of disease on the cervical biopsy, patients may safely continue with the pregnancy as long as they are willing to be assessed with frequent Pap smears and colposcopy. Stage IA2 patients have more extensive microinvasive cancer. Patients with microinvasive cancer who wish to undergo prompt therapy are usually successfully managed with a simple hysterectomy, leaving the ovaries in place. Patients who wish to have definitive surgery performed following completion of pregnancy may be delivered vaginally and have a subsequent hysterectomy or may be delivered by Cesarean section followed by an extrafascial hysterectomy.

Table 50.2 Chemotherapeutic agents and reported associated anomalies by trimester.

Chemotherapeutic agents	Mechanism of action	Reported significant anomalies by trimester*		
		1st	2nd	3rd
Alkylating agents				
Melphalan, chlorambucil, cyclophosphamide, triethylene thiophosphoramide, cisplatin, carboplatin, carmustine (BCNU), chloroethylcyclohexyl nitrosourea, methyl-CCNU, busulfan	Cell-cycle nonspecific; forms cross linkages with DNA	Yes†	No	No
Antimetabolites				
Amethopterin (methotrexate),‡ aminopterin, 5-fluorouracil,‡ cytosine arabinoside, 6-thioguanine, 5-azacytidine, hydroxyurea, hexamethylmelamine, L-asparaginase	Cell-cycle specific; structural analogue of precursor purine and pyrimidine bases; lead to nonfunctional DNA and cell death	Yes§	No	No
Antibiotics				
Actinomycin D, doxorubicin, daunorubicin, bleomycin, mitomycin C, mithramycin	Cell-cycle nonspecific; interferes with DNA-dependent RNA synthesis; cell death from lack of RNA and an inability to produce cell proteins	No	No	No
Vinca alkaloids				
Vincristine, vinblastine, etoposide (VP-16), teniposide (VM-26)	Cell phase specific	Yes	No	No
Glucocorticoids				
Cortisone, prednisolone, prednisone, methylprednisolone, dexamethasone	Inhibition of DNA, RNA, and protein synthesis	Yes¶	No	No

*Reports of anomalies are limited and should be viewed with caution.

†Chlorambucil syndrome: renal aplasia, cleft palate, skeletal abnormalities.

‡Abortifacients in first trimester.

§Aminopterin syndrome: cranial dysostosis, hypertelorism, anomalies of the external ears, micrognathia, cleft palate.

¶Cleft lip, cleft palate.

Table 50.3 International Federation of Gynecology and Obstetrics (FIGO) cervical cancer staging classification.

0	Carcinoma *in situ*, intraepithelial carcinoma; cases of stage 0 should not be included in any therapeutic statistics for invasive carcinoma
I	Carcinoma is strictly confined to the cervix (extension to the corpus should be disregarded)
Ia	Preclinical carcinoma of the cervix, i.e., those diagnosed only by microscopy
Ia1	Minimal microscopically evident stromal invasion
Ia2	Lesions detected microscopically that can be measured; the upper limit of the measurement should not show a depth of invasion of more than 5 mm taken from the base of the epithelium, either surface or glandular, from which it originates; a second dimension, the horizontal spread, must not exceed 7 mm; larger should be staged as Ib
Ib	Lesions of greater dimension than stage Ia2, whether seen clinically or not; preformed space involvement should not alter the staging but should be specifically recorded so as to determine whether it should affect treatment decisions in the future
II	Carcinoma extends beyond the cervix but has not extended onto the pelvic wall; the carcinoma involves the vagina, but not as far as the lower third
IIa	No obvious parametrial involvement
IIb	Obvious parametrial involvement
III	Carcinoma has extended onto the pelvic wall; on rectal examination there is no cancer-free space between the tumor and the pelvic wall; the tumor involves the lower third of the vagina; all cases with a hydronephrosis or nonfunctioning kidney should be included, unless they are known to be due to another cause
IIIa	No extension onto the pelvic wall, but involvement of the lower third of the vagina
IIIb	Extension onto the pelvic wall or hydronephrosis or nonfunctioning kidney
IV	Carcinoma has extended beyond the true pelvis or has clinically involved the mucosa of the bladder or rectum
IVa	Spread of the growth to adjacent organs
IVb	Spread to distant organs

Reprinted from Staging Announcement: FIGO Cancer Committee. *Gynecol Oncol* 1986;25:383, with permission.

Invasive cancer of the cervix

The identification of invasive cancer of the cervix requires prompt treatment, except for patients in the third trimester, when one may briefly delay therapy until fetal viability is established. Patients with stage IB and stage IIA cervical cancer recognized in the first trimester of pregnancy are routinely recommended to be treated with a type III radical hysterectomy and bilateral deep pelvic lymphadenectomies. Patients with more advanced cervical cancer are treated with concurrent chemoradiation therapy.

Breast cancer

The breast is the second most common site for invasive cancers in pregnant women. It is estimated that approximately 1 in 3000 pregnancies will be associated with breast cancer. Breast self-examination as well as physician examinations should be a routine part of prenatal care. The diagnosis of cancer in pregnancy is complicated by the physiologic enlargement of the breast and associated hyperemia. Mammography may be employed safely in pregnancy, provided the abdomen is shielded. Suspicious breast masses in pregnancy must be biopsied. Excisional biopsy is the best way to confirm the nature of a breast mass. The biopsy can be done under either local anesthesia or general anesthesia. The frequencies of the histologic types of breast cancer occurring in pregnancy are similar to those in the nonpregnant state. Stage for stage, the prognosis for breast cancer patients in pregnancy is similar to that in the nonpregnant state.

Ovarian cancer

Most ovarian cancers in the United States are epithelial in origin and occur in women over age 35 years. Most ovarian cancers complicating pregnancy are either borderline malignant potential epithelial cancers or germ cell malignancies. Invasive epithelial cancers are rare in pregnancy, and sex cord–stromal tumors occur extremely infrequently. Ovarian malignancies occurring in pregnancy are estimated to complicate 1 in 9000 to 1 in 25 000 pregnancies. Ovarian neoplasms are usually observed in the first trimester and are operated upon in the second trimester.

Surgical staging

Surgical staging for ovarian cancer in pregnancy should be the same as that recommended for surgical staging in the nonpregnant state. A vertical incision should be used. On entering the abdomen, any free fluid should be aspirated and sent for cytology. If no free fluid is present, washings of the paracolic spaces, the pelvis, and subdiaphragmatic spaces should be obtained. The ovarian lesion should then be removed and sent for frozen section. Every effort should be made to remove the tumor intact. The remaining ovary should be inspected carefully. Any peritoneal abnormalities should be sampled. Any retroperitoneal nodularities should also be sampled. Sampling of periaortic lymph nodes should be attempted. Germ cell ovarian malignancies are almost invariably unilateral. Removing the contralateral ovary does not affect prognosis for the patient. The current FIGO staging system for ovarian cancer is presented in Table 50.4.

Uterine carcinoma

Adenocarcinoma of the endometrium is an extremely unusual disease in pregnant women, and only 8% of endometrial cancers have been reported to recur in women under age 40 years.

Table 50.4 International Federation of Gynecology and Obstetrics (FIGO) ovarian cancer staging classification.

I	Growth limited to the ovaries
Ia	Growth limited to one ovary; no ascites; no tumor on the external surface; capsule intact
Ib	Growth limited to both ovaries; no ascites; no tumor on the external surfaces; capsule intact
Ic	Tumor either stage Ia or Ib, but with tumor on the surface of one or both ovaries; or with the capsule ruptured; or with ascites containing malignant cells; or with positive peritoneal washings
II	Growth involving one or both ovaries with pelvic extension
IIa	Extension, metastases, or both to the uterus, tubes, or both
IIb	Extension to other pelvic tissue
IIc	Tumor either stage IIa or IIb but with tumor on the surface of one or both ovaries; or with the capsule ruptured; or with ascites present containing malignant cells; or with positive peritoneal washings
III	Tumor involving one or both ovaries with peritoneal implants outside the pelvis and/or positive retroperitoneal or inguinal nodes; superficial liver metastases equals stage III; tumor is limited to the true pelvis but with histologically proven malignant extension to the small bowel or omentum
IIIa	Tumor grossly limited to the true pelvis with negative nodes but with histologically confirmed microscopic seeding of abdominal peritoneal surfaces
IIIb	Tumor involving one or both ovaries with histologically confirmed implants of abdominal peritoneal surfaces, none exceeding 2 cm in diameter; nodes are negative
IIIc	Abdominal implants greater than 2 cm in diameter and/or positive retroperitoneal or inguinal nodes
IV	Growth involving one or both ovaries with distant metastases. If pleural effusion is present, there must be positive cytology to allot a case to stage IV; parenchymal liver metastasis equals stage IV

Reprinted from Staging Announcement: FIGO Cancer Committee. *Gynecol Oncol* 1986;25:383, with permission.

Vulvar cancer

Vulvar carcinoma *in situ* has been increasing, according to data from the Connecticut Tumor Registry. Forty percent of patients with vulvar carcinoma *in situ* are under age 40 years. Thus, it can be anticipated that more women will be diagnosed in pregnancy as having vulvar carcinoma *in situ*. The management of a vulvar lesion in pregnancy is a local excision.

Vaginal cancer

Carcinoma of the vagina occurs infrequently and is usually a squamous carcinoma presenting in a peri- or postmenopausal woman. Its management is similar to that of cervical cancer.

Table 50.5 Ann Arbor staging classification for Hodgkin's disease.

I	Involvement of a single lymph node region (I) or a single extralymphatic organ or site (I_E)
II	Involvement of two or more lymph node regions on the same side of the diaphragm (II) or localized involvement of an extralymphatic organ or site (II_E)
III	Involvement of lymph node regions on both sides of the diaphragm (III) or localized involvement of an extralymphatic organ or site (III_E), spleen (III_S), or both (III_{SE})
IV	Diffuse or disseminated involvement of one or more extralymphatic organs with or without associated lymph node involvement. The organ(s) involved should be identified by a symbol
	A = Asymptomatic
	B = Fever, sweats, weight loss >10% of body weight

Reprinted from DeVita VT Jr, Hellman S, Rosenberg SA, eds. *Cancer: principles and practice of oncology*, 3rd edn. Philadelphia, PA: Lippincott–Raven, 1989; with permission.

Hodgkin's disease

Hodgkin's disease generally occurs during the reproductive years, the peak incidence being between ages 18 and 30 years. It is estimated that one-third of women with Hodgkin's disease are pregnant or have delivered within 1 year of the diagnosis. As with almost all malignancies associated with pregnancy, Hodgkin's disease has not been reported to be affected by the pregnancy. It is a disease that is extremely sensitive to therapy; the cure rate for localized disease treated with radiation therapy is 80%, and patients with advanced disease treated with chemotherapy can anticipate a long-term disease-free survival of 65%. Selection of local radiation or systemic chemotherapy is based on the staging system (Table 50.5).

Non-Hodgkin's lymphoma

Fewer than 50 cases of non-Hodgkin's lymphomas during pregnancy have been published. The mean age of patients with non-Hodgkin's lymphoma is 42 years.

Acute leukemia

Acute leukemia rarely complicates pregnancy, the incidence being less than 1 case in 75 000 pregnancies. The disease is usually first recognized in the second or third trimester. Pregnancy does not influence the natural history of acute leukemia.

Chronic myelocytic leukemia

Chronic myelocytic leukemia makes up 90% of the chronic leukemias complicating pregnancy. Pregnancy does not adversely affect the natural history of chronic myelocytic leukemia. Treatment is palliative.

Melanoma

Pregnancy frequently induces a darkening in the appearance of pigmented nevi, but a bluish or slightly gray appearance to a nevus requires immediate excisional biopsy. Indeed, pigmented nevi that have become darker or irregular in outline and elevated should always be promptly excised in pregnancy under local anesthesia. Pregnancy does not change the natural history of melanoma.

Gastrointestinal cancer

Colorectal cancers

Cancers of the gastrointestinal tract rarely complicate pregnancy. There is no evidence that pregnancy changes the natural history of colorectal cancer, the most common of these neoplasms. Most pregnant patients with gastrointestinal cancers have rectal carcinomas. Approximately 20% of patients have carcinoma presenting in the sigmoid colon.

Pancreatic tumors, stomach tumors, liver tumors

These carcinomas rarely complicate pregnancy.

Endocrine tumors

Thyroid cancer

The thyroid is an infrequent site for cancer to develop in pregnancy. Patients at high risk of thyroid cancer include women exposed to radiation therapy to the head, neck, or chest during childhood. Most cancers of the thyroid present as solitary nodules. Pregnancy changes should not result in the misdiagnosis of thyroid cancer. The most common type of thyroid cancer to be diagnosed in pregnancy is the papillary carcinoma or mixed papillary follicular carcinoma. Fine needle aspiration biopsies are used to diagnose thyroid cancer in pregnancy. Radionuclide scans are contraindicated in pregnancy because of the theoretical risk of destroying the fetal thyroid. As the overwhelming number of thyroid cancers presenting in pregnancy are histologically well differentiated, there is no reason to terminate pregnancy or avoid future pregnancies. Pregnancy does not appear to influence the course of thyroid cancer.

Adrenal tumors

Pheochromocytoma is the most common tumor arising in the adrenal gland in pregnancy. The management of pheochromocytoma has been surgical in the first two trimesters and delivery by Cesarean section followed by tumor resection in the third trimester.

Urinary tract malignancies

Kidney tumors

Renal cell carcinoma is the most common malignancy arising in the urinary tract in pregnancy. Hematuria is the most common presenting symptom. Nephrectomy with or without radiation therapy is the standard treatment.

Bladder cancers

Bladder cancers have been reported infrequently in pregnancy. The histologic distribution is similar to that in the nonpregnant state, with an overwhelming majority being transitional cell carcinoma followed by squamous cell and adenocarcinomas.

Central nervous system tumors

Central nervous system tumors rarely complicate pregnancy. Patients present with headaches and visual disturbances. Magnetic resonance imaging allows for rapid evaluation without radiation exposure. The overall maternal mortality for patients with central nervous system tumors is 60%.

Further reading

ACOG Practice Bulletin. Diagnosis and treatment of cervical carcinoma. No. 35, May 2002. *Int J Gynecol Obstet* 2002; 78(1):79.

Anderson BO, Petrek JA, Byrd DR, et al. Pregnancy influences breast cancer stage at diagnosis in women 30 and younger. *Ann Surg Oncol* 1996;3:204.

Cappell MS. Colon cancer during pregnancy. *Gastroenterol Clin North Am* 2003;32(1):34.

Jabiry-Zieniewicz Z, Gajewska M. The pregnancy and delivery course with pregnant women with uterine myomas. *Ginekol Pol* 2002;73(4):271.

Jemal A, Tiwari RC, Murray T, et al. Cancer statistics, 2004. *Cancer* 2004;54:8.

Kaplan KJ, Dainty LA, Dolinsky B, et al. Prognosis and recurrence risk for patients with cervical squamous intraepithelial lesions diagnosed during pregnancy. *Cancer* 2004;102(4): 228.

Lolis DE, Kalantoridou SN, Makrydimas G, et al. Successful myomectomy during pregnancy. *Hum Reprod* 2003;18(8):1699.

Rose PG. Combined-modality therapy of locally advanced cervical cancer. *J Clin Oncol* 2003; 21(10 Suppl):211.

Sood AK, Sorosky JI, Krogman S, et al. Surgical management of cervical cancer complicating pregnancy: a case–control study. *Gynecol Oncol* 1996;63:294.

Streffer C, Shore R, Konermann G, et al. Biological effects after prenatal irradiation (embryo and fetus). A report of International Commission on Radiological Protection. *Ann ICPP* 2003;33(1–2):5.

Suzuki S. Comparison between spontaneous ovarian hyperstimulation syndrome and hyper-reactio luteinalis. *Arch Gynecol Obstet* 2004;269(3):227.

Part XI

Medicosocial Considerations in Pregnancy

51 Pregnancy before age 20 years and after age 35 years

Helen H. Kay

Young and older maternal age are considered to be suboptimal for childbearing, but it is uncertain whether that adversity results from age itself, biologic factors, or socioeconomic factors. The relative risk of maternal mortality by age in the United States from 1979 to 1986 is demonstrated in a J-shaped distribution with slightly increased risk mortality for those less than 20 years of age and for those beyond 24 years of age, rising exponentially. Pregnancy complications kill 70 000 teenagers a year worldwide. At higher age greater than 40 years, the risk of mortality is 8.6 times that for women between the ages of 20 and 24 years. Pregnancy for women at the extremes of reproductive potential may be more hazardous, and physicians should be aware when they are counseling patients regarding the optimal timing of pregnancy. It is important to determine whether adverse outcomes are related to physiology, genetics, or psychosocial behaviors. Many epidemiologic studies have not been able to control for a multitude of variables such as smoking, education, socioeconomic status, and race. Consequently, only associations have been identified without direct cause and effect relationships.

Adolescent pregnancies

Many resources have been spent on preventing and reducing the incidence of teenage births. The primary reason for doing so is the high-risk nature of these pregnancies, resulting in physical and psychosocial ill-effects to the young mothers. In addition, there are long-term socioeconomic burdens to society from the offspring of these often unplanned pregnancies.

Incidence

Over one million teenagers become pregnant in the USA each year. This is a very high rate for an advanced society and underscores the inadequate educational efforts that have been put forth. The incidence of unplanned and unwanted pregnancies among the black teenage population is 51.2%. Approximately half are aborted. In

2002, Hispanic teenagers had the highest pregnancy rate (82.9/1000) compared with other ethnic groups, surpassing black women for the first time.

The teenage birth rate for women aged 15–19 years was 61.8/1000 women in 1991, but declined to 43.0/1000 women in 2002. This is a 30% decrease. In 2002, the teenage birth rate decreased by 50% among the highest risk ages of 15–17 years; the rate for black teenagers decreased by 40%. According to recent statistics from national surveys in 2001, sexual activity decreased by 16% from 1991 (54.1%) to 2001 (45.6%); the prevalence of multiple partners decreased by 24%; condom use increased; and sexually transmitted diseases decreased.

Health risk behaviors

Risk behaviors and social factors leading to teenage pregnancies

In contrast with older women, who often obtain prepregnancy consultation, teenagers rarely seek advice prior to getting pregnant. Therefore, abusive habits such as alcohol, cigarette, and drug use are not addressed and resolved prior to conception. Illegal drug use is prevalent among adolescents and may account for some adverse outcomes. There is no increase in preterm deliveries, preterm rupture of membranes, or poor neonatal outcomes.

Low socioeconomic status

Low socioeconomic status promotes adolescent pregnancies because it is a vicious cycle. Poverty leads to adverse behavior such as drug and alcohol abuse as well as poor self-esteem. These contribute to a lack of incentive to avoid parenthood.

Support from family

Teenagers with strong parental and community support as well as support from the father of the baby are less likely to become teenage parents, whereas those whose parents do not openly discuss contraception and sexual behavior with their children tend not to use contraception and are more likely to be teenage parents.

Poor self-esteem and poor achievement in school

Women with low self-esteem also tend to be poor achievers or underachievers at school. They also tend to have a higher rate of drug, alcohol, and tobacco use. Such individuals are more likely to be influenced by their surroundings and engage in destructive behaviors, leading to a higher pregnancy rate. Many girls with poor self-esteem have had a prior history of sexual or physical abuse, as high as 33%. Health-care providers should routinely inquire about a history of abuse when taking care of pregnant adolescents.

Racial factors

Half of all teenage births are to non-Hispanic whites, but blacks and Hispanic teenagers have almost twice the pregnancy rates of whites. Blacks have a higher proportion of preterm and low birthweight births compared with whites or

Hispanics. At the same time, however, blacks also have a higher mortality rate among term, post-term, normal birthweight, and macrosomic infants. Hispanics have the lowest risk of neonatal mortality at term.

Adverse outcomes of teenage pregnancies

Adverse outcomes in teenagers result from poor psychosocial environments rather than biologic risks inherent in the adolescent. In other words, adverse outcomes are more a reflection of a social problem than a medical problem.

Teenage mortality

Mortality to a teenager secondary to pregnancy is extremely low.

Perinatal mortality

In California, USA, teenagers had a higher rate of infant and neonatal deaths than an older control group of white women irrespective of race, except that Asians had a similar rate to the control group. However, in another study, the perinatal mortality rate was not increased in adolescents compared with older women and, in some reports, the data are inconsistent.

Preterm labor

The incidence of preterm labor does not seem to be increased in a teenage population. There is no difference between young or older women compared with women over 20 years of age.

Preterm birth

In subgroups of teenagers with good access to tertiary care centers, as well as social and medical support, the incidence of preterm birth is not increased compared with older patients. It appears that the data for preterm delivery risk are mixed and most likely reflect a lack of control in some studies of factors that influence the access to, or quality of, medical care.

Preterm ruptured membranes

Despite being high-risk pregnancies, teenage pregnancies do not appear to have an increased risk of preterm premature rupture of membranes.

Low birthweight

Most studies, but not all, report a higher risk of low birthweight and very low birthweight infants from teenage women. However, other studies do not show an increased rate of low birthweight infants in populations in which there was a commitment to prenatal care.

Preeclampsia/eclampsia

Rates of preeclampsia (6.3%) were higher in teenagers than in adult black (2.5%)

and white women (2.2%) in an inner city, black population on the east coast of the USA. This was not true in studies from the west coast. It appears that adolescents, if given proper care, may not be at increased risk of hypertensive disorders of pregnancy compared with older women of similar race. Until the etiology of preeclampsia is identified, we may not be able to assess the risks unique to the age of a population because of many confounding variables.

Cesarean section

Although it has been reported that the pelvises of girls at menarche have room to grow, it is not certain that this leads to an obstructed pelvis. Therefore, Cesarean section is not increased, and there does not appear to be an anatomic risk associated with adolescent childbearing. Even in studies from Africa, where some episiotomies are performed for obstructive labor, the procedure was not performed in a higher percentage of adolescents, suggesting that an immature pelvis is not responsible for obstructive labor. Therefore, the concern for an increased risk of dystocia or cephalopelvic disproportion among adolescents may need to be revisited, perhaps with imaging studies.

Risk factors contributing to adverse pregnancy outcomes among teenagers

Anemia

Anemia among adolescents is rampant, most likely secondary to poor nutrition. However, adverse pregnancy outcomes have been inconsistently demonstrated.

Poor nutrition

Nutritional intake is clearly a significant problem among teenagers. Anorexia is more common among white adolescents than among blacks or Hispanics. Excess weight gain may induce further hazards to the fetus if macrosomia is present, and there is an increased risk of long-term health problems and obesity for the mothers.

Late prenatal care

Factors influencing late entry to care include unemployment, lower educational level, and race. There is a clear racial difference, with white women usually reporting more prenatal visits than black women. Understanding and accepting these risk factors will enable the medical and social community to better design clinics that would successfully encourage adolescents to seek prenatal care, i.e., school-based clinics.

Drug use

Cigarettes, alcohol, and illegal drug use among teenagers contributes to adverse pregnancy outcomes for a variety of reasons, including bleeding in pregnancy, fetal alcohol syndrome, and the socioeconomic issues related to the drug scene. Although use has declined since the 1970s, a large number of teenagers still admit to partaking, 17% by questionnaire self-report and 11% by urine screening.

Infection

One of the more common complications is pyelonephritis. Teenagers have a high rate of sexually transmitted diseases. At the first prenatal visit, as many as 23.5% tested positive for *Neisseria gonorrhoeae* (1.2%), *Chlamydia trachomatis* (13%), *Trichomonas vaginalis* (8.9%), and *Treponema pallidum* (1.2%). One sobering reason to work toward educating adolescents against unplanned childbearing is the very real issue that human immunodeficiency virus (HIV)-positive adolescents are becoming pregnant. This will be an increasing concern as the number of parentless adolescents continues to increase worldwide.

What can be done about reducing the incidence of teenage pregnancies?

Sex education

School sex education is one of the best means of preventing teenage pregnancies and their recurrence. One of the reasons for failure is the timing of this education. Investigators have reported that 52% of 15-year-old girls have already initiated coitus before taking sex education classes.

School-based clinics

The school environment is one of the best locations to establish classes to educate teenagers about responsibilities related to sexual freedom. It is an environment that reaches those in the neediest age groups within an atmosphere of learning and training. Within that environment, interventions may be undertaken in the form of additional education, counseling, or introduction to prevention programs. The success of these programs needs further testing. Specialized teenage pregnancy clinics have also been suggested as effective and successful in educating teenagers. Although there are few randomized trials, such clinics appear to be successful through close direct educational efforts with adolescents.

Emergency contraception

Although it is debated whether access to emergency contraception promotes unprotected intercourse, the provision of emergency contraception may actually encourage young teenagers to seek pelvic examinations and Pap smear screening. Emergency contraception is most effective when taken within 72 hours of unprotected intercourse.

Abortion

Abortion has been practiced as a very effective means of contraception for teenagers. Abortion rates increased dramatically from the mid-1970s to the mid-1980s. The proportion of black and white adolescents who obtain abortions is similar but, because there is a higher pregnancy rate among blacks, the rate of abortion is higher among blacks than among whites.

Contraception

Teenagers should be educated regarding their reproductive options and childbearing options. Older studies support the fact that adolescents are capable of using contraception effectively provided that there is a supportive environment from the mothers and from the fathers of the babies.

Pregnancy in older women aged more than 35 years

Within the past decade, there has been a rise in the number of births to women aged over 35 years, and it is now not uncommon to see women over the age of 40 years having pregnancies. There is even an increasing number of pregnant women over the age of 50 years. The primary reasons for this increase in older gravidas are social changes that have taken place over the past four decades including the acceptance of oral contraceptive technologies, the legalization of abortions, the availability of prenatal diagnosis, and the improvements in medical care overall, such that women with diabetes or hypertension are now well controlled and able to consider pregnancy options.

Risks to older women having pregnancies

There are some unique risks to pregnancy at an older age. Physicians should recognize that these women will enter pregnancy with more medical complications. Women older 35 years of age have a higher incidence of hypertension (2.7%), pre-existing diabetes (0.7%), and obesity (6.9%) at the beginning of pregnancy. Gestational diabetes was also identified in 6.9% of older women. However, in a setting in which women have access to good medical care, adverse pregnancy outcomes may not be increased.

Declining fertility

Older women should be aware that their fertility is expected to decline. Options for an older woman desiring fertility have increased through assisted reproductive technologies.

Risk of aneuploidy

A woman's risk of an aneuploid conceptus increases with increasing age. They should be counseled regarding prenatal diagnosis options.

Multiple gestations

Dizygotic multiples are increased among gestations from older women. This is influenced by a higher incidence of women undergoing assisted reproductive technologies.

Mortality

Maternal mortality for women over 40 years was 50/100 000 in 1954, 10/100 000 in 1985, and 8.9/100 000 live births in the year 2002. Recent medical advances have significantly decreased maternal mortality. Mortality does rise with an increase in maternal age. Mortality is also influenced by race, with black women having a higher mortality rate than white women aged over 40 years. For older black women, the most common cause of death is hypertensive disorders of pregnancy followed by hemorrhage and embolism.

Maternal obstetric complications due to advanced age

Cesarean sections

Cesarean sections are increased among women aged over 40 years. The reasons for the increased rate are not fully understood. There is a higher incidence of birth asphyxia, fetal growth restriction, malpresentation, and gestational diabetes that may explain the higher rates of surgical delivery. Other reasons could include higher rates of hypertensive diseases, fetal growth restriction leading to a higher incidence of fetal distress, or more dysfunctional labor because of higher parity. A higher incidence of infertility also generates the recognition that these may be "premium" pregnancies and, hence, may contribute to the higher incidence of Cesarean sections.

Increased operative vaginal deliveries

Operative vaginal deliveries are higher among older women. There is also a higher need for oxytocin augmentation. The cause of these findings is uncertain, but may be due to a higher rate of dysfunctional labor. They may also be related to a higher incidence of maternal exhaustion, but that variable is difficult to quantify.

Preeclampsia/eclampsia

Older women tend to have a higher incidence of preeclampsia and eclampsia. Older women also tend to have a higher incidence of chronic hypertension, which contributes to the incidence of preeclampsia and eclampsia.

Postpartum hemorrhage

The odds ratios for postpartum hemorrhage are higher for women aged 35 years and older, most often due to uterine atony.

Dysfunctional labor

It is equivocal whether older women have a higher incidence of dysfunctional labor.

Induction of labor

The odds of labor induction are higher for older women than for younger women. However, the causes cannot be defined, but may be influenced by physicians' desire to deliver older women by their due date.

Preterm labor/preterm delivery

Very preterm delivery was found to be increased among older women. Some have a higher risk of preterm labor and preterm rupture of membranes, which may contribute to the preterm delivery. However, in other studies among educated women with access to good healthcare, there was no increased risk of preterm delivery or preterm labor.

Placenta previa
The incidence of placenta previa is increased for women aged over 40 years. This reflects a higher incidence of multiparity, uterine myomas, or uterine scarring from prior surgeries.

Antepartum bleeding
Antepartum bleeding is more frequent for women aged over 40 years because of a higher incidence of abruptions and placenta previa.

Adverse perinatal outcomes due to advanced maternal age
Early and late fetal loss
Early pregnancy loss is more common among older women because of the increased risk of aneuploidy. Fetal death rates are increased with increasing maternal age. The cause of the increase in fetal death is uncertain, but may be related to increasing maternal vascular disease.

Low birthweight
Low birthweight is an adverse perinatal outcome for older women. Some have reported a rate of 10.1% for low birthweight infants among older women versus 5.9% for women aged less than 40 years. This is not surprising because older women tend to have a higher incidence of medical complications; whether this is enhanced by age itself is somewhat controversial.

Fetal death
Perinatal mortality rates are increased in older women compared with younger women, 28.6/1000 live births versus 10.8/1000 for younger women.

Further reading

Ananth CV, Wilcox AJ, Savitz DA, et al. Effect of maternal age and parity on the risk of utero-placental bleeding disorders in pregnancy. *Obstet Gynecol* 1996;88:511–516.

Ananth CV, Balasubramanian B, Demissie K, Kinzler WL. Small-for-gestational-age births in the United States: an age-period-cohort analysis. *Epidemiology* 2004;15(1):28–35.

Berkowitz GS, Skovron ML, Lapinski RH, Berkowitz RL. Delayed childbearing and the outcome of pregnancy. *N Engl J Med* 1990;322(10):659–664.

Canterino JC, Ananth CV, Smulian J, et al. Maternal age and risk of fetal death in singleton gestations: United States, 1995–2000. *J Matern Fetal Neonatal Med* 2004;15:193–197.

Eure CR, Lindsay MK, Graves WL. Risk of adverse pregnancy outcomes in young adolescent parturients in an inner-city hospital. *Am J Obstet Gynecol* 2002;186(5):918–920.

Fraser AM, Brockert JE, Ward RH. Association of young maternal age with adverse repro-ductive outcomes. *N Engl J Med* 1995;332(17):113–117.

Gortzak-Uzan L, Hallak M, Press F, et al. Teenage pregnancy: risk factors for adverse peri-natal outcome. *J Matern Fetal Med* 2001;10(6):393–397.

Heffner LJ. Advanced maternal age—how old is too old? *N Engl J Med* 2004;351(19): 1927–1929.

Hemminki E, Gissler M. Births by younger and older mothers in a population with late and regulated childbearing: Finland 1991. *Acta Obstet Gynecol Scand* 1996:75(1):19–27.

Olausson PM, Cnattingius S, Goldenberg RL. Determinants of poor pregnancy outcomes among teenagers in Sweden. *Obstet Gynecol* 1997;89(3):451–457.

52 Essentials in biostatistics and perinatal epidemiology

Paula K. Roberson and Benjamin P. Sachs

Epidemiology

Basic definitions

Understanding the strengths and weaknesses of study design and the quality of evi-dence provided is critical when evaluating a research article. *Epidemiology* is con-cerned with the assessment of exposure and outcome. The basic design strategies used in epidemiologic research can be broadly classified as either descriptive or ana-lytic. The three main types of *descriptive* study are correlational studies, case reports, and cross-sectional studies. *Analytic epidemiology* explicitly compares exposure and outcome by means of either observational or interventional studies. *Observational studies* can be further divided into case–control and cohort studies (Table 52.1). A clinical trial is an example of an *interventional study*.

Both precision and validity are important concepts when performing a critical lit-erature review. *Validity* refers to the extent that the outcome variable actually meas-ures the effect of interest. High validity implies a lack of systematic error or *bias*. *Precision* refers to the consistency or closeness of repeated measurements of outcome to each other.

Confounding is a form of bias that can occur in both case–control and cohort studies, leading to inaccurate conclusions. A *confounding factor* (or *confounder*) can be defined as a risk factor for disease, other than the exposure under study, that is unequally distributed between the cases and the comparison or control groups.

In both diagnostic testing and disease screening, the term *sensitivity* refers to the probability of correctly identifying a sick individual, whereas *specificity* is the prob-

Table 52.1 Relative strengths and weaknesses of observational study designs.

	Cohort studies	Case–control studies
Strengths	Enable direct estimation of disease rates Less subject to recall bias	More economical Can be completed in shorter time-frame
Weaknesses	More likely to be biased in determining disease frequency Require large sample size, particularly if disease is rare More expensive May require very long time if induction time for disease development is long May pose ethical dilemmas if exposure could be removed Subject to losing subjects to follow-up	Greater risk of recall bias Identification of appropriate control group may be more difficult

Table 52.2 Relationship of sensitivity, specificity, and predictive values.

Risk factors	Disease	No disease
Yes	a	b
No	c	d

Predictive value negative = d/(c + d); predictive value positive = a/(a + b); sensitivity = a/(a + c); specificity = d/(d + b).

ability of correctly identifying a healthy individual (Table 52.2.) Positive and negative *predictive values* depend not only on the sensitivity and specificity of the test but also on the disease prevalence of the population under study, and thus are not measures of test accuracy.

Statistics

The *null hypothesis* is the focus of statistical testing in biomedical research. This hypothesis generally stipulates that there is no difference between the groups being compared with respect to the mean of a variable of interest. Rejection of the null hypothesis implies an identifiable difference in the group means beyond that attributable to chance. The null hypothesis is evaluated via the *P*-value, i.e., the probability that a difference at least as great as that observed would occur by chance if the null hypothesis were true. Table 52.3 defines the possible errors in decision-making that can occur. The level of either error depends on the cutoff value chosen

Table 52.3 Possible types of error associated with hypothesis testing.

Statistical testing decision	Truth (null hypothesis true)	Truth (null hypothesis false)
Do not reject null hypothesis	No error	Type II error (β)
Reject null hypothesis	Type I error (α)	No error ($1 - \beta$ = power)

Table 52.4 Factors relating to power and required sample size of a specific statistical test.

Alpha level (type I error)	Standard deviation
Power (1 – type II error)	Sample size
Difference to detect at specified power	

Table 52.5 Alternative univariate and multivariate statistical methods used in hypothesis testing of continuous and/or categorical data.

Exposure (explanatory) variables	Outcome (response) variables	
	Categorical	Continuous
Single		
Categorical	Contingency table (chi-squared or Fisher's exact text) or normal approximation (Z-statistic)	Z-statistic, Student's t-test, ANOVA, or nonparametric analogs
Continuous	Z-statistic, Student's t-test, ANOVA, or nonparametric	Linear regression, correlation coefficient
Multiple*		
Categorical	Stratification or loglinear analysis or logistic regression	ANOVA
Continuous	Logistic regression	Multiple regression
Mixed	Logistic regression	ANCOVA

ANCOVA, analysis of covariance; ANOVA, analysis of variance.

*Adapted from Louis T, Fineberg H, Mosteller F. *Annu Rev Public Health* 1985;6:1.

to define significance. Thus, the type II error is larger if the type I error is reduced and vice versa.

The *power* of a statistical test is its ability to detect a difference between the groups at a given level of significance. For a given statistical probability distribution, the five factors listed in Table 52.4 are related such that, given four of the five, one can solve for the fifth. Thus, power is a (nonlinear) function of sample size (and vice versa). As sample size is increased, it is possible to detect smaller differences with a given power. The failure to consider statistical power is one of the most frequent errors in study design.

Table 52.5 outlines the categories of statistical tests that are commonly used to examine various combinations of exposure (explanatory) and outcome (response) variables. The appropriate use of statistical tests is not a trivial task and investigators should work closely with a biostatistician.

Some investigators prefer to report measures of effect and confidence intervals rather than P-values from hypothesis testing. These are often more informative than P-values alone but, given the point estimate and standard error, it is possible to calculate confidence intervals of whatever confidence limit is desired.

Multivariate procedures can control for a large number of variables simultaneously and facilitate the exploration of interrelationships between covariates. The methods encountered frequently in the clinical and epidemiological literature include multiple linear regression, logistic regression, loglinear analysis, mixed effects models and generalized estimating equations (GEE) for longitudinal data, and the (Cox) proportional hazards model for censored time-to-event data. General information about the appropriate application and interpretation of each of these procedures is discussed in van Belle and colleagues. Care is needed when assessing the adequacy of data to meet the assumptions underlying the various methods as well as when evaluating model fit and interpreting the results.

Further reading

Bailar III JC, Mosteller F. *Medical uses of statistics*, 2nd edn. Boston, MA: NEJM Books, 1995.
van Belle G, Fisher LD, Heagerty PJ, et al. *Biostatistics: a methodology for the health sciences*, 2nd edn. Hoboken, NJ: John Wiley & Sons, 2004.
Cummings SR, Browner WS, Grady D, et al. *Designing clinical research: an epidemiologic approach*, 2nd edn. Philadelphia, PA: Lippincott Williams & Wilkins, 2001.
Dawson-Saunders B, Trapp RG. *Basic and clinical biostatistics*, 4th edn. New York: McGraw-Hill, 2004.
Fleiss JL, Levin B, Paik MC. *Statistical methods for rates and proportions*, 3rd edn. Hoboken, NJ: John Wiley & Sons, 2003.
Friedman LM, Furberg CD, DeMets DL. *Fundamentals of clinical trials*, 3rd edn. New York: Springer-Verlag, 1998.
Gordis L. *Epidemiology*, 3rd edn. Philadelphia, PA: Elsevier Saunders, 2004.
Matthews DE, Farewell VT. *Using and understanding medical statistics*, 3rd edn. Basel: S Karger AG, 1996.
Rosner B. *Fundamentals of biostatistics*, 6th edn. Pacific Grove, CA: Duxbury Press, 2005.
Sackett DL. Bias in analytic research. *J Chronic Dis* 1978;32:51.

53 Sexuality in pregnancy and the postpartum period

Kirsten von Sydow

Sex is of little relevance for most new breastfeeding mothers during the first 3 months postpartum because adaptation to motherhood requires all of their energy, involves profound psychosocial and hormonal changes, and results in a lack of sleep. Male sexual activity is also reduced during this phase of life but to a lesser degree. Although this seems to be universal, there is a remarkable variation in female and male sexual behavior during pregnancy and the later postpartum stages (months 4–12). On average, all heterosexual activity tends to decline during pregnancy and reaches a point near zero in the immediate postpartum period; it then slowly starts to increase again.

Sexual problems and dysfunctions are relatively common during pregnancy and the first year postpartum, but some women experience an intensification of their sexuality during pregnancy or postbirth. Many women experience an increase in their sexual desire and enjoyment, especially during the second trimester of pregnancy. During pregnancy, sexual problems are often related to fear of harming the fetus, the man's fear of harming his partner, female dyspareunia, and fatigue (Table 53.1). Intercourse and/or orgasm should be avoided by expectant mothers who have certain pregnancy complications (Table 53.2). Common postpartum problems are lack of sexual interest (in women and in men), painful intercourse, and vaginal dryness (Table 53.3). Sexual problems are caused by the complex interplay of bio-medical, psychological, and marital–social factors. Important biomedical aspects are perineal lesions, especially resulting from episiotomy and assisted vaginal delivery, and breastfeeding long term. Additionally, mental symptoms of the mother (and perhaps the father), pre-existing sexual problems, and problems in the couple's relationship contribute to postpartum sexual problems.

A reduction in the use of episiotomies and an improvement in the training of doctors and other medical professions in sexual counseling is very important for the prevention and treatment of sexual problems in pregnancy and during the postpartum period (Table 53.4). Medical staff rarely discuss sexual issues with their patients during pregnancy or the postpartum stage, although the great majority of (expectant) mothers (and fathers) think that this would be helpful. Postbirth discussions focus only on contraception, and many sexual and perineal problems are not even mentioned (e.g., painful intercourse, incontinence).

Table 53.1 Factors associated with decreased sexual interest, activity, and enjoyment and increased sexual problems during pregnancy.

Biomedical factors
Tiredness
Worry that the fetus could be hurt during intercourse
Dyspareunia
Backache
Woman's low physical attractiveness (self and partner evaluation)

Psychosocial factors
Mental symptoms (depressed mood, emotional lability)
Prepregnancy sexual history and sexual symptoms (e.g., dyspareunia)
Negative or ambivalent feelings about the pregnancy

Couple/relationship factors
Low relationship satisfaction

Table 53.2 Indications for coital and orgasm abstinence during pregnancy.

Vaginal bleeding
Abdominal pains
Rupture of the membranes
Premature dilation of the cervix
History of premature delivery, heightened risk of premature labor
Placenta previa
Placental insufficiency
Incompetent cervix
Multiple pregnancy

Table 53.3 Factors associated with decreased sexual interest, activity, and enjoyment and increased sexual problems during the postpartum period.

Biomedical factors
Degree of perineal birth trauma (tears, episiotomy)
Assisted vaginal delivery
Tiredness
Kegel exercises not performed.
No reliable method of contraception

Psychosocial factors
Mental symptoms (depressed mood, emotional lability)
Prepregnancy sexual history and sexual symptoms (e.g., dyspareunia)
Poor childhood relationship with father (e.g., good relationship only with mother)

Couple/relationship factors
Low relationship satisfaction (in women and men)

Attributes of the baby and the mother–child relationship
Male babies: mothers of boys are perceived by their partners as being less tender during the postpartum months than mothers of girls
Mothers with a rigid and overprotective relationship to their baby
Breastfeeding

Table 53.4 Recommendations for taking a sexual history and giving the patient sexual information.

If possible, include the partner

Put open questions and listen to the answers
Pregnancy: the current emotional, marital, and sexual situation, and the information needs of the woman and her partner
Postpartum: sexual interest, behavior, coital pain, or incontinence

Give information about normal changes during the transition to parenthood
Pregnancy: some women (and men) have no sexual interest, whereas, in others, sexual interest is intensified
Postpartum: some mothers experience erotic feelings during breastfeeding and some fathers are jealous about breastfeeding. Vaginal dryness may be associated with breastfeeding

Acknowledge patients' and partners' fears and uncertainties and respect their inner limitations
The aim is a sexual life that both partners and, from the medical and parental point of view, the baby are contented with. This also includes the option of sexual abstinence

Give technical advice about the range of sexual options
Tenderness, noncoital sexual activities (e.g., manual and oral stimulation, masturbation) and, during pregnancy, alternative coital positions (female superior, rear entry/"spoon," use of pillows)

Instruct the patient in self-help
Postbirth: self-inspection of the vulva with a hand mirror and insertion of a finger to test for healing; vaginal muscle-toning (Kegel) exercises

Be sensitive for sexual and nonsexual domestic violence

Further reading

Avery MD, Duckett L, Frantzich CR. The experience of sexuality during breastfeeding. *J Midwifery Wom Health* 2000;45:227–237.

Barrett G, Victor C. Incidence of postnatal dyspareunia. *Br J Sex Med* 1996;23:6–8.

Berghella V, Klebanoff M, McPherson C, et al. Sexual intercourse association with asymptomatic bacterial vaginosis and *Trichomonas vaginalis* treatment in relationship to preterm birth. *Am J Obstet Gynecol* 2002;187:1277–1282.

Glazener CMA. Sexual function after childbirth: women's experiences, persistent morbidity and lack of professional recognition. *Br J Obstet Gynaecol* 1997;104:330–335.

Klein MC, Gauthier RJ, Robbins JM, et al. Relationship of episiotomy to perineal trauma and morbidity, sexual dysfunction, and pelvic floor relaxation. *Am J Obstet Gynecol* 1994; 171:591–598.

Signorello LB, Harlow BL, Chekos AK, et al. Postpartum sexual functioning and its relationship to perineal trauma: a retrospective cohort study of primiparous women. *Am J Obstet Gynecol* 2001;184:881–890.

von Sydow K. Sexuality during pregnancy and after childbirth: a meta-content-analysis of 59 studies. *J Psychosom Res* 1999;47:27–49.

von Sydow K. Sexual enjoyment and orgasm postpartum: sex differences and perceptual accuracy concerning partners' sexual experience. *J Psychosom Obstet Gynecol* 2002;23: 147–155.

von Sydow K. Female sexual dysfunction: pregnancy, childbirth and postpartum period. In: Goldstein I, Meston CM, Davis SR, et al. (eds). *Women's sexual function and dysfunction*. London: Taylor & Francis, 2006.

von Sydow K, Ullmeyer M, Happ N. Sexual activity during pregnancy and after childbirth: results from the Sexual Preferences Questionnaire. *J Psychosom Obstet Gynecol* 2001;22: 29–40.

54 Psychiatric problems during pregnancy and the puerperium

Linda L.M. Worley and Jennifer L. Melville

Psychiatric disorders are common in pregnant and postpartum women, yet they often go undiagnosed and untreated. Women suffering from a severe depressive illness or psychosis are also at risk for suicide, the leading cause of maternal death through the first postpartum year.[1] All women should be asked early in their pregnancy for a history of psychiatric disorders and screened for current psychiatric disorders. When present, management plans should be initiated to decrease both complications from the illness and the high risk of recurrence following delivery. Management of psychiatric disorders is complicated by pregnancy and the potential risk to the fetus, but collaboration between obstetric providers and psychiatrists can provide effective treatments.

Table 54.1 Depressive disorders.

Syndrome	Onset/course	Possible features	Management
Antenatal depression: 9–23% of pregnant women	Before conception or during pregnancy May progress to postpartum depression	Must have depressed mood or anhedonia lasting at least 2 weeks Loss of interest and pleasure, sleep disturbance, appetite change, guilt, decreased concentration, suicidal ideation	For mild to moderate depression with minimal role impairment, refer for counseling or bright light therapy For depression with significant role impairment, add treatment with an antidepressant
Postpartum blues: 50–70% of postpartum women	Peaks 3–5 days after delivery Resolves < 2 weeks	Crying spells, emotional lability, irritability, anxiety,[47] hypochrondriasis[47]	Reassure and educate Monitor for resolution[47] Encourage family to offer emotional and social support
Postpartum depression: 12–16% of postpartum women[8,9]	Within 6 months of delivery Insidious onset	Classic depression symptoms lasting at least 2 weeks (same as antenatal depression above) May also include intrusive thoughts or fears of harming infant	For mild to moderate depression with minimal role impairment, refer for counseling or bright light therapy For depression with significant role impairment, add treatment with an antidepressant Hospitalization when warranted
Postpartum psychosis:* 0.5% of postpartum women	Within 3 weeks of childbirth Abrupt onset Women with bipolar disorder are at high risk	Delusions, confusion, hallucinations, agitation, insomnia, disorganized thinking	Emergency referral to psychiatrist Medical workup to rule out underlying etiology

*See section on psychiatric emergencies.

Depressive disorders affect 9–23% of antepartum women[2-7] and 12–16% of postpartum women[8,9] (Table 54.1). There are common risk factors for the development of antenatal and postpartum depression (Table 54.2), with additional risks for postpartum depression based on prior depressive episodes. Women with a history of

Table 54.2 Risk factors for developing antenatal and postpartum depression.[15]

Family or personal history of depression, anxiety disorder, or bipolar disorder
Limited social support
History of physical, emotional, or sexual abuse
Cigarette smoking, alcohol, or substance use
Current financial, occupational, health, or relationship stressors
Abrupt discontinuation of an antidepressant before completing a full treatment course

Table 54.3 Risks of untreated depression.

Antepartum risks
Increased physical pain and discomfort[48]
Increased use of cigarettes, alcohol, and other drugs[49,50]
Inadequate self-care and poor compliance with prenatal care[21]

Peripartum risks
Low birthweight (< 2500 g)[51,52] and SGA infants[52]
Preeclampsia[53]
Preterm delivery (< 37 weeks)[52]
Operative delivery[54]

Postpartum risks
Difficulty breastfeeding[55]
Poor growth and failure to thrive[56,54]
Decreased IQ in infants and children[27]
Missed pediatric outpatient appointments and increased emergency room visits[58]
Marital and relationship difficulties[59]
Depression in children[28]

SGA, small for gestational age.

depression have a 25% risk of developing postpartum depression,[6] whereas those with a history of postpartum depression have a 50% chance for recurrence and should be monitored closely throughout pregnancy and the postpartum period. Untreated antenatal and postpartum depression have been shown to have a detrimental effect on both maternal and fetal outcomes (Table 54.3). Direct and indirect mechanisms of association have been hypothesized. Maternal psychosocial factors have been shown to affect neuroendocrine activity[10,11] and uterine blood flow,[12] both of which may play a direct role in adverse outcomes such as low birthweight, prematurity, and preeclampsia. Both maternal depression and anxiety have been linked to adverse health behaviors (e.g., poor nutrition and smoking),[13] which in turn contribute to adverse pregnancy outcomes.

The high prevalence of depressive disorders warrants screening of all pregnant and postpartum women. Self-report screening instruments, such as the PRIME-MD Patient Health Questionnaire 9-item (PHQ-9), shown in Fig. 54.1A and B, can be

(A)

Over the *last 2 weeks*, how often have you been bothered by any of the following problems?
Please check the box that corresponds to your response:

	Not at all <0>	Several days <1>	More than half the days <2>	Nearly every day <3>
a. Little interest or pleasure in doing things	☐	☐	☐	☐
b. Feeling down, depressed, or hopeless	☐	☐	☐	☐
c. Trouble falling or staying asleep, or sleeping too much	☐	☐	☐	☐
d. Feeling tired or having little energy	☐	☐	☐	☐
e. Poor appetite or overeating	☐	☐	☐	☐
f. Feeling bad about yourself – or that you are a failure or have let yourself or your family down	☐	☐	☐	☐
g. Trouble concentrating on things, such as reading the newspaper or watching television	☐	☐	☐	☐
h. Moving or speaking so slowly that other people could have noticed? Or the opposite – being so fidgety or restless that you have been moving around a lot more than usual	☐	☐	☐	☐
i. Thoughts that you would be better off dead or of hurting yourself in some way	☐	☐	☐	☐

Scoring instructions:
*If at least one of 3a and 3b in dark gray area is checked <☐ YES> **and** at least five total of 3a through 3i in total shaded area are checked <☐ YES> 'you' may benefit from treatment for depression.*

*PHQ-9 Copyright © 1999 Pfizer Inc. All rights reserved. Reproduced with permission.
PRIME MD TODAY is a trademark of Pfizer Inc.*

(B)

If you checked off any problems on questions above, how difficult have these problems made it for you to do your work, take care of things at home, or get along with other people?

Not difficult at all	Somewhat difficult	Very difficult	Extremely difficult
☐	☐	☐	☐

Figure 54.1 PHQ-9 depression screen (A) and role impairment screen (B).

easily incorporated into obstetric care to facilitate diagnosis and treatment or refer-ral. When establishing a diagnosis, potential underlying etiologies such as hypothy-roidism, nicotine withdrawal, substance use, and current abuse must be considered.

Management of depression during pregnancy depends on both the severity of symptoms and degree of impairment. The optimal treatment for antenatal and post-partum depression minimizes the risk to the fetus and neonate while limiting mor-bidity from untreated psychiatric illness in the mother.[14] For mild depression with minimal impairment, support groups and interpersonal psychotherapy have been found to be effective.[9,15–17] Additionally, bright light therapy (e.g., sitting in front of a broad spectrum light each morning for approximately 15–60 min) may be bene-ficial; the exposure dose can be reduced[18–20] if side-effects of hypomania or nausea emerge. Social support for the patient is also very important, with the involvement of family and friends if possible.

For major depression with impaired role functioning, antidepressant treatment may be necessary. Selective serotonin reuptake inhibitors (SSRIs) are widely used in pregnancy; prescribing information for commonly used SSRIs, for which antenatal exposure data are available, are listed in Table 54.4. Sufficient prospective data on

Table 54.4 Administration schedule for selected SSRI antidepressants.

Antidepressants	Dose range (mg/day)	Initial suggested dose	Characteristics and administration schedule
Fluoxetine (Prozac)	10–40	10–20 mg every morning with food (10 mg if ↑ anxiety)	Activating; not first choice in patients with ↑ anxiety, but can be beneficial for patients with fatigue Increase in 10-mg increments at intervals of 7 days Maintain 20 mg for 4–6 weeks before dose increase Monitor maternal and neonatal weight gain; decrease dose in week prior to delivery to aid in neonatal clearance
Sertraline (Zoloft)	50–150	25–50 mg q.d. with food (25 mg if ↑ anxiety)	Increase in 25–50 mg increments at intervals of 7 days as tolerated Maintain 100 mg for 4–6 weeks before dose increase Extensively studied for use in breastfeeding; minimal amounts transfer into breast milk, and milk can be discarded 8–9 h after dose to further minimize exposure[60]
Paroxetine (Paxil)*	10–50	10–20 mg q.d. with food (10 mg if ↑ anxiety every morning)	The most anticholinergic of the SSRIs Avoid first-trimester exposure when possible* Sedating: good choice for patients with ↑ anxiety Increase in 10-mg increments at intervals of 7 days up to a maximum of 40 mg/day Maintain 20 mg for 4–6 weeks before dose increase Monitor the newborn for transient neonatal discontinuation syndrome[61,62] Of the SSRIs, this passes least into breastmilk and is virtually undetectable[63]
Citalopram (Celexa)	10–40	10–20 mg every morning with food (10 mg if ↑ anxiety)	Increase in 10-mg increments every 7 days as tolerated Maintain 20 mg for 4–6 weeks before dose increase This medication has been widely prescribed in Europe during pregnancy and lactation

*FDA, FDA Alert. *Increase in the risk of birth defects. Paroxetine hydrochloride (marketed as Paxil) information.* US Food and Drug Administration. Center for Drug Evaluation and Research, 2005.

the use of buproprion, mirtazapine, nefazodone, trazodone, and escitalopram are not currently available.[21] Monoamine oxidase inhibitors (MAOIs) are generally avoided during pregnancy because of their potential to precipitate a hypertensive crisis in the event that tocolytic medications are necessary.[21] Severely depressed patients with acute suicidality or psychosis, or women who wish to avoid extended exposure to psychotropic medications during pregnancy, may also be effectively treated with electroconvulsive therapy.[22,23]

For women taking antidepressants at term, a rare transient neonatal discontinuation syndrome has been reported.[24] Although rare, it is recommended that newborns with recent *in utero* antidepressant exposure be monitored for symptoms of tachypnea, respiratory distress, desaturation upon feeding, hypoglycemia, poor tone, and weak or absent cry for at least 48 h after birth[24,25] and that supportive care be appropriately administered.

Decisions regarding breastfeeding while taking an antidepressant should be discussed with the patient prior to delivery. Minimal concentrations of sertraline, paroxetine, and nortriptyline in breast milk make them the preferred antidepressants while breastfeeding.[26]

Treatment with antidepressant medication may be initiated and monitored by the obstetrician or the consulting psychiatrist (see Table 54.5). Treatment choices must balance the risks associated with untreated depression[27,28] against the potential risks from treatment with antidepressants. It is the healthcare provider's responsibility to provide accurate and up-to-date information on the reproductive safety of pharmacological treatment and to help the patient make an informed decision regarding treatment.[21] A resource list below gives registries which maintain up-to-date information on antidepressant use in pregnancy. If medication is initiated, depressive symptoms should be reassessed at each appointment and the dose adjusted accordingly (Table 54.4). Once the depression is in remission, treatment should be continued for a full 6–9 months.[29,30] After full treatment, the medication should be gradually tapered and discontinued over 2–4 weeks with careful observation for reemergence of symptoms. A patient who has experienced more than two major depressive episodes may require maintenance antidepressant treatment to remain depression free.[31,32]

Bipolar disorder is a serious, recurrent psychiatric illness with a lifetime prevalence of above 1% for women and men.[33] There have been no studies examining the specific prevalence of this disorder in pregnancy. The postpartum period presents the

Table 54.5 Antidepressant treatment tips.

Rule out bipolar disorder (e.g., episodes of high energy, little need for sleep, excessive spending); if present, refer to psychiatry for management
For *anxious* patients, begin with lowest possible dose and increase *very* slowly
Resume a medication that worked previously (*if safe in pregnancy*)
Use a *single* antidepressant medication[46]
Use the same medication in pregnancy and lactation[64]

Table 54.6 Pharmacological treatment considerations in bipolar disorder.

Medication	Organ dysgenesis	Clinical management	Breastfeeding[34]
Lithium: considered first-line treatment option in pregnancy[35,65]	Ebstein's anomaly occurs in 1 in 20000 of the general population, and 1 or 2 in 1000 offspring of lithium users, although the absolute risk remains small[66,67]	High-resolution ultrasound with fetal echocardiography at 16–18 weeks to aid in decision-making[68]	Expert opinion ranges from strong statements against breastfeeding while taking lithium to supporting a mother's informed choice[44]
		Increase dose in second trimester	Many have breast fed without complication with careful monitoring of infant's and mother's blood levels, complete blood count (CBC) and thyroid status, and a rapid reduction in dose exposure when infant has fever, dehydration, or diarrhea[69]
		Decrease dose in labor	
		Maintain adequate hydration	
		Observe the neonate for signs of toxicity,[68] and "floppy baby" syndrome, and manage supportively	
Valproate: avoid in pregnancy if possible	First-trimester exposure associated with neural tube defect (5–9%)	4mg of folic acid per day before and during pregnancy[40]	Usually compatible with breastfeeding[69,75]
	Effect occurs 17–30 days post conception	Measure B12 level before folate supplementation[35]	Infant serum levels range from undetectable to 40% of maternal serum levels
	Risk is dose related	Observe neonate for heart rate decelerations;[70] withdrawal symptoms of irritability, jitteriness, feeding difficulties, abnormal tone;[71] liver toxicity;[72] hypoglycemia,[73] and low fibrinogen levels[74]	Half-life in neonates is 47h; in infants from 10 days to 2 months, half-life is 9–22h[76]

(*Continued*)

Table 54.6 *Continued*

Medication	Organ dysgenesis	Clinical management	Breastfeeding[34]
Carbamazepine: avoid in pregnancy if possible	Neural tube defect (0.5–1%),[78,79] craniofacial defects (11%), fingernail hypoplasia (26%), and developmental delay (20%)[78] Risk worse when co-administered with valproate[79]	20 mg of oral vitamin K per day in the last month of pregnancy[79] Can cause fetal vitamin K deficiency; administer 1 mg i.m. of vitamin K to exposed neonates[35]	Usually compatible with breastfeeding[69,75] Infant serum levels range from 6% to 65% of maternal serum concentrations[34] Monitor for hepatic dysfunction[69,80,81]
Lamotrigine: approved as a maintenance therapy for bipolar disorder	Risk for major malformation appears to be similar to the general population rate (~2%)	Increase dose in second trimester Decrease dose in labor[82] Observe neonate for hepatotoxicity and skin rash	Infant serum levels range from 23% to 33% of maternal serum concentrations
Gabapentin	More research is needed before safety in pregnancy and breastfeeding can be clarified[83]		
Oxcarbazepine	More research is needed before safety in pregnancy and breastfeeding can be clarified[83]		

Table 54.7 Associated risks in bipolar disorder.[35]

Potential risks of pharmacotherapy in pregnancy
Neural tube defects (window of risk: 17–30 days after conception)
Heart defects (window of risk: 21–56 days after conception)
Lip/palate defects (window of risk: 8–11 weeks after conception)
Craniofacial defects (window of risk: 8–20 weeks after conception)
Neurobehavioral teratogenicity from exposure after the first trimester

Pregnancy and recurrence risks
Abrupt discontinuation of a mood stabilizer (1–14 days) led to a 100% relapse of illness
Slow taper over more than 2 weeks (15–30 days) led to a 62% risk for relapse

---

highest risk for symptom exacerbation, and 40% of women with bipolar disorder experience postpartum mania or depression.[34,35] A history of postpartum exacerbation increases the risk of postpartum episodes in subsequent pregnancies. Recent studies have shown that puerperal prophylaxis with a mood stabilizer reduces the rate of recurrence to 10%.[36–38] Given the risks associated with a postpartum bipolar episode for both the mother and newborn, the use of prophylactic mood stabilizers is advised.[34] Suicide is also a grave concern, with actual suicide carried out by 10–15% of individuals with the most severe form of bipolar disorder.[39] The management of bipolar disorder in pregnancy and postpartum is challenging and should be carried out by a psychiatrist with expertise in women's mental health in close collaboration with an obstetrician. Several of the medications routinely prescribed to manage bipolar disorder are neurotoxic[40,41] (Tables 54.6 and 54.7).

Psychiatric emergencies are most likely to occur in the first month postpartum,[42,43] but may arise at any point in the course of obstetric care. Four major conditions should be regarded as emergencies requiring immediate psychiatric consultation: psychosis, delirium, suicidal ideation, and homicidal ideation.

The following websites can be accessed to obtain further information:
1 AED (Antiepileptic Drug) Pregnancy Registry, Genetics & Teratology Unit.[34] Registry for pregnant women who are using antiepileptic drugs. World Wide Web URL: http://www.aedpregnancyregistry.org.
2 The Motherisk Program.[44,45] A counseling service for pregnant and lactating mothers on the safety and risk of drugs, chemicals, radiation, and infections to the fetus and neonate. World Wide Web URL: http://www.motherisk.org.
3 Emory Women's Program.[46] A website with links to many support groups, reproductive safety registries or other women's health websites. World Wide Web URL: http://www.emorywomensprogram.org.

References

1 Oates M. Perinatal psychiatric disorders: a leading cause of maternal morbidity and mortality. *Br Med Bull* 2003;67:219–229.

2 Holcomb WL, Jr, et al. Screening for depression in pregnancy: characteristics of the Beck Depression Inventory. *Obstet Gynecol* 1996;88:1021–1025.

3 Johanson R, et al. The North Staffordshire Maternity Hospital prospective study of pregnancy-associated depression. *J Psychosom Obstet Gynecol* 2000;21:93–97.

4 Spitzer RL, et al. Validity and utility of the PRIME-MD patient health questionnaire in assessment of 3000 obstetric–gynecologic patients: the PRIME-MD Patient Health Questionnaire Obstetrics–Gynecology Study. *Am J Obstet Gynecol* 2000;183:759–769.

5 Kelly R, et al. The detection and treatment of psychiatric disorders and substance use among pregnant women cared for in obstetrics. *Am J Psychiatry* 2001;158:213–219.

6 Smith M, et al. Screening for and detection of depression, panic disorder, and PTSD in public-sector obstetric clinics. *Psychiatr Serv* 2004;55:407–414.

7 Andersson L, et al. Neonatal outcome following maternal antenatal depression and anxiety: a population-based study. *Am J Epidemiol* 2004;159:872–881.

8 O'Hara MW, et al. Rates and risk of postpartum depression: a meta-analysis. *Int Rev Psychiatry* 1996;8:37–54.

9 Wisner KL, et al. Clinical practice. Postpartum depression (see Comment). *N Engl J Med* 2002;347:194–199.

10 Wadhwa PD, et al. Prenatal psychosocial factors and the neuroendocrine axis in human pregnancy. *Psychosom Med* 1996;58:432–446.

11 Hobel CJ, et al. Maternal plasma corticotropin-releasing hormone associated with stress at 20 weeks' gestation in pregnancies ending in preterm delivery. *Am J Obstet Gynecol* 1999;180:S257–S263.

12 Teixeira JM, et al. Association between maternal anxiety in pregnancy and increased uterine artery resistance index: cohort based study (see Comment). *Br Med J* 1999;318:153–157.

13 Martin JA, et al. Births: final data for 2002. *Natl Vital Stat Rep* 2003;52:1–113.

14 Newport DJ, et al. Maternal depression: a child's first adverse life event. *Semin Clin Neuropsychiatry* 2002;7:113–119.

15 Altschuler LL, et al. Treatment of depression in women: a summary of the expert consensus guidelines. *J Psychiatr Pract* 2001:185–208.

16 Stuart S, et al. The prevention and psychotherapeutic treatment of postpartum depression. *Arch Wom Ment Health* 2003;6(Suppl.2):57–69.

17 Spinelli MG. Interpersonal psychotherapy for depressed antepartum women: a pilot study. *Am J Psychiatry* 1997;154:1028–1030.

18 Oren DA, et al. An open trial of morning light therapy for treatment of antepartum depression. *Am J Psychiatry* 2002;159:666–669.

19 Epperson CN, et al. Randomized clinical trial of bright light therapy for antepartum depression: preliminary findings. *J Clin Psychiatry* 2004;65:421–425.

20 Freeman MP, et al. Selected integrative medicine treatments for depression: considerations for women. *J Am Med Wom Assoc* 2004;59:216–224.

21 Nonacs R, et al. Assessment and treatment of depression during pregnancy: an update. *Psychiatr Clin North Am* 2003;26:547–562.

22 Ferrill MJ, et al. ECT during pregnancy: physiologic and pharmacologic considerations. *Convulsive Ther* 1992;8:186–200.

23 Miller LJ. Use of electroconvulsive therapy during pregnancy. *Hosp Community Psychiatry* 1994;45:444–450.

24 Chambers D, et al. Birth outcomes in pregnant women taking fluoxetine. *N Engl J Med* 1996;335:1010–1015.

25 Koren G. Discontinuation syndrome following late pregnancy exposure to antidepressants. *Arch Pediatr Adolesc Med* 2004;158:307–308.

26 Weissman AM, et al. Pooled analysis of antidepressant levels in lactating mothers, breast milk, and nursing infants. *Am J Psychiatry* 2004;161:1066–1078.

27 Hay DF, et al. Intellectual problems shown by 11-year-old children whose mothers had postnatal depression. *J Child Psychol Psychiatry Allied Disciplines* 2001;42:871–889.

28 Halligan SL, et al. Exposure to postnatal depression predicts elevated cortisol in adolescent offspring. *Biol Psychiatry* 2004;55:376–381.

29 Schulberg HC, et al. Treating major depression in primary care practice. Eight-month clinical outcomes. *Arch Gen Psychiatry* 1996;53:913–919.

30 Kocsis JH, et al. Stability of remission during tricyclic antidepressant continuation therapy for dysthymia. *Psychopharmacol Bull* 1995;31:213–216.

31 Keller MB, et al. Maintenance phase efficacy of sertraline for chronic depression: a randomized controlled trial (see Comment). *JAMA* 1998;280:1665–1672.

32 Kocsis JH, et al. Maintenance therapy for chronic depression: a controlled clinical trial of desipramine. *Arch Gen Psychiatry* 1996;53:769–774.

33 Kessler RC, et al. Lifetime and 12-month prevalence of DSM-III-R psychiatric disorders in the United States. Results from the National Comorbidity Survey. *Arch Gen Psychiatry* 1994;51:8–19.

34 Chaudron LH, et al. Mood stabilizers during breastfeeding: a review. *J Clin Psychiatry* 2000;61:79–90.

35 Yonkers KA, et al. Management of bipolar disorder during pregnancy and the postpartum period. *Am J Psychiatry* 2004;161:608–620.

36 Cohen LS, et al. Postpartum prophylaxis for women with bipolar disorder (see Comment). *Am J Psychiatry* 1995;152:1641–1645.

37 Stewart DE, et al. Prophylactic lithium in puerperal psychosis. The experience of three centres. *Br J Psychiatry* 1991;158:393–397.

38 Austin MP. Puerperal affective psychosis: is there a case for lithium prophylaxis? (see Comment). *Br J Psychiatry* 1992;161:692–694.

39 Dell DL, et al. Suicide in pregnancy. *Obstet Gynecol* 2003;102:1306–1309.

40 Crawford P, et al. Best practice guidelines for the managment of women with epilepsy. *Seizure* 1999;8:201–217.

41 Baldessarini RJ, et al. Is lithium still worth using? An update of selected recent research. *Harvard Rev Psychiatry* 2002;10:59–75.

42 Paffenbarger RS. Epidemiological aspects of mental illness associated with childbearing. In: Brockington IF, Kumar R, eds. *Motherhood and Mental Illness*. London, UK: Academic Press; 1982:21–36.

43 Kendell RE, et al. Epidemiology of puerperal psychoses [erratum appears in *Br J Psychiatry* 1987;151:135]. *Br J Psychiatry* 1987;150:662–673.

44 Moretti ME, et al. Monitoring lithium in breast milk: an individualized approach for breast-feeding mothers. *Ther Drug Monitoring* 2003;25:364–366.

45 Einarson A, et al. How physicians perceive and utilize information from a teratogen information service: the Motherisk Program. *BMC Med Educ* 2004;4:5.

46 Levey L, et al. Psychiatric disorders in pregnancy. *Neurol Clin* 2004;22:863–893.

47 O'Hara MW, et al. Prospective study of postpartum blues. Biologic and psychosocial factors. *Arch Gen Psychiatry* 1991;48:801–806.

48 Kelly RH, et al. Somatic complaints among pregnant women cared for in obstetrics: normal pregnancy or depressive and anxiety symptom amplification revisited? *Gen Hosp Psychiatry* 2001;23:107–113.

49 Zuckerman B, et al. Depressive symptoms during pregnancy: relationship to poor health behaviors. *Am J Obstet Gynecol* 1989;160:1107–1111.

50 Ludman EJ, et al. Stress, depressive symptoms, and smoking cessation among pregnant women. *Health Psychol* 2000;19:21–27.
51 Paarlberg KM, et al. Psychosocial predictors of low birthweight: a prospective study. *Br J Obstet Gynaecol* 1999;106:834–841.
52 Steer RA, et al. Self-reported depression and negative pregnancy outcomes. *J Clin Epidemiol* 1992;45:1093–1099.
53 Kurki T, et al. Depression and anxiety in early pregnancy and risk for preeclampsia. *Obstet Gynecol* 2000;95:487–490.
54 Chung TK, et al. Antepartum depressive symptomatology is associated with adverse obstetric and neonatal outcomes. *Psychosom Med* 2001;63:830–834.
55 Henderson JJ, et al. Impact of postnatal depression on breastfeeding duration [erratum appears in *Birth* 2004;31:76]. *Birth* 2003;30:175–180.
56 Rahman A, et al. Impact of maternal depression on infant nutritional status and illness: a cohort study. *Arch Gen Psychiatry* 2004;61:946–952.
57 O'Brien LM, et al. Postnatal depression and faltering growth: a community study. *Pediatrics* 2004;113:1242–1247.
58 Flynn HA, et al. Rates of maternal depression in pediatric emergency department and relationship to child service utilization. *Gen Hosp Psychiatry* 2004;26:316–322.
59 Burke L. The impact of maternal depression on familial relationships. *Int Rev Psychiatry* 2003;15:243–255.
60 Stowe ZN, et al. The pharmacokinetics of sertraline excretion into human breast milk: determinants of infant serum concentrations. *J Clin Psychiatry* 2003;64:73–80.
61 Nordeng H, et al. Neonatal withdrawal syndrome after in utero exposure to selective serotonin reuptake inhibitors. *Acta Paediatr* 2001;90:288–291.
62 Dahl ML, et al. Paroxetine withdrawal syndrome in a neonate. *Br J Psychiatry* 1997;171:391–392.
63 Stowe ZN, et al. Paroxetine in human breast milk and nursing infants (see Comment). *Am J Psychiatry* 2000;157:185–189.
64 Stowe Z. *Ob/gyn grand rounds: depression and anxiety disorders in women across the reproductive life: identification and treatment.* Little Rock, AR:2004.
65 Cohen L. Bipolar disorder in pregnancy. *Clin Psychiatry News* 2002;30:20.
66 Jacobson SJ, et al. Prospective multicentre study of pregnancy outcome after lithium exposure during first trimester (see Comment). *Lancet* 1992;339:530–533.
67 Cohen LS, et al. A reevaluation of risk of in utero exposure to lithium (see Comment) [erratum appears in *JAMA* 1994;271:1485]. *JAMA* 1994;271:146–150.
68 Pinelli JM, et al. Case report and review of the perinatal implications of maternal lithium use. *Am J Obstet Gynecol* 2002;187:245–249.
69 AAP, American Academy of Pediatrics Committee on Drugs. Transfer of drugs and other chemicals into human milk (see Comment). *Pediatrics* 2001;108:776–789.
70 Jager-Roman E. Fetal growth, major malformations and minor anomalies in infants born to women receiving valproic acid. *J Pediatr* 1986;108:997–1004.
71 Kennedy D, et al. Valproic acid use in psychiatry: issues in treating women of reproductive age. *J Psychiatry Neurosci* 1998;23:223–228.
72 Felding I, et al. Congenital liver damage after treatment of mother with valproic acid and phenytoin. *Acta Paediatr Scand* 1984;73:565–568.
73 Thisted E, et al. Malformations, withdrawal manifestations, and hypoglycaemia after exposure to valproate in utero. *Arch Dis Child* 1993;69:288–291.
74 Majer R, et al. Neonatal afibrinogenaemia due to sodium valproate. *Lancet* 1987;2:740–741.

75 AAP, American Academy of Pediatrics Committee on Drugs. The transfer of drugs and other chemical into human milk. *Pediatrics* 1994;93:137–150.

76 Nau H, et al. Anticonvulsants during pregnancy and lactation. Transplacental, maternal and neonatal pharmacokinetics. *Clin Pharmacokinetics* 1982;7:508–543.

77 Jones K, et al. Pattern of malformations in the children of women treated with carbamazepine during pregnancy. *N Engl J Med* 1989;320:1661–1666.

78 Rosa F. Spina bifida in infants of women treated with carbamazepine during pregnancy. *N Engl J Med* 1991;324:674–677.

79 Karceski S, et al. The expert consensus guideline series: treatment of epilepsy. *Epilepsy Behav* 2001;2:A1–A50.

80 Merlob P, et al. Transient hepatic dysfunction in an infant of an epileptic mother treated with carbamazepine during pregnancy and breastfeeding. *Ann Pharmacother* 1563;26: 1563–1565.

81 Frey B, et al. Transient cholestatic hepatitis in a neonate associated with carbamazepine exposure during pregnancy and breast-feeding. *Eur J Pediatr* 1990;150:136–138.

82 Tran T, et al. Lamotrigine clearance during pregnancy. *Neurology* 2002;59:251–255.

83 Dodd S, et al. The pharmacology of bipolar disorder during pregnancy and breastfeeding. *Expert Opinion Drug Safety* 2004;3:221–229.

Further reading

Andersson, L, et al. Point prevalence of psychiatric disorders during the second trimester of pregnancy: a population-based study. *Am J Obstet Gynecol* 2003;189:148–154.

Baldessarini RJ, et al. Is lithium still worth using? An update of selected recent research. *Harvard Rev Psychiatry* 2002;10:59–75.

Chaudron LH, et al. Mood stabilizers during breastfeeding: a review. *J Clin Psychiatry* 2000;61:79–90.

Dodd S, et al. The pharmacology of bipolar disorder during pregnancy and breastfeeding. *Expert Opinion Drug Safety* 2004;3:221–229.

Hay DF, et al. Intellectual problems shown by 11-year-old children whose mothers had postnatal depression. *J Child Psychol Psychiatry Allied Disciplines* 2001;42:871–889.

Kelly RH, et al. Somatic complaints among pregnant women cared for in obstetrics: normal pregnancy or depressive and anxiety symptom amplification revisited? *Gen Hosp Psychiatry* 2001;23:107–113.

Levey L, et al. Psychiatric disorders in pregnancy. *Neurol Clin* 2004;22:863–893.

Levine RE, et al. Anxiety disorders during pregnancy and postpartum. *Am J Perinatol* 2003;20:239–248.

Nair S, et al. The evaluation of maternal competency. *Psychosomatics* 2000;41:523–530.

Nonacs R, et al. Assessment and treatment of depression during pregnancy: an update. *Psychiatr Clin North Am* 2003;26:547–562.

Pinelli JM, et al. Case report and review of the perinatal implications of maternal lithium use. *Am J Obstet Gynecol* 2002;187:245–249.

Weissman AM, et al. Pooled analysis of antidepressant levels in lactating mothers, breast milk, and nursing infants. *Am J Psychiatry* 2004;161:1066–1078.

Yonkers KA, et al. Management of bipolar disorder during pregnancy and the postpartum period. *Am J Psychiatry* 2004;161:608–620.

55 Ethical and legal dimensions of medicine of the pregnant woman and fetus

Judith L. Chervenak, Frank A. Chervenak, and Laurence B. McCullough

Medical ethics

Ethics is the disciplined study of morality. Medical ethics is the disciplined study of morality in medicine and concerns the ethical obligations of physicians and health-care organizations to patients as well as the obligations of patients themselves. The approach to medical ethics has been secular since the eighteenth-century European and American Enlightenments; it makes no reference to God or revealed tradition but focuses on what rational discourse requires and produces. Therefore, medical ethics apply to all physicians, regardless of their personal religious and spiritual beliefs.

Informed consent

The process of informed consent involves three sequential autonomy-based behaviors on the part of the patient: (1) absorbing and retaining information about her condition, and the alternative diagnostic and therapeutic responses to it; (2) understanding the information (i.e., evaluating and rank-ordering those responses, and appreciating that there may be benefits and risks of treatment); and (3) expressing a value-based preference.

The legal obligations of the physician regarding informed consent include disclosure of information sufficient to enable patients to make informed decisions about whether to say "yes" or "no" to medical intervention. There are two legal standards for such disclosure. The professional community standard defines adequate disclosure in the context of what the relevantly trained and experienced physician tells patients. The reasonable person standard, which has been adopted by most states, goes further and requires the physician to disclose "material" information, i.e., what any patient in that particular condition needs to know and what the lay person of average sophistication should not be expected to know. This reasonable person standard has emerged as the ethical standard.

Malpractice law

Black's Law Dictionary defines malpractice as "an instance of negligence on the part of a professional." Negligence is a tort or civil wrong whose elements are

(1) a duty recognized by the law; (2) a failure on the part of the person to conform to the standard required; (3) a reasonably close connection between the conduct and the resulting injury, known as the "proximate or legal cause;" and (4) actual loss or damage to the interests of another. The court provides a remedy for this civil wrong in the form of equity or monetary damages.

The duty to the patient arises from the physician–patient relationship and is generally considered to be a contractual duty implied from the actions of the parties rather than one expressed in written form. This relationship ends with the consent of both parties, dismissal of the physician, or when the services of the physician are no longer required.

In a medical malpractice action, the standard of conduct for the physician is usually expressed as "the minimum knowledge, skill and care ordinarily possessed and employed by members of the profession in good standing." For those who hold themselves out to be specialists, the standard is modified accordingly. Therefore, a physician who has met the applicable legal standard will not be liable for an honest mistake in judgment even if the clinical outcome is poor.

Further reading

1 American College of Obstetricians and Gynecologists. *Ethics in obstetrics and gynecology.* Washington, DC: American College of Obstetricians and Gynecologists, 2002

2 Association of Professors of Gynecology and Obstetrics. *Exploring medical–legal issues in obstetrics and gynecology.* Washington, DC: APGO Medical Education Foundation, 1994.

3 FIGO Committee for the Study of Ethical Aspects of Human Reproduction. *Recommendations of ethical Issues in obstetrics and gynecology.* London: International Federation of Gynecology and Obstetrics, 1997.

4 McCullough LB, Chervenak FA. *Ethics in obstetrics and gynecology.* New York: Oxford University Press, 1994.

5 Engelhardt HT Jr. *The foundations of bioethics,* 2nd edn. New York: Oxford University Press, 1995.

6 Beauchamp TL, Childress JF. *Principles of biomedical ethics,* 5th edn. New York: Oxford University Press, 2001.

7 Faden RR, Beauchamp TL. *A history and theory of informed consent.* New York: Oxford University Press, 1986.

8 American College of Obstetricians and Gynecologists. 2005 Legislative Program: District II website. info@nyacog.org.

9 Abrams, FR, Barclay, ML, Cain, JM et al (eds). *APGO Task Force on Medical Ethics, Exploring medical–legal issues in obstetrics and gynecology.* Washington, DC: Association of Professors of Gynecology and Obstetrics, 1994.

10 Strunk AL, Esser L. (Editorial) Overview of the 2003 ACOG Professional Liability Survey *ACOG Clin Rev* 2004;9:1–13.

56 Bleeding in the third trimester

Lawrence W. Oppenheimer and the late Carl A. Nimrod

Bleeding in the third trimester is common. The most important cause is placental abruption (also called *abruptio placentae*), which has an incidence of approximately 0.6% in the USA and an associated risk of stillbirth of 12%. Placenta previa, which can also cause third-trimester bleeding, occurs with a frequency of 0.3%. Cesarean section is significantly associated with placenta previa and placenta accreta: the risk is 25% for one previous Cesarean section and 40% for two. Vasa previa, which occurs in 1 in 3000 to 5000 pregnancies, is a rare but important cause of vaginal bleeding. However, in approximately 50% of cases of vaginal bleeding, the etiology is either unexplained or assumed to occur from local lesions. Notable points concerning placenta previa, placenta previa/accreta, vasa previa, and placental abruption are given below:

Placenta previa

• Placenta previa is defined as a placenta implanted in the lower segment of the uterus presenting ahead of the leading pole of the fetus.
• The "gold standard" for diagnosis is transvaginal sonography (TVS; see Figs 56.1 and 56.2). The data suggest that a placental edge that overlaps the internal os by less than 10 mm at any time before 24 weeks on TVS is highly unlikely to be associated with a placenta previa at term.
• Vaginal delivery is possible when the distance from the placental edge to internal os is greater than 20 mm on TVS at any gestational age.
• A placenta overlapping the internal os by any amount after approximately 35 weeks' gestation requires delivery by Cesarean section.
• A placental edge lying within 20 mm of the os but not overlapping requires individualized management, but vaginal delivery is possible (Table 56.1).
• The clinical outcomes of placenta previa are highly variable and cannot be predicted confidently from antenatal events.
• For selected patients, outpatient management appears to be an acceptable alternative.

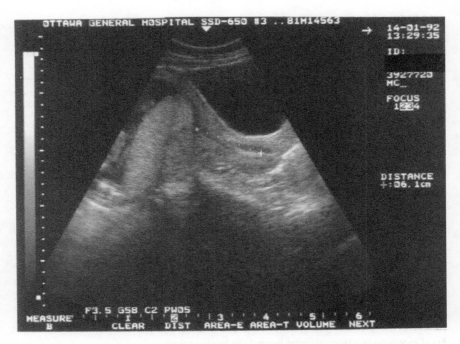

Figure 56.1 Transabdominal scan of placenta covering cervical os at 28 weeks' gestation. Note full bladder at top right.

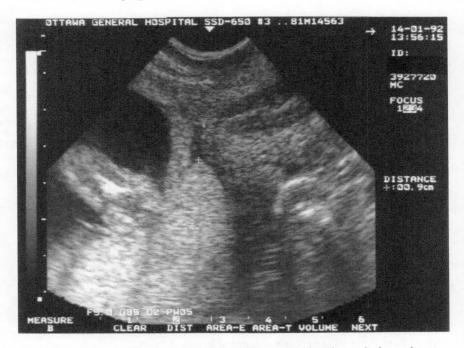

Figure 56.2 Transvaginal scan of above case with empty bladder. Placental edge no longer covers os. At follow-up, the placental edge moved further away and resulted in vaginal delivery.

Table 56.1 Likelihood of Cesarean section based on placental-edge to internal-os distance on last scan prior to delivery performed at an average of 35 weeks' gestation.

Distance	Cesarean section
Overlapping	100%
< 10 mm	84%
> 10 mm and < 20 mm	40%
> 20 mm	16%

Table 56.2 Ultrasound features of placenta accreta.

Hypoechoic zone between myometrium and placenta less than 2 mm
Disruption of the hyperechoic uterine serosa–bladder interface
Lacunar spaces (Swiss cheese) in placental parenchyma
Prominent vessels extending from placental base to uterine wall
Dilated blood vessels and turbulent blood flow in lacunae
Abnormal blood vessels linking the placenta and bladder with diastolic flow
Focal extension of placental tissue beyond the uterine serosa

Placenta previa/accreta

• The relative risk of placenta accreta in the presence of placenta previa is 2065-fold higher than in women who have a normally situated placenta. In any pregnancy, the risk of placenta accreta in the presence of placenta previa increases dramatically with the number of previous deliveries by Cesarean section, with a 25% risk for one previous Cesarean section, and more than a 40% risk for two.
• In suspected cases, prenatal diagnosis of placenta accreta by ultrasound (Table 56.2; Fig. 56.3) or magnetic resonance imaging (MRI; Fig. 56.4) may be beneficial in preparing for delivery (Table 56.3).

Vasa previa

• Vasa previa occurs when the fetal vessels cross within the membranes between the internal os and the presenting part. It is strongly associated with a low-lying placenta and color Doppler with TVS now offers the possibility of prediction of vasa previa well before the onset of delivery (Table 56.4).
• In two large case series, the specificity and sensitivity of a prenatal diagnosis was excellent. The survival rates of infants with a prenatal diagnosis was 97% compared with 44% in those who were not diagnosed before delivery.

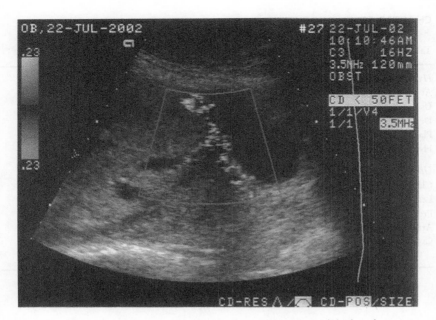

Figure 56.3 Transabdominal scan of placenta accreta. There is loss of the hypolucent zone between placenta and myometrium, multiple lacunae (Swiss cheese appearance), and abnormal vasculature extending into the bladder wall. The case was managed by classical Cesarean section, the placenta was left *in situ* and resorbed spontaneously.

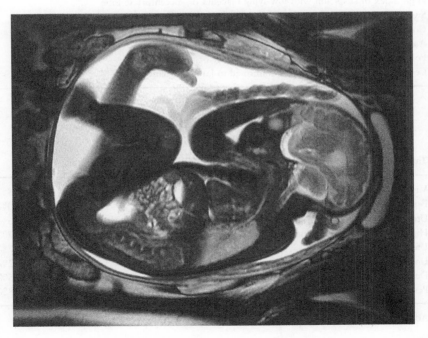

Figure 56.4 MRI of anterior placenta with loss of the retroplacental space and invasion of the placenta into the myometrium superior to the bladder.

Table 56.3 Management options in placenta accreta/percreta.

Hysterectomy
Avoid incision of placenta or attempted removal
Use of cell saver
Deliberate cystotomy to assist bladder mobilization
Placement of ureteral stents
Hypogastric artery ligation or embolization/balloon occlusion

Uterine conservation
Classical Cesarean section avoiding placenta
Leave placenta *in situ* if no hemorrhage
Prophylactic radiological hypogastric artery embolization/balloon occlusion
Attempt placental removal if bleeding occurs
Control bleeding by: circumferential sutures over placental site; prostaglandin F2-alpha
    myometrial injection; ligating uterine pedicles and/or ovarian vessels; uterine packing

---

Table 56.4 Protocol for diagnosis of vasa previa.

Attempt to visualize cord insertion in all cases
High index of suspicion with low-lying placenta or succenturiate lobe
Sweep across the lower uterine segment to look for velamentous vessels
Color or power Doppler with TVS to further investigate suspicious cases
Ascertain whether pulse rate maternal or fetal on Doppler
Follow-up sonograms if vessels identified over or near the cervix
Cesarean delivery if vasa previa confirmed in later pregnancy

---

Table 56.5 Clinical presentation in 59 cases of moderate to severe abruption.

Vaginal bleeding	78%
Fetal distress	50%
Uterine tenderness/back pain	66%
High-frequency contractions	17%
Uterine hypertonus	17%
Unexplained preterm labor	22%
Dead fetus at admission	15%
Perinatal death of fetus alive at admission	18%

Adapted from ref. 108.

Table 56.6 Management principles for severe abruption.

Fetal assessment for viability, welfare, and size (growth restriction is common)

Estimate severity of abruption (uterine tone, hardness, pain, amount of vaginal bleeding)

Maternal assessment for hypovolemia and coagulation status

Early aggressive treatment of suspected disseminated intravascular coagulation

Kleihauer–Betke test and Rhesus status should be checked as fetal–maternal hemorrhage is present in up to 30% of cases, particularly in traumatic abruption

Expedite delivery of a live fetus with a low threshold for Cesarean section

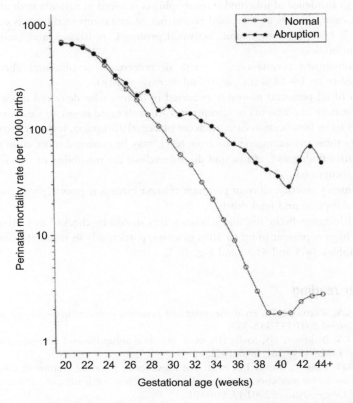

Figure 56.5 Gestational age-specific perinatal mortality rate (plotted on a logarithmic scale) in pregnancies with and without abruption, USA, 1995 and 1996 (reproduced from Ananth and Wilcox (2001), with permission).

Placental abruption

- Placental abruption is defined as complete or partial separation of the placenta prior to delivery and is accompanied by hemorrhage into the decidua basalis.
- Abruption is associated with a nearly ninefold increase in the risk of stillbirth compared with pregnancies without abruption. The case fatality rate, expressed as the number of abruptio-stillbirth cases per 100 total placental abruption cases, is reported to be 5.3–7%. Abruption accounts for more than 8% of all cases of perinatal mortality.
- Major risk factors for placental abruption include: cocaine use (OR 3.9), chorioamnionitis (2.6), chronic hypertension (OR 2.8), severe preeclampsia (OR 4.1), twins (OR 2.1), and smoking (OR 2). In total, 15–25% of placental abruption episodes could be prevented if women stopped smoking cigarettes during their pregnancies.
- A high incidence of inherited thrombophilias is noted in patients with abruption. In particular, there is an increased prevalence of mutations in the genes coding for Factor V Leiden, homocysteine, activated protein C resistance, and antiphospholipid antibodies.
- In subsequent pregnancies, the risk of recurrence of placental abruption is observed to be 10–15% (i.e., a 30-fold increase in risk).
- 70% of all perinatal mortality occurred in infants who delivered more than 2 h from the time of diagnosis of abruption. Although rapid resort to Cesarean section appears to be beneficial in cases of acute placental abruption, less severe cases, particularly those presenting remote from term, may be managed more conservatively.
- Negative findings on ultrasound do not exclude the possibility of significant placental abruption.
- The injury severity score in pregnant trauma victims is poorly predictive of placental abruption and fetal death.
- The Kleihauer–Betke test and Rhesus status should be checked as fetal–maternal hemorrhage is present in up to 30% of cases, particularly in traumatic abruption.
- See Tables 56.5 and 56.6, and Fig. 56.5.

Further reading

Ananth CV, Wilcox AJ. Placental abruption and perinatal mortality in the United States. *Am J Epidemiol* 2001;153:332–337.

Ananth CV, Berkowitz GS, Savitz DA, et al. Placental abruption and adverse perinatal outcomes. *JAMA* 1999;282:1646–1651.

Becker RH, Vonk R, Mende BC, et al. The relevance of placental location at 20–23 gestational weeks for prediction of placenta previa at delivery: evaluation of 8650 cases. *Ultrasound Obstet Gynecol* 2001;17:496–501.

Bhide A, Prefumo F, Moore J, et al. Placental edge to internal os distance in the late third trimester and mode of delivery in placenta previa. *Br J Obstet Gynaecol* 2003;110:860–864.

Faiz AS, Ananth CV. Etiology and risk factors for placenta previa: an overview and meta-analysis of observational studies. *J Maternal–Fetal Neo Med* 2003;13:175–190.

Glantz C, Purnell L. Clinical utility of sonography in the diagnosis and treatment of placental abruption. *J Ultrasound Med* 2002;21:837–840.

Hurd WW, Miodovnik M, Hertzberg V, et al. Selective management of abruptio placentae: a prospective study. *Obstet Gynecol* 1983;61:467–473.

Miller DA, Chollet JA, Goodwin TM. Clinical risk factors for placenta praevia/placenta accreta. *Am J Obstet Gynecol* 1997;177:210–214.

Nelson JP. Interventions for suspected placenta praevia. *Cochrane Database Syst Rev* 2003:2. Oxford: Update Software.

Oppenheimer L, Farine D, Ritchie K, et al. What is a low-lying placenta? *Am J Obstet Gynecol* 1991;165:1036–1038.

Oyelese Y, Catanzarite V, Prefumo F, et al. Vasa previa: the impact of prenatal diagnosis on outcomes. *Obstet Gynecol* 2004;103:937–942.

Normal and abnormal labor

Wayne R. Cohen

An assessment of labor requires a graphic analysis of the relationships among cervical dilation, fetal descent, and elapsed hours in labor. This approach, in conjunction with information about pelvic architecture, uterine contractility, fetal position and attitude, and the state of fetal oxygenation is the basis for clinical decision-making in labor.

Normal cervical dilation

The relationship between cervical dilation and elapsed time in labor is described by a sigmoid curve (Fig. 57.1). The *latent phase* extends from labor onset to the upward inflection in the curve. Enhanced dilation occurs in the *active phase*. The short acceleration phase initiates the active phase and leads to rapid linear dilation. During the terminal portion of the active phase, the deceleration phase, dilation appears to slow. Labor patterns differ in nulliparas and multiparas (Table 57.1). The labors of multiparas who have had all previous babies by Cesarean section are judged by nulliparous criteria.

Latent phase
The latent phase is shorter in multiparas than in nulliparas, a consequence in part of the fact that multiparas tend to begin labor with more cervical dilation. The cervix dilates at a maximal rate of 0.5 cm/h during the latent phase.

Active phase
The rate at which the cervix dilates during the active phase is used to assess normality. When two observations of dilation have been plotted on a graph, the slope of the dilation line can be calculated. If the labor is normal, dilation continues at the same rate until the deceleration phase. Abnormalities of active phase are defined

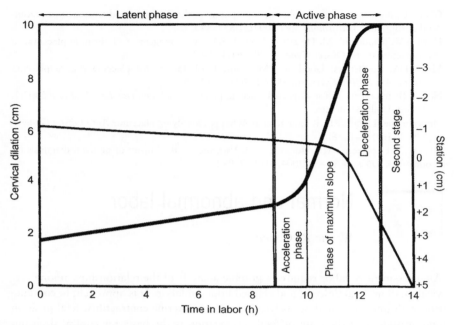

Figure 57.1 Composite of normal cervical dilation and fetal descent curves showing their interrelations and components. From Cohen WR, Friedman EA, eds. *Management of labor.* Rockville, MD: Aspen Publishers, 1983.

Table 57.1 Dysfunctional labor patterns.

Dysfunction	Nulliparas	Multiparas
Disorders of dilation		
Prolonged latent phase	> 20 h duration	> 14 h duration
Protracted active phase	Dilation at < 1.2 cm/h	Dilation at < 1.5 cm/h
Arrest of dilation	2 h without progress in active phase	2 h without progress in active phase
Prolonged deceleration phase	> 3 h duration	> 1 h duration
Disorders of descent		
Protracted descent	Descent at < 1 cm/h	Descent at < 2 cm/h
Arrest of descent	1 h without progress after active descent has begun	1 h without progress after active descent has begun
Failure of descent	No descent by deceleration phase or second stage onset	No descent by deceleration phase or second stage onset

by deviations from this projected rate of dilation. Cervical retraction to the widest diameter of the presenting part defines full cervical dilation and is the end of the active phase.

Normal fetal descent

Descent usually becomes linear by the time of complete cervical dilation and, during the second stage, normally proceeds in this manner until the presenting part encounters the pelvic floor. The rate of descent is used to judge its normality (Fig. 57.1).

Uterine activity in labor

Contractions often begin as mild and irregular and become progressively more intense, frequent, and regular in the latent phase. During the active phase, contractions are generally more frequent and of greater amplitude and duration than in the latent phase. However, a large spectrum of contractile patterns exists during normal labor and there is no reliable means of identifying abnormal dilation or descent by observing uterine activity.

Abnormal labor

Latent phase dysfunction

Prolonged latent phase (Figs 57.2 and 57.3; Table 57.1) is diagnosed when the latent phase exceeds 20 h in nulliparas or 14 h in multiparas. It is most likely to occur when labor begins with the cervix minimally effaced and dilated. The latent phase is susceptible to prolongation by narcotics and anesthetics. Prolonged latent phase is not a predictor of active phase disorders, nor does it have a strong association with cephalopelvic disproportion. Treatment consists of maternal sedation or stimulating uterine contractility (Fig. 57.3). When a fetal or maternal condition exists

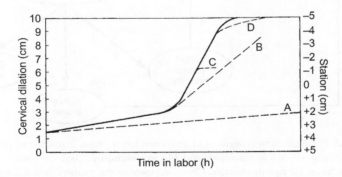

Figure 57.2 Schematic showing various disorders of dilation (broken lines) compared to a normal pattern of dilation (solid line). (A) prolonged latent phase; (B) protracted active phase; (C) arrest of dilation; (D) prolonged deceleration phase.

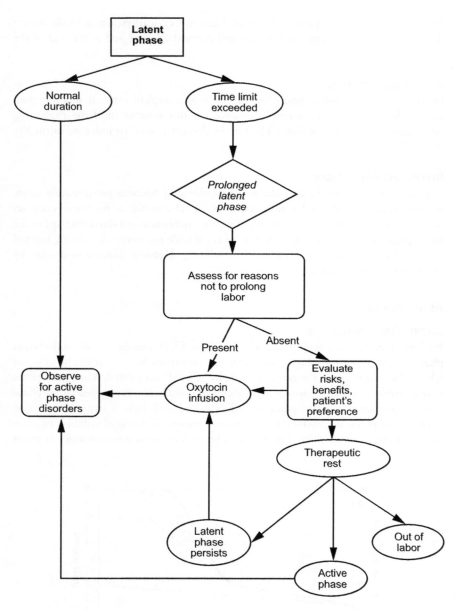

Figure 57.3 Paradigm for management of prolonged latent phase, diagnosed when the latent phase exceeds 20 h in a nullipara and 14 h in a multipara. Oxytocin stimulation and narcotic sedation are equally effective. Choice depends on the patient's preference and the presence of risks that would accrue if the labor were prolonged.

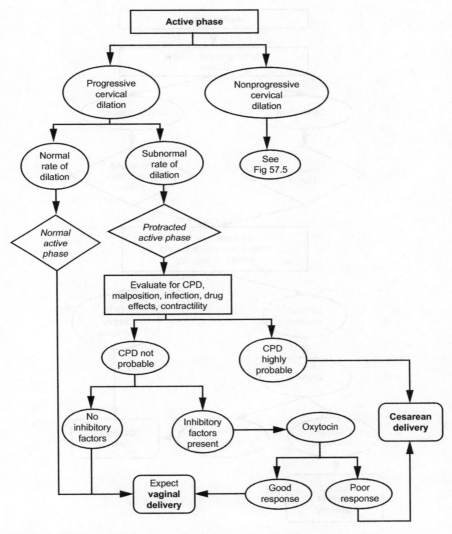

Figure 57.4 Paradigm for management of protracted active phase, diagnosed when advancement in dilation is progressive but < 1.2 cm/h in nulliparas and < 1.5 cm/h in multiparas. A good response to oxytocin is defined as one in which dilation is maintained at the same or an improved rate. Oxytocin is useful in this disorder when the slow progress is related to the presence of factors that may inhibit contractility (e.g., infection, drug effects). CPD, cephalopelvic disproportion.

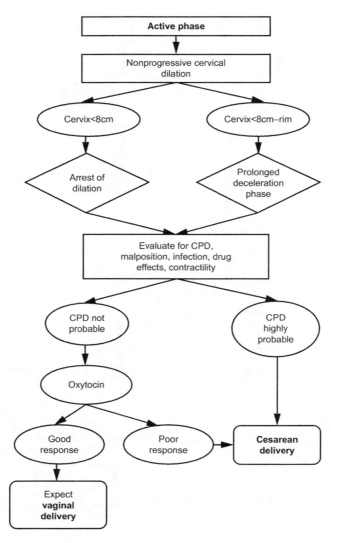

Figure 57.5 Paradigm for management of arrest of dilation, defined as an absence of progress in dilation for 2 h once the active phase has begun. When progress is abnormally slow at the end of the active phase, prolonged deceleration phase is diagnosed (> 3 h in nulliparas; > 1 h in multiparas). There is a strong association with cephalopelvic disproportion (CPD). A good response to oxytocin is defined as a postarrest slope that is equal to or greater than the prearrest slope. A poor response usually requires Cesarean delivery.

that could be jeopardized by prolonging the labor (e.g., prolonged rupture of membranes, preeclampsia, early intrauterine infection, or certain acute maternal illnesses), active intervention should generally be used. The mother's wishes are important; some women prefer oxytocin stimulation, whereas others prefer the interposition of some rest into the arduous experience of childbirth.

Active phase dysfunction

Three abnormalities of the active phase can occur (Figs 57.2, 57.4, and 57.5; Table 57.1). In a *protracted active phase*, cervical dilation progresses linearly after commencement of the active phase but at a rate below the limits of normal. *Arrest of dilation* occurs when dilation ceases for 2 h during the active phase. The term *prolonged deceleration phase* describes protracted or arrested labor during the terminal period of cervical dilation. The time limits for the duration of the deceleration phase are 3 h in nulliparas and 1 h in multiparas. The obstetric conditions associated with protraction and arrest disorders are similar (Table 57.2), but therapeutic approaches differ. All active phase disorders commonly occur in association with cephalopelvic disproportion, malpositions (persistent occiput posterior or transverse), excessive sedation or anesthesia, chorioamnionitis, or deciduitis. Myometrial dysfunction, which may be primary or a consequence of these other factors, also contributes.

In the evaluation of active phase dysfunction, it is necessary to carry out a thorough examination of the patient to identify any predisposing conditions. Clinical cephalopelvimetry is useful in ascertaining the likelihood of disproportion. If disproportion seems unlikely and fetal head position is normal, it is necessary to assess uterine contractility and search for infection and possible pharmacological inhibition of labor.

Table 57.2 Conditions associated with protraction and arrest disorders.

Cephalopelvic disproportion
Intrauterine infection
Malpositions
Excess anesthesia or analgesia
Insufficient uterine contractility

When protraction disorders arise *de novo*, they are not amenable to correction by stimulating uterine contractions. If a protraction disorder has resulted from an inhibitory influence (e.g., conduction anesthesia), oxytocin may restore normal dilation. Protraction disorders are sensitive to many inhibitory factors and may be exacerbated or even converted to arrest disorders under some circumstances. Deliberate rupture of the fetal membranes has not been proved beneficial as a treatment for protraction disorders.

Arrest of dilation may evolve during a protracted or previously normal active phase. This dysfunction requires a similar evaluation as for protraction disorders and is associated with cephalopelvic disproportion in about 40% of cases. Arrest disorders may respond to oxytocin augmentation of uterine activity. If there is considerable evidence for fetopelvic disproportion in the presence of an arrest, especially if uterine activity is normal, it may be appropriate to deliver by Cesarean section. It is reasonable to consider stimulation of uterine activity if the pelvis is deemed probably adequate.

About 85% of the patients who respond to oxytocin do so within about 3 h. The likelihood of vaginal delivery is high if cervical dilation is at least as rapid as before the arrest. If dilation resumes at a rate slower than before the arrest (or does not resume), it is likely that disproportion or an insurmountable problem with uterine contractility is present.

The second stage of labor

The first stage of labor (from onset to full cervical dilation) serves to ready the parturient for expulsion of the fetus from the uterus. The second stage, from full dilation to delivery, encompasses that expulsive process. The rate at which active fetal descent occurs is influenced by several factors (Table 57.3).

Three descent disorders have been identified: protracted descent, arrest of descent, and failure of descent (Figs 57.6 and 57.7; Table 57.1). All are associated with

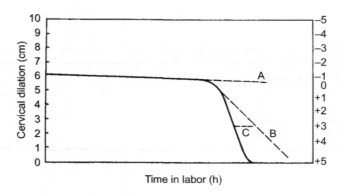

Figure 57.6 Schematic showing possible disorders of descent. (A) failure of descent; (B) protracted descent; (C) arrest of descent.

Table 57.3 Factors that influence the rate of fetal descent.

Uterine contractile force	Deformability of the fetal head
Voluntary maternal expulsive efforts	Pelvic architecture
Fetal size, position, and attitude	Characteristics of the pelvic floor

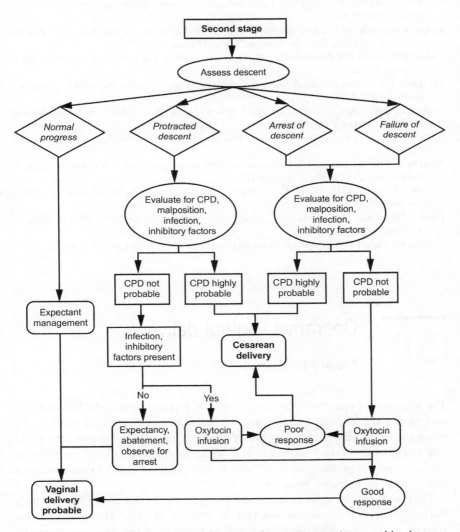

Figure 57.7 Paradigm for management of the second stage. Progress is assessed by the rate of descent rather than elapsed time. Fetal position, station, attitude, and molding should be assessed at each examination. A good response to oxytocin given for arrest of descent is defined as a postarrest slope equal to or greater than the prearrest slope.

similar obstetric conditions and are analogous to the protraction and arrest disorders of dilation. To determine the significance of descent abnormalities it is necessary to carry out a serial assessment of the factors listed in Table 57.3.

Further reading

Chazotte C, Madden R, Cohen WR. Labor patterns in women with previous cesareans. *Obstet Gynecol* 1990;75:350.

Cohen WR, Friedman EA. The assessment of labor. In: Kurjak A, Chervenak F, eds. *Textbook of perinatal medicine*, 2nd edn. London: Taylor & Francis, 2005.

Cohen WR, Acker DB, Friedman EA. *Management of labor*, 2nd edn. Rockville, MD: Aspen Publishers, 1989.

Friedman EA. *Labor: clinical evaluation and management*, 2nd edn. New York: Appleton-Century-Crofts, 1978.

Garrett K, Butler A, Cohen WR. Cesarean delivery in the second stage: characteristics and diagnostic accuracy. *J Maternal–Fetal Neonat Med* 2005;17:49.

Mahon T, Chazotte C, Cohen WR. Short labor: characteristics and outcome. *Obstet Gynecol* 1994;84:47.

Murphy K, Shah L, Cohen WR. Labor and delivery in nulliparas who present with an unengaged fetal head. *J Perinatol* 1998;18:122.

Peisner DB, Rosen MG. Latent phase of labor in normal patients: a reassessment. *Obstet Gynecol* 1985;66:644.

Peisner DB, Rosen MG. Transition from latent to active phase labor. *Obstet Gynecol* 1985;68:448.

Schifrin BS, Cohen WR. Labor's dysfunctional lexicon. *Obstet Gynecol* 1989;74:123.

58 Operative vaginal delivery

Edward R. Yeomans

The frequency of operative vaginal delivery (OVD) is declining in the United States and worldwide. Multiple factors are contributing to this trend. One factor is the rising Cesarean delivery rate. The fear of litigation may be driving down the OVD rate and driving up the Cesarean rate. If we are to maintain a place for OVD in modern obstetric practice, we must provide high-quality training in our obstetrics and gynecology residency programs.

The popularity of vacuum extraction is rising as forceps use diminishes. In 1980, the ratio of forceps to vacuum was 18:1; in 2000, it was 1:2.[1] The reason for this reversal is not clear. Short-term neonatal[2] and long-term maternal and neonatal[3] consequences are comparable for each type of procedure.

A multifaceted approach to training that allows residents to develop their skills, knowledge, and judgment is mandatory. Forceps deliveries can first be rehearsed on

Table 58.1 Prerequisites for forceps application.

Experienced operator in attendance	Completely dilated cervix
Engagement of the fetal head	Clinically adequate pelvis
Knowledge of the position of the fetal head	Adequate anesthesia

Table 58.2 Indications for forceps or vacuum delivery.

Fetal indications	Maternal indications
Nonreassuring fetal heart rate pattern	Protracted second stage
Premature separation of placenta	Maternal exhaustion
Prolapsed cord	Certain maternal medical conditions

manikins,[4] and then easy outlet deliveries can be supervised by experienced practitioners. The physician in training can progress at his or her own pace to deliveries that require greater skills. For all OVD, prerequisites must be met (Table 58.1), and appropriate indications (Table 58.2) should be observed. The same prerequisites, indications, and classification system should be used for both vacuum and forceps deliveries.[5] Randomized controlled trials (RCTs) comparing these two different methods of OVD have been conducted and published.[6] The instrument of "first choice" cannot be determined from the existing literature.[7] Instead, the choice of methods should depend on the skill and comfort level of the physician and be acceptable to the woman.

As with all surgeries, these vaginal operations are associated with unique complications.[5,8] Whether Cesarean delivery should replace OVD is not clear, for there are no RCTs comparing these two approaches to childbirth. Retrospective studies[9] indicate that the morbidity of OVD is low. The American College of Obstetricians and Gynecologists (ACOG)[5] has taken the position that forceps and vacuum deliveries are "safe in appropriate circumstances."

References

1 Kozak LJ, Weeks JD. US trends in obstetric procedures, 1990–2000. *Birth* 2002;29: 157–161.

2 Towner D, Castro MA, Eby-Wilkens E, Gilbert WM. Effect of mode of delivery in nulliparous women on neonatal intracranial injury. *N Engl J Med* 1999;341:1709–1714.

3 Johanson RB, Heycock E, Carter J, et al. Maternal and child health after assisted vaginal delivery: five-year follow up of a randomized controlled study comparing forceps and ventouse. *Br J Obstet Gynaecol* 1999;106:544–549.

4 Dennen EH. *Forceps deliveries*. Philadelphia: F.A. Davis Company, 1955.

5 ACOG Practice Bulletin. *Clinical management guidelines for obstetrician–gynecologists. Operative vaginal delivery*. No. 17, June 2000.

6 Bofill JA, Fust OA, Schorr SJ, et al. A randomized prospective trial of the obstetric forceps versus the M-cup vacuum extractor. *Am J Obstet Gynecol* 1996;175:1325–1330.

7 Drife JO. Choice and instrumental delivery. *Br J Obstet Gynaecol* 1996;103:608–611.

8 Leung WC, Lam HS, Lam KW, et al. Unexpected reduction in the incidence of birth trauma and birth asphyxia related to instrumental deliveries during the study period: was this the Hawthorne effect? *Br J Obstet Gynaecol* 2003;110:319–322.

9 Murphy DJ, Leibling RE, Patel R, et al. Cohort study of operative delivery in the second stage of labour and standard of obstetric care. *Br J Obstet Gynaecol* 2003;110:610–615.

59 Preterm labor

Erol Amon and Thomas D. Myles

Epidemiology and demography

Definitions

According to the World Health Organization, a preterm birth is any birth, regardless of birthweight, that occurs before 37 menstrual weeks' gestation. The lower gestational age limit for a preterm birth, whether the infant is born alive or dead, is 20 weeks' gestation.

Importance of subject

Preterm birth is one of the most important issues in reproductive medicine. In 2002, the preterm delivery rate was 12.0%.[1] Preterm birth is directly responsible for 75–90% of all neonatal deaths that are not due to lethal congenital malformations.[2,3] It also accounts for the vast majority of perinatal mortality and both short- and long-term neonatal morbidity. The major diseases of the preterm infant result from organ immaturity, and their incidence and severity are inversely related to gestational age.[4] The break-even or 50% survival rate is about 24 weeks or a weight of 600 g.[5,6] Although the overall handicap rate of these infants is high, the severe handicap rate in survivors is about 30%.[6]

Epidemiology

The concepts of preterm birth and low birthweight (LBW) differ in their pathogenesis but share many predisposing factors (Table 59.1) and, as such, these phenomena are often considered together. Impaired fetal growth does not exert the same force on neonatal and infant mortality as early gestational age.

Nearly 85% of preterm births occur at 32 weeks or more,[7] a time when uncorrected gestational age-specific mortality is 4% or less. Neonatal mortality and severe morbidity tend to concentrate in the late second trimester and early third trimester, a period that accounts for less than one in six preterm births.

Table 59.1 Categories of maternal risk for low birthweight.

Economic	*Biological–genetic–medical*
Poverty	Previous low birthweight infant
Unemployment	Mother low weight at birth
Maternal father's poor socioeconomic	Black race*
status	Low weight for height
Uninsured, underinsured	Short stature
Poor access to prenatal care	Poor nutrition
Poor access to food	Chronic medical illness
	Inbreeding (autosomal recessive?)
Cultural–behavioral	Intergenerational effects
Low educational status	
Poor healthcare attitudes	*Reproductive*
No or inadequate prenatal care	Multiple gestation
Cigarette, alcohol, drug abuse	Premature rupture of membranes
Age of < 16 years or > 35 years	Infections (systemic, amniotic,
Unmarried	extra-amniotic, cervical)
Short interpregnancy interval	Preeclampsia or eclampsia
Lack of support group (husband,	Uterine bleeding (placental abruption,
family, church)	placenta previa)
Stress (physical, psychological)	Parity (0 or > 5)
Poor weight gain during pregnancy	Uterocervical anomalies
Black race*	Fetal disease
	Anemia or high hemoglobin
	Idiopathic premature labor
	Iatrogenic prematurity

From ref. 173, with permission.

* Black race is a risk factor for both growth retardation and premature birth. The risk is twice that for white people and remains present when confounding social and economic variables are controlled. Classification of risk for black people as cultural and biological is due to the uncertainty of the role of these variables.

The incidence of LBW infants has risen from a low of 6.7% in 1984 to its current rate of 8%, whereas the rate of very LBW (VLBW) births has increased from 1.2% to 1.5%. The national preterm birth rate has risen steadily from 10.2% to 12%.[1]

Racial disparity between black people and white people

The rates of LBW and VLBW births differ substantially between black people and white people.[7] The incidence of preterm birth is 17.4% in black people and 11.0% in white people,[7] and this racial disparity increases as gestational age at delivery decreases (Fig. 59.1). Differences in the incidence of urogenital tract infections may account for up to 35% of the racial difference in preterm birth rates. These differences in infection rates cannot be accounted for by racial differences in reported sexual behavior.

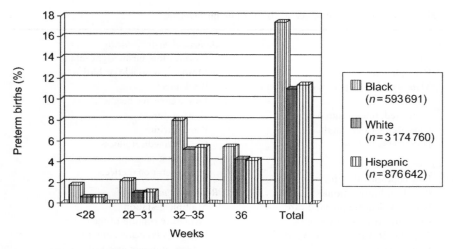

Figure 59.1 Percentage of preterm births by race. Created from data from ref. 7.

Etiology

Table 59.2 lists the identifiable causes most proximate to preterm birth. Most spontaneous preterm births are not idiopathic; only after known or suspected causes are eliminated should patients be diagnosed with idiopathic preterm labor. Most high-risk infants (those with a weight less than or equal to 1000 g) are born prematurely because of etiological factors that are currently not preventable.[3] If a comprehensive evaluation (including placental pathology, immunopathology, and intrauterine infection) is combined with clinical factors, up to 96% of patients have a potentially identifiable etiology and more than 50% of patients have two or more proximate causes.[8]

Pathophysiology

The pathophysiology of preterm labor is unknown. Factors produced locally within the placenta, chorioamniotic membranes, and decidua, together with biochemical messages from the fetus, act in some complex manner to initiate normal spontaneous labor.

During labor, and perhaps before, prostaglandin production increases in all mammalian species that have been tested. In many species, the three most temporally related uterine events antecedent to the onset of spontaneous labor are cervical ripening, formation of gap junctions, and an increase in oxytocin receptors. Fundamentally, these mechanisms must bring about myometrial contractions by regulating the free intracellular cytosolic calcium concentration in myometrial cells. When this concentration increases, myometrial cells contract; the cells relax when the concentration decreases.

Table 59.2 Proximate factors and causes associated with preterm birth.

Iatrogenic preterm delivery
  Physician error
	Amniotic fluid causes
	  Oligohydramnios with intact
	    membranes

Maternal causes
  Significant systemic medical illness
  Significant nonobstetric abdominal
    pathology
  Illicit drug abuse
  Severe preeclampsia or eclampsia
  Trauma
	Preterm rupture of chorioamniotic
	    membranes
	  Polyhydramnios
	  Subclinical intra-amniotic infection
	  Clinical chorioamnionitis

	Fetal causes
	  Fetal malformation
	  Multifetal gestation
	  Fetal hydrops
	  Fetal growth retardation
	  Fetal distress
	  Fetal demise

Uterine causes
  Malformation
  Acute overdistention
  Large myomata, degenerating myomata
  Deciduitis, decidual thrombosis and
    hemorrhage
  Idiopathic uterine activity	

Placental causes
  Placental abruption
  Placenta previa
  Marginal placental bleeding
  Large chorioangioma
	Cervical causes
	  Cervical incompetence
	  Cervical foreshortening
	  Acute cervicitis or vaginitis

Infection may precipitate up to 30% of preterm labor. Preterm labor and delivery may result from dysregulation of the normal host defense inflammatory response.[9] However, placental histology indicates that inflammation accounts for only 30–40% of cases. The most common noninflammatory lesion of the placenta in the setting of preterm labor is decidual thrombosis and acute atherosis, which may lead to uteroplacental ischemia and subsequent initiation of preterm labor.[10] This may explain the subset of patients complicated by fetal growth restriction and placental abnormalities. Preterm labor *per se* is not a disease in itself but an aberration of timing with diverse underlying heterogeneity.

Clinical antecedents to preterm labor and delivery

Many risk factors antedate the diagnosis of preterm labor, but unfortunately these factors are not very specific. This lack of specificity is further compounded by the inability to accurately diagnose preterm labor.

Table 59.3 Major and minor risk factors of the modified scoring system for spontaneous preterm labor.

Major factors*		More than one second-trimester abortion
Multiple gestation		Cervical dilation (> 1 cm) at 32 weeks
Previous preterm delivery		Cervical effacement (< 1 cm) at 32 weeks
Previous preterm labor, term delivery		
Abdominal surgery during pregnancy		*Minor factors†*
Diethylstilbestrol exposure		Febrile illness during pregnancy
Hydramnios		Bleeding after 12 weeks
Uterine anomaly		History of pyelonephritis
History of cone biopsy		Cigarette smoking (> 10 per day)
Uterine irritability (admission to rule out		One second-trimester abortion
preterm labor)		More than two first-trimester abortions

From ref. 12, with permission.

* Presence of one or more indicates high risk.

† Presence of two or more indicates high risk.

Traditional risk factor scoring

In general, risk scoring quantitatively screens a population for factors associated with a given outcome or disease. Individual patients identified as being at high risk can then receive specialized care.

In the USA, Creasy and colleagues[11] first popularized a scoring system of risk factors to predict spontaneous preterm birth. Holbrook and associates[12] (Table 59.3) modified the Creasy system so that the calculation of a risk score was not required; twelve factors were defined as major (any one indicating high risk) and six as minor (two or more indicating high risk). In a more complex screening process that also included race, low prepregnant body mass index (BMI; underweight), and a poor work environment, the positive predictive values for spontaneous preterm birth for nulliparous and multiparous patients were 28% and 33% respectively.[13]

Despite the limitations of risk scoring for the prevention of spontaneous preterm labor and birth, it is an inexpensive index that can be readily used in clinical practice to identify individual pregnant women at risk. After identification, these women can be given a more intense workup and ongoing individualized medical attention.

Recurrence risk for preterm labor and preterm birth

In a middle-class population, a second-trimester abortion was associated with an increased risk of preterm labor (14%).[12] In a study of an indigent population,[14] if the second-trimester loss occurred between 19 and 24 weeks, the subsequent preterm delivery rate was approximately 50%. After one previous preterm birth, the recurrence risk for preterm birth varied from 15% to 40%.[15,16–19] An intervening term pregnancy markedly decreased the risk of a subsequent preterm birth,

Table 59.4 Risk for recurrent preterm labor.

First birth preterm	Second birth preterm	Risk for preterm birth
No	–	4.6
No	No	2.6
No	Yes	11.1
Yes	–	17.2
Yes	No	5.7
Yes	Yes	28.4

Modified from ref. 21.

whereas the risk significantly increased with two or more previous preterm births (Table 59.4).[20] The more preterm the delivery, the less likely the subsequent pregnancy was to deliver at term.[21]

Digital cervical examination

Asymptomatic cervical dilation may represent silent preterm labor, cervical incompetence, or normal anatomic variation. In the general obstetric population, the frequency of preterm asymptomatic cervical dilation increases as gestation advances.

A large multicenter randomized controlled trial in seven European countries compared the use of "routine" cervical examination at every prenatal visit with a "clinically indicated" examination. There were no significant differences between the two groups in any of the following measurements: preterm birth, LBW, premature rupture of membranes, admission to neonatal intensive care units, or perinatal mortality. Therefore, this powerful clinical study does not support routine digital cervical evaluation.

Sonographic cervical evaluation

Digital examination is prone to subjectivity and variation between examiners. Funneling at the internal os cannot be evaluated digitally if the cervix is closed. If the cervix is dilated, placement of the examining finger next to the fetal membranes may increase the risk of infection or membrane rupture. Transvaginal sonography is more reproducible and accurate, relatively noninvasive, and provides a quantitative description of cervical anatomy. The biological variation in the endocervical length of the cervix resembles a normal bell-shaped curve. A length of 35 mm represents the 50th percentile, whereas 25 and 45 mm represent the 10th and 90th percentiles respectively. The relative risk of spontaneous preterm delivery before 35 weeks is inversely related to transvaginal sonographic cervical length.[22] A more thorough ultrasound description of the cervix includes the parameters depicted in Fig. 59.2.[23] In practice, it is rare to see a clinically significant funnel if the functional (residual) cervical length is 30 mm or more.[24] Thus, measurement of the degree of

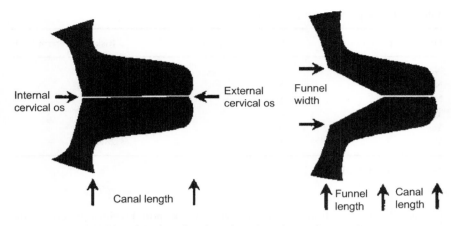

Figure 59.2 Cervical length with and without funneling (from ref. 23, with permission).

funneling becomes more important as the sonographically apposed endocervical length shortens. For reviews of cervical sonography, see Iams[24] and Doyle and Monga.[25]

Home uterine activity monitoring

Home uterine activity monitoring (HUAM) allows the patient at risk to be physically monitored at home with external tocodynamometers. The data are transmitted to a central viewing station by telephone, where the pattern of uterine activity is assessed by a nursing service. The nursing service contacts the patient once or twice daily and prepares a detailed history on the patient's current status. If the service detects any abnormalities, the physician is notified immediately. The clinical recommendations for HUAM use, and its role in outpatient management remain controversial. However, neither the bulk of scientific evidence nor the American College of Obstetricians and Gynecologists Committee Opinion[26] recommends HUAM as the standard of care.

Fetal fibronectin

Fetal fibronectin (fFN) is a unique fibronectin found in the basement membrane near the choriodecidual interface. It is produced by fetal membranes and is likely to function as an adhesive binding the placenta and membranes to the decidua. fFN is commonly found in cervicovaginal secretions before 20 weeks' gestation and at term. Its clinical detection at 22–34 weeks, at concentrations greater than 50 mg/mL, is considered abnormal and indicates choriodecidual disruption. Because fFN is also found in amniotic fluid, its presence in the vagina may indicate the presence of amniotic fluid in cervicovaginal secretions.

Three categories of patients were evaluated for fFN: symptomatic patients hospitalized for evaluation of preterm labor, high-risk asymptomatic patients, and

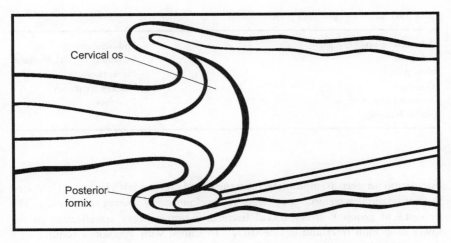

Figure 59.3 Specimen collection for fFN testing. Lightly rotate swab across either the posterior fornix of the vagina or the ectocervical region of the external cervical os for 10 seconds. This must be done prior to digital examination; alternatively, wait another 24 h.

asymptomatic patients from the general obstetric population.[27-30] From a clinical viewpoint, it is unclear how clinical management should be affected: with a negative result, the odds of delivering within a week were extremely low and numerous false-positive results were produced. Lukes and colleagues[31] found that cervical dilation or manipulation (specifically, recent sexual intercourse, vaginal bleeding, recent cervical examination, and uterine contractions) could explain some of these false-positive results. To improve the accuracy of a positive result, specimens should therefore be obtained before cervical manipulation and before advanced dilation or increased uterine activity has occurred. Faron and colleagues[32] noted that test results were more frequently positive among multiparae than nulliparae. The collection technique is illustrated in Fig. 59.3.

In low-risk populations, the overall rate of fFN positivity was found to be 3–4%.[33] More than one-half of spontaneous preterm births occurring before 28 weeks had a positive fFN test result at 24 weeks.[33] However, there was also an extremely high false-positive rate: out of the patients who tested positive for fFN at 24 weeks, 83% delivered after 28 weeks and 75% after 34 weeks.[33] fFN has also been proposed as a marker for upper genital tract infections. However, asymptomatic women with a positive cervical or vaginal fFN test between 21 and 25 weeks' gestation who were treated with metronidazole plus erythromycin did not have a decreased risk of spontaneous delivery or show an improvement in neonatal outcome.[34]

Urogenital tract infections
There is increasing evidence that urogenital tract infection, inflammation, or both are associated with and causative of many cases of preterm labor.[35] The

Table 59.5 Chief symptoms of preterm labor.

Abdominal pain	Pinkish staining
Back pain	Increased vaginal discharge
Pelvic pain	Pelvic pressure
"Gas pain"	Urinary frequency
Menstrual-like cramps	Diarrhea
Vaginal bleeding	

association between asymptomatic bacteriuria and preterm birth is clear.[36] Untreated asymptomatic bacteriuria may lead to pyelonephritis during pregnancy. The presence of group B streptococcal bacteria indicates heavy colonization of the lower urogenital tract and in one study[37] treatment with antibiotics resulted in a decreased incidence of preterm birth. However, in a further study,[38] prenatal treatment of group B streptococci with erythromycin was ineffective in preventing preterm birth.

In a study by Hillier and colleagues,[39] the association between bacterial vaginosis and preterm birth was clearly demonstrated; the relative risk of preterm delivery was 1.5–3 times higher than in patients without bacterial vaginosis. However, a recent systematic review of *all* the literature[40] found no evidence to support antibiotic treatment of bacterial vaginosis or *Trichomonas vaginalis* in pregnancy to reduce the risk of preterm birth or its associated morbidities in low- or high-risk women. In fact, for women with *T. vaginalis*, the use of metronidazole reduced the risk of persistent infection but increased the incidence of preterm birth.

Major symptoms of preterm labor

A host of complaints may herald preterm labor (Table 59.5); these often relate to painless uterine activity described as "balling up" and tightening of the uterus. Some symptoms are misinterpreted and consequently misreported by the patient, thus misleading both physician and patient. These include "gas pains," intestinal cramps, constipation, and an increase in fetal movements, any of which may represent undiagnosed actual preterm labor. Vague constitutional symptoms relating to the abdomen and pelvis may also indicate preterm labor. It is generally a good idea to instruct patients, especially those at increased risk, about the vague signs and symptoms of preterm labor. A bloody vaginal discharge (bright red, pink, brown, or other discoloration) may well be the signal of a cervical change. Patients with any of these symptoms should be encouraged to contact the physician as soon as possible.

Diagnosis

Preterm labor can be classified as threatened or actual. The basis for such a classification is the difference in prognosis; approximately 85% of patients with threat-

Table 59.6 Creasy criteria for diagnosing preterm labor.

Gestation of 20–37 weeks
Documented uterine contractions (4 in 20 min or 8 in 60 min)
Documented cervical change or cervical effacement of 80% or cervical dilation of 2 cm (or
  more)
Intact membranes

Adapted from information in ref. 111.

ened preterm labor deliver at term, whereas 40–50% of patients in actual preterm labor deliver at term.

The hallmark of threatened preterm labor is uterine activity; a diagnosis of threatened preterm labor is given when there is uterine activity but no evidence of cervical changes. In any pregnancy, the recurrence rate of threatened preterm labor is approximately 30%; of these women, approximately one-half deliver preterm.[41]

The diagnostic criteria for preterm labor in nulliparous women are described in Table 59.6. It is generally agreed that the same criteria can be used for multiparous women, although the prognostic value may be less. Documenting cervical change requires serial documentation of cervical status, ideally by the same examiner and under similar circumstances (e.g., during a contraction). One method of determining cervical change is by noting changes in the Bishop score.[42] Dilation of the internal cervical os or effacement of cervical length are the most significant values. Although not part of the diagnostic criteria for actual preterm labor, fetal station has prognostic value; the lower the station, the greater the risk of spontaneous preterm delivery.

The use of cervical sonography and measurement of fFN levels may further define who could benefit from tocolysis as the combination of a positive fFN and short cervix is strongly associated with preterm delivery (Fig. 59.4), whereas a negative fFN or normal cervical length have a strong negative predictive value.

Managing preterm labor

After a diagnosis of preterm labor is made, an appropriate evaluation is carried out and an initial management plan instituted. The evaluation phase has two major parts. First, an assessment is made of the need for tocolytic therapy, focusing on the specific nature of the agents to be used and, second, an etiological diagnostic workup is conducted.

During the evaluation, the physician seeks contraindications to substantially prolonging the pregnancy (Table 59.7). Temporary efforts to inhibit uterine activity (to enable a treatment course of antenatal corticosteroids to be administered, to transport the mother to a tertiary care centre, and to optimize conditions for maternal and fetal well-being) must be weighed against the relative urgency and necessity of

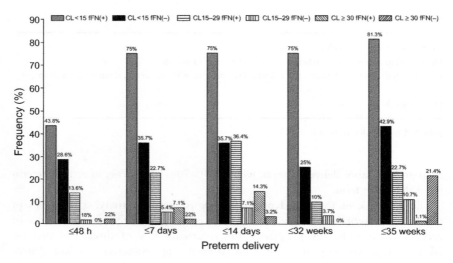

Figure 59.4 Frequency of spontaneous preterm delivery according to cervical length (CL), categorized as < 15 mm, 15–29 mm, and ≥ 30 mm, and vaginal fFN measurement. (From ref. 74.)

Table 59.7 Contraindications to tocolysis.

Absolute contraindications	Relative contraindications
Fetal demise	Fetal heart rate abnormalities
Lethal fetal anomaly	Fetal growth restriction
Severe preeclampsia or eclampsia requiring immediate delivery	Preeclampsia not requiring immediate delivery
Chorioamnionitis	Stable late second or third trimester vaginal bleeding
Severe hemorrhage	Significant maternal disease
	Cervical dilation ≥ 5.0 cm
	Progressive structural but nonlethal fetal anomalies

delivery. The fundamental issue underlying the use of tocolytic agents is whether the odds of delivery and its attendant maternal and perinatal risks outweigh the odds of prolonging the pregnancy with medical interventions and its attendant maternal and perinatal risks. Testing for fFN and evaluating the cervix for anatomical changes with digital and sonographic examinations may help exclude patients from prolonged surveillance and unneeded tocolysis.

The lower fetal age limit for initiating tocolysis in a favorable candidate is approximately 17–20 weeks. Different opinions exist as to what are the upper limits of fetal age and weight for appropriate tocolytic therapy. However, few data exist to support an overly aggressive tocolytic approach at tertiary care centers beyond the beginning of the 35th week or above an estimated fetal weight of 2000 g,

Table 59.8 Agent-specific contraindications.

Beta-agonist	*Prostaglandin synthesis inhibitors*
New York Heart Classification 2 or higher	Maternal:
Cardiac arrhythmias or maternal tachycardia	Hepatic insufficiency
Severe hypertension	Coagulation disorder
Thyrotoxicosis	Peptic ulcer disease
Asymmetric septal hypertrophy	Uncontrolled hypertension
Uncontrolled diabetes mellitus	Renal disease
Adrenal tumors	Aspirin sensitivity
Neurological thromboembolic phenomena	Fetal:
	Oligohydramnios
Magnesium sulfate	Gestational age > 32–34 weeks
Myasthenia gravis	Monozygotic twins
Heart block	Discordant twins
Certain cardiac rhythm disturbances	Ductal dependent cardiac defect
Myocardial damage	
Severe renal disease (may be used with specific precautions)	

particularly if fetal lung maturity is present. If therapy is appropriate, the physician must weigh up a number of factors in deciding which tocolytic agents to use (Table 59.8).

During the initial evaluation period, some authors also recommend analyzing microbiological cultures (including from amniotic fluid) and performing urine toxicology and baseline maternal cardiac, hematological, and electrolyte measurements. While these test results are pending and the mother and fetus are deemed stable, a thorough ultrasound examination is carried out to complete the etiological and prognostic evaluation. Factors to be assessed are listed in Table 59.9; many have a tremendous influence on clinical management.

Fetal age, weight, and growth status

Routine fetal biometric measurements should be made including the biparietal diameter (BPD), head circumference, occipitofrontal diameter (OFD), cephalic index, abdominal circumference (AC), and femur length (FL). Once the gestational age is assigned, the estimated fetal weight (EFW) should be calculated. The measurement of EFW is also important at the lower limits of viability. As with assigning gestational age, estimating fetal weight by sonography carries an inherent error. A 10% error in predicting birthweight usually represents less than 75 g at the lower limits of viability. This is equivalent to ± 5 days of average fetal growth assuming a fetal weight gain of 15 g per day at 24–25 weeks' gestation. Despite some cases of marked fetal growth restriction, birthweight is still the most important factor in immediate neonatal prognosis, particularly for infants weighing less than 1000 g.[43] Accordingly, a determination of fetal weight is useful for predelivery counseling

Table 59.9 Fetal and maternal assessment via ultrasonography.

Fetal evaluation	Placental and funic evaluation
Age, weight, and growth status	Previa
Life and fetal number	Abruption
Lie, presentation, and position	Marginal bleed with membrane separation
Well-being	Location, internal anatomy, contour,
Behavior	thickness, and grade
Anatomy and sex	Umbilical cord insertion sites
Blood and sampling (funicentesis) for	Funic presentation
rapid karyotype, blood gases,	Umbilical artery Doppler
disease-specific hematologic profiles	
	Uterine and cervical evaluation
Amniotic fluid evaluation	Defective uterine scar
Polyhydramnios	Uterine septum
Oligohydramnios	Weak lower uterine segment
Amniocentesis for infection, fetal	Cervical length
pulmonary maturation, fetal	Cervical dilation
hemolysis	Myomatous uterus

regarding prognosis and, at times, is superior to standard determinations of gestational age as a predictor for survival.[44]

After assigning fetal age and weight, intrauterine growth status should be assessed. Several investigators have suggested that fetal growth restriction is more common than expected in the setting of preterm labor.[45,46] A finding of fetal growth restriction at the lower limits of fetal viability (i.e., 22–25 weeks) is of great importance in clinical management. In these situations, sonographic measurements may erroneously underestimate fetal age secondary to suboptimal growth and the infant may be declared previable. In cases of fetal growth restriction at the other end of the prematurity spectrum (32–36 weeks), it is not uncommon to find fetal pulmonary maturity when performing transabdominal amniocentesis.

Fetal number

In multiple pregnancies, the risk of preterm labor is at least 12 times higher than in singleton pregnancies.[2] In the USA, the likelihood that a multiple gestation will be delivered before 37 weeks is over 50%.[1] More than 50% of all twins and 90% of all triplets deliver with LBWs compared with 6% of all singletons.[1]

In addition, multiple pregnancies have a higher incidence than singleton pregnancies of many maternal and fetal complications that strongly influence the management of preterm labor and delivery. These include maternal complications such as preeclampsia (incidence of 20–33%), severe polyhydramnios, fetal growth restriction, fetal malformation, nonimmune hydrops, and twin–twin transfusion syndrome. A complete sonographic evaluation is required for appropriate decision making and choice of drug therapy in multiple gestations complicated by preterm labor. When using tocolysis combined with fluid therapy, the risk of pulmonary edema is higher in multiple gestations than in singleton pregnancies. To prevent pulmonary edema, the total fluid intake should be restricted to 3000 mL of salt-free or salt-poor solution per 24 h.

Malpresentation

The incidence of malpresentation is inversely related to gestational age. In cases of malpresentation it is possible to detect associated uterine malformation, placental abnormality, polyhydramnios, oligohydramnios, or fetal abnormality using sonography. There must be a high index of suspicion for a fetal malformation or genetic syndrome because of the higher incidence of fetal malformation in the preterm breech infant. When faced with preterm delivery (25–34 weeks) of a breech-presenting fetus in the absence of other clinically pertinent maternal or fetal complications, most specialists in maternal–fetal medicine usually perform a Cesarean section despite the fact that there is little scientific evidence to support such an approach.[47,48]

It is appropriate to consider performing a Cesarean section for singleton breech-presenting fetuses estimated to weigh between 600 and 1500 g with a gestational age of 24–32 weeks. Individualization of care is necessary regarding the method of delivery of the extremely LBW preterm breech infant. Head entrapment has been shown to occur in both vaginal and Cesarean deliveries with a reported incidence of 5–10%.[49] However, management of this complication appears to be easier with a Cesarean delivery than with a vaginal delivery.

Fetal well-being

Fetal well-being during preterm labor is most commonly assessed using the non-stress test. A classically reactive test is most widely defined as being at least two accelerations of fetal heart rate of 15 beats per minute (b.p.m.) for 15 s during a 20-min monitoring period. These classical criteria for a reactive test have been modified in the setting of preterm labor by defining reactivity as three accelerations of 10 b.p.m.; in this case, almost all fetuses tested at 26 weeks were reactive at the end of a 60-min period, and approximately 90% of the 24-week-old fetuses were reactive. Because the contraction stress test is strongly contraindicated in the presence of preterm labor, the test of choice for further fetal evaluation is the biophysical profile. Fetal tone, movement, amniotic fluid volume, and fetal breathing movements (FBMs) all become normally manifest weeks before classic fetal heart reactivity;[50] fetal oxygenation is sufficient if these four parameters are present.

Fetal malformation

There is an increased incidence of fetal malformations in patients with preterm labor.[51] Often, these patients have advanced preterm labor, spontaneous rupture of membranes, or vaginal bleeding. Overall, there is a relative risk of 2.0 that an infant with a congenital malformation will be born preterm.

It is important, therefore, to perform a complete fetal malformation screen during preterm labor. If sonographic evidence suggests aneuploidy, a rapid fetal karyotype may be useful for optimal medical and obstetric management of labor, mode and place of delivery, and neonatal resuscitation.[52] If a lethal karyotype is found, tocolysis should be discontinued.

Polyhydramnios

Polyhydramnios is an important cause of preterm labor resulting from uterine overdistention. Polyhydramnios is suspected when uterine enlargement is greater than expected for gestational age and there is an inability to palpate fetal parts. Maternal respiratory compromise and postrenal obstruction may result from massive uterine overdistention. As many as 40% of patients with polyhydramnios experience preterm labor and delivery.[53] Sonography is used to confirm the diagnosis, to help determine the proximate cause, and to guide therapeutic mechanical relief via reduction amniocentesis. The cause of polyhydramnios may be maternal, fetal, placental, or a combination of these factors.

Oligohydramnios

Oligohydramnios, a significant reduction in amniotic fluid volume, can be easily diagnosed using ultrasound. In the setting of preterm labor, this may result from premature rupture of the membranes, maternal intake of nonsteroidal anti-inflammatory agents, severe intrauterine growth retardation, or a genitourinary malformation in which fetal urination into the amniotic cavity is absent.

The diagnosis of lethal renal diseases is important because, during preterm labor, many of these cases may present with fetal distress or malpresentation, two of the most common fetal indications for Cesarean section. In these situations, Cesarean section is performed solely for maternal indications. Tocolysis is not indicated except to allow a diagnostic evaluation and maternal transfer.

Fetal gender

A curiosity of preterm birth is the presence of an excess of male fetuses. These results suggest the existence of a mechanism of preterm birth which is influenced by fetal gender. Fetal gender has important prognostic significance. Female fetuses have a significant survival advantage over male fetuses at weights of less than 1000 g.[43] In female fetuses, the lecithin–sphingomyelin (L/S) ratio reaches 2:1 at 33.7 weeks, 1.4 weeks earlier than in male fetuses. Phosphatidylglycerol first appears at 34 weeks in female fetuses and at 35 weeks in male fetuses.

Amniocentesis and neonatal outcome

In experienced hands, amniocentesis in the late second or third trimester carries a minimal risk; there is no scientific evidence that it stimulates labor. One-third of the patients at 31–32 weeks' and 50% of those at 33 weeks' gestation or more had mature L/S ratios.

The amniotic cavity is normally sterile; thus, isolation of any organism indicates microbial invasion. Microorganisms can gain access to the cavity by ascending from the lower genital tract, maternal hematogenous spread, retrograde fallopian tube spread, and iatrogenic introduction during invasive prenatal diagnostic and therapeutic procedures. The most common organisms found in amniotic fluid are *Ureaplasma urealyticum*, *Mycoplasma hominis*, and *Fusobacterium* species.

In a review of studies of transabdominal amniocentesis in patients with preterm labor and intact membranes, a positive culture rate of 16% has been quoted. Out of these patients, 65% were refractory to tocolysis, 58% had clinical chorioamnionitis, and 40% had rupture of the membranes. The respective rates in patients with negative culture results were 16%, 7%, and 4%. Although a large percentage of the microbes recovered were anaerobic, neonates rarely developed significant anaerobic infections. A review of preterm labor patients with intact membranes found an incidence of amniotic fluid infection of approximately 13%.[54] Approximately 10–15% of neonates in the positive culture group developed sepsis compared with approximately 2% in the negative culture group.[55]

Despite pulmonary maturity, respiratory distress syndrome (RDS) and other morbidities still occur as an inverse function of gestational age. Hence, prolongation of pregnancy should still be attempted even in the presence of mature amniotic fluid indices for selected patients at less than 34 weeks' gestation. At 34–36 weeks' gestation, testing of fetal lung maturity is a cost-effective procedure.

Testing of fetal lung maturity is biochemically comparable between twin and singleton pregnancies and has the same neonatal prognostic value for a given gestational age.

Uterine malformations

Didelphia and all types of bicornuate uteri are associated with an incidence of preterm labor of more than 20%. Fedele and colleagues[56] found that preterm labor occurred in up to 37.5% of patients with unicornuate uteri. The best fetal survival rate (86%) was found in women with complete septate uteri, whereas the worst rates were found in women with complete bicornuate uteri (50%) and unicornuate uteri (40%). Uterine anomalies may be associated with cervical incompetence, malpresentation, and maternal genitourinary malformations.

Management decisions at the lower end of viability

Managing preterm delivery at the lower limits of viability (22–24 weeks' gestation at present) is a vexing problem. It is optimal for delivery to occur in the immediate proximity to a neonatal intensive care center.[57] When conditions permit, decisions regarding the delivery of a severely preterm fetus (i.e., 22–26 weeks' gestation by best obstetric estimate) are ideally made after the mother has been transported to a tertiary care center. Highly coordinated predelivery family counseling by obstetricians and neonatal physicians is recommended to discuss the prognosis and plan management, thereby minimizing anxiety, confusion, and fear.

Survival rates increase as a function of gestational age and birthweight. The survival rate is 50% at 24 weeks' gestation, 60–70% at 25 weeks, and 70–80% at 26 weeks. Consideration of Cesarean section for fetal distress should begin at an estimated gestational age of 24 weeks, an estimated weight of 600 g, or both. An obstetric willingness to perform a Cesarean delivery for fetal indications is associated with an increased rate of survival and a virtual absence of intrapartum stillbirth.[58]

Because of the inherent inaccuracies in estimating fetal age and weight, survival considerations on behalf of the fetus should begin between 22 and 23 weeks' gestation and 450–500 g. The likelihood for survival in these instances is very low (i.e., less than 10–20%), therefore Cesarean section for fetal indications is best avoided; if the infant survives, it usually survives regardless of the delivery mode. To protect the mother from an undue risk of Cesarean section, which has very little potential benefit for the newborn, the mother should be offered all other available options including: transfer to a tertiary care center, family counseling, standard hydration, fetal monitoring, maternal positioning, maternal oxygenation, controlled sterile delivery, and the presence of one or two neonatologists at delivery. Additional measures include transcervical amnioinfusion and acute tocolysis for uterine relaxation.[59,60]

Tocolytic agents

Beta-sympathomimetic agents

Beta-1 receptors predominate in the heart, small intestine, and adipose tissue, whereas beta-2 receptors predominate in the uterus, blood vessels, bronchioles, and liver. Some agents (e.g., ritodrine) are thought to have selective beta-2 activity.[61] Beta-2 selective sympathomimetic amines are structurally related to catecholamines and stimulate all beta receptors throughout the entire body.[62] With continued use, tachyphylaxis is seen.[63,64]

The side-effects of these agents are represented by an exaggeration of their physiological effects. In the cardiovascular system, they cause peripheral vasodilation with a decrease in diastolic blood pressure, a positive chronotropic effect with decreased ventricular filling time, a positive inotropic effect, and a tendency toward arrhythmogenesis. With parenteral administration, chest pain is not uncommon. These drugs increase oxygen demand and decrease coronary artery perfusion, and may cause myocardial ischemia; however, levels of cardiac isoenzymes are not increased. These clinical and electrocardiographic findings may relate directly to drug therapy or indirectly to electrolyte disturbance *per se*, rather than to ischemia.[65] Maternal cardiac death has also been reported.[66–68]

Pulmonary edema may occur in a small percentage of patients treated with parenteral beta-sympathomimetic agents.[69] This life-threatening complication has several predisposing factors: multiple gestation, a positive fluid balance, blood transfusion, anemia, infection, associated hypertension, polyhydramnios, and underlying cardiac disease. These findings highlight the importance of refraining from using isotonic fluids throughout ritodrine therapy, restricting total fluids to less than 3000 mL/day, and maintaining a meticulous fluid intake and output record.

Metabolic complications, such as hypokalemia resulting from increases in glucose and insulin, hyperglycemia resulting from glucagon stimulation and glycogenolysis, and an increase in free fatty acids resulting from lipolysis, are common with intravenous therapy.[70,71] Less common metabolic complications include lactic acidosis and ketosis,[72] and occasionally there have been cases of diabetic ketoacidosis.[73]

The common effects on the neonate have been limited primarily to hypoglycemia, occasional ileus, hypocalcemia, and hyperbilirubinemia.[74] Apgar scores are not significantly affected,[75] and long-term follow-up studies have revealed no significant problems in child development.[76-80]

Ritodrine

Favorable reports in 1980 by Barden and colleagues[66] and Merkatz and colleagues[81] promulgated the clinical use of ritodrine in the USA. Ritodrine became the first drug approved by the Food and Drug Administration (FDA) for the inhibition of preterm labor.

In a meta-analysis of ritodrine efficacy there were significantly fewer deliveries in the beta-mimetic group during the first 24–48 h of therapy. There was a slight reduction in the percentage of preterm deliveries in the group receiving beta-mimetic therapy. However, there was no significant reduction in the incidence of LBW infants, respiratory distress morbidity, or perinatal mortality. A Canadian trial[82] found a statistically significant 48-h delay in delivery in women receiving ritodrine as opposed to placebo. There was a trend toward improved neonatal survival in women receiving ritodrine who were randomized between 24 and 27 weeks.

To date, beta-agonists have not been shown to be effective when given as a prophylactic agent. In fact, one meta-analysis indicated the lack of tocolytic efficacy of standard oral beta-agonist maintenance therapy.[83]

Terbutaline

Terbutaline is commonly used in the management of preterm labor. Initially, its efficacy was thought to be quite significant, but subsequent studies have found it to be limited. Terbutaline has significant, potentially life-threatening side-effects similar to those of ritodrine, especially when given intravenously.[69,84]

When given subcutaneously, the effect is rapid and there are fewer side-effects.[85-87] The ease of administration and the avoidance of intravenous hydration makes the subcutaneous route a reasonable alternative. In a commonly used regimen, 0.25 mg of terbutaline is given subcutaneously every 20–60 min until contractions have subsided. Common daily doses range from 10 to 30 mg, with the maximum daily dose approximately 40 mg. To prevent serious complications, close attention must be paid to the maternal heart rate and other symptoms. Cardiovascular collapse and peripartum heart failure have been rarely associated with oral terbutaline therapy.[88,89]

Prostaglandin synthetase inhibitors

Prostaglandin synthetase inhibitors are among the most effective drugs known for inhibiting preterm labor.[90] They are easily administered and well tolerated by the mother; however, they have only a limited window of human application on account of fetal safety.

Of all the traditional tocolytic agents available, indomethacin is likely to have the greatest efficacy. The daily dose ranges from 100 to 200 mg. More recent trials have indicated that these agents are similar to beta-agonists[91–93] and magnesium sulfate[94] in terms of their efficacy.

Maternal side-effects are minimal; the primary side-effect is a gastrointestinal upset, which may require the use of calcium carbonate (Maalox). Indomethacin is contraindicated in patients with hematological dysfunction, peptic ulcer disease, and known allergy; it appears to increase the bleeding time. It is relatively contraindicated in maternal renal disease.

The most significant potential complications in the fetus relate to the premature closure of the ductus arteriosus, right-sided heart failure, and fetal death.[95] It is therefore important to carry out a sonographic evaluation of structural fetal anatomy to rule out a ductal-dependent lesion both before and during therapy of preterm labor with indomethacin. Use for more than 72 h should prompt further evaluation of the ductus and an investigation to rule out fetal heart failure.

The most feared complication in the neonate is persistent pulmonary hypertension.[96] Fetal and neonatal oliguria is not uncommon. Sonographic surveillance for oligohydramnios is indicated when indomethacin is used for more than 72 h. There are case reports of neonatal bowel perforation,[97] and hyperbilirubinemia may occur because indomethacin can displace bilirubin from the binding sites of albumin.[98] Indomethacin use may also predispose users to necrotizing enterocolitis (NEC) and intraventricular hemorrhage (IVH).[99,100] Because of the variance in fetal safety one could consider these agents as second-line therapy, using proper precautions to minimize fetal and neonatal effects.

Selective use of indomethacin before 32 weeks' gestation and for less then 72 h causes no substantial and permanent side-effects to the fetus or neonate. Additional data are being accumulated using cyclo-oxygenase-2-selective inhibitors (COXIBs).

Magnesium sulfate

Magnesium sulfate has become the first-line agent of choice for continuous intravenous tocolytic therapy in the USA. Used properly, magnesium sulfate is safe for both tocolysis and seizure prophylaxis. Most clinicians monitor reflexes, respiration, urine output, and intermittent serum magnesium levels to prevent serious complications of hypermagnesemia. A diminished glomerular filtration rate diminishes the excretion of magnesium, and continued administration of parenteral magnesium sulfate may result in toxicity as serum levels rise. Fortunately, a fast-acting and safe antidote is readily available: intravenous injection of calcium gluconate or chloride rapidly antagonizes the actions of excessive magnesium.

Pharmacology

Only 30% of the normal daily intake of magnesium is absorbed; this takes place in the upper small bowel and occurs by an active process. The National Research Council's recommended daily dietary allowance of magnesium for pregnant women is 450 mg. Dietary sources of magnesium are meat, milk, dark-green vegetables, seafood, and chocolate. The kidney is the major regulator of the serum magnesium concentration because magnesium is principally excreted in the urine.[101]

The mechanism by which hypermagnesemia exerts its relaxant effects on smooth muscle differs from that of skeletal muscle. Smooth muscle undergoes pharmaco-mechanical coupling mediated by various agonists rather than the electromechanical coupling characteristic of skeletal muscle. Excess magnesium depresses the peripheral neuromuscular system by inhibiting acetylcholine release and reducing the sensitivity of the motor end plate potential. Acetylcholine is unnecessary for spontaneous contractility of smooth muscle. The exact mechanism by which magnesium diminishes or abolishes uterine activity remains unclear. The extracellular excess of magnesium causes an increase of 50% in the intracellular magnesium concentration. The inhibition of calcium channel currents appears to be related to magnesium-induced tocolysis.[102]

Maternal magnesium sulfate-induced hypermagnesemia is associated with increased urinary excretion of both magnesium and calcium. Three-fourths of the infused elemental magnesium is excreted during the infusion and 90% within 24 h of the end of the infusion.[103] The urinary excretion of calcium is three times that observed in control subjects. The mean total maternal serum calcium decreases by 12% and the mean serum ionized calcium by 25%.

Maternal side-effects

Table 59.10 summarizes the major clinical side-effects of maternal hypermagnesemia, and Table 59.11 provides the critical serum levels of magnesium needed for some of these effects to occur. Clinically, respiratory depression from hypermagnesemia does not occur before the disappearance of the deep tendon reflexes, and the absence of the reflex arc should therefore serve as a warning sign of impending magnesium toxicity. However, for patients who inadvertently receive high doses of magnesium intravenously over a short period, the initial clinical presentation may be respiratory or cardiac arrest.[104–106]

One of the most important side-effects encountered during standard tocolytic therapy with magnesium sulfate is chest pain, possibly due to myocardial ischemia. This uncommonly occurs as a result of magnesium sulfate therapy alone but, more often, there are additional factors. A higher incidence of cardiorespiratory side-effects occurs in patients undergoing supplemental drug therapy after failed single-agent therapy.[107,108]

Table 59.10 Potential maternal effects of hypermagnesemia.

Common side-effects	Lengthening of the P-R and QRS interval
Loss of deep tendon reflexes	Controversial effect on the T wave
Warmth during infusion	Chest pain
Mild central hypothermic effects	Puimonary edema
Increase in skin temperature	
Cutaneous vasodilation	*Effects seen at very high serum*
Nausea, possible emesis	*concentrations*
	Respiratory depression
Not uncommon side-effects seen with	Cardiac arrest
moderately elevated serum levels	Profound muscular paralysis
Somnolence, lethargy, lightheadedness	Amnesia
Visual blurring, diplopia	Decreased rate of impulse formation of
Dysarthria	the sinoatrial node
Nystagmus	
Constipation and dyspepsia	*Rare side-effects*
	Profound hypotension
Uncommon side-effects	Maternal tetany
Potentiation of other neuromuscular	Hypersensitivity: urticarial reaction
blockers	Paralytic ileus

Table 59.11 Critical serum levels for magnesium sulfate.

Therapeutic range	6–8 mg/dL
Loss of deep tendon reflexes	8–12 mg/dL
Respiratory paralysis	12–15 mg/dL
Cardiac arrest	> 20 mg/dL

Based in part on information obtained from ref. 103.

A potentially lethal side-effect encountered during magnesium sulfate tocolytic therapy is pulmonary edema. It occurs with an incidence of approximately 1%, compared with 5% in patients receiving beta-sympathomimetics.[109,110] Generally, these cases are complicated by other factors associated with pulmonary edema: multiple gestation, polyhydramnios, preeclampsia, anemia, blood transfusion, chorioamnionitis, positive fluid balance, operative delivery, dual-agent therapy, and prolonged therapy.[111-113] With proper patient selection, judicious therapy, and close monitoring, the risk of pulmonary edema can be minimized.[82]

Perinatal side-effects
The neonatal and fetal side-effects of hypermagnesemia are summarized in Table 59.12.[114] None of the neonatal effects appears to be due to magnesium alone but may be related to confounding variables such as maternal illness, fetal growth retar-

Table 59.12 Potential fetal and neonatal effects of hypermagnesemia.

Controversial effects on fetal heart rate variability
Lack of significant effect on fetal umbilical Doppler studies
Fetal breathing movements decrease
Mean baseline fetal heart rate decreases
Flaccidity, hyporeflexia
Need for assisted ventilation
Weak or absent cry
Transient decreased active tone of neck extensors
Possible transient radiographic bony changes

Modified from ref. 115.

dation, and prematurity. A decreased bone density is seen in magnesium-treated patients when compared with control subjects.[115]

Because of both maternal heat loss from peripheral vasodilation and a blunted shivering ability, a maternal central hypothermic effect can occur with temperatures dropping as low as 94°F (34.4°C). Being very sensitive to maternal temperature, the baseline fetal heart rate changes accordingly, and a temporary benign fetal bradycardia occurs. Concomitant accelerations are reassuring and delivery is not indicated.

Efficacy and relative safety

In 1966, Rusu and colleagues[116] performed the first therapeutic trials of magnesium as a tocolytic agent. In 1977, Steer and Petrie[117] were the first investigators to publish the results of a clinical trial evaluating such therapy in English; they concluded that magnesium sulfate might become an alternate method of controlling preterm labor.

Multiple studies over the years have found that magnesium sulfate is as effective as other tocolytic agents and safer than beta-agonists. However, a 1990 study concluded that magnesium sulfate is ineffective in preventing preterm birth. This was not a blind study, the dosages used were lower than average, and many in the control group remained undelivered; these findings therefore render their conclusions as speculative at best.

Higher dosing is not required in twin gestations; however, tocolysis in higher order multifetal gestations appears to require higher doses.[118] Also, when a hospitalized patient who has responded to intravenous magnesium therapy is converted to outpatient therapy, a 'weaning-off' period from magnesium sulfate is not necessary.

Empirical drug combinations containing magnesium sulfate have been used quite successfully and safely in our hands (e.g., magnesium sulfate and either intermittent oral or subcutaneous terbutaline or oral nifedipine). We and others have found that the combination of magnesium sulfate and indomethacin is relatively safe and have advocated its use in patients with advanced cervical dilation.[119,120]

Long-term therapy

In 1989, Dudley and colleagues[121] concluded that there is no time limit for magnesium sulfate therapy and that tocolysis may be continued as clinically indicated. However, some reports have implicated the long-term continuous infusion of magnesium sulfate in the genesis of transient neonatal radiographic bony lesions.[114,122]

Oral magnesium as prophylaxis for preterm delivery

Serum magnesium levels are usually lower in pregnancy than in the nonpregnant state and, during preterm labor, levels appear to drop still further.[123,124] Some authors have suggested an etiological relationship between low magnesium concentration and preterm delivery.[125–127] Oral tocolysis with magnesium oxide and gluconate has been used.[124] The mean serum concentration of magnesium may increase from 1.44 ± 0.22 mg per 100 mL before therapy to 2.16 ± 0.32 mg per 100 mL after oral therapy.[128] Most studies have shown no improvement in pregnancy outcome after oral magnesium supplementation.

Recommended clinical protocol

Most reported studies use a loading dose of 4 g of intravenous magnesium sulfate followed by administration of 2 g/h; however, some studies[129–132] have advocated a 6-g loading dose. The clinical protocol in Table 59.13, modified from Petrie,[130] allows for fine-tuning of infusion rates with decreased potential for fluid overload, and is well tolerated by most patients. Paying careful attention to contraindications (Table 59.8) and to fluid intake and output diminishes the risk of pulmonary edema and magnesium toxicity.

Nifedipine

Nifedipine inhibits uterine activity and has less of an effect on the cardiac conduction system than verapamil, another calcium channel antagonist. The mechanism of action of nifedipine appears to be limited to the inhibition of the slow voltage-dependent channels regulating calcium influx. Adverse pharmacological effects include vasodilation, negative inotropism, and sinoatrial or atrioventricular node conduction disturbances. Because it is a potent vasodilator, nifedipine may cause dizziness, lightheadedness, flushing, headache, and peripheral edema.[133] Although the overall incidence of side-effects is 17%, severe effects necessitating discontinuation of therapy only occur in 2–5% of patients.[134] The negative inotropic and dromotropic (affecting cardiac nodal conduction) effects of nifedipine are minimal. This is largely because of the heart's baroreflex response to peripheral vasodilation. Idiosyncratic reactions to nifedipine are rare.

Nifedipine is rapidly and almost completely absorbed from the gastrointestinal tract. Absorption after sublingual administration was rapid but less complete, with levels being measurable in the plasma within 5 min.[135] The rate of absorption of oral and sublingual capsules varies widely among patients. The mean elimination half-life was about 80 min, and levels were undetectable in most patients receiving a 10-mg dose by 360 min. The mean ratio of fetal cord to maternal serum

Table 59.13 A clinical recipe to administer magnesium sulfate.

1. 100 mL of a 50% solution of magnesium sulfate is easily obtained from readily available products. This volume contains 50 g of magnesium sulfate.
2. 100 mL is sterilely removed from a 500-mL bag of 5% dextrose in water. Fifty grams of magnesium sulfate is injected into the remaining 400 mL of fluid for intravenous infusion. It should be noted that 10 mL of this final solution equals 1 g of magnesium sulfate.
3. A loading dose of 6 g is infused over 30 min. Perspiration and flushing are observed and occur with a feeling of warmth due to vasodilatation. These findings are usually noted early during the intravenous infusion and continue to a greater or lesser degree throughout the infusion. The face, neck, and hands are particularly affected. Nausea and emesis may occur.
4. The initial continuous maintenance rate is 2–3 g/h for 60 min. One or two doses of subcutaneous terbutaline 0.25 mg per dose, may be used during this interval if there are no contraindications and rapid diminution in uterine activity is desired.
5. Complete and rapid uterine quiescence is unnecessary.
6. The infusion rate is increased in increments of 0.5 g/h every 30 min until uterine activity begins to decrease or signs and symptoms of hypermagnesemia occur. These findings include lethargy, somnolence, diplopia, dysarthria, blurred vision, dry mouth, dizziness, and nystagmus. These effects generally occur at a dose of greater than 2 g/h (2.5–4.0 g/h). Downward adjustments in the rate by half-gram increments are generally all that is needed; discontinuation of therapy for side-effects is rarely needed. If necessary, intravenous injection of 1 g of calcium gluconate can be used in the symptomatic patient; this will be followed by rapid symptomatic relief.
7. The infusion is continued at the lowest effective rate of 2 g/h, whichever is greater, for at least 12 h of relative uterine quiescence.
8. Oral beta-sympathomimetic therapy is administered and the magnesium infusion is discontinued. Should uterine activity begin to increase during this interval, magnesium sulfate infusion should be increased to the effective rate.
9. If the patient cannot be successfully weaned from intravenous magnesium therapy, continuous short-term therapy (24–72 h) may be safely administered, usually at rates of 2–3 g/h. During this interval, another attempt at weaning may be attempted.
10. If uterine activity recurs coincident with the conversion from intravenous magnesium therapy to oral beta-sympathomimetic, attempts to use other tocolytic agents may be instituted.
11. Should discontinuation of magnesium infusion and conversion to an oral tocolytic agent fail to abate increasing uterine activity, continuous intermediate-term to long-term therapy with magnesium sulfate may be given. In general, cervical dilation will not change significantly during these therapeutic maneuvers. During long-term magnesium sulfate infusion therapy, the patient can be managed safely in a step-down unit. The healthcare team should be ready to provide emotional and moral support for patients requiring long-term hospitalization.
12. Most true failures of magnesium sulfate therapy and progressive preterm labor are due to cervical dilatation of > 4 cm, placental abruption, or chorioamnionitis.

(Continued)

489

Table 59.13 *Continued*

---

13. The occasional patient continues to have increased uterine activity, yet has no associated cervical changes while on magnesium sulfate therapy. Other tocolytic agents may be tried in these cases in an attempt to quiet the uterus.
14. Patients who are refractory to treatment for preterm labor are likely to have an identifiable pathophysiologic process, most notably amniotic infection or abruptio placentae. An amniocentesis for studies of infection and pulmonary maturity are indicated.
15. Dual-agent combination therapy with intravenous magnesium sulfate and intravenous beta-sympathomimetic agents is not recommended due to a significantly increased risk of side-effects. However, dual therapy magnesium with oral or subcutaneous tocolytic agents is reasonable. Combined use of magnesium with nifedipine, indomethacin, or oxytocin analogs may be used but needs further study.
16. In the severely preterm gestation with inevitable delivery due to advanced cervical dilation (4–8 cm), aggressive magnesium tocolysis alone or in combination with other tocolytic agents may be extremely useful in delaying delivery for 24–48 h to improve the neonatal survival advantage by giving antenatal betamethasone.

Modified from ref. 115.

nifedipine was 0.93 ± 0.20, whereas the mean amniotic fluid concentration was $53\% \pm 15\%$ that of simultaneously obtained maternal vein samples.

Clinical experience

Recent studies have supported the use of nifedipine in tocolysis; it has been found to be as effective as more commonly used tocolytic agents and to have fewer cardiovascular side-effects than beta-agonists. In normotensive patients, nifedipine caused a statistical decrement in blood pressure but one of unlikely clinical significance. However, nifedipine was associated with more flushing.

In a study comparing nifedipine with magnesium sulfate, patients in the magnesium sulfate group experienced chest pain more often and drug therapy was discontinued. However, more patients in the nifedipine group experienced episodes of transient hypotension, although none was clinically significant. The authors stressed the need for adequate hydration before administering nifedipine for tocolysis. Initially, a 10-mg capsule was given sublingually; if uterine activity persisted, this dose was repeated every 20 min up to a maximum of 40 mg during the first hour. If tocolysis was successful, oral therapy was initiated for 48 h, with a dose of 20 mg every 4 h. Patients were then maintained on oral nifedipine, with a 10-mg dose every 8 h.

Similarly to terbutaline and ritodrine, nifedipine has been associated with drug-induced hepatitis.[136] Nifedipine (in combination with magnesium) has been rarely associated with neuroblockade, an effect that can be reversed with calcium administration and discontinuation of magnesium.[137,138] Hypocalcemia can also rarely occur.[139] Combined usage with magnesium is not contraindicated.

Clinical implications

Nifedipine has an efficacy profile which is at least as effective as beta-agonists and magnesium sulfate. More recently, it has been reported that nifedipine is more effective than ritodrine.[140] Its safety profile renders it quite favorable in comparison with other tocolytic agents.

Progestational agents

Progestational agents have been widely used to prolong pregnancy in women who are judged to be at an increased risk of miscarriage or preterm birth. The most commonly used agent is 17α-hydroxyprogesterone caproate (17P).

Meis and colleagues[141] noted a significant reduction in preterm delivery when a weekly intramuscular injection of 250 mg of 17P was administered (summarized in Fig. 59.5). Therapy was initiated at 16–20 weeks' gestation in multiparous single-

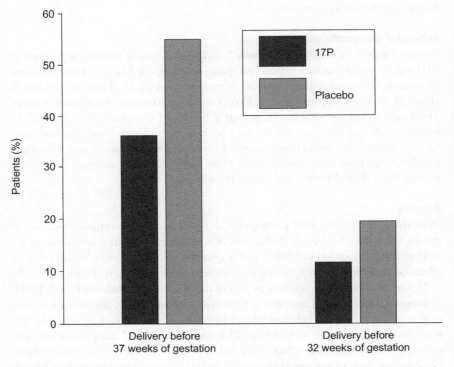

Figure 59.5 Effects of 17P on preterm delivery at 32 and 37 weeks' gestation. Patients had a previous history of spontaneous preterm delivery, and were given weekly injections of 250 mg of 17P. There was a decreased incidence of preterm delivery at < 37 weeks [RR 0.66 (0.54–0.81)] and < 32 weeks [RR 0.58 (0.37–0.91)]. Decreased incidences of both LBW births and IVH [(RR 0.25 (0.08–0.82)] were observed. (From ref. 175.)

ton patients with a history of spontaneous preterm delivery. Treatment was more useful for prophylaxis than for inhibiting active preterm labor. In a similar study of high-risk patients by da Fonseca and colleagues,[142] treatment with a daily 100-mg progesterone suppository resulted in a decrease in uterine activity and preterm birth.

Oxytocin receptor blockade and nitroglycerin

The concentration of oxytocin receptors in uterine tissues increases dramatically just before and during labor.[143] Augmented uterine sensitivity to constant serum levels of oxytocin may result in increases in uterine activity. Oxytocin receptors are also found in the decidua, and stimulation produces prostaglandins. Consequently, the potential role of oxytocin antagonists (e.g., atosiban) as tocolytic agents has been studied; theoretically, they may offer greater specificity with fewer side-effects than agents in use at present.[144-146]

Nitric oxide is a potent smooth muscle relaxant. However, recent studies have found that nitroglycerin, although better than placebo, is less effective than either magnesium sulfate or beta-agonists.[147,148]

Antenatal glucocorticoids

An initial report by Liggins and Howie[149] in 1972 revealed a significant decrease in RDS and neonatal death in patients receiving two doses of 12 mg of betamethasone 24 h apart. The optimal glucocorticoid preparation and the ideal dose are unknown, although most subsequent studies have used betamethasone or dexamethasone. These two agents are identical except for a 16-methyl group which is in the alpha position in dexamethasone and the beta position in betamethasone. Neither agent has significant mineralocorticoid activity (as opposed to hydrocortisone or methyl-prednisolone). Both drugs have elevated plasma glucocorticoid activities for approximately 60–72 h and both readily cross the placenta.

Benefits

Data from more than 3000 participants demonstrated that corticosteroids could reduce the incidence of RDS. Reductions in respiratory morbidity were also associated with reductions in IVH, NEC, and neonatal death. Fortunately, these beneficial effects occurred in the absence of strong evidence for adverse effects of corticosteroids.

This meta-analysis was updated as part of the National Institutes of Health (NIH) Consensus Conference. There was a 50% reduction in RDS in the group receiving antenatal corticosteroids between 29 and 34 weeks. The most dramatic effects (70% reduction) were noted in infants born 24 h after but within 7 days of the last dose of corticosteroids. A lesser effect (30% reduction) was noted in those infants delivering within 24 h of the initial treatment. Neonatal mortality appeared to be substantially reduced (40% reduction), and both male and female infants benefited. Reductions in the rates of periventricular and intraventricular hemorrhage (50% reduction) and NEC (65% reduction) were also noted. Randomized data indicated a decrease in the severity of RDS before 28 weeks, but not a decrease in incidence.[150]

Risks

Controversial findings from five large observational databases in the multicenter network (more than 30 000 patients) revealed that antenatal corticosteroid exposure was associated with a significant increase (30–50%) in neonatal sepsis and NEC;[151] this finding is at odds with the meta-analysis and with two early randomized trials, one of which was in patients with membrane rupture.

Data from trials with long-term follow-up for up to 12 years have indicated that antenatal corticosteroids do not adversely affect physical growth or psychomotor development.[152] Short-term effects of transient adrenal suppression by feedback inhibition of adrenocorticotropic hormone have been demonstrated in the mother and newborn after prenatal exposure to a single course of corticosteroids.[153] Maternal cortisol levels return to normal within 48 h of the last dose, while fetal cortisol levels return to baseline within 6 days.

Clinical caveats

In higher order multifetal gestations, antenatal corticosteroids are associated with an increase in uterine contractions.[154] In patients with premature rupture of membranes, the benefit of antenatal corticosteroids has been demonstrated but the benefit–risk ratio is controversial. In general, in the reduction of RDS and mortality, the benefits of corticosteroids were additive to those of surfactant. However, it should be noted that the absence of pulmonary maturity was not used in any of these trials as a basis for the administration of corticosteroids; rather, the basis for administration was gestational age. The risk for RDS varied greatly with gestational age even in the presence of fetal lung maturity (Table 59.14).[155]

The NIH consensus statement concluded that all fetuses between 24 and 34 weeks' gestation at risk for preterm delivery are candidates for antenatal corticosteroid therapy.[152] However, some important caveats are suggested. In general, corticosteroid injections are not indicated for high-risk pregnant women whose pregnancy is stable enough to be managed in an outpatient setting. For hospitalized patients at an increased risk for emergent preterm delivery, initial corticosteroids are indicated, but repeat courses are not generally indicated. However, for patients who received their steroids in the remote past, a single rescue dose may be of benefit.[156] For patients who may deliver precipitously, a benefit has been shown if steroids are given as little as 4 h prior to delivery.[157] Patients with active peptic ulcer disease, active viral infection, active tuberculosis, and either active or suspected chorioamnionitis should probably not receive antenatal corticosteroids.

Thoughtful consideration must be exercised in gestational and pregestational diabetic women. Glucocorticoid therapy is likely to provoke insulin resistance and a deterioration in diabetic control. The combination of beta-agonists and corticosteroids may well have an even more marked effect. As such, fetal hyperinsulinism due to hyperglycemia may actually block surfactant production of type 2 pneumocytes.[158] Moreover, there has been a report of glucocorticoid-induced ketoacidosis in a patient with gestational diabetes in the setting of preterm labor.[159] Glucose values should be closely monitored and insulin should be either added or

Table 59.14 Absolute risk of RDS (%) based on TDx-FLM (fetal lung maturity) II ratio and gestational age*.

TDx-FLM II ratio (mg/g)	Gestational age (weeks)										
	29	30	31	32	33	34	35	36	37	38	39
10	98	97	96	95	92	89	85	80	73	–	–
20	94	92	89	85	80	73	65	57	47	38	–
30	85	79	73	65	56	47	38	30	23	17	12
40	64	55	46	37	29	22	17	12	8.7	6.2	4.4
50	37	29	22	16	12	8.5	6.1	4.3	3.0	2.1	1.5
60	16	12	8.4	6.0	4.2	3.0	2.1	1.4	1.0	0.70	0.49
70	5.8	4.1	2.9	2.0	1.4	0.98	0.68	0.47	0.33	0.23	0.16
80	2.0	1.4	0.96	0.67	0.46	0.32	0.22	0.16	0.11	0.07	0.05
90	–	0.45	0.31	0.22	0.15	0.11	0.07	0.05	0.04	0.02	0.02
100	–	–	0.10	0.07	0.05	0.03	0.02	0.02	0.01	< 0.01	< 0.01

From ref. 153, with permission.

*These risk estimates reflect the prevalence pattern of RDS across the gestational age range observed in the current study data. The overall prevalence of RDS in a clinical setting depends on both the prevalence of RDS at each gestational age and the distribution of gestational ages encountered.

significantly increased to cover the acute effects of antenatal corticosteroids, which last approximately 72 h.

Adjunctive therapy

Outside the accepted standard antibiotic regimen for intrapartum chemoprophylaxis for group B streptococci, administering antenatal antibiotics to patients in preterm labor, to prolong "subclinically" infected pregnancies and prevent neonatal sepsis, is still controversial and not established practice. Several large multicenter studies have failed to demonstrate a benefit of prophylactic antibiotics in the prevention of preterm labor in at-risk patients.[160-162]

Operative delivery of the very preterm fetus using procedures such as episiotomy, prophylactic forceps, and prophylactic Cesarean section has not been shown to prevent neonatal birth trauma and IVH.[163-167] Major surgical maneuvers strictly on behalf of the fetus are best reserved for established indications such as nonreassuring fetal heart rate patterns and malpresentation. Even though Cesarean section for the preterm breech fetus is commonly practiced, no randomized studies have shown benefits from operative delivery.[47,48,168,169]

Preventing preterm birth

Most preterm births are due to spontaneous but not idiopathic preterm labor. Preterm labor predictions based on risk scoring systems, biochemical markers, and cervical examination are still of limited value. Prophylaxis with bedrest, cerclage, tocolytic agents, and progestational agents is also of limited value, and HUAM remains highly controversial, with the bulk of evidence not being very supportive.

Advances in risk factor assessment have identified several of the strongest known predictors of spontaneous preterm birth.[170] These are multifetal gestation, a previous spontaneous preterm birth, black race, low BMI (thinness), a positive fFN test result, and a foreshortened cervical length on sonographic evaluation.

Factors that decrease the risk of preterm birth are also important. At 24–26 weeks' gestation, a cervical length of more than 35 mm retrospectively identified a group of 34 women with a low-risk twin pregnancy. Only one delivered before 34 weeks, indicating the high predictive value (97%) of a normal cervical length.

Prevention strategies and policies

Primary prevention focuses on the entire reproductive age population and seeks to eliminate known factors associated with preterm birth. Some of these are summarized in Table 59.15.

A study by Miller and Merritt[171] is a prime example of the potential impact of behavior modification on prematurity. They studied six modifiable behavioral risk factors that are significantly related to LBW: low prepregnant maternal weight for height, low maternal weight gain, lack of prenatal care, age younger than 17 or older than 35 at delivery, cigarette smoking, and the use of drugs/alcohol. Among white women, if three of these variables were present, the risk of a LBW birth was 29%; with two variables, the risk was 10%; with one variable, it was 6.7%; and with none of these variables it was 1%.

Secondary prevention identifies pregnant patients at increased risk for preterm labor and provides education, detection of uterine activity and cervical changes, ready access to medical care, and medical interventions, as necessary, to prolong gestation, including the use of progesterone prophylaxis. Some of these strategies are identified in Table 59.16.

Table 59.15 Primary prevention strategies.

Delay childbearing until age 17 years
Delay interpregnancy interval
Eliminate low maternal weight for height
Smoking prevention and cessation
Prevent and detect sexually transmitted diseases, and treat to cure
Detect bacteriuria and treat to cure
Manage fertility to avoid multifetal gestation
Provide or refer for preconceptional counseling
Detect and treat iron-deficiency anemia
Provide or refer for drug abuse prevention and treatment

Table 59.16 Secondary prevention strategies.

Risk assessment in prenatal care
Improved sufficiency of the content of prenatal care
Repeated education regarding warning signs and symptoms of preterm labor
Early-diagnosis programs
Home uterine activity monitoring, cervical length, oncofetal fibronectin
Early medical intervention
Medications, surgery, early referral
Reduced maternal physical activity
Maternal work leave
Eliminate barriers to care (access, access, access)
Education, education, education

Tertiary prevention focuses on eleventh-hour intensive perinatal care. This includes the use of tocolytics, antibiotics, and corticosteroids, maternal transport to a tertiary care center, emergency cerclage, appropriate mode of delivery, and neonatal intensive care.

Most proximate causes of preterm birth remain unpreventable despite scientific advances and the implementation of prevention and treatment programs. Even if all of the appropriately eligible patients (ideally, previous spontaneous preterm birth presenting for prenatal care between 16 and 20 weeks) were treated with 17P, there would only be a very modest reduction in prematurity.[172] Therefore, it is not reasonable to expect a large reduction in premature births in the foreseeable future in the USA. In the USA, most premature births still occur in low-risk pregnant women as a result of factors which are not yet identifiable. Therefore, prevention strategies may provide the greatest benefit for these low-risk women.

References

1 Arias E, MacDorman MF, Strobino DM, et al. Annual summary of vital statistics, 2002. *Pediatrics* 2003;112:1215.

2 Rush RW, Keirse MJNC, Howat P, et al. Contribution of preterm delivery to perinatal mortality. *Br Med J* 1976;2:965.

3 Amon E, Anderson GD, Sabai BM, et al. Factors responsible for a preterm delivery of the immature newborn infant (< 1000 gm). *Am J Obstet Gynecol* 1987;156:1143.

4 Robertson PA, Sniderman SH, Laros RK, et al. Neonatal morbidity according to gestational age and birthweight from five tertiary care centers in the United States, 1983–1986. *Am J Obstet Gynecol* 1992;166:1629.

5 Amon E, Steigerwald J, Winn HN. Obstetric factors associated with survival of the borderline viable liveborn infant (500–750 gm) (Abstract). *Am J Obstet Gynecol* 1995;172: 418.

6 Lemons JA, Bauer CR, Oh W, et al. Very low birth weight outcomes of the National Institute of Child Health And Human Development Neonatal Research Network, January 1995 through December 1996. NICHD Neonatal Research Network. *Pediatrics* 2001;107(1):E1.

7 Martin JA, Hamilton BE, Sutton PD, et al. Births: final data for 2002. *Natl Vital Stat Rep* 2003;52(10):1.

8 Lettieri L, Vintzileos AM, Rodis JF, et al. Does "idiopathic" preterm labor resulting in preterm birth exist? *Am J Obstet Gynecol* 1993;168:1480.

9 Dudly DJ. Preterm labor: an intrauterine inflammatory response syndrome? *J Reprod Immunol* 1997;36:93.

10 Arias F, Rodriguez L, Rayne SC, et al. Maternal placental vasculopathy and infection: two distinct subgroups among patients with preterm labor and preterm ruptured membranes. *Am J Obstet Gynecol* 1993;168:585.

11 Creasy RK, Gummer BA, Liggins GC. System for predicting spontaneous preterm birth. *Obstet Gynecol* 1980;55:692.

12 Holbrook RH, Laros RK, Creasy RK. Evaluation of a risk-scoring system for prediction of preterm labor. *Am J Perinatol* 1989;6:62.

13 Mercer BM, Goldenberg RL, Das A, et al. The preterm birth prediction study: a clinical risk assessment system. *Am J Obstet Gynecol* 1996;174:1885.

14 Goldenberg RL, Mayberry SK, Copper RL, et al. Pregnancy outcome following a second trimester loss. *Obstet Gynecol* 1993;81:444.

15 Fedrick J, Anderson ABM. Factors associated with spontaneous preterm birth. *Br J Obstet Gynaecol* 1976;83:342.

16 Funderburk S, Guthrie D, Meldrum D. Suboptimal pregnancy outcome among women with prior abortions and premature births. *Am J Obstet Gynecol* 1976;126:55.

17 Carr-Hill RA, Hall MH. The repetition of spontaneous preterm labour. *Br J Obstet Gynaecol* 1985;92:921.

18 Bakketeig LS, Hoffman HJ. The epidemiology of preterm birth: results from a longitudinal study of births in Norway. In: Elder MG, Hendricks CH, eds. *Preterm labor*. London: Butterworth, 1981.

19 Keirse M, Rush R, Anderson A, et al. Risk of preterm delivery in patients with previous preterm delivery and/or abortion. *Br J Obstet Gynaecol* 1978;85:81.

20 Mercer BM, Goldenberg RL, Moawad AH, et al. The Preterm Prediction Study: effect of gestational age and cause of preterm birth on subsequent obstetric outcome. *Am J Obstet Gynecol* 1999;181:1216.

21 Bakketeig LS, Hoffman HJ, Harley EE. The tendency to repeat gestational age and birth weight in successive births. *Am J Obstet Gynecol* 1979;135:1086.

22 Iams JD, Golderberg RL, Meis PJ, et al. The length of the cervix and the risk of spontaneous delivery. *N Engl J Med* 1996;334:567.

23 Gomez R, Galasso M, Romero R, et al. Ultrasonographic examination of the uterine cervix is better than cervical digital examination as a predictor of the likelihood of premature delivery in patients with preterm labor and intact membranes. *Am J Obstet Gynecol* 1994;171:956.

24 Iams JD. Opinion: cervical ultrasonography. *Ultrasound Obstet Gynecol* 1997;10:156.

25 Doyle NM, Monga M. Role of ultrasound in screening patients at risk for preterm delivery. *Obstet Gynecol Clin North Am* 2004;31:125.

26 American College of Obstetricians and Gynecologists. ACOG Committee Opinion no. 172. Home uterine activity monitoring. *Int J Gynecol Obstet* 1996;54:71.

27 Chien PF, Kahn KS, Ogston S, et al. The diagnostic accuracy of cervico-vaginal fetal fibronectin in predicting preterm delivery: an overview. *Br J Obstet Gynaecol* 1997;104:436.

28 Peaceman AM, Andrews WW, Thorp JM, et al. Fetal fibronectin as a predictor of preterm birth in patients with symptoms: a multicenter trial. *Am J Obstet Gynecol* 1997;177:13.

29 Ascarelli MH, Morrison JC. Use of fetal fibronectin in clinical practice. *Obstet Gynecol Surv* 1997;52:S1.

30 Tekesesin I, Marek S, Hellmeyer L, et al. Assessment of rapid fetal fibronectin in predicting preterm delivery. *Obstet Gynecol* 2005;105:280.

31 Lukes AS, Thorp JM, Eucker BSN, et al. Predictors of positivity for fetal fibronectin in patients with symptoms of preterm labor. *Am J Obstet Gynecol* 1997;176:639.

32 Faron G, Boulvain M, Lescrainier JP, et al. A single fetal fibronectin screening test in a population at low risk for preterm delivery: an improvement on clinical indicators? *Br J Obstet Gynaecol* 1997;104:697.

33 Goldenberg RL, Mercer BM, Meis PJ, et al. The preterm prediction study: fetal fibronectin testing and spontaneous preterm birth. *Obstet Gynecol* 1996;87:643.

34 Andrews WW, Sibai BM, Thom EA, et al. Randomized clinical trial of metronidazole plus erythromycin to prevent spontaneous preterm delivery in fetal fibronectin-positive women. *Obstet Gynecol* 2003;101:847.

35 Gibbs RS, Romero R, Hillier SL, et al. A review of premature birth and subclinical infection. *Am J Obstet Gynecol* 1992;166:1515.

36 Romero R, Oyarzun E, Mazor M, et al. Meta-analysis of the relationship between symptomatic bacteriuria and preterm delivery/low birthweight. *Obstet Gynecol* 1989;73:576.

37 Thomsen AC, Morup L, Hansen KB. Antibiotic elimination of group B streptococci in urine in prevention of preterm labor. *Lancet* 1987;1:591.

38 Klebanoff MA, Regan JA, Rao AV, et al. Outcome of the vaginal infections and prematurity study: results of a clinical trial of erythromycin among pregnant women colonized with group B Streptococci. *Am J Obstet Gynecol* 1995;172:1540.

39 Hillier SL, Nugent RP, Eschenbach DA, et al. Association between bacterial vaginosis and preterm delivery of a low birth weight infant. *N Engl J Med* 1995;333:1737.

40 Okun N, Gronau KA, Hannah ME. Antibiotics for bacterial vaginosis or Trichomonas vaginalis in pregnancy: a systematic review. *Obstet Gynecol* 2005;105:857.

41 Valenzuela G, Cline S, Hayashi R. Follow-up of hydration and sedation in the pretherapy of premature labor. *Am J Obstet Gynecol* 1983;147:396.

42 Catalano PM, Ashikaga T, Mann LI. Cervical change and uterine activity as predictors of preterm delivery. *Am J Perinatol* 1989;6:185.

43 Amon E, Sibai BM, Anderson GD, et al. Obstetric variables predicting survival of the immature newborn (< 1000gm.): a five year experience at a single perinatal center. *Am J Obstet Gynecol* 1987;156:1380.

44 Smith RS, Bottoms SF. Ultrasonographic prediction of neonatal survival in extremely low birth weight infants. *Am J Obstet Gynecol* 1939;169:490.

45 Tamura RK, Sabbagha RE, Depp R, et al. Diminished growth in fetuses born preterm after spontaneous labor or rupture of membranes. *Am J Obstet Gynecol* 1984;148:1105.

46 Weiner CP, Sabbagha RE, Visrub N, et al. A hypothetical model suggesting suboptimal intrauterine growth in infants delivered preterm. *Obstet Gynecol* 1985;65:323.

47 Amon E, Sibai BM, Anderson GD. How perinatologists manage the problem of the presenting breech fetus. *Am J Perinatol* 1988;5:247.

48 Penn ZJ, Steer PJ. How obstetricians manage the problem of preterm delivery with special reference to the preterm breech. *Br J Obstet Gynaecol* 1991;98:531.

49 Robertson PA, Foran CM, Croughan-Minimane MS, et al. Head entrapment and neonatal outcome by mode of delivery in breech deliveries from 24 to 27 weeks of gestation. *Am J Obstet Gynecol* 1995;173:1171.

50 Vintzileos AM, Campbell WA, Nochimson DJ, et al. The use and misuse of the fetal biophysical profile. *Am J Obstet Gynecol* 1987;156:527.

51 Stubblefield PG. Causes and prevention of premature birth: an overview. In: Fuchs AR,

Fuchs F, Stubblefield PG, eds. *Preterm birth: causes, prevention, and management,* 2nd edn. New York: McGraw-Hill; 1993:3.

52 Donnenfeld AE, Mennuti MT. Sonographic findings in fetuses with common chromosome abnormalities. *Clin Obstet Gynecol* 1988;31:80.

53 Kirbinen P, Jouppila P. Polyhydramnios: a clinical study. *Ann Chir Gynaecol* 1978;67:117.

54 Harlow BL, Frigoletto FD, Cramer DW, et al. Determinants of preterm delivery in low-risk pregnancies. *J Clin Epidemiol* 1996;49:441.

55 Romero R, Munoz H, Gomez R, et al. Does infection cause preterm labor and delivery? *Semin Reprod Endocrinol* 1994;12:227.

56 Fedele L, Zamberletti D, Vercellini P, et al. Reproductive performance of women with unicornuate uterus. *Fertil Steril* 1987;47:416.

57 Morrison JJ, Rennie JM. Clinical scientific and ethical aspects of fetal and neonatal care at extremely preterm periods of gestation. *Br J Obstet Gynaecol* 1997;104:1341.

58 Yu VYH, Wong PY, Bajuk B, et al. Outcome of extremely low birthweight infants. *Br J Obstet Gynaecol* 1986;93:196.

59 Miyazaki FS, Taylor NA. Saline amnioinfusion for relief of variable or prolonged decelerations. *Am J Obstet* 1983;146:670.

60 Mendez-Bauer C, Shekarloo A, Cook V, et al. Treatment of acute intrapartum fetal distress by beta2 sympathomimetics. *Am J Obstet* 1987;156:638.

61 Lipshitz J, Bailie P. Uterine and cardiovascular effects of beta2-selective sympathomimetic drugs administered as an intravenous infusion. *S Afr Med J* 1976;50:1973.

62 Grospietsch G, Kuhn W. Effects of β-mimetics on maternal physiology. In: Fuchs F, Stubblefield PG, eds. *Preterm birth: causes, prevention, and management.* New York: Macmillan; 1984:171.

63 Caritis SN, Chiao JP, Moore JJ, et al. Myometrial desensitization after ritodrine infusion. *Am J Physiol* 1987;253:E410.

64 Berg G, Anderson RGG, Ryden G. β-adrenergic receptors in human myometrium during pregnancy. Changes in the numbers of receptors after β-mimetic treatment. *Am J Obstet Gynecol* 1985;151:392.

65 Hendricks SK, Keroes J, Katz M. Electrocardiographic changes associated with ritodrine-induced maternal tachycardia and hypokalemia. *Am J Obstet Gynecol* 1986;154:921.

66 Barden TP, Peter JB, Merkatz IR. Ritodrine hydrochloride: a betamimetic agent for use in preterm labor. I. Pharmacology, clinical history, administration, side effects, and safety. *Obstet Gynecol* 1980;56:1.

67 Milliez S, Blot PH, Sureau C. A case report of maternal death associated with betamimetic and betamethasone administration in premature labor. *Eur J Obstet Gynecol Reprod Biol* 1980;2:95.

68 Hudgens DR, Conradi SE. Sudden death associated with terbutaline sulfate administration. *Am J Obstet Gynecol* 1993;172:416.

69 Benedetti TJ. Maternal complications of parenteral beta-sympathomimetic therapy for preterm labor. *Am J Obstet Gynecol* 1983;145:1.

70 Spellacy WN, Cruz AC, Buhi WC, et al. The acute effects of ritodrine infusion on maternal metabolism: measurements of levels of glucose, insulin, glucagons, triglycerides, cholesterol, placental lactogen, and chronic gonadotropin. *Am J Obstet Gynecol* 1978;131:637.

71 Lipshitz J, Vinik AI. The effects of hexoprenaline, a beta2-sympathomimetic drug, on maternal glucose, insulin, glucagons, and free fatty acid levels. *Am J Obstet Gynecol* 1978;130:761.

72 Lenz S, Kuhl C, Wang P, et al. The effect of ritodrine on carbohydrate and lipid metabolism in normal and diabetic pregnant women. *Acta Endocrinol* 1979;92:669.

73 Wager J, Fredholm B, Lunell N, et al. Metabolic and circulatory effects of intravenous and oral salbutamol in late pregnancy in diabetic and non-diabetic women. *Acta Obstet Gynecol Scand* 1982;108(Suppl.):41.

74 Huisjes JH, Touwen BC. Neonatal outcome after treatment with ritodrine: a controlled study. *Am J Obstet Gynecol* 1983;147:250.

75 Hancock PJ, Setzer ES, Beydoun SN. Physiologic and biochemical effects of ritodrine therapy in the mother and perinate. *Am J Perinatol* 1985;2:1.

76 Brazy JE, Eckerman CO, Gross SJ. Clinical and laboratory observations. Follow-up of infants of < 1500 gram birth weight with antenatal isoxsuprine exposure. *J Pediatr* 1983;102:611.

77 Haddengra M, Touwen BCL, Huisjes JH. Longterm follow-up of children prenatally exposed to ritodrine. *Br J Obstet Gynaecol* 1986;1:156.

78 Freysz H, Williard D, Lehr A, et al. A long term evaluation of infants who received a beta-mimetic drug while in utero. *J Perinat Med* 1977;5:94.

79 Svenningsen NW. Follow-up studies on preterm infants after maternal beta-receptor agonist treatment. *Acta Obstet Gynecol Scand* 1982;108(Suppl.):67.

80 Polowczyk D, Tejani N, Laursen N, et al. Evaluation of seven-to-nine-year old children exposed to ritodrine in utero. *Obstet Gynecol* 1984;64:485.

81 Merkatz IR, Peter JB, Barden TP. Ritodrine hydrochloride: a betamimetic agent for use in preterm labor. II. Evidence of efficacy. *Obstet Gynecol* 1980;56:7.

82 Canadian Preterm Labor Investigators Group. Treatment of preterm labor with the beta-adrenergic agonist ritodrine. *N Engl J Med* 1992;327:308.

83 Macones GA, Berlin M, Berlin JA. Efficacy of oral beta-agonist maintenance therapy in preterm labor: a meta-analysis. *Obstet Gynecol* 1995;85:313.

84 Caritis SN, Tolg G, Heddinger LA, et al. A double-blind study comparing ritodrine and terbutaline in the treatment of preterm labor. *J Obstet Gynecol* 1984;150:7.

85 Stubblefield PG, Heyl PS. Treatment of premature labor with subcutaneous terbutaline. *Obstet Gynecol* 1982;59:457.

86 Moise KJ, Dorman K, Giebel R, et al. A randomized study of intravenous versus subcutaneous/oral terbutaline in the treatment of preterm labor (Abstract 276). Presented at the Seventh Annual Meeting of the Society of Perinatal Obstetricians, Lake Buena Vista, FL, February 1987.

87 Leferink JG, Lamont H, Wagenmaker-Engles I, et al. Pharmacokinetics of terbutaline after subcutaneous administration. *Int J Clin Pharmacol Biopharmacol* 1979;17:181.

88 Carpenter RJ, Jr, Decuir P. Cardiovascular collapse associated with oral terbutaline tocolytic therapy. *Am J Obstet Gynecol* 1984;146:821.

89 Lampert MB, Hibbard J, Weinert L, et al. Peripartum heart failure associated with prolonged tocolytic therapy. *Am J Obstet Gynecol* 1993;168:493.

90 Repke JR, Niebyl JR. Role of prostaglandin synthetase inhibitors in the treatment of preterm labor. *Semin Reprod Endocrinol* 1985;3:29.

91 Morales WJ, Smith SG, Angel JL, et al. Efficacy and safety of indomethacin versus ritodrine in the management of preterm labor: a randomized study. *Obstet Gynecol* 1989;74:567.

92 Kurki T, Eronen M, Lumme R, et al. A randomized double-dummy comparison between indomethacin and nylidrin in threatened preterm labor. *Am J Obstet Gynecol* 1991;164:981.

93 Besinger RE, Niebyl JR, Keyes WG. Randomized comparative trial of indomethacin and ritodrine for the long-term treatment of preterm labor. *Am J Obstet Gynecol* 1991;164:981.

94 Morales WJ, Madhav H. Efficacy and safety of indomethacin compared with magnesium

sulfate in the management of preterm labor: a randomized study. *Am J Obstet Gynecol* 1993;169:97.

95 Moise KJ, Huhta JC, Ddawod S, et al. Indomethacin in the treatment of preterm labor: effects on the human fetal ductus arteriosus. *N Engl J Med* 1988;319:327.

96 Itskovitz J, Abramovich H, Brandes JM. Oligohydramnios, meconium and perinatal death concurrent with indomethacin treatment in human pregnancy. *J Reprod Med* 1980;24:137.

97 Vanhaesebrouck P, Thiery M, Leroy JG, et al. Oligohydramnios, renal insufficiency, and ileal perforation in preterm infants after uterine exposure to indomethacin. *J Pediatr* 1988;113:737.

98 Rasmussen LF, Wennberger RP. Displacement of bilirubin from albumin binding sites by indomethacin. *Clin Res* 1977;25:2.

99 Norton ME, Merrill J, Cooper BAB, et al. Neonatal complications after the administration of indomethacin for preterm labor. *N Engl J Med* 1993;329:160.

100 Major CA, Lewis DF, Harding JA, et al. Tocolysis with indomethacin increases the incidence of necrotizing enterocolitis in the low birth weight neonate. *Am J Obstet Gynecol* 1994;170:102.

101 Altura BM, Altura BT, Carella A, et al. Mg^{+2}-Ca^{+2} interacts in contractility of smooth muscle: magnesium versus organic calcium channel blockers on myogenic tone and agonist-induced responsiveness of blood vessels. *Can J Physiol Pharmacol* 1987; 65:729.

102 Cruikshank DP, Pitkin RM, Donnelly E, et al. Urinary magnesium, calcium, and phosphate excretion during magnesium sulfate infusion. *Obstet Gynecol* 1981;58:430.

103 Hoff HE, Smith PK, Winkler AW. Effects of magnesium on nervous system in relation to its concentration in serum. *Am J Physiol* 1940;130:292.

104 Winkler AW, Smith PK, Hoff HE. Intravenous magnesium sulfate in the treatment of nephritic convulsions in adults. *J Clin Invest* 1942;21:207.

105 Chesley LC. Parenteral magnesium sulfate and the distribution, plasma levels, and excretion of magnesium. *Am J Obstet Gynecol* 1979;133:1.

106 McCubbln JH, Sibai BM, Abdella TN, et al. Cardiopulmonary arrest due to acute maternal hypermagnesaemia. *Lancet* 1981;1:1058.

107 Wilkins IA, Lynch L, Mehalek KE, et al. Efficacy and side effects of magnesium sulfate and ritodrine as tocolytic agents. *Am J Obstet Gynecol* 1988;159:685.

108 Wilkins IA, Goldberg JD, Phillips RN, et al. Long-term use of magnesium sulfate as a tocolytic agent. *Obstet Gynecol* 1986;67:385.

109 Ferguson JE, II, Hensleigh PA, Kredenster D. Adjunctive use of magnesium sulfate with ritodrine for preterm labor tocolysis. *Am J Obstet Gynecol* 1984;148:166.

110 Katz M, Robertson PA, Creasy RK. Cardiovascular complications associated with terbutaline treatment for preterm labor. *Am J Obstet Gynecol* 1981;139:605.

111 Ogburn PL, Hansen CA, Williams PP, et al. Magnesium sulfate and β-mimetic dual-agent tocolysis in preterm labor after single-agent failure. *J Reprod Med* 1985;30:583.

112 Diamond MP, Mulloy MK, Entman SS. Combined use of ritodrine and magnesium sulfate for tocolysis of preterm labor (Letter). *Am J Obstet Gynecol* 1985;148:827.

113 Amon E, Petrie RH. Magnesium sulfate, nifedipine, and other calcium antagonists. In: Fuchs AR, Fuchs F, Stubblefield PG, eds. *Preterm birth: causes, prevention, and management*, 2nd edn. New York: McGraw-Hill; 1993:333.

114 Holcomb WL, Schackelford GD, Petrie RH. Magnesium tocolysis and neonatal bone abnormalities. *Obstet Gynecol* 1991;78:611.

115 Smith LG, Burns PA, Schanler RF. Calcium homeostasis in pregnant women receiving long-term magnesium sulfate therapy for preterm labor. *Am J Obstet Gynecol* 1992;167:45.

116 Rusu O, Lupan C, Baltescu V. MagnezivI serie in sarcina normala la termen si nasterea

prematura. Rolvl magneziterapiei in combatera nasterii premature. *Obstet Gynecol* 1966;14:215.

117 Steer CM, Petrie RH. A comparison of magnesium sulfate and alcohol for the prevention of premature labor. *Am J Obstet Gynecol* 1977;129:1.

118 Elliott JP, Radin TG. Serum magnesium levels during magnesium sulfate tocolysis in high-order multiple gestations. *J Reprod Med* 1995;40:450.

119 Amon E, Midkiff C, Winn HN, et al. Tocolysis with advanced cervical dilatation. *Obstet Gynecol* 2000;95:358.

120 Lewis DF, Grimshaw A, Brooks G, et al. A comparison of magnesium sulfate and indomethacin to magnesium sulfate to magnesium sulfate only for tocolysis in preterm labor with advanced cervical dilatation. *South Med J* 1995;88:737.

121 Dudley D, Gagnon D, Varner M. Long-term tocolysis with intravenous magnesium sulfate. *Obstet Gynecol* 1989;73:373.

122 Cumming WA, Thomas VJ. Hypermagnesemia. A cause of abnormal metaphyses in the neonate. *Am J Roentgenol* 1989;152:1071.

123 Hall DG. Serum magnesium in pregnancy. *Obstet Gynecol* 1957;9:158.

124 Martin RW, Martin IN, Pryor JA, et al. Comparison of oral ritodrine and magnesium gluconate for ambulatory tocolysis. *Am J Obstet Gynecol* 1988;158:1440.

125 Kiss D, Stoke B. Rolle des Magnesiums bei der verhuttung des frühgeburt. *Zentralb Gynakol* 1975;97:924.

126 Kiss V, Balasz M, Morvav F, et al. Effect of maternal magnesium supply on spontaneous abortion and premature birth and on intrauterine foetal development: experimental epidemiological study. *Mag Bull* 1988;3:73.

127 Spatling L, Spading G. Magnesium supplementation in pregnancy: a double-blind study. *Br J Obstet Gynaecol* 1988;95:120.

128 Martin RW, Gaddy DK, Martin JN, et al. Tocolysis with oral magnesium. *Am J Obstet Gynecol* 1987;156:433.

129 Sibai BM. The use of magnesium sulfate in preeclampsia-eclampsia. In: Petrie RH, ed. *Perinatal pharmacology.* Oradell, NJ: Medical Economics, 1989.

130 Petrie RH. Tocolysis using magnesium sulfate. *Semin Perinatol* 1981;5:266.

131 Elliott JP. Magnesium sulfate for tocolysis. In: Petrie RH, ed. *Perinatal pharmacology.* Oradell, NJ: Medical Economics. 1989.

132 Amon E, Petrie RH. Magnesium as a tocolytic agent. *Clin Consult Obstet Gynecol* 1991;3:231.

133 Lewis JG. Adverse reactions to calcium antagonists. *Drugs* 1983;25:196.

134 Talbert RL, Bussey HI. Update on calcium channel blocking agents. *Clin Pharmacol* 1983;2:403.

135 Raemsch KD, Sommer J. Pharmacokinetics and metabolism of nifedipine. *Hypertension* 1983;5(Suppl.2):18.

136 Sawaya GE, Robertson PA. Hepatotoxicity with the administration of nifedipine for treatment of preterm labor. *Am J Obstet Gynecol* 1992;167:512.

137 Snyder SW, Cardwell MS. Neuromuscular blockade with magnesium sulfate and nifedipine. *Am J Obstet Gynecol* 1989;161:35.

138 Ben-ami M, Giladi Y, Shalev E. The combination of magnesium sulfate and nifedipine: a cause of neuromuscular blockade. *Br J Obstet Gynaecol* 1994;101:262.

139 Koontz SL, Friedman SA, Schwartz ML. Symptomatic hypocalcemia after tocolytic therapy with magnesium sulfate and nifedipine. *Am J Obstet Gynecol* 2004;190:1773.

140 Papatsonis DN, Van Geijn HP, Ader HJ, et al. Nifedipine and ritodrine in the management of preterm labor: a randomized multicenter trial. *Obstet Gynecol* 1997;90:230.

141 Meis PJ, Klebanoff M, Thom E, et al. Prevention of recurrent preterm delivery by 17 alpha-hydroxyprogesterone caproate. *N Engl J Med* 2003;348:2379.

142 da Fonseca EB, Bittar RE, Carvalho MH, et al. Prophylactic administration of progesterone by vaginal suppository to reduce the incidence of spontaneous preterm birth in women at increased risk: a randomized placebo-controlled double blind study. *Am J Obstet Gynecol* 2003;188:419.

143 Fuchs AR, Fuchs F, Husslein P, et al. Oxytocin receptors in the human uterus during pregnancy and parturition. *Am J Obstet Gynecol* 1984;150:734.

144 Akerlund M, Stromberg P, Hauksson A, et al. Inhibition of uterine contractions of premature labour with an oxytocin analogue. Results from a pilot study. *Br J Obstet Gynaecol* 1987;94:1040.

145 Wilson L, Parsons MT, Quano L, et al. A new tocolytic agent: development of an oxytocin antagonist for inhibiting uterine contractions. *Am J Obstet Gynecol* 1990;163:195.

146 Andersen LF, Lyndrup J, Akerlund M, et al. Oxytocin receptor blockade: a new principle in the treatment of preterm labor? *Am J Perinatol* 1989;6:196.

147 El-Sayed YY, Riley ET, Holbrook RH, Jr, et al. Randomized comparison of intravenous nitroglycerin and magnesium sulfate for treatment of preterm labor. *Obstet Gynecol* 1999;93:79.

148 Smith GN, Walker MC, McGrath MJ. Randomized, double-blind, placebo controlled pilot study assessing nitroglycerin as a tocolytic. *Br J Obstet Gynaecol* 1999;106:736.

149 Liggins GC, Howie RN. A controlled trial of antepartum glucocorticoid treatment for prevention of the respiratory distress syndrome in premature infants. *Pediatrics* 1972;50:515.

150 Garite TJ, Rumney PJ, Briggs GG, et al. A randomized placebo controlled trial of betamethasone for the prevention of respiratory distress syndrome at 24 to 28 weeks gestation. *Am J Obstet Gynecol* 1992;166:646.

151 Wright LL, Horbar JD, Gunkel H, et al. Evidence from the multicenter networks on the current use and effectiveness of antenatal corticosteroids in low birth weight infants. *Am J Obstet Gynecol* 1995;173:263.

152 NIH Consensus Statement. Effect of corticosteroids for fetal maturation on prenatal outcomes, February 28 to March 2, 1994. *Am J Obstet Gynecol* 1995;173:246.

153 Ballard PL, Ballard RA. Scientific basis and therapeutic regimens for use of antenatal glucocorticoids. *Am J Obstet Gynecol* 1995;173:253.

154 Elliott JP, Radin TG. The effect of corticosteroid administration on uterine activity and preterm labor in high-order multiple gestations. *Obstet Gynecol* 1995;85:250.

155 Parvin CA, Kaplan LA, Chapman JF, et al. Predicting respiratory distress syndrome using gestational age and fetal lung maturity by fluorescent polarization. *Am J Obstet Gynecol* 2005;192:199.

156 Vermillion ST, Bland ML, Soper DE. Effectiveness of a rescue dose of antenatal betamethasone after an initial single dose. *Am J Obstet Gynecol* 2001;185:1086.

157 Sen S, Reghu A, Ferguson SD. Efficacy of a single dose of antenatal steroid in surfactant-treated babies under 31 weeks' gestation. *J Maternal Fetal Neonatal Med* 2002;12:298.

158 Crowley PA. Antenatal corticosteroid therapy: a meta analysis of the randomized trials, 1972–1994. *Am J Obstet Gynecol* 1995;173:322.

159 Bedalov A, Balasubramanyarn A. Glucocorticoid-induced ketoacidosis in gestational diabetes: a sequela of the acute treatment of preterm labor. *Diabetes Care* 1997;20:922.

160 Vermeulen GM, Bruinse HW. Prophylactic administration of clindamycin 2% vaginal cream to reduce the incidence of spontaneous preterm birth in women with an increased recurrence risk: a randomised placebo-controlled double-blind trial. *Br J Obstet Gynaecol* 1999;106:652.

161 Carey JC, Klebanoff MA, Hauth JC, et al. Metronidazole to prevent preterm delivery in pregnant women with asymptomatic bacterial vaginosis. National Institute of Child Health and Human Development Network of Maternal-Fetal Medicine Units. *N Engl J Med* 2000;342:534.

162 Huff DL, Thurnau GR, Sheldon R. The outcome of protective forceps deliveries of 26–33 week infants (Abstract 45). *Proc Soc Perinatal Obstet* 1987.

163 Anderson GC, Bada HS, Sibai BM, et al. The relationship between labor and route of delivery in the preterm infant. *Am J Obstet Gynecol* 1988;158:1382.

164 Tejani N, Verma U, Hameed C, Chayen B. Method and route of delivery in the low birth weight vertex presentation correlated with early periventricular/intraventricular hemorrhage. *Obstet Gynecol* 1987;69:1.

165 Schwartz D, Miodovnik M, Lavin J. Neonatal outcome among low birth weight infants delivered spontaneously or by low forceps. *Obstet Gynecol* 1983;62:283.

166 Died J, Arnold H, Mentzel H, et al. Effect of cesarean section on outcome in high- and low-risk very preterm infants. *Arch Gynecol Obstet* 1989;246:91.

167 Grant A, Glazener CM. Elective caesarean section versus expectant management for delivery of the small baby. *Cochrane Database Syst Rev* 2001;2:CD000078.

168 Penn ZJ, Steer PJ, Grant A. A multicentre randomised controlled trial comparing elective and selective caesarean section for the delivery of the preterm breech infant. *Br J Obstet Gynaecol* 1996;103:684.

169 Grant A, Penn ZJ, Steer PJ. Elective or selective caesarean delivery of the small baby? A systematic review of the controlled trials. *Br J Obstet Gynaecol* 1996;103:1197.

170 Goldenberg RL, Iams JD, Mercer BM, et al. The preterm birth prediction study: the value of new vs old risk factors in predicting early and all spontaneous preterm births. *Am J Public Health* 1998;88:233.

171 Miller HC, Merritt TA. *Fetal growth in humans.* Chicago, IL: Year Book Medical Publishers, 1977.

172 Petrini KR, Callaghan WM, Klebanoff M, et al. Estimated effect of 17 alpha-hydroxyprogesterone caproate on preterm birth in the United States. *Obstet Gynecol* 2005;105:267.

173 Kliegman RM, Rottman CJ, Behrman RE. Strategies for the prevention of low birth weight infants. *Am J Obstet Gynecol* 1990;162:1073.

174 Utter GO, Dooley SL, Tamura RK, et al. Awaiting cervical change for the diagnosis of preterm labor does not compromise the efficacy of ritodrine tocolysis. *Am J Obstet Gynecol* 1990;163:882.

175 Moretti M, Fairle FM, Aki S, et al. The effect of nifedipine therapy on fetal and placental Doppler waveforms in preeclampsia remote from term. *Am J Obstet Gynecol* 1990;163:1844.

Further reading

Crowther CA, Hiller JE, Doyle LW, et al. Effect of magnesium sulfate given for neuroprotection before preterm birth: a randomized controlled trial. *JAMA* 2003;26;2669.

Guinn DA, Atkinson MW, Sullivan L, et al. Single vs weekly courses of antenatal corticosteroids for women at risk of preterm delivery: A randomized controlled trial. *JAMA* 2001;286:1581.

Myers ER, Alvarez JG, Richardson DK. Cost-effectiveness of fetal lung maturity testing in preterm labor. *Obstet Gynecol* 1997;90:824.

Papiernik E, Breart G. Should a prevention program be proposed to high risk patients or all patients? *Am J Obstet Gynecol* 1994:171:1676.

Sawdy RJ, Lye S, Fisk NM,. A double-blind randomized study of fetal side effects during and after the short-term maternal administration of indomethacin, sulindac, and nimesulide for the treatment of preterm labor. *Am J Obstet Gynecol* 2003;188:1046.

Prelabor rupture of the membranes

Joaquin Santolaya-Forgas, Roberto Romero,
Jimmy Espinoza, Offer Erez, Lara A. Friel,
Juan Pedro Kusanovic, Ray Bahado-Singh, and
Jyh Kae Nien

Prelabor rupture of the membranes (PROM) refers to rupture of the chorioamniotic membranes before the onset of labor.[1] The "latency period" is the interval between PROM and the onset of labor. Term PROM occurs in approximately 10% of patients, while the frequency of preterm PROM is 2–3.5%.[2–7] Preterm PROM accounts for 30–40% of preterm deliveries and, therefore, is a leading clinically identifiable cause of preterm birth and a major contributor to perinatal morbidity and mortality.

The term "fetal membranes" is applied to an anatomical structure that includes amnion and chorion (of fetal origin) and portions of decidua (of maternal origin). Examination of the chorioamniotic membranes from patients undergoing elective Cesarean delivery at term with intact membranes has demonstrated that membranes apposed to the cervix have localized morphologic changes that have been referred to as a "zone of altered morphology" (ZAM).[8] ZAM is proposed to encompass an area of about $119 \pm 21 \, cm^2$ [9] and is characterized by marked swelling and disruption of the connective tissue, thinning of the trophoblast layer, and thinning or absence of the decidua.[8] Membranes that rupture before labor have decreased elasticity.[10,11] It has been proposed that these membranes have focal areas of weakness rather than a generalized weakening.[12–16]

Matrix metalloproteinases (MMPs) are proteases that can degrade several components of the chorioamniotic membranes. The amnion, chorion, and decidua are sources of MMPs and their tissue inhibitors (TIMP-1 and TIMP-2).[17–27] Evidence supports the role of MMPs in both preterm and term PROM. Indeed, preterm PROM has been associated with high amniotic fluid concentrations of immunoreactive MMP-1, MMP-8,[22,25] and the active form of MMP-9,[23] but with low amniotic fluid concentrations of the active form of MMP-2[23] and immunoreactive TIMP-2. PROM at term has been associated with high amniotic fluid concentrations of the active form of MMP-9,[23] but not of other MMPs.

Intra-amniotic infection/inflammation has been implicated in term and preterm PROM. Indeed, preterm PROM is associated with positive amniotic fluid cultures in approximately 30% of cases.[28] However, when amniocenteses are performed at the time of the onset of labor, 75% of patients have microbial invasion of the amniotic cavity.[29] Moreover, histologic examination of the placenta of women who delivered with preterm PROM identified two major subclusters of patients: those with acute histologic chorioamnionitis and those with vascular lesions of the placenta.

Vaginal bleeding, a short cervix ($\leq 25\,mm$), a history of previous spontaneous preterm delivery (with intact or ruptured membranes), and smoking are risk factors for preterm PROM in the index pregnancy. The risk of PROM in a subsequent pregnancy is 4% if the patient's first pregnancy went to term and was not complicated by PROM. In contrast, the recurrence rate of preterm PROM is 21%, whereas that of term PROM is 26%.[30]

The main consequences of preterm PROM are: (1) spontaneous onset of labor leading to prematurity;[31-33] (2) infection;[28] (3) abruptio placentae;[34] (4) fetal death;[35] and (5) the oligohydramnios sequence. Gestational age at the time of PROM and the presence of oligohydramnios, but not the latency period, are independent predictors of the subsequent development of pulmonary hypoplasia.[36] The risk of pulmonary hypoplasia when PROM occurs at 19 weeks is 50%, whereas this risk is only 10% when the membranes rupture at 25 weeks.[37]

The prevalence of positive amniotic fluid cultures in women with preterm and term PROM are 32.4% (473/1462)[28] and 34.3% (11/32)[38] respectively. Of interest, fetal blood cultures can yield positive results in about 10% of cases with preterm PROM.[39] In preterm PROM, genital mycoplasmas (*Ureaplasma urealyticum* and *Mycoplasma hominis*) are the most frequent isolates from the amniotic fluid, followed by *Streptococcus agalactiae*, *Fusobacterium* species, and *Gardnerella vaginalis*. Polymicrobial infection is found in 26.7% (43/161) of cases.[29,40-45]

The most common microorganisms isolated from women with term PROM are *U. urealyticum*, *Peptostreptococcus*, *Lactobacillus*, *Bacteroides* species, and *Fusobacterium*.[38] Microorganisms isolated from the amniotic fluid in women with term and preterm PROM are qualitatively similar.

Amniotic fluid, when put on a slide and allowed to dry, will show arborization ("ferning") under the microscope at low magnification.[46] This method has an overall accuracy of 95% in identifying membrane rupture.[47] Inspection for pooling and nitrazine tests are also frequently performed. When the diagnosis of preterm PROM is not clear, a transabdominal injection of dye (indigo carmine, Evans blue, fluorescein) into the amniotic cavity may be used for confirmation.[48-51] Methylene blue should not be used, as it may cause fetal methemoglobinemia.[52-54] A tampon in the vagina can document subsequent dye leakage in cases of PROM.

The major objection to a digital examination in the setting of PROM is that it may unnecessarily increase the risk of ascending infection, and the information it provides can be obtained by sterile speculum examination. Indeed, visual examination underestimated actual cervical dilation by only 0.6 cm (95% CI 0.58–0.62).[55-57]

The initial evaluation of a patient with preterm PROM includes: (1) accurate assessment of gestational age; (2) estimation of fetal weight and presentation; (3) evaluation of the risk of infection; (4) determination of lung maturity; (5) assessment of fetal well-being; and (6) exclusion of occult cord prolapse. The available evidence indicates that fetal lung maturity studies can be performed on amniotic fluid obtained from the vagina, and that a mature lecithin-to-sphingomyelin (L/S) ratio or the presence of phosphatidylglycerol (PG) is associated with a very low risk of respiratory distress syndrome. Moreover, this noninvasive, low-risk approach

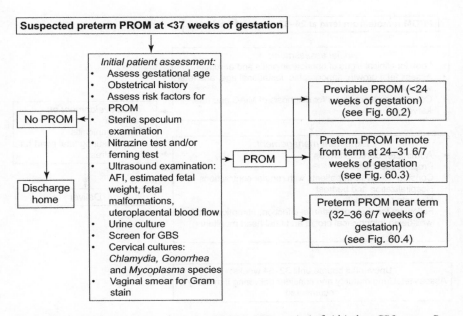

Figure 60.1 Initial assessment of preterm PROM. AFI, amniotic fluid index; GBS, group B *Streptococcus*. Modified from Mercer BM. *Clin Perinatol* 2004;31:765–782.

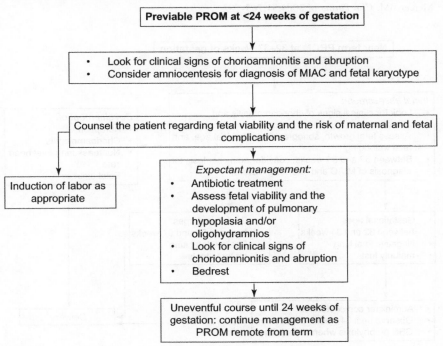

Figure 60.2 Management of previable PROM (before 24 weeks of gestation). MIAC, microbial invasion of the amniotic cavity. Modified from Mercer BM. *Clin Perinatol* 2004;31:765–782.

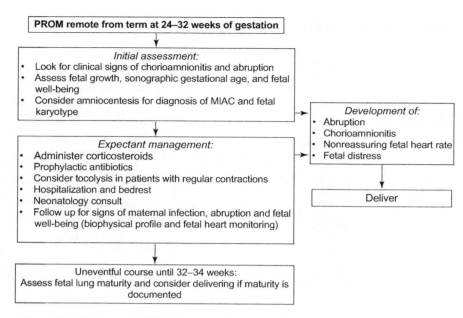

Figure 60.3 Management of PROM remote from term (between 24 weeks and 31 weeks and 6 days of gestation). MIAC, microbial invasion of the amniotic cavity. Modified from Mercer BM. *Clin Perinatol* 2004;31:765–782.

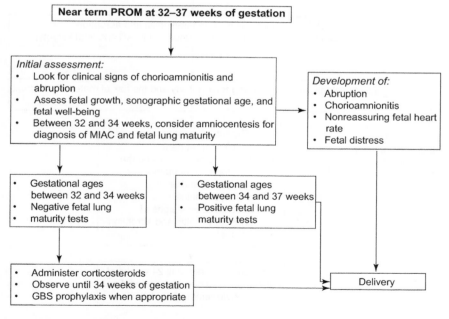

Figure 60.4 Management of near term PROM (between 32 and 37 weeks of gestation). MIAC, microbial invasion of the amniotic cavity; GBS, group B *Streptococcus*. Modified from Mercer BM. *Clin Perinatol* 2004;31:765–782.

allows for serial L/S and PG determinations. See Figs 60.1–60.4 on the management of preterm PROM.

The management of patients with PROM at term includes: (1) exclusion of cord prolapse; (2) detection of infection; and (3) evaluation of fetal well-being. Expectant management at home of patients with PROM at term is not recommended. This recommendation is based upon the report by Hanna et al. that home care was associated with an increased risk of neonatal infections (OR 1.97, 95% CI 1.00–3.90) and Cesarean delivery in patients not colonized with group B *Streptococcus* (OR 1.48, 95% CI 1.03–2.14).[58]

References

1 Keirse MJ, Ohlsson A, Treffers PE, Kanhani HHH. Prelabour rupture of the membranes preterm. In: Chalmers I, Enkin M, Keirse MJ, eds. *Effective care in pregnancy and childbirth*. Oxford: Oxford University Press; 1989:666.

2 Lebherz TB, Hellman LP, Madding R, et al. Double-blind study of premature rupture of the membranes. A report of 1,896 cases. *Am J Obstet Gynecol* 1963;87:218–225.

3 Sachs M, Baker TH. Spontaneous premature rupture of the membranes. *Am J Obstet Gynecol* 1967;97:888.

4 Gunn GC, Mishell DR, Jr, Morton DG. Premature rupture of the fetal membranes. A review. *Am J Obstet Gynecol* 1970;106:469–483.

5 Christensen KK, Christensen P, Ingemarsson I, et al. A study of complications in preterm deliveries after prolonged premature rupture of the membranes. *Obstet Gynecol* 1976;48: 670–677.

6 Fayez JA, Hasan AA, Jonas HS, Miller GL. Management of premature rupture of the membranes. *Obstet Gynecol* 1978;52:17–21.

7 Daikoku NH, Kaltreider DF, Khouzami VA, et al. Premature rupture of membranes and spontaneous preterm labor: maternal endometritis risks. *Obstet Gynecol* 1982;59: 13–20.

8 Malak TM, Bell SC. Structural characteristics of term human fetal membranes: a novel zone of extreme morphological alteration within the rupture site. *Br J Obstet Gynaecol* 1994;101:375–386.

9 McParland PC, Taylor DJ, Bell SC. Mapping of zones of altered morphology and chorionic connective tissue cellular phenotype in human fetal membranes (amniochorion and decidua) overlying the lower uterine pole and cervix before labor at term. *Am J Obstet Gynecol* 2003;189:1481–1488.

10 Artal R, Sokol RJ, Neuman M, et al. The mechanical properties of prematurely and non-prematurely ruptured membranes. Methods and preliminary results. *Am J Obstet Gynecol* 1976;125:655–659.

11 Parry-Jones E, Priya S. A study of the elasticity and tension of fetal membranes and of the relation of the area of the gestational sac to the area of the uterine cavity. *Br J Obstet Gynaecol* 1976;83:205–212.

12 Lavery JP, Miller CE. The viscoelastic nature of chorioamniotic membranes. *Obstet Gynecol* 1977;50:467–472.

13 Lavery JP, Miller CE. Deformation and creep in the human chorioamniotic sac. *Am J Obstet Gynecol* 1979;134:366–375.

14 Bou-Resli MN, Al Zaid NS, Ibrahim ME. Full-term and prematurely ruptured fetal membranes. An ultrastructural study. *Cell Tissue Res* 1981;220:263–278.

15 Ibrahim ME, Bou-Resli MN, Al Zaid NS, Bishay LF. Intact fetal membranes. Morphological predisposal to rupture. *Acta Obstet Gynecol Scand* 1983;62:481–485.
16 Parry S, Strauss JF, III. Premature rupture of the fetal membranes. *N Engl J Med* 1998;338:663–670.
17 Vadillo-Ortega F, Gonzalez-Avila G, Furth EE, et al. 92-kd type IV collagenase (matrix metalloproteinase-9) activity in human amniochorion increases with labor. *Am J Pathol* 1995;146:148–156.
18 Fortunato SJ, Menon R, Swan K, Baricos W. Expression of matrix degrading enzymes and tissue inhibitors of metalloproteinases (TIMP) in human fetal membranes. 15th Annual Meeting of the Society of Perinatal Obstetricians, Atlanta. *Am J Obstet Gynecol* 1995;170.
19 Lei H, Vadillo-Ortega F, Paavola LG, Strauss JF, III. 92-kDa gelatinase (matrix metalloproteinase-9) is induced in rat amnion immediately prior to parturition. *Biol Reprod* 1995;53:339–344.
20 Vadillo-Ortega F, Hernandez A, Gonzalez-Avila G, et al. Increased matrix metalloproteinase activity and reduced tissue inhibitor of metalloproteinases-1 levels in amniotic fluids from pregnancies complicated by premature rupture of membranes. *Am J Obstet Gynecol* 1996;174:1371–1376.
21 Fortunato SJ, Menon R, Lombardi S. Induction of MMP-9 and normal presence of MMP-2, TIMP-1 and -2 in human fetal membranes. 17th Annual Meeting of the Society of Perinatal Obstetricians, Anaheim. *Am J Obstet Gynecol* 1997;176:1.
22 Maymon E, Romero R, Pacora P, et al. Human neutrophil collagenase (matrix metalloproteinase 8) in parturition, premature rupture of the membranes, and intrauterine infection. *Am J Obstet Gynecol* 2000;183:94–99.
23 Maymon E, Romero R, Pacora P, et al. Evidence of *in vivo* differential bioavailability of the active forms of matrix metalloproteinases 9 and 2 in parturition, spontaneous rupture of membranes, and intra-amniotic infection. *Am J Obstet Gynecol* 2000;183:887–894.
24 Maymon E, Romero R, Pacora P, et al. Matrilysin (matrix metalloproteinase 7) in parturition, premature rupture of the membranes, and intrauterine infection. *Am J Obstet Gynecol* 2000;182:1545–1553.
25 Maymon E, Romero R, Pacora P, et al. Evidence for the participation of interstitial collagenase (matrix metalloproteinase 1) in preterm premature rupture of membranes. *Am J Obstet Gynecol* 2000;183:914–920.
26 Maymon E, Romero R, Pacora P, et al. A role for the 72 kDa gelatinase (MMP-2) and its inhibitor (TIMP-2) in human parturition, premature rupture of membranes and intra-amniotic infection. *J Perinat Med* 2001;29:308–316.
27 Fortunato SJ, LaFleur B, Menon R. Collagenase-3 (MMP-13) in fetal membranes and amniotic fluid during pregnancy. *Am J Reprod Immunol* 2003;49:120–125.
28 Goncalves LF, Chaiworapongsa T, Romero R. Intrauterine infection and prematurity. *Ment Retard Dev Disabil Res Rev* 2002;8:3–13.
29 Romero R, Quintero R, Oyarzun E, et al. Intraamniotic infection and the onset of labor in preterm premature rupture of the membranes. *Am J Obstet Gynecol* 1988;159:661–666.
30 Naeye RL. Factors that predispose to premature rupture of the fetal membranes. *Obstet Gynecol* 1982;60:93–98.
31 Wilson JC, Levy DL, Wilds PL. Premature rupture of membranes prior to term: consequences of nonintervention. *Obstet Gynecol* 1982;60:601–606.
32 Cox SM, Williams ML, Leveno KJ. The natural history of preterm ruptured membranes: what to expect of expectant management. *Obstet Gynecol* 1988;71:558–562.
33 Nelson LH, Anderson RL, O'Shea TM, Swain M. Expectant management of preterm premature rupture of the membranes. *Am J Obstet Gynecol* 1994;171:350–356.

34 Ananth CV, Oyelese Y, Srinivas N, et al. Preterm premature rupture of membranes, intrauterine infection, and oligohydramnios: risk factors for placental abruption. *Obstet Gynecol* 2004;104:71–77.

35 Barfield WD, Tomashek KM, Flowers LM, Iyasu S. Contribution of late fetal deaths to US perinatal mortality rates, 1995–1998. *Semin Perinatol* 2002;26:17–24.

36 Vergani P, Ghidini A, Locatelli A, et al. Risk factors for pulmonary hypoplasia in second-trimester premature rupture of membranes. *Am J Obstet Gynecol* 1994;170:1359–1364.

37 Rotschild A, Ling EW, Puterman ML, Farquharson D. Neonatal outcome after prolonged preterm rupture of the membranes. *Am J Obstet Gynecol* 1990;162:46–52.

38 Romero R, Mazor M, Morretti R, et al. Infection and labor VII. Microbial invasion of the amniotic cavity in spontaneous rupture of membranes at term. *Am J Obstet Gynecol* 1992;166:129.

39 Carroll SG, Ville Y, Greenough A, et al. Preterm prelabour amniorrhexis: intrauterine infection and interval between membrane rupture and delivery. *Arch Dis Child Fetal Neonatal Ed* 1995;72:F43–F46.

40 Averbuch B, Mazor M, Shoham-Vardi I, et al. Intra-uterine infection in women with preterm premature rupture of membranes: maternal and neonatal characteristics. *Eur J Obstet Gynecol Reprod Biol* 1995;62:25–29.

41 Carroll SG, Papaioannou S, Ntumazah IL, et al. Lower genital tract swabs in the prediction of intrauterine infection in preterm prelabour rupture of the membranes. *Br J Obstet Gynaecol* 1996;103:54–59.

42 Cotton DB, Hill LM, Strassner HT, et al. Use of amniocentesis in preterm gestation with ruptured membranes. *Obstet Gynecol* 1984;63:38–43.

43 Coultrip LL, Grossman JH. Evaluation of rapid diagnostic tests in the detection of microbial invasion of the amniotic cavity. *Am J Obstet Gynecol* 1992;167:1231–1242.

44 Garite TJ, Freeman RK, Linzey EM, Braly P. The use of amniocentesis in patients with premature rupture of membranes. *Obstet Gynecol* 1979;54:226–230.

45 Zlatnik FJ, Cruikshank DP, Petzold CR, Galask RP. Amniocentesis in the identification of inapparent infection in preterm patients with premature rupture of the membranes. *J Reprod Med* 1984;29:656–660.

46 Reece EA, Chervenak FA, Moya FR, Hobbins JC. Amniotic fluid arborization: effect of blood, meconium, and pH alterations. *Obstet Gynecol* 1984;64:248–250.

47 Friedman ML, Mcelin TW. Diagnosis of ruptured fetal membranes. Clinical study and review of the literature. *Am J Obstet Gynecol* 1969;104:544–550.

48 Atlay RD, Sutherst JR. Premature rupture of the fetal membranes confirmed by intra-amniotic injection of dye (Evans blue T-1824). *Am J Obstet Gynecol* 1970;108:993–994.

49 Diaz-Garzon J. Indigocarmine test of preterm rupture of membranes. *Rev Columb Obstet Gynecol* 1969;20:373.

50 Fujimoto S, Kishida T, Sagawa T, et al. Clinical usefulness of the dye-injection method for diagnosing premature rupture of the membranes in equivocal cases. *J Obstet Gynaecol* 1995;21:215–220.

51 Meyer BA, Gonik B, Creasy RK. Evaluation of phenazopyridine hydrochloride as a tool in the diagnosis of premature rupture of the membranes. *Am J Perinatol* 1991;8:297–299.

52 Cowett RM, Hakanson DO, Kocon RW, Oh W. Untoward neonatal effect of intraamniotic administration of methylene blue. *Obstet Gynecol* 1976;48:74S–75S.

53 McEnerney J, McEnerney L. Unfavourable neonatal outcomes after intraamniotic injection of methylene blue. *Obstet Gynecol* 1983;1983:351.

54 Troche BI. Methylene blue baby. *N Engl J Med* 1989;320:1756–1757.

55 Munson LA, Graham A, Koos BJ, Valenzuela GJ. Is there a need for digital examination in patients with spontaneous rupture of the membranes? *Am J Obstet Gynecol* 1985;153: 562–563.

56 Brown CL, Ludwiczak MH, Blanco JD, Hirsch CE. Cervical dilation: accuracy of visual and digital examinations. *Obstet Gynecol* 1993;81:215–216.

57 Morgan MA, de Veciana M, Rumney PJ, Schlinke S. Cervical assessment: visual or digital? *J Perinatol* 1996;16:103–106.

58 Hannah ME, Hodnett ED, Willan A, et al. Prelabor rupture of the membranes at term: expectant management at home or in hospital? The TermPROM Study Group. *Obstet Gynecol* 2000;96:533–538.

59 Mercer BM. Preterm premature rupture of the membranes: diagnosis and management. *Clin Perinatol* 2004;31:765–782, vi.

Further reading

ACOG Technical Bulletin No. 15. *Premature rupture of the membranes*. Washington, DC: ACOG, 1988.

Bell SC, Malak TM. Structural and cellular biology of the fetal membranes. In: Elder M, Romero R, Lamont R, eds. *Preterm labor*. New York: Churchill Livingstone; 1997:401–428.

Gomez R, Romero R, Ghezzi F, et al. The fetal inflammatory response syndrome. *Am J Obstet Gynecol* 1998;179:194–202.

Hannah ME, Ohlsson A, Farine D, et al. Induction of labor compared with expectant management for prelabor rupture of the membranes at term. TERMPROM Study Group. *N Engl J Med* 1996;334:1005–1010.

Kenyon SL, Taylor DJ, Tarnow-Mordi W. Broad-spectrum antibiotics for preterm, prelabour rupture of fetal membranes: the ORACLE I randomised trial. ORACLE Collaborative Group. *Lancet* 2001;357:979–988.

Mercer BM. Preterm premature rupture of the membranes. *Obstet Gynecol* 2003;101: 178–193.

Mercer BM, Miodovnik M, Thurnau GR, et al. Antibiotic therapy for reduction of infant morbidity after preterm premature rupture of the membranes. A randomized controlled trial. National Institute of Child Health and Human Development Maternal–Fetal Medicine Units Network. *JAMA* 1997;278:989–995.

Pacora P, Chaiworapongsa T, Maymon E, et al. Funisitis and chorionic vasculitis: the histological counterpart of the fetal inflammatory response syndrome. *J Matern Fetal Neonatal Med* 2002;11:18–25.

Parry S, Strauss JF, III. Premature rupture of the fetal membranes. *N Engl J Med* 1998; 338:663–670.

Romero R, Yoon BH, Mazor M, et al. A comparative study of the diagnostic performance of amniotic fluid glucose, white blood cell count, interleukin-6, and gram stain in the detection of microbial invasion in patients with preterm premature rupture of membranes. *Am J Obstet Gynecol* 1993;169:839–851.

61 Prolonged pregnancy

Curtis L. Lowery and Paul Wendel

Prolonged pregnancy is identified by a number of terms: postterm, prolonged, post-dates, and postmature, to name a few. Because of the lack of continuity in the use of these terms, comparison between studies has proved exceedingly difficult. For the purposes of clarity, postterm or prolonged pregnancy should be the preferred terminology for the pregnancy extending beyond 42 weeks. Postmaturity is a neonatal diagnosis and should be used to described the infant with recognizable clinical features associated with postmaturity including peeling, parchment-like skin, meconium staining of skin, membranes, and the umbilical cord, and possibly overgrown nails, well-developed creases on the palms and soles, abundance of scalp hair, little vernix or lanugo hair, scaphoid abdomen, and minimal subcutaneous fat.[1,2]

Confusion regarding the dating of the pregnancy complicates the determination of the prolonged pregnancy. Many women cannot remember their last menstrual period, thus making the estimated date of delivery (EDD) difficult to determine accurately. The most important way to minimize the incorrect diagnosis of postterm pregnancy is to establish accurate pregnancy dating as early as possible. An ultrasound in the first or second trimesters should be obtained, from which the crown–rump length can determine gestational age to within 5 days.

Prolonged pregnancy presents significant maternal and fetal risks. Maternal risks associated with the prolonged pregnancy include the increased need for operative delivery in both spontaneous and induced labor. Furthermore, multiple studies have demonstrated an increased risk of perinatal mortality after 42 weeks.[3–20] Perinatal mortality reaches its nadir at 39–40 weeks and then increases as pregnancy exceeds 41 weeks.[21]

While there is an increased incidence of stillbirth with increasing gestational age beyond 40 weeks, most studies have shown no clear benefit from the induction of labor versus conservative management with aggressive fetal assessment. Most of the excessive perinatal mortality associated with the prolonged pregnancy occurs in the intrapartum and neonatal periods.[22] Conditions associated with prolonged pregnancy include intrapartum asphyxia, meconium aspiration, neonatal seizures,[22] fetal macrosomia resulting in dystocia and associated brachioplexus injuries and fractures, anencephaly, and adrenal hypoplasia with pituitary insufficiency.[23,24]

In an attempt to avoid stillbirth, many physicians concerned about adverse events in patients beyond 40 weeks lean toward induction of labor. Assuming that induction of labor does not carry increased perinatal risk, planned induction of labor at any gestational age should always result in fewer adverse perinatal outcomes and testing strategies. Based on current evidence, induction of labor at 41 weeks should be effective in reducing mortality. While there is no universally agreed upon method for induction of labor, as a general rule, the more effective these agents are in initiating labor and shortening induction to delivery times, the more likely are these agents to produce uterine hyperstimulation and the subsequent associated fetal distress.[25] Prostaglandin E_2 (PGE_2) appears to be more effective than oxytocin, and misoprostol is more effective than PGE_2. The use of castor oil and the procedure of sweeping the membranes may be useful in decreasing the frequency and maximum dose of inducing agents in the management of the prolonged pregnancy.

References

1 Culikova V, Culik J, Topolsky L. [Amnioscopy, Clifford's syndrome and serologic conflict.] *Cesk Gynekol* 1974;39(1):34–35.

2 Clifford SH. Postmaturity with placental dysfunction: clinical syndrome and pathologic findings. *J Pediatr* 2005;44:1–13.

3 Kolonja S. [Possible effect of prolonged pregnancy on perinatal fetal mortality.] *Riv Ostet Ginecol Prat* 1957;39(7):583–587.

4 Kolonja S. [Does prolonged pregnancy really increase perinatal mortality.] *Wien Med Wochenschr* 1957;107(48):989.

5 Stamm O, Mattern L. [V. Perinatal mortality in prolonged pregnancy.] *Bull Fed Soc Gynecol Obstet Lang Fr* 1957;9(1, bis):133–142.

6 Bach HG. [Postmaturity syndrome, prolonged pregnancy and perinatal mortality.] *Gynaecologia* 1960;150:197–204.

7 Backer JE. [Perinatal mortality in relation to duration of pregnancy and weight of infant at birth.] *Tidsskr Nor Laegeforen* 1968;88(22):2106–2111.

8 Lattanzi WE. Perinatal morbidity and mortality committee. Case history and commentary. *Conn Med* 1974;38(5):251–252.

9 Harper RG, Sokal MM, Sokal S, et al. The high-risk perinatal registry. A systematic approach for reducing perinatal mortality. *Obstet Gynecol* 1977;50(3):264–268.

10 Naeye RL. Causes of perinatal mortality excess in prolonged gestations. *Am J Epidemiol* 1978;108(5):429–433.

11 Stubblefield PG, Berek JS. Perinatal mortality in term and post-term births. *Obstet Gynecol* 1980;56(6):676–682.

12 Kumari S, Jain S, Pruthi PK, et al. Perinatal risks in postdated pregnancy. *Indian Pediatr* 1984;21(1):21–27.

13 Eden RD, Seifert LS, Winegar A, Spellacy WN. Perinatal characteristics of uncomplicated postdate pregnancies. *Obstet Gynecol* 1987;69(3 Pt 1):296–299.

14 Eden RD, Seifert LS, Winegar A, Spellacy WN. Postdate pregnancies: a review of 46 perinatal deaths. *Am J Perinatol* 1987;4(4):284–287.

15 Papiernik E, Alexander GR, Paneth N. Racial differences in pregnancy duration and its implications for perinatal care. *Med Hypotheses* 1990;33(3):181–186.

16 Iffy L, Apuzzio JJ, Mitra S, et al. Rates of cesarean section and perinatal outcome. Perinatal mortality. *Acta Obstet Gynecol Scand* 1994;73(3):225–230.

17 Hogberg U, Larsson N. Early dating by ultrasound and perinatal outcome. A cohort study. *Acta Obstet Gynecol Scand* 1997;76(10):907–912.

18 Bastian H, Keirse MJ, Lancaster PA. Perinatal death associated with planned home birth in Australia: population based study (see comment). *Br Med J* 1998;317(7155): 384–388.

19 Onah HE. Effect of prolongation of pregnancy on perinatal mortality. *Int J Gynaecol Obstet* 2003;80(3):255–261.

20 Kallen K. Increased risk of perinatal/neonatal death in infants who were smaller than expected at ultrasound fetometry in early pregnancy. *Ultrasound Obstet Gynecol* 2004;24(1):30–34.
21 Cnattingius S, Taube A. Stillbirths and rate of neonatal deaths in 76,761 postterm pregnancies in Sweden, 1982–1991; a register study. *Acta Obstet Gynecol Scand* 1998;77(5): 582–583.
22 Curtis PD, Matthews TG, Clarke TA, et al. Neonatal seizures: the Dublin Collaborative Study. *Arch Dis Child* 1988;63(9):1065–1068.
23 O'Donohoe NV, Holland PD. Familial congenital adrenal hypoplasia. *Arch Dis Child* 1968;43(232):717–723.
24 Roberts G, Cawdery JE. Congenital adrenal hypoplasia. *J Obstet Gynaecol Br Commonw* 1970;77(7):654–656.
25 Agency for Healthcare Research and Quality. *Management of prolonged pregnancy (summary).* US Department of Health and Human Services Public Health Service 2005, No. 53. Available at: URL: www.AHRQ.gov.

Further reading

American College of Obstetricians and Gynecologists (ACOG). Management of postterm pregnancy. *ACOG Practice Patterns* 1997;6.
American College of Obstetricians and Gynecologists (ACOG). ACOG practice patterns. Management of postterm pregnancy. No. 6, October 1997. *Int J Gynaecol Obstet* 1998;60(1): 86–91.
Crowley P. Interventions for preventing or improving the outcome of delivery at or beyond term. *Cochrane Database Syst Rev* 2000;2:CD000170.
Hannah ME, Hannah WJ, Hellmann J, et al. Induction of labor as compared with serial antenatal monitoring in post-term pregnancy. A randomized controlled trial. The Canadian Multicenter Post-term Pregnancy Trial Group. *N Engl J Med* 1992;326(24):1587–1592.
Hilder L, Costeloe K, Thilaganathan B. Prolonged pregnancy: evaluating gestation-specific risks of fetal and infant mortality. *Br J Obstet Gynaecol* 1998;105(2):169–173.
Myers ER Blumrick R, Christian AL, et al. *Management of prolonged pregnancy.* Evidence Report/Technology Assessment No. 53 (Prepared by Duke Evidence-based Practice Center, Durham, NC, under Contract No. 290-97-0014). Rockville, MD: Agency for Healthcare Research and Quality, 2002. AHRQ Publication No. 02-E018.
O'Reilly-Green CP, Divon MY. Receiver operating characteristic curves of sonographic estimated fetal weight for prediction of macrosomia in prolonged pregnancies. *Ultrasound Obstet Gynecol* 1997;9(6):403–408.
Sanchez-Ramos L, Olivier F, Delke I, Kaunitz AM. Labor induction versus expectant management for postterm pregnancies: a systematic review with meta-analysis. *Obstet Gynecol* 2003;101(6):1312–1318.
The National Institute of Child Health and Human Development Network of Maternal–Fetal Medicine Units. A clinical trial of induction of labor versus expectant management in postterm pregnancy. *Am J Obstet Gynecol* 1994;170(3):716–723.
Vrouenraets FP, Roumen FJ, Dehing CJ, et al. Bishop score and risk of cesarean delivery after induction of labor in nulliparous women (see comment). *Obstet Gynecol* 2005;105(4): 690–697.

62 Anesthesia in the high-risk patient

Danny Wilkerson and Richard B. Clark

Pregnant patients present a challenge to the anesthesiologist because of the changes imposed on maternal physiology. Respiration, circulation, and the gastrointestinal tract are particularly affected. Perhaps the most significant advance in obstetric anesthesia in the past 50 years has been the substitution of regional anesthesia for general anesthesia in both abdominal and vaginal delivery. The leading cause of maternal death from anesthesia was aspiration; now, trauma is the leading non-obstetric cause of maternal death.

The problems of pregnancy are compounded considerably by maternal complications such as obesity, hypertensive disease, prematurity, cardiac disease, neurological disease, substance abuse, asthma, diabetes, seizure disorders, sickle cell anemia, AIDS, sexually transmitted diseases (STDs), incompetent cervix, renal disease, chorioamnionitis, and thyroid disease. Such complications make a successful pregnancy outcome much more difficult.

Obesity is a common problem in the USA and many pregnant patients are overweight. Obesity is defined as a body mass index of $30 \, kg/m^2$ or more. The work of breathing is increased and these patients become hypoxemic very quickly when apneic. Regional anesthesia is preferred for vaginal or abdominal delivery. If a Cesarean section is performed on a morbidly obese patient and regional anesthesia is contraindicated, a difficult airway can be anticipated. A thorough evaluation of the airway should precede a rapid sequence induction followed by intubation.

Hypertensive disorders in pregnancy include gestational hypertension, preeclampsia, eclampsia, preeclampsia superimposed on chronic hypertension, and chronic hypertension. The first three conditions were previously known as pregnancy-induced hypertension (PIH). All of these disorders exhibit a decrease in blood volume; therefore, the administration of spinal or epidural anesthesia is likely to result in hypotension. This can usually be prevented by the administration of a balanced salt solution preoperatively. Magnesium sulfate is commonly used to prevent seizures in these hypertensive disorders. If general anesthesia is used for delivery, special attention should be given to utilizing drugs to abate the hypertensive response to endotracheal intubation. Magnesium potentiates muscle relaxants.

About 1% of pregnancies are complicated by heart disease. These patients are most likely to develop heart failure postpartum or during labor. Heart disease can present enormous challenges to the anesthesiologist; regional anesthesia, particularly epidural, is often the best choice. Previously, primary pulmonary hypertension, cyanotic heart disease, and aortic stenosis were considered to be contraindications to regional anesthesia; however, at present, regional anesthesia is relatively contraindicated only in cyanotic heart disease and severe aortic stenosis. With all of these conditions, extreme care must be exercised with regional anesthesia or the outcome can be disastrous. Invasive monitoring must be considered in critically ill patients.

Neurological diseases, such as multiple sclerosis, myasthenia gravis, seizure disorder, amyotrophic lateral sclerosis, residual poliomyelitis, muscular dystrophy, polyneuritis, and spinal cord injury, may complicate pregnancy. In general, neurological disease does not contraindicate regional anesthesia.

Many pregnancies are complicated by substance abuse, for example opioids, cocaine, LSD, and amphetamines. Infants born to opioid-dependent women are at great risk of opioid addiction and/or withdrawal. Cocaine can cause maternal hypertension, vasoconstriction, placental abruption, premature labor, and uteroplacental insufficiency leading to emergency Cesarean section.

Further reading

Birnbach DJ. *Ostheimer's manual of obstetric anesthesia*, 3rd edn. New York: Churchill Livingstone, 2000.

Chestnut DH. *Obstetric anesthesia principles and practice*, 3rd edn. Philadelphia, PA: Elservier Mosby, 2004.

Datta S. *The obstetric anesthesia handbook*, 3rd edn. New York: Hanley & Belfus, 2000.

Datta S. *Anesthetic and obstetric management of high-risk pregnancy*, 3rd edn. New York: Springer-Verlag, 2004.

Gambling DR, Douglas MJ. *Obstetric anesthesia and uncommon disorders*. Philadelphia: WB Saunders Co., 1998.

Hood DD, Curry R. Spinal versus epidural anesthesia for cesarean section in severely preeclamptic patients: a retrospective survey. *Anesthesiology* 1999;90:1276–1292.

Hughes SC, Levinson G, Rosen MA. *Shnider and Levinson's anesthesia for obstetrics*. Philadelphia, PA: Lippincott, Williams & Wilkins, 2002.

Miller RD, ed. *Anesthesia*, 5th edn. Philadelphia, PA: Churchill Livingstone, 2000.

Stoelting RE, Dierdorf SF. *Anesthesia and co-existing disease*, 4th edn. Philadelphia: Churchill Livingstone, 2002.

Tsen LC. The Gerald W. Ostheimer "What's new in obstetric anesthesia" lecture. *Anesthesiology* 2005;102:672–679.

63 Puerperium and lactation: physiology of the reproductive system

Judy M. Hopkinson, Pamela D. Berens, and E. Albert Reece

Reproductive system

Uterus and lochia

Twenty-four hours postpartum, the uterine fundus is typically palpable near the umbilicus. By 2 weeks postpartum, the uterus is no longer palpated on abdominal examination. Total lochial volume is estimated at 200–500 mL.[1] The mean duration of lochia is 33 days with 15% of women continuing to experience lochial discharge at 6 weeks postpartum.[2] Painful postpartum uterine contractions are more problematic in multiparous women.[3] Nonsteroidal anti-inflammatory agents such as ibuprofen may be used for analgesia.

Over the first week postpartum, the cervix assumes a more typical gross appearance, although it may remain slightly dilated for the first few days. Persistent heavy bleeding and a continued open cervical os should alert the physician to the possibility of retained placental fragments. The vagina may initially appear relatively estrogen deficient in postpartum lactating women or women using progesterone-only contraception. A vaginal lubricant may be beneficial if dyspareunia occurs.

Hormonal regulation

Nonlactating mothers experience ovulation on average 45 days after delivery with return of menses in many by 7–9 weeks postpartum. Lactating mothers experience a delayed and much more variable return to both ovulation and menstruation, which may relate to specific breastfeeding practices.[4–6] During the first 6 months postpartum, women who experience amenorrhea and breastfeed without giving supplements have a less than 2% risk of pregnancy.[7–13]

Lactation

Exclusive breastfeeding during approximately the first 6 months of life with continued breastfeeding through at least the second half of infancy is associated with reduced risk of adverse outcomes in mother and infant.[14] Environmental factors have a marked influence on breastfeeding success. Obstetric practices must be evaluated for their potential impact on lactation performance.

Mammary anatomy and physiology

Figure 63.1 illustrates the general anatomic structures of the developed human breast. By 16 weeks' gestation, the breast is fully competent to produce milk. This is prevented by high levels of circulating progesterone, which block prolactin activation of alfa-lactalbumin formation within the alveolus. Onset of copious milk production (lactogenesis stage II or LS-II) begins after delivery of the placenta and subsequent fall in progesterone.[15] The mean time for LS-II is 50–73 h postpartum.[16] Early lactation failure or partial inhibition of milk production can result from primary glandular insufficiency, retained placenta,[15] and severe postpartum hemorrhage resulting in ischemic pituitary necrosis and Sheehan's syndrome.[17]

Regulation of milk production

Following LS-II, milk production increases to a mean of 750 mL/day by 2–4 weeks after delivery and remains there throughout exclusive breastfeeding.[18] Milk volume increases or declines in response to alterations in the frequency of suckling or pumping and the degree of breast emptying. Prolactin is the primary endocrine

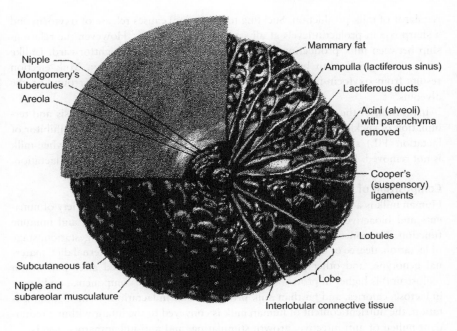

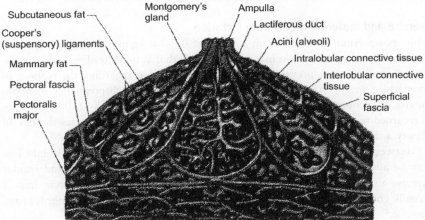

Figure 63.1 Anatomy of the human breast. Copyright 1980 Ciba-Geigy Corporation. Reproduced with permission from the Clinical Symposia by Frank H. Netter, MD.

regulator of milk production. Suckling (or pumping) causes release of oxytocin and a sharp rise in prolactin levels at all stages of lactation.[19-22] However, the relationship between milk production and prolactin levels is not straightforward. Unlike prolactin, oxytocin can be released through a conditioned reflex. Milk ejection results from oxytocin-induced contraction of myoepithelial cells surrounding the alveolus.

Involution of the mammary gland is triggered by prolonged milk stasis and termination of suckling. Peaker and Wilde[23] identified a protein, feedback inhibitor of lactation (FIL), synthesized in each mammary gland, which accumulates when milk is not removed. FIL blocks the secretion of milk constituents and disrupts lactation.

Composition of human milk

Human milk is a complex, highly structured fluid containing a wide variety of nutrients and bioactive factors that impact infant growth, development, and immune function. The concentration of components varies with duration of gestation, stage of lactation, degree of breast emptying, exposure to pathogens, maternal diet, maternal genotype, and other particulars. The initial milk produced after parturition (colostrum) is higher in protein and immunologically active components, and lower in lactose, calories, and fat than milk produced later in lactation.[24] Throughout lactation, the nutrient content of human milk is conveyed to the infant within a redundant milieu of anti-infective, growth-stimulating, and anti-inflammatory agents.

Exercise and maternal diet during lactation

While postpartum women lose an average of 0.5–1.0 kg/month after postpartum diuresis,[25,26] individual weight loss varies. The myth that breastfeeding assures postpartum weight loss is prevalent, and prenatal education regarding the realities of postpartum weight management is advisable. In the US, each pregnancy increases the risk of becoming overweight by 60% and the risk of obesity by 110%.[27] Failure to returned to prepregnancy weight by 6 months postpartum increases the risk of obesity a decade later.[28]

Overweight breastfeeding women who desire to initiate or increase weight loss may be advised to begin moderate calorie restriction (500 kcal/day) and regular exercise after breastfeeding is well established. Exercise has no apparent impact on milk composition, excluding a temporary rise in lactate after prolonged, heavy exercise.[29]

Women should be advised to consume a balanced diet during the postpartum period to protect their own health and body stores. In well-nourished women, maternal stores provide critical nutrients to maintain milk quality during temporary fluctuations in nutrient intake. Two nutrients may not be supplied in adequate amounts in milk from normal, well-nourished women: vitamin K[30] and vitamin D.[31] Routine intramuscular injection of vitamin K1 at birth provides all the vitamin K needed. The American Academy of Pediatrics recommends daily supplementation with 200 IU of vitamin D to all infants unless they consume at least 500 mL/day vitamin D-fortified formula or milk.[32] Without supplements, strict vegetarians will eventually develop vitamin B12 deficiencies and produce milk deficient in vitamin B12.[33,34] Infants may become symptomatic before the mother.[34] Although infant symptoms can be partially reversed with B12 shots, neurologic deficits can be irreversible. Strict vegetarians should consume B12 supplements, particularly during lactation.

Prenatal and perinatal practices that affect breastfeeding

Breastfeeding should be recommended at the initial prenatal examination. Further education can be offered during prenatal and postpartum care. During an uncomplicated pregnancy and delivery, the infant can be given to the mother at delivery, and breastfeeding initiation should be encouraged within the first hour. Newborn interventions can be delayed until after this time. The family should be encouraged to room in and breastfeed on demand. Having staff trained in lactation support can mitigate potential obstacles to breastfeeding that may present with complicated pregnancies and/or medical interventions associated with delivery. Patient-controlled analgesia with morphine or continuous extradural anesthesia in the initial period after Cesarean is preferred over the use of meperidine because of the association of meperidine with an adverse effect on infant suckling behavior.[35]

Latch and milk transfer during feeding should be assessed by trained personnel within 8 h prior to hospital discharge. Predischarge teaching should include the elements listed in Table 63.1. Parents should be advised to report promptly deviations from normal urine and stool patterns or concerns about low milk production to the healthcare provider.

Drugs and medications

Healthy lifestyle choices such as avoiding smoking and alcohol consumption are ideal; however, their use is not an absolute contraindication for breastfeeding.

Table 63.1 Breastfeeding information for new parents.

1 Normal milk production is quite low until after the onset of lactogenesis stage II between the first and fifth days postpartum
2 Most infants nurse 8–14 times/day in the first 1–2 weeks. This decreases to 7–10 times/day by 4 weeks
3 Each infant's "demand" breastfeeding frequency reflects his own developmental status and nursing skill as well as the mother's milk flow
4 After the third day of life, exclusively breastfed infants usually soak six or more diapers and have three or more stools of 1 tablespoon or greater/day
5 Infant stools normally change from dark (green or brown) to mustard yellow by the fifth day. This happens after the mother's milk "comes in" and the baby begins to receive larger volumes of milk, which clears the meconium from the gastrointestinal tract
6 Healthcare provider should be notified promptly if urine or stool patterns deviate from norms indicated in items 4 and 5 or if parents are concerned about adequacy of infant intake or maternal milk production

Substances of abuse are contraindicated during pregnancy and lactation. The exception to this is the woman who is in a successful methadone maintenance program.

Specific advice regarding the use of a medication in a breastfeeding mother should be done after reviewing information on that particular medication, exploring alternative treatments, which may be better researched in lactation, and discussing the individual situation with the parents. The age, weight, and health of the child, in addition to the amount of breast milk in the diet and any medications the child is taking, should all be considered when choosing which medication is best.

Mastitis

Signs and symptoms of mastitis include an erythematous, tender breast, fever, and flu-like symptoms such as myalgia, nausea, and headache. A new localized tender knot in the breast in the absence of symptoms of infection suggests a plugged duct, which can be managed with frequent nursing and warm compresses. More diffuse firmness in both breasts is suggestive of engorgement, and is usually associated with normal or low-grade fever. The presence of a fluctuant, palpable, and tender mass in the mastitic breast is suggestive of a breast abscess.

Mastitis is treated with a penicillinase-resistant antibiotic such as Dicloxicillin or a cephalosporin for 10–14 days. If symptoms do not improve after 24–48 h of therapy, milk should be cultured for resistant organisms and/or the breast should be re-examined for possible abscess. Breastfeeding the healthy, term infant during treatment of mastitis should be continued. Abrupt weaning increases the risk of abscess.

Contraception

If a hormonal contraceptive is chosen, a progesterone-only alternative has less potential impact on milk supply. In breastfeeding mothers, estrogen-containing contraceptive options have the theoretical concern of adversely affecting milk supply.

Low milk production

If a mother expresses concern about low milk production in the early postpartum period, the infant should be evaluated and the mother assessed for possible causes of failed LS-II (see above). If infant status is normal and the child is exclusively breastfed, maternal concerns likely reflect misinterpretation of infant behavior. If the infant is not thriving or is receiving formula supplements, it suggests that maternal milk volume is low. Medications and over-the-counter drugs should be reviewed for potential impact on milk production. If no medical or pharmacologic cause is apparent, milk volume usually increases in response to increased frequency of breast stimulation (nursing or pumping) and/or the increased degree of breast emptying (improved infant latch or breast massage during nursing).

References

1 Sherman D, Lurie S, Frenkel E, et al. Characteristics of normal lochia. *Am J Perinatol* 1999;16(8):399–402.

2 Oppenheimer LW, Sherriff EA, Goodman JD, et al. The duration of lochia. *Br J Obstet Gynaecol* 1986;93(7):754–757.

3 Murray A, Holdcroft A. Incidence and intensity of postpartum lower abdominal pain. *Br Med J* 1989;298(6688):1619.

4 McNeilly AS, Friesen HG. Presence of a nonlactogenic factor in human serum which synergistically enhances prolactin-stimulated growth of Nb2 rat lymphoma cells in vitro. *J Clin Endocrinol Metab* 1985;61(3):408–411.

5 Howie PW, McNeilly AS. Breast-feeding and postpartum ovulation. *IPPF Med Bull* 1982;16(2):1–3.

6 Rogers IS. Lactation and fertility. *Early Hum Dev* 1997;49(Suppl.):S185–190.

7 Lactation amenorrhea: experts recommend full breastfeeding as a child spacing method. *Network* 1988;10(2):12.

8 Short RV, Lewis PR, Renfree MB, Shaw G. Contraceptive effects of extended lactational amenorrhoea: beyond the Bellagio Consensus. *Lancet* 1991;337(8743):715–717.

9 Kennedy KI, Visness CM. Contraceptive efficacy of lactational amenorrhoea. *Lancet* 1992;339(8787):227–230.

10 Perez A, Labbok MH, Queenan JT. Clinical study of the lactational amenorrhoea method for family planning. *Lancet* 1992;339(8799):968–970.

11 Gross BA. Is the lactational amenorrhea method a part of natural family planning? Biology and policy. *Am J Obstet Gynecol* 1991;165(6 Pt 2):2014–2019.

12 World Health Organization Task Force on Methods for the Natural Regulation of Fertility. The World Health Organization multinational study of breast-feeding and lactational amenorrhea. III. Pregnancy during breast-feeding. *Fertil Steril* 1999;72(3):431–440.

13 Labbok MH, Hight-Laukaran V, Peterson AE, et al. Multicenter study of the Lactational Amenorrhea Method (LAM): I. Efficacy, duration, and implications for clinical application. *Contraception* 1997;55(6):327–336.

14 Gartner LM, Morton J, Lawrence RA, et al. Breastfeeding and the use of human milk. *Pediatrics* 2005;115(2):496–506.

15 Neifert MR, McDonough SL, Neville MC. Failure of lactogenesis associated with placental retention. *Am J Obstet Gynecol* 1981;140(4):477–478.

16 Perez-Escamilla R, Chapman DJ. Validity and public health implications of maternal perception of the onset of lactation: an international analytical overview. *J Nutr* 2001;131(11): 3021S–3024S.

17 Kelestimur F. Sheehan's syndrome. *Pituitary* 2003;6(4):181–188.

18 Butte NF, Garza C, Stuff JE, et al. Effect of maternal diet and body composition on lactational performance. *Am J Clin Nutr* 1984;39(2):296–306.

19 Lawrence RA, Lawrence R. *Breastfeeding: a guide for the medical profession*, 6th edn. St Louis, MO: Mosby (Elsevier Inc.); 2005:77.

20 Diaz S, Seron-Ferre M, Cardenas H, et al. Circadian variation of basal plasma prolactin, prolactin response to suckling, and length of amenorrhea in nursing women. *J Clin Endocrinol Metab* 1989;68(5):946–955.

21 Freeman ME, Kanyicska B, Lerant A, Nagy G. Prolactin: structure, function, and regulation of secretion. *Physiol Rev* 2000;80(4):1523–1631.

22 Stern JM, Reichlin S. Prolactin circadian rhythm persists throughout lactation in women. *Neuroendocrinology* 1990;51(1):31–37.

23 Peaker M, Wilde CJ. Feedback control of milk secretion from milk. *J Mammary Gland Biol Neoplasia* 1996;1(3):307–315.

24 Garza C, Hopkinson J. Physiology of lactation. In: Tsang RC, Nichols BL, eds. *Nutrition during infancy*. Philadelphia: Hanley & Belfus; 1988:20.

25 Prentice AM, Prentice A. Energy costs of lactation. *Annu Rev Nutr* 1988;8:63–79.

26 Butte NF, Hopkinson JM. Body composition changes during lactation are highly variable among women. *J Nutr* 1998;128(2 Suppl.):381S–385S.

27 Keppel KG, Taffel SM. Pregnancy-related weight gain and retention: implications of the 1990 Institute of Medicine guidelines. *Am J Public Health* 1993;83(8):1100–1103.

28 Rooney BL, Schauberger CW. Excess pregnancy weight gain and long-term obesity: one decade later. *Obstet Gynecol* 2005;100(2):245–252.

29 Larson-Meyer DE. Effect of postpartum exercise on mothers and their offspring: a review of the literature. *Obes Res* 2002;10(8):841–853.

30 Canfield LM, Hopkinson JM, Lima AF, et al. Vitamin K in colostrum and mature human milk over the lactation period – a cross-sectional study. *Am J Clin Nutr* 1991;53(3):730–735.

31 Lammi-Keefe CJ. Vitamins D and E in human milk. In: Jensen RG, ed. *Handbook of milk composition (food science and technology international)*. San Diego, CA: Academic Press (Division of Harcourt Brace & Co.); 1995:706–717.

32 Gartner LM, Greer FR. Prevention of rickets and vitamin D deficiency: new guidelines for vitamin D intake. *Pediatrics* 2003;111(4 Pt 1):908–910.

33 Specker BL, Black A, Allen L, Morrow F. Vitamin B-12: low milk concentrations are related to low serum concentrations in vegetarian women and to methylmalonic aciduria in their infants. *Am J Clin Nutr* 1990;52(6):1073–1076.

34 Hamosh M, Dewey KG, Garza C, et al. Infant outcomes. In: Tsang RC, Nichols BL, eds. *Nutrition during lactation*, 1st edn. Washington, DC: National Academy Press; 1991:153–196.

35 Wittels B, Glosten B, Faure EA, et al. Postcesarean analgesia with both epidural morphine and intravenous patient-controlled analgesia: neurobehavioral outcomes among nursing neonates. *Anesth Analg* 1997;85(3):600–606.

Part XIII The Newborn Infant

64 Premature birth and neurological complications

Alan Hill

With the improved survival of more than 85% of very low birthweight infants, prematurity has become a major risk factor for neurological sequelae in survivors. Specific patterns of hemorrhagic and hypoxic–ischemic brain injury relate directly to unique anatomic and physiological features of the premature brain.

Germinal matrix–intraventricular hemorrhage (GMH–IVH) originates from fragile vessels in the subependymal germinal matrix that rupture through the adjacent wall of the lateral ventricle to cause IVH. The incidence of GMH–IVH has declined to less than 20% of premature infants. It is diagnosed clinically in only 50%, and definitive diagnosis requires ultrasonography, often performed between 7 and 14 days of age. Serial scanning is required to identify the major complications of GMH–IVH, i.e., posthemorrhagic hydrocephalus (PHH) and periventricular hemorrhagic infarction (PVI).

Progressive PHH usually develops over weeks and may arrest or resolve spontaneously in 35–65% of cases, usually in approximately 4–6 weeks. Temporizing measures, e.g., serial lumbar punctures, subcutaneous reservoir, subgaleal shunt, or a permanent ventriculoperitoneal shunt, may be required in the remainder. Progressive PHH must be distinguished from ventriculomegaly related to cerebral atrophy.

Periventricular hemorrhagic infarction (PVI) represents unilateral hemorrhagic venous infarction in white matter secondary to obstruction of the terminal vein by large GMH.

Periventricular leukomalacia (PVL) is the principal pattern of hypoxic–ischemic injury in the premature and is usually bilateral. Major pathogenetic factors involve the watershed zones of arterial supply in the periventricular white matter, impaired cerebrovascular autoregulation, vulnerability of oligodendrocyte precursors to free radicals, and white matter injury from inflammatory mediators. Long-term sequelae include spastic diplegia and visual impairment.

The central nervous system toxicity of unconjugated hyperbilirubinemia is not well defined in premature newborns, and hearing loss may be a major manifestation. Similarly, the threshold and duration of significant hypoglycemia remain unclear.

Major interventional strategies to reduce premature brain injury include prevention of premature delivery, administration of antenatal steroids, avoidance of prolonged labor, and postnatal correction of hemodynamic disturbances in the premature newborn.

There is a high risk of neurological morbidity in survivors of prematurity: approximately 5–15% develop cerebral palsy, and an additional 25–50% have cognitive and behavioral difficulties that may not be recognized until later in childhood.

Further reading

De Vries LS, Roelants-van Rijn AM, Rademaker KJ, et al. Unilateral parenchymal hemorrhagic infarction in the preterm infant. *Eur J Pediatr Neurol* 2001;5:139.

Dubowitz LMS, Dubowitz V, Palmer PG, et al. Correlation of neurologic assessment in the preterm infant with outcome at one year. *J Pediatr* 1984;105:452.

Ferreiro DM. Neonatal brain injury. *N Engl J Med* 2004;351:1985.

Kalhan S, Peter-Wohl S. Hypoglycemia: what is it for the neonate? *Am J Perinatol* 2000;17:11.

Oh W, Tyson JE, Fanaroff AA, et al. Association between peak serum bilirubin and neurodevelopmental outcome in extremely low birth weight infants. *Pediatrics* 2003;112:773.

du Plessis AJ. Posthemorrhagic hydrocephalus and brain injury in the preterm infant: dilemmas in diagnosis and management. *Semin Pediatr Neurol* 1998;5:161.

Roland EH, Hill A. Germinal matrix–intraventricular hemorrhage in the premature newborn. Management and outcome. *Neurol Clin North Am* 2003;21:833.

Torrioli MG, Fisone MF, Bonvini L, et al. Perceptual-motor, visual and cognitive ability in very low birthweight preschool children without neonatal ultrasound abnormalities. *Brain Dev* 2000;22:163.

Volpe JJ. Neurobiology of periventricular leukomalacia in the premature infant. *Pediatr Res* 2001;50:553.

Volpe JJ. *Neurology of the newborn.* Philadelphia, PA: W.B. Saunders, 2001.

65 Common problems of the newborn

Fernando R. Moya and Matthew Laughon

Overall mortality and morbidity of the preterm infant

Over the past 15 years, the survival of preterm infants has been increasing at the lowest end of gestational age, that is around 23–26 weeks. However, clinicians generally underestimate the chances of survival and overestimate the chances of serious morbidity, which may lead to restricting potentially beneficial or life-saving therapies.

In preterm infants, decreasing birthweight and gestational age are the most important determinants of mortality and morbidity (Table 65.1). At a given birthweight, infants who are more mature have a lower mortality. Similarly, at a given gestational age, infants with higher birthweight have a lower mortality. Acute morbidities increase with decreasing birthweight, as shown in Table 65.2. There is also substantial variability between centers in the frequency of these complications. The long-term morbidities associated with preterm birth include cerebral palsy, neurodevelopmental delay, chronic lung disease, short bowel syndrome, poor growth, and visual and hearing deficits.

Common problems of term and preterm neonates

Asphyxia and neonatal resuscitation

Asphyxia occurs primarily in high-risk pregnancies, but can present without warning. At birth, if an infant appears depressed, then the initial steps of resuscitation include providing warmth, drying, positioning the infant to open the airway

Table 65.1 Mortality by gestational age and birthweight, 1995–1997.

Mortality (%)

Weeks of gestation	22–23	24–25	26–27	28–29	30–31	32–33	Total
Total	63.7	27.0	12.0	5.0	2.2	1.0	
Weight (g)							
1750–1999				1.8	1.5	1.2	1.4
1500–1749			4.5	2.7	2.0	1.1	2.2
1250–1499		3.7	3.4	2.7	2.1	2.0	2.8
1000–1249	12.8	7.9	5.3	3.5	3.2	4.5	4.5
750–999	17.4	14.0	8.5	6.6	5.8		10.2
500–749	61.5	31.9	23.7	19.6	23.3		40.0
250–499	87.3	70.5	62.7				84.2

Adapted from Alexander GR, Kogan M, Bader D, et al. US birth weight/gestational age-specific neonatal mortality: 1995–1997 rates for whites, hispanics, and blacks. *Pediatrics* 2003;111:e61–66.

and clearing it as necessary, and stimulating plus giving oxygen as needed. Respirations, heart rate, and color are more useful in assessing the neonatal status and need for intervention initially. Subsequent steps depend on the infant's response and may include providing positive pressure ventilation, chest compressions, and endotracheal intubation, and are all outlined in the *Neonatal Resuscitation Manual* jointly produced by the American Academy of Pediatrics and the American Heart Association. A good response is indicated by rapid increases in heart rate, improvements in color, and initiation of spontaneous respiratory efforts. Endotracheal intubation and suctioning for infants born through meconium-stained amniotic fluid is now reserved primarily for nonvigorous infants.

Respiratory problems

Signs of respiratory distress (tachypnea, retractions, nasal flaring, end-expiratory grunting, and cyanosis) may be the result of many diseases (Table 65.3). Respiratory distress syndrome (RDS) due to surfactant deficiency and lung immaturity is one of the most common causes of neonatal respiratory difficulty. Its incidence varies inversely with gestational age. Infants with RDS have lower amounts of surfactant phospholipids and proteins in the airway than control subjects. Surfactant deficiency and structural lung immaturity lead to decreased pulmonary compliance and atelectasis. Hypoxemia develops as a consequence of the resulting right-to-left intrapulmonary shunting. Hypercarbia may also occur. The diagnosis of RDS is based on the presence of clinical signs and radiographic findings of diffuse reticulogranular pattern, poor lung expansion, and air bronchograms. Specific measures to treat infants with RDS are oxygen therapy and the use of positive airway pressure, either

Table 65.2 Common morbidities of infants 501–1500 g as reported by centers of the Vermont Oxford Network in 2004.

	Birthweight (g)				
	501–1500	501–750	751–1000	1001–1250	1251–1500
Respiratory					
RDS	74 (65, 85)	94 (91, 100)	87 (82, 100)	72 (63, 88)	54 (40, 71)
Pneumothorax	5 (2, 6)	10 (0, 14)	6 (0, 10)	3 (0, 5)	3 (0, 4)
Chronic lung disease					
Oxygen at:					
28 days	53 (41, 61)	92 (88, 100)	74 (63, 88)	43 (28, 57)	22 (9, 30)
36 weeks	36 (21, 45)	70 (50, 92)	49 (25, 65)	27 (8, 38)	15 (0, 22)
Symptomatic PDA	37 (26, 45)	57 (40, 71)	51 (33, 65)	33 (20, 44)	19 (8, 25)
NEC	6 (2, 8)	10 (0, 16)	8 (0, 11)	5 (0, 7)	3 (0, 4)
GI perforation	2 (0, 3)	5 (0, 8)	3 (0, 5)	1 (0, 0)	1 (0, 0)
Intraventricular hemorrhage (IVH)	26 (18, 33)	46 (30, 59)	32 (19, 43)	21 (10, 28)	16 (6, 21)
Ultrasound grade					
0	74 (67, 82)	54 (41, 70)	68 (57, 81)	79 (72, 90)	84 (79, 94)
1	11 (5, 15)	12 (0, 18)	12 (0, 18)	11 (0, 15)	10 (0, 14)
2	6 (2, 8)	11 (0, 15)	7 (0, 11)	5 (0, 7)	3 (0, 5)
3	4 (1, 6)	9 (0, 14)	6 (0, 9)	3 (0, 5)	2 (0, 2)
4	5 (2, 7)	14 (0, 21)	7 (0, 11)	2 (0, 3)	1 (0, 0)
Cystic PVL	3 (0, 5)	5 (0, 7)	4 (0, 6)	3 (0, 5)	2 (0, 3)
Retinopathy of prematurity					
ROP (any)	41 (26, 51)	79 (67, 100)	56 (38, 73)	28 (11, 41)	13 (0, 20)
ROP stage					
0	59 (49, 74)	21 (0, 33)	44 (27, 62)	72 (59, 89)	87 (80, 100)
1	18 (8, 23)	19 (0, 28)	24 (8, 33)	18 (0, 25)	10 (0, 14)
2	13 (5, 18)	28 (6, 40)	19 (4, 29)	8 (0, 11)	3 (0, 0)
3	9 (4, 13)	29 (10, 42)	12 (0, 17)	3 (0, 3)	1 (0, 0)
4	1 (0, 0)	2 (0, 0)	1 (0, 0)	0 (0, 0)	0 (0, 0)

Numbers are percentiles (Network Quartiles).

continuously (CPAP) or by assisted ventilation. Administration of exogenous surfactant is standard therapy for infants with RDS who are intubated. This can be at birth (prophylactic) or after RDS has been diagnosed (rescue/treatment). Therapy with surfactant results in decreases in neonatal mortality and air leaks. However, the occurrence of complications such as intraventricular hemorrhage (IVH) and bronchopulmonary dysplasia (BPD) is not decreased with surfactant replacement therapy.

Table 65.3 Common causes of respiratory distress in the newborn.

I. Respiratory disorders:

    A. Pulmonary diseases
       Respiratory distress syndrome
       Meconium aspiration syndrome
       Transient tachypnea
       Pneumonia
       Pneumothorax and other air leaks
       Developmental anomalies (congenital lobar emphysema, chylothorax, pulmonary hypoplasia)

    B. Airway obstruction
       Choanal atresia
       Pierre Robin syndrome

    C. Rib cage abnormalities
       Asphyxiating thoracic dystrophy

    D. Diaphragmatic disorders
       Diaphragmatic hernia
       Phrenic nerve injury

II. Extrarespiratory disorders:

    A. Congenital heart disease

    B. Acid–base abnormalities (inherited disorders of metabolism, other causes of metabolic acidosis)

    C. Central nervous system disorders (cerebral edema, hemorrhage, infection)

Bronchopulmonary dysplasia (BPD)

Some preterm neonates develop a form of chronic respiratory disease called BPD. Its diagnosis is based on the need for supplemental oxygen at 28 days after birth or preferably at 36 weeks adjusted gestational age. Radiographic findings in BPD include interstitial fibrosis, cystic changes, hyperinflation, and segmental atelectasis. The incidence of BPD is also inversely proportional to gestational age. Its pathogenesis is multifactorial and includes oxygen toxicity, volutrauma, pulmonary immaturity, acute lung injury (air leaks, pulmonary edema), acquired infections, and poor nutrition. Treatment includes chronic administration of oxygen, aggressive nutritional support, fluid restriction, use of chronic diuretics, bronchodilators, and environmental measures to minimize the risk of respiratory infection.

Meconium aspiration syndrome and persistent pulmonary hypertension of the newborn

Of all infants delivered through meconium-stained amniotic fluid, between 1% and 9% may develop meconium aspiration syndrome (MAS), most of whom delivered through thick meconium. In MAS, airway resistance is increased, and there can be a mix of alveolar overdistention and collapse. Air leaks are frequent, particularly in those on mechanical ventilation. There are ventilation–perfusion abnormalities and intrapulmonary shunting with resulting hypoxemia and respiratory acidosis. The diagnosis of MAS is based on the presence of clinical signs of respiratory distress and radiographic findings of hyperexpansion combined with asymmetric areas of atelectasis. Pneumothorax and pneumomediastinum are frequent findings. Management of infants with MAS is aimed at maintaining adequate oxygenation, correction of metabolic acidosis, and support of the circulation in order to minimize the stimuli for pulmonary vasoconstriction. Infants with MAS often develop a condition known as persistent pulmonary hypertension of the newborn (PPHN). In PPHN, there is right-to-left shunting through the foramen ovale and/or ductus arteriosus with significant systemic hypoxemia. Besides MAS, PPHN may develop in infants with acute asphyxia, pneumonia, or other respiratory problems, and in pulmonary hypoplasia (congenital diaphragmatic hernia). Besides the general measures described before, high-frequency ventilation, inhaled nitric oxide, and extracorporeal membrane oxygenation (ECMO) are additional therapies used to treat infants with PPHN.

Transient tachypnea of the newborn

This respiratory problem results from delayed lung fluid reabsorption. It is seen mostly in term or near-term infants, but may also affect premature infants. Delivery by Cesarean section without labor is a common risk factor. Clinical signs of respiratory distress and radiologic features of mild hyperinflation, increased interstitial and vascular markings (primarily around the hilar areas), and fluid in the horizontal fissure suggest the diagnosis of transient tachypnea. There can be hypoxemia and respiratory acidosis. Treatment consists of supportive therapy and the administration of supplemental oxygen. Some infants may require the use of CPAP or mechanical ventilation for significant respiratory distress or blood gas derangements.

Hematologic problems

Anemia

Anemia (Hb < 13 g/dL) in term infants can be the result of hemorrhage, hemolysis, or decreased red cell production (Table 65.4). Helpful clinical and laboratory findings for the differential diagnosis of neonatal anemia are listed in Table 65.5. Acute anemia secondary to hemorrhage frequently presents at birth or soon thereafter with signs of hypovolemia including lethargy, poor capillary refill, tachycardia, weak pulses, hypotension, and pallor. Significant blood loss may lead to poor response to

Table 65.4 Common causes of anemia in the newborn.

Hemorrhage	Hemolysis	Decreased RBC production
External	*Immune*	Diamond–Blackfan syndrome
Placenta abruptio	ABO	Transcobalamin II deficiency
Placenta previa	Rh	Congenital leukemia
Tumors	Minor groups	
Cord	Maternal autoimmune	
Nuchal cord	Drug-induced	
Velamentous insertion	*Nonimmune*	
Fetoplacental	Infection	
Fetomaternal	RBC membrane defects	
Twin–twin transfusion	Glucose-6-phosphate dehydrogenase deficiency	
Internal	Pyruvate kinase deficiency	
Cephalhematoma	Hemoglobinopathies	
Intracranial		
Ruptured liver, spleen		
Adrenal		
Retroperitoneal		
Iatrogenic		

RBC, red blood cell.

Table 65.5 Differential diagnosis of anemia in the newborn: clinical and laboratory findings.

	Hemorrhage		Hemolysis	Decreased RBC production
	Acute	Chronic		
Clinical				
Pallor	(−) to +++	+ to +++	+ to +++	+ to +++
Hepatosplenomegaly	(−)	(−) to +++	++ to +++	(−)
Early jaundice	(−)	(−)	++ to +++	(−)
Hypovolemia	+ to +++	(−)	(−)	(−)
Laboratory				
Cord hemoglobin	Nl or ↓	↓ to ↓↓↓	↓ to ↓↓↓	↓ to ↓↓↓
Bilirubin (cord or day 1)	Nl	Nl	↑ to ↑↑↑	Nl
Direct Coombs' test	(−)	(−)	(−) to +++	(−)
Reticulocytes	Nl to ↑↑↑	↑ to ↑↑↑	↑ to ↑↑↑	Low

↓, mild decrease; ↑, mild increase; ↓↓↓, marked decrease; ↑↑↑, marked increase; (−), absent; +, mild; +++, severe; Nl, normal; RBC, red blood cell.

resuscitative maneuvers. The main presenting sign of chronic blood loss is pallor. If the hemorrhage is external, there is no additional bilirubin load to the liver once the postnatal breakdown of Hb begins. In contrast, internal hemorrhages (e.g., cephalhematoma) contribute to elevations in the serum bilirubin beyond the first 24–48 h after birth. External bleeding may be apparent by history (vaginal bleeding in the mother in placenta previa) or physical examination (ruptured umbilical cord). However, it may be occult and thus more difficult to diagnose (fetal–maternal hemorrhage).

Anemia secondary to hemolysis

It usually manifests with pallor and early onset of jaundice, but without signs of hypovolemia. ABO or Rh incompatibility and infection are the most common causes of hemolytic anemia in the newborn. ABO hemolytic disease can vary from immune hemolysis only, demonstrated by a decreased red blood cell (RBC) survival, to severe anemia and, rarely, hydrops fetalis. In contrast, Rh isoimmunization frequently results in more significant degrees of anemia and hyperbilirubinemia. The severity of the hemolysis increases with subsequent pregnancies of Rh-positive fetuses. Other causes of immune hemolysis should be suspected in the presence of a positive direct Coombs' test but compatible ABO and Rh types between mother and infant. Viral or bacterial infections are the most common cause of nonimmune hemolysis.

Decreased RBC production

Neonatal anemia due to decreased RBC production is very uncommon and usually features a low reticulocyte count (< 2%) not explained by other obvious causes.

Polycythemia

Polycythemia is defined as a spun peripheral venous hematocrit (Hct) above 65%. The most common signs associated with polycythemia are plethora, lethargy, tachypnea, feeding difficulties, hypotonia, and jitteriness. Polycythemia may result from either a chronic increase in the RBC mass or an acute expansion of the circulating blood volume with subsequent increases in Hct when transudation to the interstitial compartment occurs. *In utero*, hypoxia stimulates erythropoietin production, which in turn promotes erythropoiesis [small for gestational age (SGA) infants, postmaturity]. These infants are generally not hypervolemic and can have elevated reticulocyte counts. Conversely, infants with polycythemia due to transfusion may be hypervolemic. Treatment of polycythemia is usually initiated for infants with central venous Hct above 70% or those with Hct above 65% if they are symptomatic. Treatment consists of a partial exchange transfusion to lower the Hct to a range at which blood viscosity will also be much lower. The volume to exchange is calculated as: volume (mL) = blood volume × (observed Hct–desired Hct)/observed Hct, where blood volume is 80–100 mL/kg body weight. Normal saline, lactated Ringer's, or albumin can be used for the isovolemic exchange. The long-term benefits of this intervention are not entirely clear.

Hyperbilirubinemia

The definitions of physiologic and pathologic jaundice are given in Table 65.6. Pathologic jaundice most commonly results from excess RBC mass, as in polycythemia, or excess RBC destruction. Examples of excess destruction include hemolysis (as in hemolytic disease of the newborn), RBC defects (e.g., spherocytosis), and internal hemorrhages (e.g., cephalhematoma). Decreased conjugation of bilirubin is seen in neonatal hypoglycemia and hypothyroidism. Decreased excretion occurs with certain infections (e.g., transplacental infections, bacterial sepsis, urinary tract infections), genetic enzymatic defects (e.g., Dubin–Johnson), biliary atresia, cystic fibrosis, galactosemia, and with prolonged use of parenteral nutrition. Regardless, the jaundiced infant should be carefully evaluated prior to the institution of therapy. A complete blood count (CBC) should be performed to ascertain red cell number and morphology. A high reticulocyte count indicates rapid RBC turnover. Blood type determination and a Coombs' test should be performed on the mother and infant, looking for incompatibility of ABO or Rh blood group systems. If the direct fraction of bilirubin is elevated, transplacental viral and parasitic infections should be considered. If no etiology is ascertained, a urinalysis and urine culture (urinary tract infection) and, possibly, a urine-reducing substance test (galactosemia) and a serum T_4 (hypothyroidism) should be performed, even though these etiologies usually present with jaundice either after feedings (lactose) have been introduced or beyond the first several days.

The goal of treatment is to reduce the likelihood of bilirubin encephalopathy. Phototherapy is the main therapy for hyperbilirubinemia. It causes photoisomerization of bilirubin molecules into structural isomers that are excreted through the liver and urine. It slows the rate of rise of bilirubin but, once it is discontinued, there tends to be a 1–2 mg/dL rebound in the next 12–24 h. Exchange transfusion is usually reserved for infants in whom phototherapy was not sufficient as it has many complications (thrombosis, arrhythmias, electrolyte disturbances, problems of coagulation, and infections).

Table 65.6 Physiologic and pathologic jaundice.

	Physiologic	Pathologic
Time of onset	> 24 h	< 24 h or > 1 week
Peak bilirubin level	8–12 mg/dL	> 12 mg/dL (term)
		> 12 mg/dL (preterm)
		> 5 mg/dL/day
Timing of peak	3–4 days	> 1 week (term)
		> 2 weeks (preterm)

Metabolic problems

Hypoglycemia

In normal term neonates delivered vaginally to healthy mothers, there is a rapid fall in plasma glucose to 56 ± 19 mg/dL (mean ± standard deviation) at 1 h and 70 ± 13 mg/dL at 3 h after birth. Then, plasma glucose values remain fairly stable for the first week after birth. Normal glucose values in preterm infants are slightly less than those in term infants. The definition of hypoglycemia remains controversial but is generally placed at glucose concentrations < 40–50 mg/dL. Plasma glucose is usually between 10% and 15% higher than whole blood values. Use of rapid reagent strips is acceptable for screening and follow-up of blood glucose levels. However, low values must be confirmed by laboratory determination of true glucose concentrations. The causes of neonatal hypoglycemia are listed in Table 65.7. Lower endogenous glucose production due to lack of glycogen storage is common in preterm and SGA infants. Hypoglycemia may also result from endocrine or metabolic disorders that lead to decreased hepatic glucose output. Infants with panhypopituitarism are of normal weight and length at birth, but hypoplastic genitalia in male infants (small phallus and scrotum, undescended testes) may suggest this diagnosis. Hepatomegaly, jaundice, and metabolic acidosis are all findings suggestive of a metabolic disorder. Hypoglycemia due to an insulin excess is most often a result of maternal diabetes. Excessive maternal glucose administration during labor and

Table 65.7 Common causes of neonatal hypoglycemia.

I. Altered glucose production:	II. Excess glucose utilization:

A. Lack of glycogen stores
  Prematurity
  Small for gestational age
 	
B. Failure of glucose mobilization
  Endocrine disorders
    Panhypopituitarism
    Cortisol deficiency
    Glucagon deficiency
  Metabolic disorders
    Galactosemia
    Glycogen storage disease, type 1
    Hereditary fructose intolerance
    Tyrosinemia
	A. Hyperinsulinism
	  Infant of diabetic mother
	  Excess glucose administration during labor/delivery
	  Erythroblastosis fetalis
	  Beckwith–Wiedemann syndrome
	  Beta-cell hyperplasia/nesidioblastosis
	  Malposition of umbilical arterial catheter (T11–L1)
	  Leucine sensitivity
	  Maternal drugs (thiazides, beta-adrenergic tocolytics)
	
	B. Increased peripheral demands:
	  Hypoxia
	  Cold stress
	  Infection
	  Polycythemia/hyperviscosity

delivery may produce a transient neonatal hyperinsulinemia and rapid fall in glucose. However, persistently low glucose values are probably secondary to other causes of hypoglycemia. Infants of diabetic mothers are at great risk of hypoglycemia, other metabolic abnormalities (hypocalcemia, hypomagnesemia), respiratory distress, and congenital anomalies mostly involving the central nervous and cardiovascular systems. They may develop hypoglycemia soon after birth and often remain asymptomatic despite very low glucose values. Organomegaly and other anomalies (e.g., macroglossia, omphalocele, hemihypertrophy, and abnormal ear lobe grooves) are suggestive of Beckwith–Wiedemann syndrome. Hypoglycemia secondary to any form of beta-cell hyperplasia may be severe and can persist for several weeks to months. Increased peripheral use of glucose can be seen with hypoxia, cold stress, infection, and polycythemia despite the presence of adequate glycogen storage and normal insulin levels.

Early glucose screening should be done on neonates at high risk of hypoglycemia. Avoidance of maternal hyperglycemia during labor and delivery must be stressed. The treatment of neonatal hypoglycemia depends on its severity and the availability of the enteral route. In infants with borderline low values detected by reagent strip and no contraindication for feedings, a confirmatory blood or plasma glucose test must be made followed by feeding of 5% dextrose or formula. If correction to normoglycemia is observed, feedings should be advanced as tolerated, and close monitoring of glucose must be continued for at least 24–48 h. Failure to correct glucose levels with this approach or an inability to use the enteral route are indications for parenteral glucose administration. Correction of very low glucose values (< 20–25 mg/dL) is best accomplished by intravenous administration of a minibolus of 200 mg/kg of glucose followed by a constant glucose infusion of 6–8 mg/kg/min via peripheral vein or umbilical venous catheter. Use of 25–50% dextrose should be avoided. The rate of glucose infusion should be adjusted to maintain normoglycemia. Feedings should be given concomitantly with parenteral glucose whenever possible, unless they constitute the etiology of the hypoglycemia (i.e., galactosemia, tyrosinemia). A high glucose requirement to maintain normoglycemia is suggestive of hyperinsulinism. If rates in excess of 12–15 mg/kg/min of glucose are required, additional therapy is indicated. Corticosteroids (hydrocortisone, 5 mg/kg day, or prednisone, 2 mg/kg/day), glucagon (300 µg/kg), diazoxide (10–15 mg/kg/day), and epinephrine have been used for the control of hypoglycemia.

Neonates with significant seizures secondary to hypoglycemia have a risk of up to 50% of an abnormal neurologic outcome. Abnormal neurologic features observed after neonatal hypoglycemia include low IQ score, seizure disorder, and motor deficits (spasticity, ataxia).

Hypocalcemia

A steady decrease in serum calcium and ionized calcium (iCa) is observed after birth, reaching a nadir at approximately 24 h of age and remaining low for 48–72 h, which is due to interruption of the transplacental supply and predominance of hypocalcemic hormones such as calcitonin and glucagon. Neonatal hypocalcemia has been defined as a serum calcium level of < 7–8 mg/dL. Hypocalcemia has been classified as early, which occurs in the first few days after birth, and late, which presents after day 4 or 5. At term, early neonatal hypocalcemia is most commonly seen in asphyxiated neonates and infants of diabetic mothers. Infants of diabetic mothers may have decreased parathyroid hormone (PTH) secretion after birth due to fetal and neonatal magnesium deficiency secondary to the chronic maternal loss of magnesium seen with diabetes. Secretion of PTH depends on magnesium. Other infants at risk of hypocalcemia are those with rapid changes in serum pH (correction of acidosis or hyperventilation) or who undergo exchange transfusions with blood containing citrate and phosphate as anticoagulants or buffers, which can bind calcium. Late neonatal hypocalcemia may be due to primary intestinal abnormalities or deficiencies in vitamin D metabolism, ingestion of large phosphorus loads (e.g., from cow's milk), or deficient renal excretion of phosphorus (renal failure), or to parathyroid disorders such as in DiGeorge's syndrome (abnormal facies, conotruncal cardiac anomalies, and defects of T-cell function because of thymic hypoplasia). Maternal PTH excess can also result in transient suppression of neonatal parathyroid function.

Neonatal hypocalcemia is often asymptomatic. The signs suggestive of hypocalcemia are primarily jitteriness and irritability, although apnea or seizures can sometimes occur and are generally seen only when the iCa falls to very low levels. Disappearance of the symptomatology with calcium treatment supports the diagnosis of hypocalcemia. Serial determinations of serum calcium should be performed in neonates at high risk of hypocalcemia and those with suggestive signs. Persistently low serum calcium values constitute an indication for magnesium and phosphorous determinations. Treatment of hypocalcemia is reserved primarily for symptomatic infants. The therapy consists of intravenous administration of 10% calcium gluconate (9.4 mg of elemental calcium/mL) in doses of 100–200 mg/kg, followed by a continuous infusion of approximately 400–800 mg/kg/day. Whether asymptomatic preterm neonates with low serum calcium (< 7 mg/dL) should be treated is controversial as the levels usually return to normal values spontaneously after the first 3–4 days after birth. Furthermore, controlled studies to evaluate the treatment of hypocalcemia conducted in sick preterm infants with serum calcium levels of < 6–7 mg/dL have failed to show any significant benefit of parenteral calcium administration. The long-term outcome of neonates with hypocalcemia depends primarily on the associated problems (asphyxia, DiGeorge's syndrome) rather than on the presence of symptoms or serum calcium values. If seizures due to late onset hypocalcemia are recognized and treated appropriately, the prognosis is almost invariably normal.

Hypomagnesemia and hypermagnesemia

Neonatal hypomagnesemia is defined as a serum magnesium level of < 1.6 mg/dL. It has been described in 9–38% of infants of diabetic mothers and in SGA infants. Hypocalcemia often coexists in neonates with hypomagnesemia. Hypoparathyroidism, hyperphosphatemia, and exchange transfusions with citrated blood also constitute risk factors for hypomagnesemia. The signs of hypomagnesemia are similar to those of hypocalcemia. The treatment of hypomagnesemia consists of the administration of magnesium sulfate 50% (50 mg of elemental magnesium/mL) in doses of 0.05–0.25 mL/kg intravenously. Oral supplementation using the same dose can be used in neonates without severe signs such as seizures.

Neonatal hypermagnesemia at term is best defined as serum magnesium above 2.5 mg/dL in the first few days after birth. The pathogenesis of neonatal hypermagnesemia is almost invariably the use of magnesium salts in the mother. Clinically, it presents primarily as muscle weakness and lethargy. Delayed passage of stools, abdominal distention, and even meconium plug syndrome have been described in preterm neonates of hypertensive mothers with hypermagnesemia. Respiratory depression and apnea may occur at higher levels in preterm infants. The treatment of hypermagnesemia consists of support of the cardiorespiratory and renal function as serum magnesium decreases quickly in 48–72 h. More aggressive therapy, such as exchange transfusion, is not indicated unless there are signs of cardiovascular collapse and renal failure.

Sepsis/infection

The two primary modes of infection in the early neonatal period are transplacental infection of the fetus and ascending infection in the perinatal period. Nosocomial acquisition of bacteria while in the neonatal intensive care unit (NICU) is a risk factor in infections that present later on. Common signs of infection are poor temperature control and apnea; fever is very uncommon in the newborn. Other signs include respiratory distress, poor perfusion, lethargy or irritability, poor feeding tolerance, and hypoglycemia. Neonatal sepsis has been divided into "early onset infections," which usually present at birth or during the first 48–72 h after delivery, and "late onset infections," which appear beyond this period. The most common organisms causing either early or late onset bacterial or fungal sepsis in the neonatal period are listed in Table 65.8. The incidence of group B streptococcal (GBS) infection has fallen recently (to less than 1 per 1000 live births). Infections with Gram-negative bacteria are even less common than GBS infection, although the widespread use of antibiotic prophylaxis to prevent GBS disease may have led to an increase in

Table 65.8 Common organisms causing sepsis during the neonatal period.

Early onset sepsis	Late onset sepsis
Group B streptococcus	Staphylococcus coagulase negative
Escherichia coli	Escherichia coli
Klebsiella pneumoniae	Enterococcus fecalis
Listeria monocytogenes	Klebsiella pneumoniae
Staphylococcus aureus	Staphylococcus aureus
	Candida species

the rate of significant neonatal infections by Gram-negative bacteria. Nosocomial infections usually manifest beyond 5–7 days after birth and are more common among very premature infants. They are most frequently caused by coagulase-negative *Staphylococcus* species, although other Gram-positive and Gram-negative organisms are detected not infrequently. *Candida* species are most common among extremely low-birthweight infants and generally carry a poor long-term outcome.

The treatment of the neonate with a bacterial or fungal infection is relatively simple. If infection is suspected, cultures of blood, spinal fluid, and urine should be taken. Initially, the choice of antibiotics depends on the suspected organisms. Once culture results are available, they can be adjusted to the specific organisms.

Necrotizing enterocolitis

Necrotizing enterocolitis (NEC) is the most commonly acquired serious gastrointestinal disease in the NICU. It affects mainly premature infants of less than 34 weeks' gestation, with an incidence of 5–15%. The symptoms of NEC include bloody stools, decreased number of stools, abdominal distention, gastric residuals, along with variable signs of systemic involvement such as lethargy, poor perfusion, and metabolic acidosis. Abdominal radiography may reveal pneumatosis intestinalis, air in the hepatic vascular tree, and/or bowel wall edema. Free air in the peritoneal cavity due to bowel perforation may also be found. The therapy for NEC includes stopping feedings and starting intravenous fluids, while attempts are made to decompress the bowel with the use of low intermittent suction. Broad-spectrum antibiotics should be started after obtaining appropriate cultures along with general supportive care, including correction of metabolic acidosis. Only about 30–50% of cases of NEC are associated with positive blood culture results, usually for Gram-negative bacteria in the most severe cases. Should the disease progress to the point of intestinal perforation, the necrotic portion of the intestine is removed surgically, usually leaving an intestinal ostomy. Bowel perforation is the main indication for surgical intervention in infants with NEC, although a lack of clinical improvement with medical therapy, the persistence of a fixed loop of bowel on abdominal radiography (suggestive of bowel necrosis), and signs of intestinal obstruction are often the reason for surgical involvement.

The mortality still ranges from 30% to 50% for the most severe forms of NEC. Persistent neutropenia, severe thrombocytopenia, severe metabolic acidosis refractory to therapy, hypotension, shock, and disseminated intravascular coagulation carry a poor prognosis. Infants with NEC usually have a prolonged hospital course. Long-term complications in infants who recover include strictures, enterocolonic fistulas, malabsorption, and postsurgical short bowel syndrome. There may also be complications of parenteral nutrition, such as infection and cholestasis. Moreover, recent evidence suggests that infants with severe NEC are also at very high risk of poor long-term neurologic outcome.

Table 65.9 International classification for ROP*.

Zones	Zone 1 From the center of the optic nerve to twice the distance from the optic nerve to the macula in a circle Zone 2 Circle surrounding the zone 1 circle with the nasal ora serrata as its nasal border Zone 3 Crescent of the circle of zone 2 that did not encompass temporally
Stages	Stage 0 Immature retinal vasculature Stage I Mildly abnormal blood vessel growth. A line is present between the vascular and avascular region Stage II Moderately abnormal blood vessel growth. A ridge is present between the vascular and avascular region Stage III Severely abnormal blood vessels growing toward the center of the eye on or over the ridge Stage IV Partially detached retina Stage V Completely detached retina
Plus disease	Dilation and tortuosity of the peripheral retinal vessels, part of the subclassification given to the above stages

*International Committee for the Classification of Retinopathy of Prematurity. The International Classification of Retinopathy of Prematurity revisited. *Arch Ophthalmol* 2005;123:991–999.

Retinopathy of prematurity

Retinopathy of prematurity (ROP) is most common in extremely low-birthweight infants. Hyperoxia has long been implicated as a cause of ROP. Current evidence suggests that hyperoxia alone is neither a necessary nor a sufficient cause of ROP. Additional factors that have been implicated in its pathogenesis by either association or anecdotal evidence include hypercarbia, multiple transfusions, severe apnea and bradycardia, acidosis, infection, and RDS. An international classification for ROP has been developed, which allows for the assessment of its severity and consistent reporting (Table 65.9). Approximately 90% of cases of ROP regress spontaneously. The remaining 10% of cases progress to severe ROP. In infants weighing < 751 g, up to 90% develop ROP and up to 16% may develop threshold ROP (advanced stages requiring treatment). Laser surgery is now the treatment of choice for threshold or severe ROP. The risk of blindness with threshold ROP has been reduced substantially with laser treatment. However, once retinal detachment has occurred, there is little likelihood of restoring vision. Even in infants with mild or regressed ROP, the incidence of myopia, strabismus, and amblyopia is more common than in infants without ROP.

Retinopathy of prematurity

Retinopathy of prematurity (ROP) is most common in extremely low birthweight infants. Hyperoxia has long been implicated as a cause of ROP. Current evidence suggests that hyperoxia alone is rarely a relevant sufficient cause of ROP.

Index

Page numbers in *italics* and **bold** represent figures and tables respectively

breastmilk
  composition, 520
  low production, 522
  production regulation, 518, 520
breech infant, low birth weight (LBW), 479
bromocryptine, pituitary disorders in
      pregnancy, 312
bronchodilators
  aspiration of stomach contents, 283
  asthma, 280
bronchopulmonary dysplasia (BPD),
      neonates, 529
bronchoscopy, adult respiratory distress
      syndrome (ARDS), 291
butalbital, headaches, 337

cabergoline, pituitary disorders in
      pregnancy, 313
caffeine
  headaches, 337
  during pregnancy, 89, 93
  teratogenicity/toxicity, 81
CAGE instrument, 90–91
calcitonin, neonatal hypocalcemia, 536
calcium
  dietary allowances, 228
  homeostasis, 21
  metabolism, disorders in pregnancy, 315
calcium gluconate, neonatal hypocalcemia,
      536
campomelic dysplasia, 156
cancer (in pregnancy), 407–417
  benign masses, 407–408
  chemotherapy, 409–410
  incidence, 408, 409
  radiation therapy, 409
  surgery, 408–409
  see also specific malignancies
Candida spp., neonatal sepsis/infection,
      538
carbamazepine, teratogenicity/toxicity, 83
carbon monoxide, teratogenicity/toxicity, 84
cardiac anomalies, prenatal diagnosis,
      125–129
cardiac disease (during pregnancy),
      260–275
  anesthesia, 516
  counseling, 260–262
  lesions, 262–267
    acquired, 267–270
    see also specific lesions
cardiac therapy, in utero, 221

cardiomyopathy
  morbidity of infants of diabetic mothers,
      305
  peripartum, 270–271
cardiopulmonary resuscitation, 247
cardiovascular disorders, maternal mortality
      risk, 261
cardiovascular system
  beta-sympathomimetic agents, 482
  maternal adaptations, 20, 224
CD4 count, HIV infection monitoring,
      372
cefazolin, pyelonephritis, 369
cefixime, gonorrhea, 378
ceftriaxone
  gonorrhea, 378
  pyelonephritis, 369
cell division, rapid, conceptus growth, 1–2
cellular defects, fetal surgery, 218
Centers for Disease Control (CDC)
  chlamydial infection treatment guidelines,
      382
  gonorrhea treatment guidelines, 378
  HPV treatment guidelines, 383
  HSV treatment guidelines, 387
  syphilis treatment guidelines, 380
central nervous system (CNS)
  malformations
    magnetic resonance imaging (MRI),
        190
    prenatal diagnosis, 121–124
    teratogenic viruses, 94
    tumors, 417
central venous pressure (CVP), 197
cephalosporins
  gonorrhea, 378
  mastitis, 522
  use during pregnancy/lactation, 107,
      108
cerebral blood flow (fetal), 195–196, 197
  IUGR diagnosis, 196
cerebrum, congenital anomalies, 123
cervical biopsy, 410
cervical cancer (in pregnancy), 410, 412,
      412
cervical dilation
  arrest, 461, 462
  disorders, 456, 456
  normal, 455–457, 456
cervical examination, preterm birth,
      471–472
cervical intraepithelial neoplasia (CIN), 410

Printed and bound by CPI Group (UK) Ltd, Croydon, CR0 4YY

16/04/2025

14658827-0002